ADVANCES IN THE STUDY OF GENETIC DISORDERS

Edited by **Kenji Ikehara**

Advances in the Study of Genetic Disorders
Edited by Kenji Ikehara

Published by InTech
Janeza Trdine 9, 51000 Rijeka, Croatia

Publishing Process Manager Silvia Vlase

Technical Editor Teodora Smiljanic

Cover Designer InTech Design Team

Additional hard copies can be obtained from orders@intechopen.com

Advances in the Study of Genetic Disorders, Edited by Kenji Ikehara
p. cm.
ISBN 978-953-307-305-7

For EU product safety concerns:
IN TECH d.o.o., Prolaz Marije Krucifikse Kozulić 3, 51000 Rijeka, Croatia,
info@intechopen.com or visit our website at intechopen.com.

Meet the editor

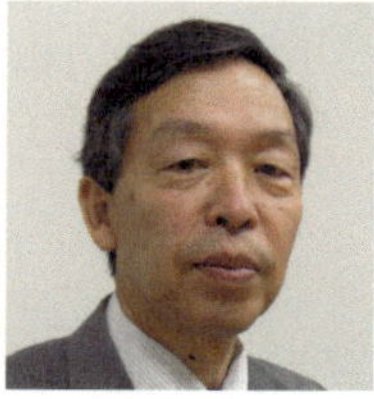

Kenji Ikehara is a professor and director in Nara Study Center of the Open University of Japan. He is also a fellow of International Institute for Advanced Studies (IIAS) of Japan and an Emeritus Professor of Nara Women's University. He graduated from Department of Industrial Chemistry, Faculty of Engineering, Kyoto University in 1968 and received his B. Eng (1968), and successively M. Eng. (1970) and D. Eng. (1976) degrees from Kyoto University. He engaged in studies on Sporulation Initiation of Bacillus subtilis and on the origins and evolutional processes of microbial genes, the genetic code, and proteins during around 30 years in Nara Women's University. Consequently, he has proposed GC-NSF(a) hypothesis on the origin of Genes, GNC-SNS hypothesis on the genetic code, protein 0th-order structure hypothesis on proteins and [GADV]-protein world hypothesis on the origin of life.

Contents

Preface

All life on the Earth, including the human race, originated from one common ancestor (comonote) which appeared on the primitive earth about 3.8~4.0 billion years ago after chemical evolutions from simple inorganic to complex organic compounds. The first life successively evolved from simple to complex organisms, such as prokaryotes, mono-cellular eukaryotes, multi-cellular micro-organisms, plants, animals and human beings. Human beings appeared on this planet between 25 and 7 million years ago and have suffered from many kinds of disease for a long time, many of which might lead to death, such as lethal viruses like smallpox and influenza and infectious bacteria like as cholera and tuberculosis. However, human beings have acquired intelligence so as to understand scientifically many concerns in various kinds of fields, including the medical sciences. Thus, human beings actually acquired the knowledge of viruses and micro-organisms to fight against diseases. Many people have seriously hoped to live as long as possible and even to get eternal life with the acquisition of intelligence. It is well-known in Asian countries that Shi Huángdì (BC259-BC210), who was an emperor in ancient China, tried to get eternal life and took various kinds of chemicals.

Human beings were protected from infection by viruses - such as the smallpox virus - by the intravenous injection of vaccines into their bodies. Owing to the medical technology of vaccines - which were first discovered by Jenner in 1796 - many lives were saved.

Furthermore, penicillin - one of the antibiotics - was first discovered by Fleming in 1881. Subsequently, many kinds of antibiotics - such as streptomycin and kanamycin - were discovered. Consequently, many people were also released from diseases caused by infectious bacteria and many lives were saved, since many patients were even cured of infectious diseases which lead to death through taking the antibiotics.

In these ways, the development of medical technologies and medicines has protected human beings from many kinds of diseases caused by the infection of viruses and bacteria, resulting in extending the life span of human beings. Currently, many Japanese people can live until between 90 and 100 years old. For example, the average life spans of females and males living in Japan had reached 86.4 and 79.6 years old by 2009, respectively, while the comparative figures in 1950 were about only 62 and 58 years old, respectively.

It is reported that the highest cause of Japanese deaths is malignant tumour or cancer. Cancers induced by genetic defects leading to deviation from the normal control of cell division can be regarded as a kind of genetic disorder. The genetic defects may occur in all organs, such as the kidney, the spleen, the stomach, the lung and the intestine etc. In addition, it is quite difficult to cure these cancers by the usual treatments such as administration of medicines (except for removal of malignant tumours by surgical operations) because at the present time it is impossible to site-specifically replace the substituted bases to the original/normal bases. This is the reason why cancers are at the top of the Japanese death causes although human beings are released from many kinds of infectious diseases.

Many genetic disorders are caused by base substitutions on double-stranded DNA, as with cancers. Although the mutated bases must be replaced with the original/normal bases in order to completely cure the disorders, it is quite difficult to achieve this purpose at the present time, again, as with the case of cancers as described above. Thus, genetic disorders remain diseases which are difficult to cure. In addition, mutations causing genetic disorders may occur in any cells carrying genetic elements or DNA and at anytime. Therefore, the organisms living on earth have been exposed to danger-generating base substitutions without exception, and genetic disorders may be induced in any organs because human beings are multi-cellular organisms.

There are two big problems with genetic disorders. One is that it is quite difficult to cure them, as described above. However, in addition to the knowledge about such mechanisms as DNA replication, transcription and the translation of genetic information, human beings have rapidly accumulated knowledge about the base substitutions or mutations occurring on chromosomal DNA which cause various genetic diseases, ever since Watson and Crick discovered the double-stranded structure of DNA in 1956. This knowledge is always significant because it may helpful in devising another medical treatment to cure genetic disorders. Surely, there exist several examples that the knowledge retrieved symptoms or succeeded even to save of patients suffered by genetic disorders. For example, many of the genetic disorders caused by abnormalities of metabolic enzymes could be relieved by going on a diet, which restricts the excess accumulation of the metabolite as a substrate of the enzyme and/or supplies a decreased metabolite as a product of the enzyme. In the case of a genetic disorder causing an excess accumulation of metabolites, it may be also useful to employ the intravenous administration of medicine, which can reduce the formation of toxic metabolites.

Another one is a problem accompanied by the recent development of genetic analysis for the diagnosis of genetic disorders, because it has made it possible to judge whether a patient is a carrier or non-carrier of an incurable genetic disease, which may lead to death after several years. A patient who has been able to confirm by their diagnosis as a non-carrier of a genetic disorder can live in peace. However, a patient, who has been proven to be a carrier of a genetic disorder must live with continual uneasiness with regard to confronting their coming death during their remaining life, since the patient must recognise themselves as being a carrier of a genetic disorder as well as their impending death. However, I believe that it is important for the patient to know whether he or she is a carrier or non-carrier of even a genetic disorder resulting in death in the future, because the patient can do their best against the disease during their remaining life based on the state of knowledge regarding the genetic disorder.

Certainly, it is quite difficult or almost impossible to cure a genetic disorder fundamentally at the present time. However, our knowledge of genetic functions has rapidly accumulated since the double-stranded structure of DNA was discovered by Watson and Crick in 1956. Therefore, nowadays it is possible to understand the reasons why genetic disorders are caused. It is probable that the knowledge of genetic disorders described in this book will lead to the discovery of an epoch of new medical treatment and relieve human beings from the genetic disorders of the future, because human beings had overcome many difficulties already (such as infectious diseases through the discovery of new medical treatment using vaccines for protection against infection form viruses and of special medicines known as antibiotics for curing diseases caused by the infection of micro-organisms). As such, I have a presentiment that a new age is now dawning with respect to the overcoming of genetic disorders. The dawn may set in suddenly upon a big discovery for a new medical treatment - which will be achieved by one genius in the future - because such kinds of big discoveries have always been carried out suddenly by geniuses, such as Jenner and Fleming. I hope that the descriptions in this book will contribute to such a discovery, of a new medical treatment for genetic disorders.

Kenji Ikehara
The Open University of Japan, Nara Study Centre,
International Institute for Advanced Studies of Japan
Japan

Part 1

Background of Genetic Disorder

1

Origin of the Genetic Code and Genetic Disorder

Kenji Ikehara
The Open University of Japan, Nara Study Center
International Institute for Advanced Studies of Japan
Japan

1. Introduction

Genetic disorders are illnesses caused by abnormalities in genetic sequences and the chromosome structures. Most base substitutions, which may lead to genetic disorders, would be repressed to a low level as affecting only one person in every thousands or millions by replication repair systems and by robustness of the genetic code, which is discussed in this Chapter. But, once persons were suffered by the genetic disorders, they would probably get serious diseases during their lives. In addition, it is quite difficult to recover the substituted bases causing the genetic diseases to original bases, after persons were suffered by the rarely occurring genetic disorders. This makes a quite big problem of the genetic disorders from a stand point of medical treatment.

The mutations causing the genetic disorders are scattered throughout genes and their neighboring regions as shown in Figure 1 (A). It is also known that many genetic diseases are induced by single-base substitutions or missense mutations including nonsense mutations in genetic regions encoding amino acid sequences of proteins. For instance, sickle-cell anemia, one of the classical genetic disorders, is caused by a one-base replacement at the sixth codon of the hemoglobin β-globin gene, from A to U, which results in one amino acid substitution from glutamic acid to valine, producing an abnormal type of hemoglobin called hemoglobin S (Figure 1 (B)). Hemoglobin S distorts the shape of red blood cells due to hemoglobin aggregation in the cells, especially when exposed to low oxygen levels, resulting in anemia giving a patient malaria resistance. Phenylketonuria (PKU), adenosine deaminase (ADA) deficiency and galactosemia are also caused by one-base replacements in genes of phenylalanine hydroxylase, adenosine deaminase and galactosidase, respectively (Table 1). Of course, deletion and insertion of a small number of bases causing frameshift mutations in a genetic sequence encoding protein may also affect normal life activities, because the frameshift mutation induce a change to different amino acid sequences following the mutation site. Base substitutions also may occur in transcriptional and translational control regions, splicing sites and so on, which affect various functions for gene expression leading to synthesis of lower or higher amounts of proteins than normal level, resulting in many kinds of genetic diseases (Figure 1 (A)).

(A)

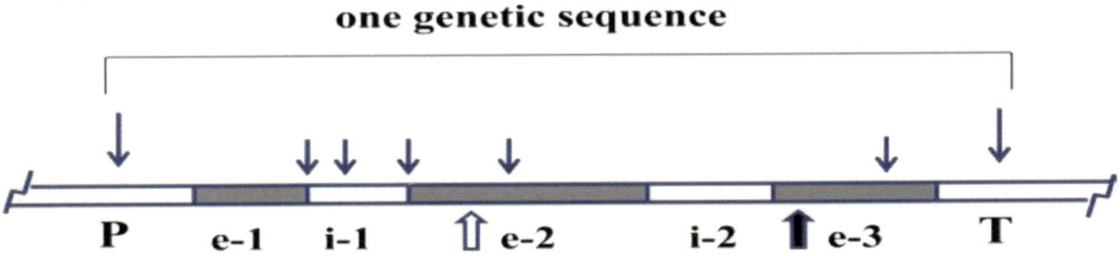

(B)

	GUG	CAU	CUG	ACU	CCU	GAG	GAG	AAG	UCU	GCC
Normal hemoglobin	1 Val	His	Leu	Thr	Pro	Glu	Glu	Lys	Ser	Ala 10
Hemoglobin S	1 Val	His	Leu	Thr	Pro	**Val**	Glu	Lys	Ser	Ala 10
	GUG	CAU	CUG	ACU	CCU	G**U**G	GAG	AAG	UCU	GCC

Fig. 1. (A) Possible mutation sites, which may affect various functions for gene expression and catalytic functions of proteins. Dark and white horizontal bars indicate exons encoding amino acid sequences of a protein and introns without genetic information for protein synthesis, respectively. Capital letters, P and T, mean a promoter for transcription initiation and a terminator required for termination of mRNA synthesis, respectively. Thick upward open and closed arrows and thin downward arrows indicate insertion and deletion of DNA sequences, and one-base substitutions, respectively. (B) Amino acid replacement observed in a classical and well-known genetic disorder, sickle cell anemia. Red letters indicate replacements of amino acid and base of the genetic mRNA sequence

Genetic Disorder	Inheritance	Gene
Hailey-Hailey Disease	Autosomal dominant	ATP2C1
Adenosine deaminase deficiency	Autosomal recessive	ADA
Thalassemia		globins
Alstrom Syndrome		ALMS1
Tangier Disease		ABCA1
Phenylketourea		PAH
Galactosemia		GALT
Aicardi-Goutieres syndrome	X-link dominant	RNAses
Bernard-Soulier syndrome		GPIs
Wiskott-Aldrich syndrome	X-link recessive	WASp
Fabry Disease		α-Gal A
Ornithine transcarbamoylase deficiency		OTC

Table 1. Examples of representative genetic disorders caused by one-base replacements on genetic sequences encoding amino acid sequences of proteins

Base substitutions might occur on every gene encoding functional proteins on a whole genome. In fact, about ten thousands genetic diseases are already known until now, out of which several genetic disorders caused by one-base replacements or monogenic disorders are described in Table 1.

In this Chapter, I will discuss on genetic disorders, which are caused by one-base replacements in coding regions, because I would like to discuss on relationships among robustness of the universal genetic code, base substitutions in codons and genetic disorders from a stand point of the origin of the genetic code. Term of "the universal genetic code", which is widely used in extant organisms, is used in this Chapter, instead of "the standard genetic code", which is used in many textbooks of in the fields of biochemistry and molecular biology since discoveries of non-universal genetic codes in mitochondria of mammals, protozoa and some bacteria. That is because I would like to emphasize that almost all organisms on this planet have actually used the genetic code. I believe that understanding on the relationship between the robustness and base substitutions will contribute to discovery of proper methods for treatments of many genetic disorders in a future.

Amino acid substitutions not largely affecting normal protein function are observed, as it is known as single nucleotide polymorohisms in the case of human beings. But, amino acid substitutions of mammals evolving at a quite slow rate due to a long generation time, such as about 25 years in the case of human, have occurred at a comparatively low frequency. On the other hand, amino acids of microbial proteins have been substituted at a high frequency without largely affecting protein functions. That is because evolution rate of microbial proteins is quite large due to the enormously large cell number and a quite short division time, such as about 20-30 minutes in the case of *Escherichia coli*. Therefore, it would be suitable to compare an amino acid sequence of a microbial protein with the homologous amino acid sequence in order to investigate amino acid substitutions occurring without largely affecting the protein function in a wide range as shown in Figure 2.

```
A. aeolicus          MLNKVFIIGRLTGDPVITYLPSGTPVVEFTLAYNRRYKNQNGEFQEESHFFDVKAYGK
C. hydrogenoformans  MFNKVILIGRLTRDPELRHTPQGTPVASITVAVDRPFTTKEG--QRETDFIDVVVWQK

A. aeolicus          MAEDWATRFSKGYLVLVEGRLSQEKWE-KEGKKFSKVRIIAENVRLINRPKGAEL-QA
C. hydrogenoformans   LAETARV-LTKGRLVMVEGRLQIRSYTDKEGQKRRVYEVVGENVRFLDKPKNAGLPAG

A. aeolicus          EEEEEVPPIEEEIEKLGKEEEKPFTDEEDEIPF
C. hydrogenoformans  NLPDEFPAVDFDPSDFGTEIEI----SDEDIPF
```

Fig. 2. Alignment of two amino acid sequences of small homologous single-stranded DNA binding proteins, from *Aquifex aeolicus* (147 amino acids) and *Carboxydothermus hydrogenoformans* (142 amino acids). Red bold and black letters indicate substituted and conserved amino acids between the two amino acid sequences, respectively. Hyphen (-) means amino acid position deleted from one amino acid sequence. Homology percent between the two single-stranded DNA binding proteins, which were obtained from GeneBank at http://www.ncbi.nlm.nih.gov/genbank/, is 38%

	A	C	D	E	F	G	H	I	K	L	M	N	P	Q	R	S	T	V	W	Y
A		0,0	4,0	6,0	0,0	1,2	2,0	2,0	1,0	2,0	2,0	4,0	1,0	2,0	3,1	6,0	2,0	4,1	0,0	3,0
C	0,0		0,0	0,0	0,0	0,0	0,0	1,0	0,0	0,0	0,0	0,0	0,0	0,0	0,0	0,0	0,0	0,0	0,0	0,0
D	0,0	1,0		5,1	1,0	1,0	0,0	0,0	4,0	1,0	2,0	2,0	0,0	3,0	0,0	2,0	2,1	0,0	0,0	0,0
E	1,0	0,0	1,5		1,1	0,1	0,0	1,1	5,0	0,1	1,0	1,1	1,1	3,0	3,2	2,3	2,1	1,0	0,0	2,0
F	0,0	0,0	0,0	0,0		0,0	0,0	2,3	0,0	1,1	0,0	0,0	0,0	1,0	1,1	0,0	0,0	1,0	0,0	5,0
G	1,0	0,0	1,0	1,0	0,0		0,0	0,0	5,0	0,0	0,0	3,1	0,0	2,1	1,1	2,0	1,0	0,0	0,0	1,0
H	1,0	0,0	1,1	1,0	0,0	1,0		0,0	0,0	0,0	0,0	2,0	0,0	0,0	0,0	0,0	0,0	0,0	0,0	1,0
I	0,0	0,0	0,0	1,0	0,0	0,0	0,0		0,0	3,3	1,0	0,0	0,1	0,0	0,0	0,0	0,0	7,3	0,0	1,0
K	2,0	0,0	2,1	4,0	1,0	0,0	1,0	1,1		0,0	0,0	0,0	2,0	0,1	3,0	0,1	0,1	1,2	0,0	1,0
L	1,0	0,0	0,0	0,0	3,3	1,0	0,0	14,0	0,0		5,1	0,0	0,0	2,0	1,0	0,0	1,2	5,1	0,0	2,0
M	0,0	0,0	0,0	0,0	0,0	0,0	0,0	3,0	0,0	5,1		0,0	0,0	1,0	0,0	0,0	0,0	2,0	0,0	1,0
N	0,0	0,0	2,2	1,1	0,0	2,0	0,0	0,0	1,0	0,0	0,0		0,0	1,0	0,0	0,0	1,1	0,0	0,0	0,0
P	1,1	0,0	1,0	1,0	0,0	2,0	0,0	1,0	1,0	1,0	0,0	2,0		0,0	2,0	2,0	1,0	1,0	0,0	1,0
Q	0,0	0,0	1,0	5,0	0,0	0,0	2,0	0,0	2,1	0,0	0,0	1,0	0,1		3,0	0,0	2,1	0,0	0,0	0,0
R	0,0	0,0	3,0	4,1	0,0	1,0	0,0	2,0	17,1	1,0	0,0	6,0	1,1	2,0		3,0	1,0	1,0	1,0	0,0
S	3,0	1,0	4,0	0,0	0,0	0,0	1,0	1,0	5,0	1,0	0,0	5,0	0,0	1,2	1,1		3,2	2,0	0,0	1,0
T	2,0	0,0	1,0	0,0	0,0	1,0	0,0	3,0	0,0	2,0	2,0	5,0	0,0	0,0	0,1	6,0		3,1	0,0	0,0
V	4,1	0,0	0,0	2,1	1,1	2,0	1,0	15,0	1,0	5,0	2,0	1,0	1,0	1,0	0,0	0,0	4,0		0,0	0,1
W	2,1	0,0	0,0	0,0	1,0	0,0	0,0	0,0	0,0	0,0	0,0	0,0	1,0	0,0	0,0	0,0	0,0	0,0		0,1
Y	1,0	0,0	1,0	0,0	3,1	1,0	1,1	1,0	0,0	0,0	0,0	0,0	0,0	0,0	0,1	0,0	0,0	0,1	0,1	

Protein	1st	2nd	3rd	1,2	1,3	others
RelA	119	93	13	10	8	154
SS-DNA.B	21	13	6	2	5	29

Fig. 3. The numbers of permissible amino acid substitutions observed between two pairs of homologous proteins, from *S. coelicolor* (left column) and to *S. aureus* (top row) RelA proteins (the numbers at the left side) and from *A. aeolicus* (left column) and to *C. hydrogenoformis* (top row) single-stranded DNA binding proteins (the numbers at the right side). Amino acid replacements upon base substitutions at the first, the second and the third codon positions are written in blue, yellow and red color boxes, respectively. Green, orange and white boxes indicate amino acid replacements induced by base substitutions at the first or the second codon positions, at the first or the third codon positions and other base substitutions, respectively. The base substitutions at the respective codon positions were deduced from amino acid replacements between two homologous proteins, which were occurred by one-base substitutions. The amino acid sequences, which were used for alignment, were obtained from GeneBank at http://www.ncbi.nlm.nih.gov/genbank/

As seen in Figure 2, many amino acid substitutions are observed between two homologous single-stranded DNA binding proteins. The amino acid substitutions caused by base substitutions at the first codon position were observed more than those caused by base substitutions at the second codon position (see the Table given in Figure 3). Similar results were obtained from amino acid substitutions between two large homologous stringent response proteins, *Streptomyces coelicolor* RelA and *Staphylococcus aureus* RelA (Figure 3). It can be interpreted as that amino acids with similar chemical and physical properties are arranged in the same column in the genetic code table at a comparably high probability (Table 2 (A), (B), (C) and (D)).
The universal genetic code is redundant and has a highly non-random structure. Typically, when nucleotide at the third codon position differs from the corresponding one, both codons encode the same amino acids at a high probability, due to the degeneracy of the genetic code at the third codon position. In addition, codons, of which nucleotide at the first codon position differs from each other, usually encode amino acids with different but rather similar chemical/physical properties.

(A)

Hydropathy

	U	C	A	G	
U	Phe	Ser	Tyr	Cys	U
	Phe	Ser	Tyr	Cys	C
	Leu	Ser	Term	Term	A
	Leu	Ser	Term	Trp	G
C	Leu	Pro	His	Arg	U
	Leu	Pro	His	Arg	C
	Leu	Pro	Gln	Arg	A
	Leu	Pro	Gln	Arg	G
A	Ile	Thr	Asn	Ser	U
	Ile	Thr	Asn	Ser	C
	Ile	Thr	Lys	Arg	A
	Met	Thr	Lys	Arg	G
G	Val	Ala	Asp	Gly	U
	Val	Ala	Asp	Gly	C
	Val	Ala	Glu	Gly	A
	Val	Ala	Glu	Gly	G

(B)

α-Helix

	U	C	A	G	
U	Phe	Ser	Tyr	Cys	U
	Phe	Ser	Tyr	Cys	C
	Leu	Ser	Term	Term	A
	Leu	Ser	Term	Trp	G
C	Leu	Pro	His	Arg	U
	Leu	Pro	His	Arg	C
	Leu	Pro	Gln	Arg	A
	Leu	Pro	Gln	Arg	G
A	Ile	Thr	Asn	Ser	U
	Ile	Thr	Asn	Ser	C
	Ile	Thr	Lys	Arg	A
	Met	Thr	Lys	Arg	G
G	Val	Ala	Asp	Gly	U
	Val	Ala	Asp	Gly	C
	Val	Ala	Glu	Gly	A
	Val	Ala	Glu	Gly	G

Table 2. Color representation of chemical/physical properties, of amino acids based on the values described in Stryer's "Biochemistry" (Berg *et al*, 2002). (A) hydrophobicities and (B) α-helix propensities of amino acids in the universal genetic code table. Letters in red, yellow and blue boxes represent amino acids with large, middle and small hydrophobicities, and the corresponding degrees of α-helix propensities, respectively

It can be seen in Table 2 that amino acids encoded by 16 codons in the same column are located in the same or two colored boxes at a high probability, such as two columns from left side of Table 2 (A) and one column at the most left side of Table 2 (D). Contrary to that, no row with the same color boxes is observed in Table 2 (A), (B), (C) and (D). This means that amino acids with similar chemical/physical properties are arranged in the same column, but those with rather different chemical/physical properties are arranged in the same rows at high probabilities. As a result, it makes the genetic code to be highly robust to the change of protein functions upon base substitutions in protein coding sequences, especially at the third and the first codon positions of genetic sequences. My original GNC-SNS primitive genetic code hypothesis on the origin and evolution of the genetic code (Ikehara, et al., 2002), which will be described in Section 3, can explain reasonably the robustness of the genetic code, which might stem from the origin and evolutionary processes. N and S mean either of four bases (A, U/T, G and C) and G or C, respectively.

(C)

β-Sheet

	U	C	A	G	
U	Phe	Ser	Tyr	Cys	U
	Phe	Ser	Tyr	Cys	C
	Leu	Ser	Term	Term	A
	Leu	Ser	Term	Trp	G
C	Leu	Pro	His	Arg	U
	Leu	Pro	His	Arg	C
	Leu	Pro	Gln	Arg	A
	Leu	Pro	Gln	Arg	G
A	Ile	Thr	Asn	Ser	U
	Ile	Thr	Asn	Ser	C
	Ile	Thr	Lys	Arg	A
	Met	Thr	Lys	Arg	G
G	Val	Ala	Asp	Gly	U
	Val	Ala	Asp	Gly	C
	Val	Ala	Glu	Gly	A
	Val	Ala	Glu	Gly	G

(D)

Turn/Coil

	U	C	A	G	
U	Phe	Ser	Tyr	Cys	U
	Phe	Ser	Tyr	Cys	C
	Leu	Ser	Term	Term	A
	Leu	Ser	Term	Trp	G
C	Leu	Pro	His	Arg	U
	Leu	Pro	His	Arg	C
	Leu	Pro	Gln	Arg	A
	Leu	Pro	Gln	Arg	G
A	Ile	Thr	Asn	Ser	U
	Ile	Thr	Asn	Ser	C
	Ile	Thr	Lys	Arg	A
	Met	Thr	Lys	Arg	G
G	Val	Ala	Asp	Gly	U
	Val	Ala	Asp	Gly	C
	Val	Ala	Glu	Gly	A
	Val	Ala	Glu	Gly	G

Table 2. (Continued). (C) β-sheet and (D) turn/coil structure propensities, of amino acids in the universal genetic code table. Letters in red, yellow and blue boxes represent large, middle, and small β-sheet and turn/coil propensities, respectively. Meanings of color boxes in Table (C) and (D) are the same as in Table (A) and (B), described above. Secondary structure (β-sheet; (C) and turn/coil; (D)) propensities of amino acids were obtained from Stryer's "Biochemistry" (Berg *et al*, 2002)

2. Significance of the Genetic Code for life

The genetic code plays a quite important role in transfer of genetic information on DNA nucleotide sequence to amino acid sequence of a protein, such as enzyme and transporter of a chemical compound, *etc* (Figure 4). But, the genetic code has been generally regarded as a simple representation of the relationship between a genetic information or a codon composed of three bases (triplet) and an amino acid in a protein sequence as described in representative text books, as Stryer's "Biochemistry" (Berg *et al*, 2002). It seems to me that the significance of the genetic code has been underestimated at the present time, judging from my original idea suggesting that protein 0th-order structures, which are specific amino acid compositions favorable for effectively producing water-soluble globular proteins even by random synthesis (see Section 4), are secretly described in the genetic code table (see Figure 7 in Section 3).

Genetic information, which is stored in base sequences or actually in codon sequences on DNA, is propagated from a parent to progeny cells through DNA replication. In parallel, the information is transformed into mRNA and successively into an amino acid sequence of a protein according to the genetic code, when necessary. Various organic molecules required to live are synthesized with enzyme proteins on metabolic pathways (Figure 4). Therefore, it is no exaggeration to say that the genetic code is much more significant for lives than genes and proteins, or that the genetic code is the most important facility in the fundamental life system. Understanding of the origin and evolutionary processes of the genetic code should be quite important to know a framework of the genetic code and a relationship between amino acid substitutions and one-base substitutions causing genetic disorders.

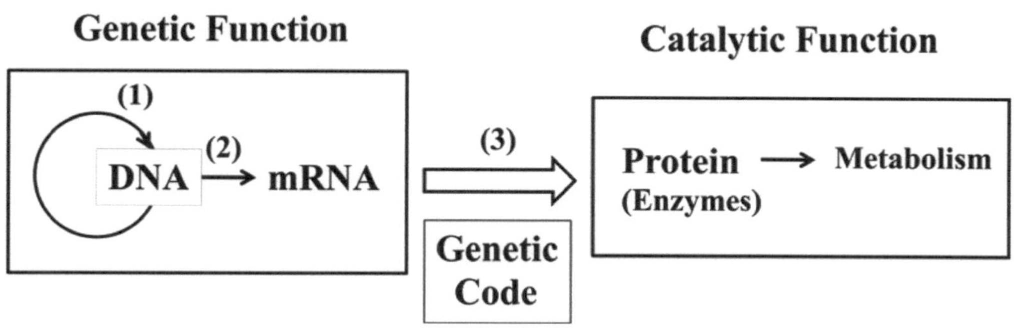

Fig. 4. Role of the genetic code playing in the fundamental life system of modern organisms, which is composed of genes, the genetic code and proteins (enzymes). Genetic code mediates between two main elements, genetic function composed of DNA (mRNA) and function carried out by proteineous catalysts (enzymes) forming chemical network or metabolism. Genetic information on DNA are transmitted to progeny cells by replication (Step 1), and transcribed into mRNA (Step 2) when necessary. Genetic information transferred into mRNA is translated to the corresponding amino acid sequence of a protein (Step 3) through genetic code mediating genetic information and catalytic function. The universal genetic code used by extant organisms on the earth is composed of 64 codons and 20 amino acids (see Table 2)

3. Origin of the Genetic Code (GNC-SNS primitive genetic code hypothesis)

Our studies on the origin of the genetic code were initiated from the search for a prospective spot on a DNA sequence, from which an entirely new gene encoding an entirely new functional protein will be created, when an extant organism using the universal genetic code has to adapt to a new environment. The spot was searched based on the six necessary conditions for producing water-soluble globular proteins as described below. The six conditions used for the search are hydropathy, α-helix, β-sheet and turn/coil formabilities, acidic amino acid and basic amino acid contents of proteins, which were obtained as average values plus/minus standard deviations of water-soluble globular proteins in extant micro-organisms. From the results, it was found that non-stop frames, which appear on anti-sense strands of GC-rich genes (GC-NSF(a)s) at a high probability, have the strongest possibility to create entirely new genes, not new modified type of genes or homologous genes (Figure 5) (Ikehara et al., 1996). Where GC-NSF(a) means nonstop frame on antisense strand of GC-rich gene. That is because hypothetical proteins encoded by GC-NSF(a)s satisfied the six conditions and because the probability of non-stop frame (NSF) appearance on the GC-rich anticodon sequences was enough high (Ikehara, 2002).

The GC-NSF(a) hypothesis on creation of the first family genes under the universal genetic code led us propose subsequent theory on the origin of the genetic code as GNC-SNS primitive genetic code hypothesis (Ikehara et al., 2002). GNC and SNS represent four codons (GUC, GCC, GAC and GGC) and 16 codons (GUC, GCC, GAC, GGC, GUG, GCG, GAG, GGG, CUG, CCG, CAG, CGG, CUC, CCC, CAC and CGC), respectively. I describe the clues briefly below, from which the hypothesis was obtained. The first one is that base sequences of the GC-NSF(a)s were rather similar to the repeating sequences of SNS. The second one is that hypothetical proteins encoded by GNC code, a part of the SNS code, satisfied the four conditions (hydropathy, α-helix, β-sheet and turn/coil formabilities of proteins) for folding polypeptide chains into water-soluble globular structures (Ikehara et al., 2002). In the following paragraphs, the progress of investigation from the discovery of origin of genes to the GNC-SNS primitive genetic code hypothesis will be describe more precisely.

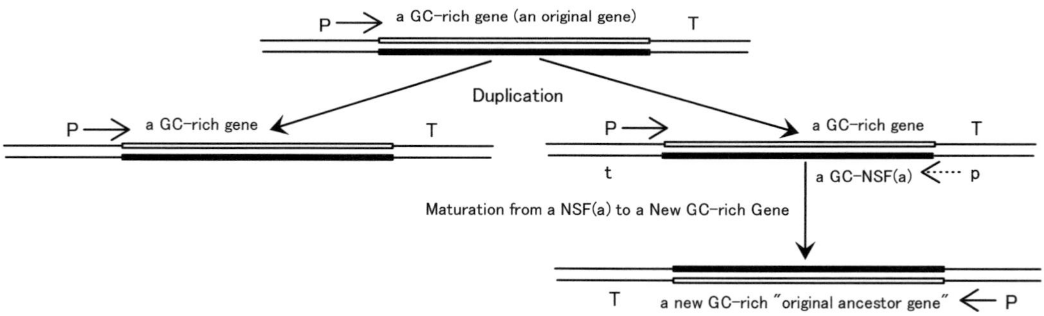

Fig. 5. GC-NSF(a) primitive gene hypothesis for creation of "original ancestor genes" under the universal genetic code. The hypothesis predicts that new "original ancestor genes" originate from nonstop frames on antisense strands of GC-rich genes (GC-NSF(a)s)

Firstly, we found that base compositions at the three codon positions of the GC-NSF(a) were similar to SNS. Actually, hypothetical polypeptide chains encoded by only SNS code, not containing A and U at the first and third codon positions, satisfied the six conditions, suggesting that polypeptides encoded by SNS code could be folded into water-soluble globular structures at a high probability (Figure 6 (A)). This indicates that SNS code has enough ability encoding proteins with definite-levels of catalytic activities. At this point, I provided SNS hypothesis on the origin of the genetic code about fifteen years ago (Ikehara & Yoshida, 1998).

But, the SNS code composed of 16 codons and 10 amino acids must be too complex to prepare as the first genetic code from the beginning. So, I further searched for which code was more primitive one than SNS by using the four more essential conditions which acidic amino acid and basic amino acid compositions were excluded from the six conditions described above. From the results, it was found that [GADV]-proteins encoded by GNC codons well satisfied the four structural conditions, when roughly equal amounts of [GADV]-amino acids were contained in the proteins (Figure 6 (B)). Where [GADV] represents four amino acids of Gly, Ala, Asp and Val, and square bracket ([ ]) was used to discriminate amino acids, especially G and A which are described by one-letter symbols of amino acids, from nucleic acid bases, G and A. It means that even the [GADV]-polypeptide chains with a quite simple amino acid composition could be folded into water-soluble structures at a high probability.

(A) (B)

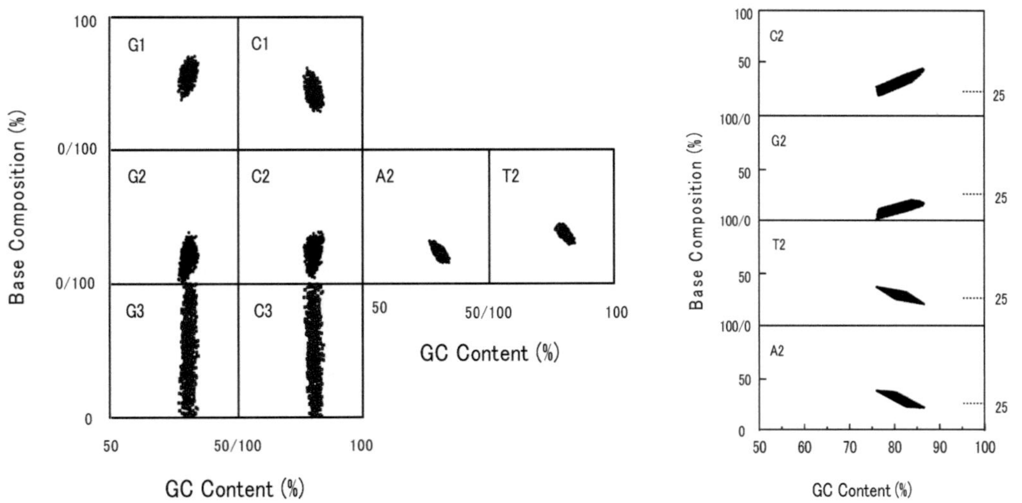

Fig. 6. (A) Dot plot analysis of SNS genetic code. Dots concentrated in the respective boxes indicate that the six conditions (hydropathy, α-helix, β-sheet and turn/coil formabilities, and acidic and basic amino acid contents) were satisfied. It means that polylpeptide chains encoded by SNS code could be folded into water-soluble globular structures when bases are contained in the respective rates at three codon positions. (B) Dot plot analysis of GNC code

On the other hand, other codes encoding four amino acids, which were picked out from the columns or rows in the universal genetic code table, did not satisfy the four structural conditions, except for GNG code, which is a modified form of the GNC code (Ikehara et al, 2002). Moreover, it was also confirmed that genetic code composed of three amino acids lined in universal genetic code table did not satisfy the four conditions for protein structure formation, suggesting that the GNC code would be used as the most primeval genetic code on the primitive earth (Ikehara et al, 2002). Then, I concluded that SNS primitive genetic code evolved from the GNC primeval genetic code by C and G introductions at the first and the third codon positions, respectively (Figure 7 (A)).

Dots concentrated in the respective boxes of Figure 6 (B) indicate that the four conditions (hydropathy, α-helix, β-sheet and turn/coil formabilities) were satisfied. It means that polylpeptide chains encoded by GNC code could be folded into water-soluble globular structures when four bases are contained in the respective rates at the second codon position.

Thus, I provided GNC-SNS hypothesis as the origin of the genetic code about ten years ago (Ikehara et al., 2002), suggesting that the universal genetic code originated from GNC code through SNS code as capturing new codons up and down in the genetic code table (Figure 7 (B)).

(A)

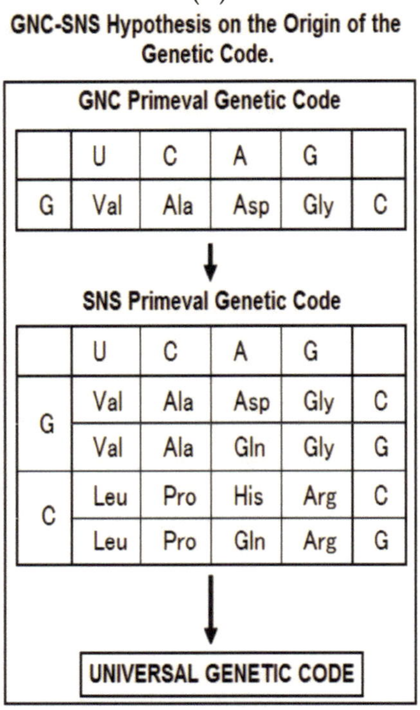

(B)

	U	C	A	G	
U	Phe	Ser	Tyr	Cys	U
	Phe	Ser	Tyr	Cys	C
	Leu	Ser	Term	Term	A
	Leu	Ser	Term	Trp	G
C	Leu	Pro	His	Arg	U
	Leu	Pro	His	Arg	C
	Leu	Pro	Gln	Arg	A
	Leu	Pro	Gln	Arg	G
A	Ile	Thr	Asn	Ser	U
	Ile	Thr	Asn	Ser	C
	Ile	Thr	Lys	Arg	A
	Met	Thr	Lys	Arg	G
G	Val	Ala	Asp	Gly	U
	Val	Ala	Asp	Gly	C
	Val	Ala	Glu	Gly	A
	Val	Ala	Glu	Gly	G

Fig. 7. GNC-SNS hypothesis on the origin and evolutionary pathway of the genetic code. (A) In the hypothesis, it is supposed that the universal genetic code originated from GNC primeval genetic code through SNS primitive genetic code. Elucidation of the most primitive GNC code made it possible to propose as GADV hypothesis on the origin of life. (B) Alternative representation of the origin and evolutionary pathway of the genetic code. The universal genetic code originated from GNC primeval genetic code (red row), successively followed by capturing codons of GNG (orange row), and CNS (yellow rows), resulting in formation of SNS code. Therefore, it is considered that the universal genetic code evolved from GNC code through the introduction of rest rows up and down

Due to the evolutionary process of the genetic code, amino acids with similar chemical/physical properties have been arranged in the same column at a high probability (Table 2). Consequently, replacements between two amino acids located in the same column have been permitted at a high probability and the robustness of the genetic code has been generated. Now I believe that the GNC code had stepped up its structure to the SNS primitive genetic code encoding ten amino acids with 16 SNS codons via GNS code (8 codons and 5 amino acids). After that, the SNS code evolved into the universal genetic code, which encodes 20 amino acids and three stop signals with 64 codons (Ikehara & Yoshida, 1998; Ikehara et al., 2002). The GNC-SNS primitive genetic code hypothesis represents that the universal genetic code (NNN: 4x4x4 = 4^3 = 64 codons), which is both formally and substantially triplet code, originated from formally triplet but substantially singlet GNC code (1x4x1 = 4^1 = 4 codons) encoding four [GADV]-amino acids, through formally triplet but substantially doublet SNS code (2x4x2 = 4^2 = 16 codons) encoding 10 amino acids (Figure 7) (Ikehara, 2009).

Evolutionary process of the genetic code from GNC code, encoding four amino acids with quite different chemical/physical properties, to the universal genetic code through SNS code arranged amino acids with similar chemical and physical properties in the same columns and with largely different properties in the same rows at high probabilities (Table 2). So, it is considered that the robustness of the genetic code originated from the evolutionary process of the genetic code as suggested by the GNC-SNS primitive genetic code hypothesis. The discussion on the robustness of the genetic code is consistent with the results of permissible amino acid substitutions, which were observed between two homologous proteins, as given in Figures 2 and 3. As described below, the finding of the GNC-SNS primitive genetic code hypothesis led to the ideas on protein 0th-order structures and on the origin of life as GADV hypothesis or [GADV]-protein world hypothesis (Ikehara, 2005; Ikehara, 2009).

4. The universal genetic code and protein 0th-order structure

Discussion on protein structure formation usually begins with primary structure or amino acid sequence of a protein, not with amino acid composition. In Stryer's textbook "Biochemistry" (Berg et al, 2002), it is described that the information needed to specify the catalytically active structure of ribonuclease is contained in its amino acid sequence. The studies on folding of polypeptide chains, which were mainly carried out with small-sized proteins, have established the generality of this central principle of biochemistry: sequence specifies conformation. One of the reasons may rely on the facts that one-dimensional base sequences on DNA or genes encode amino acid sequences or primary structure of proteins.

On the other hand, I happened to use amino acid composition for investigation of protein structure formability, the six or four conditions as described above. The utilization gave interesting results and conclusions, such as GC-NSF(a) hypothesis on creation of the first family genes and GNC-SNS primitive genetic code hypothesis as described in the previous Sections 3. During the investigation on the origin of the genetic code, I have noticed the significance of specific amino acid compositions satisfying four (hydropaty and α-helix, β-sheet and turn propensities) or six (hydropaty and α-helix, β-sheet and turn propensities plus acidic and basic amino acid compositions) conditions for folding polypeptide chains into water-soluble globular structures. The conditions were obtained as the respective average values plus/minus standard deviations of presently existing water-soluble globular proteins from seven micro-organisms carrying the genomes with widely distributed GC contents. Structure formability of one protein is the same as other proteins randomly assembled in the same amino acid composition. This means that every protein synthesized by random peptide bond formation among amino acids in the specific amino acid composition could be similarly folded into water-soluble globular structures, but into different structures, since the proteins have the same amino acid composition but different sequences from each other.

The most important point for creation of entirely new proteins encoded by the first family genes is to form water-soluble globular structure through random synthesis among amino acids in a protein 0th-order structure, because a quite large number of possible catalytic sites for an organic compound could appear on the surface of one globular protein. The number of possible catalytic sites can be estimated from combinations of amino acids locating on the protein surface as about several hundred points. I have named such a specific amino acid composition favorable for protein structure formation as protein 0th-order structure (Ikehara, 2009), for example, the compositions containing roughly equal amounts of four [GADV]-amino acids (Gly [G], Ala [A], Asp [D] and Val [V]) and ten amino acids ([GADV]-amino acids plus Glu [E], Leu [L], Pro [P], His [H], Gln [Q] and Arg [R]) encoded by GNC and SNS codes, as [GADV]- or GNC- and SNS-protein 0th-order structures, respectively. This means that the protein 0th-order structures are secretly written in the universal genetic code table (Figure 7 (B)).

Origins of genes and proteins: Genetic code plays a central role in connecting genetic function with catalytic function in the fundamental life system, as described above (Figure 4). Under the GNC code, the first genes must be composed of base sequences carrying only GNC codons, which were produced by random phosphodiester bond formation among GNC codons. Subsequently, the first double-stranded $(GNC)_n$ gene would be created by complementary strand synthesis against the single-stranded $(GNC)_n$ gene.

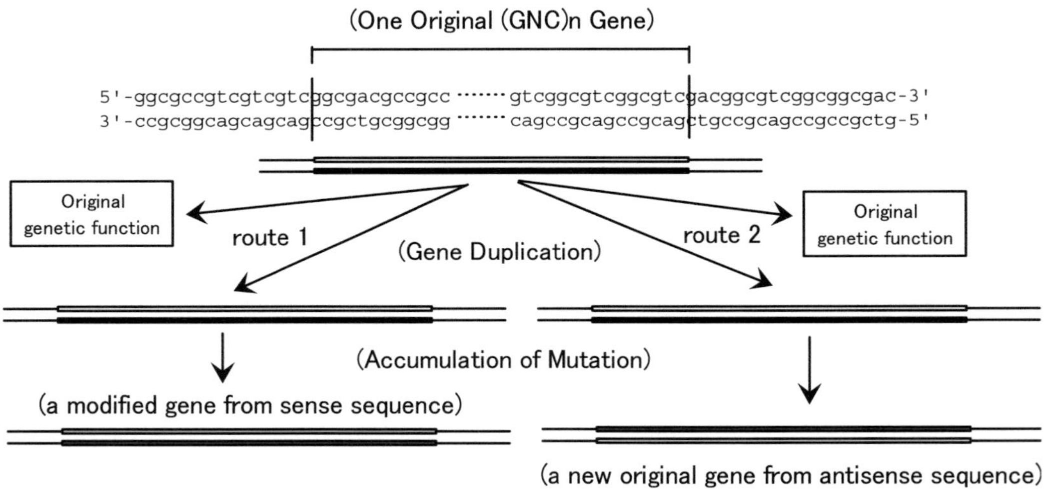

Fig. 8. Two routes for producing new genes. Once one original double-stranded $(GNC)_n$ gene was produced, new genes were easily produced by using two base sequences (one is from sense sequence and the other is from antisense sequence) of the original gene or through two routes. From route 1, new genes could be produced as modified genes of the original gene or homologous genes in a gene family and from route 2, new genes could be created as "entirely new genes" or the first family genes

Creation of the first double-stranded $(GNC)_n$ gene following establishment of the GNC primeval genetic code became the most important points leading to the emergence of life, since the invention of double-stranded genes made it possible for the first time to transmit genetic information from parents to progenies and to evolve it through accumulation of base substitutions and selection of more effective genetic sequences (Ikehara, 2009).

Base compositions at three codon positions on sense strands of $(GNC)_n$ genes are substantially same as those on anti-sense strands, due to the self-complementary structure of the double-stranded $(GNC)_n$ genes. Thus, it is easily supposed that, after creation of the first double-stranded $(GNC)_n$ gene, GNC codon sequences on anti-sense strands could be utilized as a field for creation of entirely new functional genes encoding the first ancestor proteins in homologous protein families, since GNC codon sequences on antisense strands are quite different from those on sense strands, as can be actually regarded as random arrangement of GNC codons. In addition, $(GNC)_n$ sequences on antisense strands must encode [GADV]-proteins satisfying the four conditions for producing water-soluble globular proteins at a high probability (Ikehara, 2002) (Figure. 6 (B)). Also new genetic information could be created from duplicated sense sequences, as proposed by Ohno (1970). But, the duplicated sense sequences could be utilized only for encoding homologous proteins in a family (route 1). Contrary to that, one of two antisense sequences obtained after gene duplication could give a field for production of the protein, which is quite different from all proteins existed before (route 2) (Figure 8) (Ikehara, 2009).

As seen in Figure 6 (B), [GADV]-proteins must have similar rigidity to extant proteins, when [GADV]-proteins contain less and more amounts of glycine and alanine than one quarter, respectively. Therefore, it is supposed that [GADV]-proteins, which were produced on the primitive earth in the absence of any genetic function or before creation of the first gene, were more flexible than the presently existing proteins, since the proteins should contain flexible turn/coil forming amino acid, glycine, more than rigid α-helix forming amino acid, alanine. The reason is that glycine would be pre-biotically synthesized more easily and accumulated on the primitive earth more than alanine. Therefore, [GADV]-proteins produced on the primitive earth must be more flexible than extant proteins recognizing usually one organic compound with high catalytic activities and high specificities. The flexible [GADV]-proteins would inevitably have only quite low catalytic activities. Even the low activities of the firstly appeared [GADV]-proteins would have been effective for leading to creation of the first genetic code, the first gene and the first life on the primitive earth. That is because the existence of [GADV]-proteins having the low catalytic activity must be important to develop new metabolic pathway on the primitive earth without any genetic information.

Formation of flexible but inefficient [GADV]-proteins was also essential to create newly-born proteins or the first family proteins even after the first double-stranded $(GNC)_n$ gene was produced, because the proteins, which were newly produced as ones with quite low enzymatic activities, could evolve to mature enzymes through accumulation of base substitutions and selection of more efficient enzymes with more rigid structures and higher specificities for one organic compound than before.

In fact, I believe that entirely new proteins have been created and selected from water-soluble globular proteins encoded by GC-NSF(a)s similar to $(SNS)_n$ or SNS repeating sequences, even at present, when necessary. Initially, entirely new proteins could be produced by transcription from cryptic promoters and translation of anticodon sequences on GC-rich genes if the proteins had pre-requisite catalytic functions (Figure 5). The newly-born proteins composed of 20 kinds of amino acids would evolve to mature enzyme with more rigid structure and a high specificity for one specific-organic compound through accumulation of mutations and selection of efficient enzymatic activity as similarly as the case of [GADV]-proteins encoded by $(GNC)_n$ anticodon sequences. I have now understood the important role of protein 0th-order structures or specific amino acid compositions in creation of entirely new proteins or the first family proteins. As a matter of course, mechanisms for the creation of entirely new proteins intimately related to the creation of entirely new genes. These new concepts on the origins of the genetic code, proteins and genes led to the GADV hypothesis on the origin of life.

5. GNC primeval genetic code and origin of life

In this Section, I will describe briefly GADV hypothesis on the origin of life, since the hypothesis, which I have proposed, is intimately related to the origin of the genetic code or the GNC primeval genetic code.

RNA world hypothesis has been proposed as a key idea for solving the "chicken and egg dilemma" observed between genes and proteins or the origin of life and has been widely accepted by many investigators at the present time. While I have proposed a novel hypothesis on the origin of life as GADV hypothesis, suggesting that life originated from [GADV]-protein world, which was composed of [GADV]-proteins accumulated by pseudo-replication of the proteins in the absence of any genetic function (Ikehara, 2002; Ikehara, 2005, Ikehara, 2009). In the hypothesis, it is assumed that life emerged from the world through establishment of GNC primeval genetic code followed by formation of single-stranded and double-stranded $(GNC)_n$ genes.

I believe that the most important point for solving the riddle on the origin of life would be to understand the origin and evolutionary processes of the fundamental life system, which is composed of genetic function, genetic code and catalytic function (Figure 4), not always to solve the "chicken and egg dilemma" observed between genes and protein, as considered in the RNA world hypothesis. Therefore, the GADV hypothesis would be far more rational to explain the origin of life than the RNA world hypothesis, because the former can easily explain formation processes of the fundamental life system composed of genes, the genetic code and proteins comprehensively as well as the "chicken and egg dilemma" (Ikehara, 2009). Contrary to that, the RNA hypothesis probably cannot explain the ways how the fundamental life system was created, because the hypothesis based on self-replication of RNA, which is carried out by polymerization of nucleotides one-by-one, cannot explain the origins of the genetic code and genes, which are composed of codons having triplet nucleotide sequences.

6. Robustness of the universal genetic code

Most genetic disorders are quite rare as causing the disorders at a ratio of only one person in every thousands or millions. The frequency of a genetic disorder caused by one-base substitution mainly relies on mutation rate. But, as given in Figures 2 and 3, in the cases of homologous microbial proteins belonging in the same protein family, many amino acid substitutions are observed without largely affecting protein function. The reasons are given as followings. The first one is because, utilization of many kinds of amino acids would be permissible in flexible regions of a protein at a high probability, such as turn/coil structures connecting two secondary structures and unstructured segments observed at C-terminal segment and/or at N-terminal segment at a high frequency, as can be seen in Figure 2. The second one could be attributed to the robustness of the universal genetic code, making it possible to use the same amino acids and different amino acids but with similar chemical and physical properties, when base substitutions occurred at the third and the first codon

positions, respectively. Therefore, the robustness of the genetic code could protect from destroy of protein's active state at a high probability, even if base substitutions occurred at the third and the first codon positions in genetic sequences and even when amino acid substitutions were introduced at the sites of secondary structures as α-helix and β-sheet structures. In contrast, base substitutions at the second codon positions would affect largely the protein functions, leading to the genetic disorders at a high probability, as shown in Figure 9.
According to the GNC-SNS primitive genetic code hypothesis, it is considered that the genetic code originated from GNC successively to SNS and finally to the universal genetic code as expanding the code up and down in the genetic code table as described in Section 3. From the evolutionary pathway of the genetic code, it can be understood that codons encoding amino acids with similar and with chemically different amino acids were arranged in columns and rows of the genetic code table, respectively. In other words, it is considered that the genetic code evolved as raising coding capacity to modulate the protein function, and as capturing new codons encoding new amino acids into vacant positions of the previous code table during evolutionary process. Therefore, the robustness of the genetic code could be generated from the origin and evolutionary processes of the genetic code, as described below.

1. Base substitution at the first codon position, but introducing no base change at the second position, does not destroy protein function at a high probability, since codons in the same column of the genetic code table code for amino acids with comparatively similar chemical/physical properties, because amino acids with the same color background are arranged in two and one columns out of four columns of hydrophacy and turn/coil tables, respectively. This can be also confirmed from the facts shown in Table 2.
2. Base substitution at the second codon position largely destroys protein function at a high probability, since codons located in the same row of the genetic code table encode amino acids with quite different chemical/physical properties (Table 2). Certainly, amino acids with the same color background are not observed on any row of four tables, except for one row having two termination codons in Table 2 (C). Amino acids with two different color backgrounds are arranged in eighteen out of 64 rows of the four tables of Table 2, otherwise amino acids in the same rows have three color backgrounds.
3. Base substitutions at the third codon position induce no amino acid replacement due to the degeneracy of the genetic code and substitutions between amino acids with similar chemical/physical properties, such as Phe-Leu, Asp-Glu, His-Gln and so on, are observed at a high probability.

Generally speaking, only base substitutions occurred at the second codon position, not at the first and third codon positions, induce substitutions between amino acids with largely different chemical and physical properties. The skillful location of codons in the genetic code table gives the genetic code robustness against base substitutions on genetic sequences, which is derived from the origin and evolutionary process of the genetic code, as suggested by the GNC-SNS primitive genetic code hypothesis (Ikehara et al., 2005).

7. The universal genetic code and genetic disorder

Genetic disorders are actually caused by base changes on autosomes and sex-chromosomes as X-chromosome, or on genomes in organelles as mitochondria. The genetic disorders are classified by location of genetic elements, as autosomal, X-linked, Y-linked and mitochondrial. Now, it is known that many patients are suffered from genetic disorders induced by one-base substitutions on DNA. Several representative genetic disorders are described in Table 1. For simplicity, genetic diseases induced by deletions and insertions of genetic sequences are excluded from the Table. The number of genetic disorders would be reach to the total number of genes (about from twenty to thirty thousands in human), since almost all genes are essential for organisms to live.

Besides classification by locations of genetic changes, the disorders are also classified by forms of the genetic disease appearance into descendants, as dominant and recessive. Genetic disorders caused by mutation of DNA sequences on genomes encoding metabolic enzymes, which leads to reduction of enzyme activities, such as ADA (adenosine deaminase) deficiency and PKU (phenylketonurea), are generally inherited in recessive manners. Autosomal recessive genetic disorders are not appeared into their children, if either parent has two normal genes on two chromosomes, and the disorders are inherited at a 25% chance if both parents are carriers of the disorder. Contrary to that, Huntington's disease and neurofibromatosis caused by inheritance of the abnormal genes from either parent are inherited dominant manner. Therefore, each child has a 50% chance upon inheriting the genetic disorder, if just one parent has a dominant gene defect.

Genetic disorders caused by one-base substitutions are induced when base changes in genetic sequences went across a framework of the robust genetic code or when the base changes made proteins not to satisfy the conditions for formation of water-soluble globular structures, resulting in collapsing the protein structures. As I have discussed in this Chapter, many patients would be suffered from genetic disorders upon even one-amino acid replacement at a high probability, if one-base substitution occurred at the second codon positions. As can be seen in Figure 9, ornithine transcarbamoylase deficiency (OTCD) appears, when one amino acid is replaced to other amino acid encoded by codon having different base at the second codon position, more frequently than the replacement occurring between amino acids encoded by two codons having different bases at the first codon position.

This makes a remarkable contrast with the amino acid replacements observed between homologous proteins with similarly active catalytic function as given in Figures 2 and 3. Therefore, it suggests that it is important to repress base substitutions at the second codon position in genetic sequences in order to protect from genetic diseases. It is necessary to recognize bases at the second base position of codon to accomplish the purpose. As genetic sequences or genes are codon sequences not always mere nucleotide sequences, it would be possible to discriminate the bases at the second codon position from bases at the other two codon positions, based on the differential base compositions at the three base positions in codons. The reason is that it is already known that codons in genetic sequences encoding microbial proteins have specific base compositions at the three respective base positions. For example, guanine bases are generally observed more frequently at the first codon position than other three bases, whereas relatively equal amounts of four bases are contained at the second codon position of GC-rich genes (Ikehara, et al. 1996), although it is almost impossible to find out the strategy for protection of base substitutions at the second codon position at the present time. But, it would be important to recognize the facts described above, as the first step of discovery of the strategies for repression of base replacements at the second codon position in genetic sequences. New possible genetic treatment discovered will release human beings from genetic disorders in a future.

	A	C	D	E	F	G	H	I	K	L	M	N	P	Q	R	S	T	V	W	Y
A				1									2			1	1	1		
C																				
D						2						1			1			2		2
E						1			2											
F		1								1										
G		1	2	3											6			1		
H										3			1	2	2					3
I					1						1					1	1			
K												1			1					
L					5								4	1		1		1		
M								1	1						1		2			
N								1	1							1				
P	1						1			1					1		1			
Q				1			1								1					
R		1				1	2			1			1	4			1		1	
S		1								1			1		4					
T	2							3	3		2									
V										2										
W										1										
Y		3	3																	

Protein	1st	2nd	3rd	1,2	1,3	others
OTCD	35	60	7	1	10	2

Fig. 9. Amino acid replacements observed in a genetic disorder, ornithine transcarbamoylase deficiency (OTCD). Letters written in the most left column and the top row indicate amino acids of normal ornithine transcarbamoylase described with one-letter symbols and those of mutated ornithine transcarbamoylase causing OTCD. Blue, yellow and red boxes indicate amino acid substitutions caused by base changes at the first, the second and the third codon positions, respectively. Green, orange and white boxes indicate amino acid replacements induced by base substitutions at the first or the second codon position, at the first or the third codon position and other base substitutions, respectively. Color box representation is the same as Figure 3. Data of the amino acid replacements observed in OTCD were obtained from Natural Variants in Protein Knowledgebase (UniProKB) at the address of http://www.uniprot.org/uniprot/P00480

8. Conclusion

The genetic disorders upon one-base substitutions in genes encoding amino acid sequences of proteins are induced by the base substitutions at the second codon position more frequently than those at the first codon position. The fact intimately relates to the robustness of the genetic code, which is derived from the origin and evolutionary process of the genetic code. According to the GNC-SNS primitive genetic code hypothesis, which I have proposed, it is considered that the universal genetic code originated from GNC code through SNS code as expanding the code up and down in the genetic code table. Due to the origin and evolutionary process of the genetic code, amino acids with similar chemical and physical properties have been located in the same columns. The arrangement of amino acids in the genetic code table makes it possible to repress induction of genetic disorders at a low rate, because one-base substitutions at the first codon position do not largely affect protein functions at a high probability. I would like to say that it is important to understand correctly the main cause inducing the genetic disorders as the first step for protection of the diseases, and that the recognition will release human beings from many genetic disorders someday.

9. Acknowledgment

I am grateful to Dr. Tadashi Oishi (Narasaho College) for the encouragement of our research on GNC-SNS hypothesis on the genetic code and GADV hypothesis on the origin of life.

10. References

Berg JM. Tymoczko JL, & Stryer L. (2002) Biochemistry 5th ed. New York: W. H. Freeman and Company.

Ikehara, K. (2002) Origins of gene, genetic code, protein and life: comprehensive view of life system from a GNC-SNS primitive genetic code hypothesis. *J. Biosci.* 27, 165-186.

Ikehara, K. (2005) Possible steps to the emergence of life: The [GADV]-protein world hypothesis. *Chem. Record*, 5, 107-118.

Ikehara, K. (2009) Pseudo-replication of [GADV]-proteins and origin of life. *Int. J. Mol. Sci.*, (*International Journal of Molecular Sciences*) Vol. 10, No. 4, 1525-1537.

Ikehara, K., Amada, F., Yoshida, S., Mikata, Y., & Tanaka, A. (1996) A possible origin of newly-born bacterial genes: significance of GC-rich nonstop frame on antisense strand. Nucl. Acids Res., 24, 4249-4255.

Ikehara, K., Omori, Y., Arai, R. & Hirose, A. (2002) A novel theory on the origin of the genetic code: a GNC-SNS hypothesis. *J. Mol. Evol.*, 54, 530-538.

Ikehara, K., & Yoshida, Y. (1998) SNS hypothesis on the origin of the genetic code. *Viva Origino*, 26, 301-310.

Ohno, S. (1970) Evolution by Gene Duplication, Springer: Heidelberg, Germany.

2

Inbreeding and Genetic Disorder

Gonzalo Alvarez[1], Celsa Quinteiro[2] and Francisco C. Ceballos[1]
[1]*Departamento de Genética, Facultad de Biología, Universidad de Santiago de Compostela,*
[2]*Fundación Pública Gallega de Medicina Genómica, Hospital Clínico Universitario, Santiago de Compostela*
Spain

1. Introduction

Inbreeding is usually defined as the mating between relatives and the progeny that result of a consanguineous mating between two related individuals is said to be inbred (Cavalli-Sforza & Bodmer, 1971; Hedrick, 2005; Vogel & Motulsky, 1997). As a result of inheriting the same chromosomal segment through both parents, who inherited it from a common ancestor, the individuals born of consanguineous unions have a number of segments of their chromosomes that are homozygous. Therefore, inbreeding increases the amount of homozygosity and, consequently, recessive alleles hidden by heterozygosity with dominant alleles will be expressed through inbreeding. On this basis, it is expected that recessive traits such as many human genetic disorders will occur with increased frequency in the progeny of consanguineous couples. In addition, since many recessive alleles present in natural populations have harmful effects on the organism, inbreeding usually leads to a decrease in size, vigor and reproductive fitness. In a broad sense, it is necessary to consider that inbreeding can occur under two quite different biological situations. There may be inbreeding because of restriction of population number. The degree of relationship between the individuals in a population depends on the size of that population since the individuals are more closely related to each other in a small population than in a large one. Thus, inbreeding is a phenomenon frequently associated with small populations. On the other hand, inbreeding can occur in a large population as a form of nonrandom mating when the frequency of consanguineous matings is higher than that expected by chance. In this case, the population will show a homozygote excess with respect to a random mating population in which genotypic frequencies are expected to be in Hardy-Weinberg equilibrium. The greatest extent of inbreeding is found in plants. A number of plant species are predominantly self-fertilizing which means that most individuals reproduce by self-fertilization, the most extreme form of inbreeding. In animals, inbreeding is less prevalent than in plants, even though some invertebrates have brother-sister matings as some Hymenoptera. Inbreeding also plays a very important role in animal and plant breeding because the number of breeding individuals in breeding programs is often not large. In this way, the inbreeding effects associated with small population size must be considered in the context of animal and plant breeding.

In humans, consanguineous marriage is frequent in many populations. In fact, it has been recently estimated that consanguineous couples and their progeny suppose about 10.4 % of the 6.7 billion global population of the world (Bittles & Black, 2010). First-cousin marriage and other types of consanguineous unions are frequent in a number of current populations from different parts of the world. The extent of inbreeding of an individual is usually measured in terms of his or her inbreeding coefficient. The coefficient of inbreeding (F) is the probability that an individual receives at a given autosomal locus two alleles that are identical by descent or, equivalently, the proportion of the individual´s autosomal genome expected to be homozygous by descent (autozygous) (Cavalli-Sforza & Bodmer, 1971; Hedrick, 2005). If genealogical information is available for a given individual, his or her inbreeding coefficient can be computed from pedigree analysis. The computation of the genealogical inbreeding coefficient assumes neutrality with respect to natural selection so that the transmission probabilities of alleles can be calculated from Mendelian ratios. In humans, the most extreme cases of inbreeding corresponds to incestuous unions defined as mating between biological first-degree relatives; i. e., father-daughter, mother-son and brother-sister. The progeny from an incestuous union will have an inbreeding coefficient of ¼ (0.25) in the three cases. Offspring of uncle-niece, first-cousin, and second-cousin marriages will have F = 1/8 (0.125), 1/16 (0.0625) and 1/64 (0.0156), respectively. In complex genealogies, the depth of the pedigree is very important for the computation of the inbreeding coefficient. In some cases, genealogical data from the most recent four or five generations seem to be sufficient to capture most of the information relevant to the calculation of the inbreeding coefficient (Balloux et al., 2004). This is due to the fact that recent inbreeding events have a disproportionately large influence on an individual´s inbreeding coefficient relative to events deeper in the pedigree. However, in some large and complex pedigrees, ancestral or remote consanguinity can make a substantial contribution to the inbreeding of a given individual and the exploration of pedigrees limited to a shallow depth carries the risk of underestimating the degree to which individuals are inbred (Alvarez et al., 2009; Boyce, 1983; MacCluer et al., 1983). Computation of inbreeding coefficients from extended pedigrees will be necessary in order to obtain an accurate measure of the inbreeding level in those situations in which remote consanguinity is important.

Studies on genome-wide homozygosity through the genome scan technology have opened new avenues for inbreeding research. Thus, genome-wide homozygosity may be used to estimate the inbreeding coefficient for a given individual when genealogical information is not available. Furthermore, the study of genome-wide homozygosity is very important for the identification of recessive disease genes through homozygosity mapping as well as for the investigation of homozygosity effects on traits of biomedical importance. Long homozygous chromosomal segments have been detected in human chromosomes from the analysis of polymorphic markers in whole-genome scans (Broman & Weber, 1999; McQuillan et al., 2008). These long tracts where homozygous markers occur in an uninterrupted sequence are often termed runs of homozygosity (ROH) and can arise in the genome through a number of mechanisms (Broman & Weber, 1999; Gibson et al., 2006). The most obvious explanation for such tracts is autozygosity, where the same chromosomal segment has been passed to a child from parents who inherited it from a common ancestor. The length of an autozygous segment reflects its age since haplotypes are broken up by recombination at meiosis in such a way that long tracts are expected to occur by close inbreeding whereas a short autozygous segment is likely to be the result of the mating of very distantly related individuals. Homozygous tracts are significantly more common in chromosome regions with high linkage disequilibrium and low recombination but since linkage disequilibrium is a local phenomenon would cause only short homozygous segments (Broman and Weber, 1999; Gibson et al., 2006). A genomic measure of individual autozygosity termed F_{roh} has been defined as the proportion of the autosomal genome in runs of homozygosity above a specified length threshold:

$$F_{roh} = \Sigma L_{roh} / L_{auto}$$

where ΣL_{roh} is the total length of all ROHs in the individual above a specified minimum length and L_{auto} is the length of the autosomal genome covered by the genomic markers (McQuillan et al., 2008). In a genome-wide study based on a 300,000 SNP panel, it has been found a strong correlation (r = 0.86) between F_{roh} and the genealogical inbreeding coefficient (F) among 249 individuals from the isolate population of the Orkney Isles in northern Scotland, for which complete and reliable pedigree data were available (McQuillan et al., 2008). F_{roh} values were computed for a range of minimum-length thresholds (0.5, 1.5 and 5 Mb) and the mean value of F_{roh} for 5 Mb was the closest F_{roh} to that of F computed from pedigree data. ROHs measuring less than 3 or 4 Mb were not uncommon in unrelated individuals. The size of the autozygous segments and their distribution throughout the human genome has been investigated in inbred individuals with recessive Mendelian disorders (Woods et al., 2006). Through a whole-genome scan of 10,000 SNPs, individuals affected with a recessive disease whose parents were first cousins drawn from two populations with a long history of consanguinity (Pakistani and Arab) presented, on average, 20 homozygous segments (range 7-32 homozygous segments) exceeding 3 cM and a size of the homozygous segment associated with recessive disease of 26 cM (range 5-70 cM). The proportion of their genomes that was homozygous varied from 5 to 20% with a mean value of 11%. This figure is increased about 5 % over the expected value for the offspring of a first-cousin union (F = 0.0625) but it is necessary to take into account that the proportion of the genome identical by descent has a large stochastic variation (Carothers et al., 2006). Moreover, the individuals analyzed were those children of first cousins presenting a genetic disorder so that they were a biased sample of a first-cousin progeny. Through the genome scan technology, several studies have shown that extended tracts of genomic homozygosity are globally widespread in many human populations and they provide valuable information of a population´s demographic history such as past consanguinity and population isolation (Kirin et al., 2010; Nalls et al., 2009).

Autozygosity has practical implications for the identification of human disease genes. Homozygosity mapping is the method of choice for mapping human genes that cause rare recessive Mendelian diseases (Botstein & Risch, 2003; Lander and Botstein, 1987). The method consists of searching for a region of the genome that is autozygous in individuals affected by a given disease from consanguineous families. Thus, the disease locus is detected on the basis that the adjacent region will be homozygous by descent in such inbred individuals. The method is also known as autozygosity or consanguinity mapping and has the advantage that relatively few individuals are required. Homozygosity mapping became practical with the discovery of multiple highly polymorphic markers. The first polymorphic markers used were restriction length polymorphisms, subsequently, short sequence repeats and more recently single nucleotide polymorphisms (SNPs) (Woods et al., 2004). Since 1995 until 2003, nearly 200 studies were published in which homozygosity mapping was used to map human genes causing rare recessive disease phenotypes (Botstein and Risch, 2003).

Recently, the strategy of homozygosity mapping has been extended to analyze single individuals by means of high-density genome scans in order to circumvent the limitation of the number of consanguineous families required for the analysis (Hildebrandt et al., 2009). Homozygosity mapping in single individuals that bear homozygous disease gene mutations by descent from an unknown distant ancestor may provide a single genomic candidate region small enough to allow successful gene identification. Remote consanguinity will lead in the affected individual to fewer and shorter homozygous intervals that contain the disease gene. The analysis through homozygosity mapping of 72 individuals with known homozygous mutations in 13 different recessive genes detected, by using a whole-genome scan of 250,000 SNPs, the disease gene in homozygous segments as short as 2 Mb containing an average of only 16 candidate genes (Hildebrandt et al., 2009).

2. Consanguineous marriage around the world

Studies on the prevalence and pattern of consanguineous marriages in human populations show that consanguinity is widely extended in many current populations around the world (Bittles, 2001, 2006). In demographic literature a consanguineous marriage is usually defined as a union between individuals who are related as second cousin or closer ($F \geq 0.0156$ for their progeny). This arbitrary limit is based in the perception that an inbreeding coefficient below 0.0156 has biological effects not very different from those found in the general population. At the present time, it has been estimated that the consanguineous couples and their progeny suppose 10.4% of the global population (Bittles and Black, 2010). Marriage between first cousins ($F = 0.0625$ for their progeny) is considered the most prevalent consanguineous union in human populations. Also, matrimony among two second cousins is very frequent. Globally, unions between uncle and nice or double first cousins ($F = 0.125$ for their progeny, in both cases) are less common; however it is possible to find certain populations with high incidence of uncle-nice unions. Regarding incestuous unions between biological first degree relatives (father-daughter, mother-son, brother-sister; $F = 0.25$ for their progeny, in the three cases), a universal taboo for nuclear family mating exists in all societies. Incest is illegal in many countries and specifically forbidden by the big five religions, even though incestuous practices can be found sporadically in any society. The prevalence of incest around the world is difficult to establish due to its illegality and association with social stigma (Bennett et al, 2002).
Consanguinity is not homogeneously distributed around the globe, so that it is possible to associate certain geographic areas with high consanguinity incidence. The distribution of consanguineous marriages in four continents (Europe, America, Asia and Africa) obtained from data available at the web portal Consanguinity/Endogamy Resource (consang.net) is shown in Figure 1. This web portal compiles data of global prevalence of consanguinity from more than two hundred studies performed since middle of the 20th century. These studies gathered marital information through household and school, pedigree analysis, civil registrations and census, obstetric and hospital inpatients, as well as religious dispensations for more than 450 populations from 90 countries. In this data set, 63.0% of the populations are from Asia, 19.1% from South America, 8.9% from Europe, 6.4% from Africa and just 2.6% from Central and North America. In general, a more favorable attitude towards consanguinity is found in populations from Asia and Africa. In Sub-Saharan Africa, for example, 35 to 50% of the marriages are between relatives. In Egypt, on average, 42.1% of

total marriages are consanguineous; with a preference for double first cousin and second cousin, even though there is a great heterogeneity among populations due to different beliefs and cultural backgrounds. The most consanguineous populations studied so far are found in Asia. In Afghanistan, for instance, 55.4% of the matrimonies in the country are between relatives. In the traditional nomadic *Qashqai* from Iran up to 73.5% of the marriages are consanguineous. Table 1 shows the results of a 10-year study performed in the cities of Bangalore and Mysore in the State of Karnataka, South India that involved a total number of 107,518 marriages (Bittles et al., 1991). For the entire sample, 31.4% of all unions were consanguineous and the mean consanguinity measured as the average inbreeding coefficient ($\alpha = \Sigma p_i F_i$) was 0.0299. Consanguinity was more prevalent among Hindus with 33.5% of consanguineous marriages and they had the highest average consanguinity (α = 0.0333) because the high rate of uncle-niece marriages. In the Muslim community, 23.7% of marriages were consanguineous with an average consanguinity of 0.0160. Muslims avoid uncle-niece marriage because this type of consanguineous union is proscribed by the Quran. First-cousin marriage was the most prevalent consanguineous union in the Muslim community. Christians in Karnataka presented an 18.6% of consanguineous marriages including both uncle-niece and first cousin marriages with an average consanguinity of 0.0173. Unlike Asia and Africa, Europe and America seems to have a refusal attitude over consanguinity since most populations present less than 10% of their matrimonies being consanguineous (Figure 1). In Europe, consanguinity appears to be more prevalent in Southern countries such as Spain or Italy where consanguineous unions represent 3.5% and 1.6% of total marriages respectively. North European countries appeared to have lower incidence of consanguineous marriages, for instance, 0.3% in Great Britain, 0.4 in Norway or 0.4 in Hungary. The American continent seems to be very similar to Europe. In South America, the average of consanguineous marriages in 39 Brazilian populations is 4.2%, with different preferences for union type depending on the community. In Colombia and Ecuador, data from six populations indicate that consanguineous marriages represent the 2.8% and 2.9% respectively, of total marriages. In USA, it has been estimated that only 0.2% of total marriages are consanguineous from a couple of populations from Wisconsin, a sample of all-USA of more than 130,000 people and a couple of minorities populations.

		Religion		
Type of marriage		Hindu	Muslim	Christian
Non-Consanguineous (F=0)		62.0	72.9	78.1
Beyond second cousin (F<0.0156)		4.5	3.5	3.4
Second Cousin (F=0.0156)		1.7	2.5	1.6
First cousin (F=0.0625)		10.8	17.5	6.8
Uncle-niece (F=0.125)		21.0	3.7	10.2

Table 1. Consanguineous marriages (%) and religion in Karnataka, India. The inbreeding coefficient (F) of the offspring for each type of marriage is given. (Form Bittles et al. 1991)

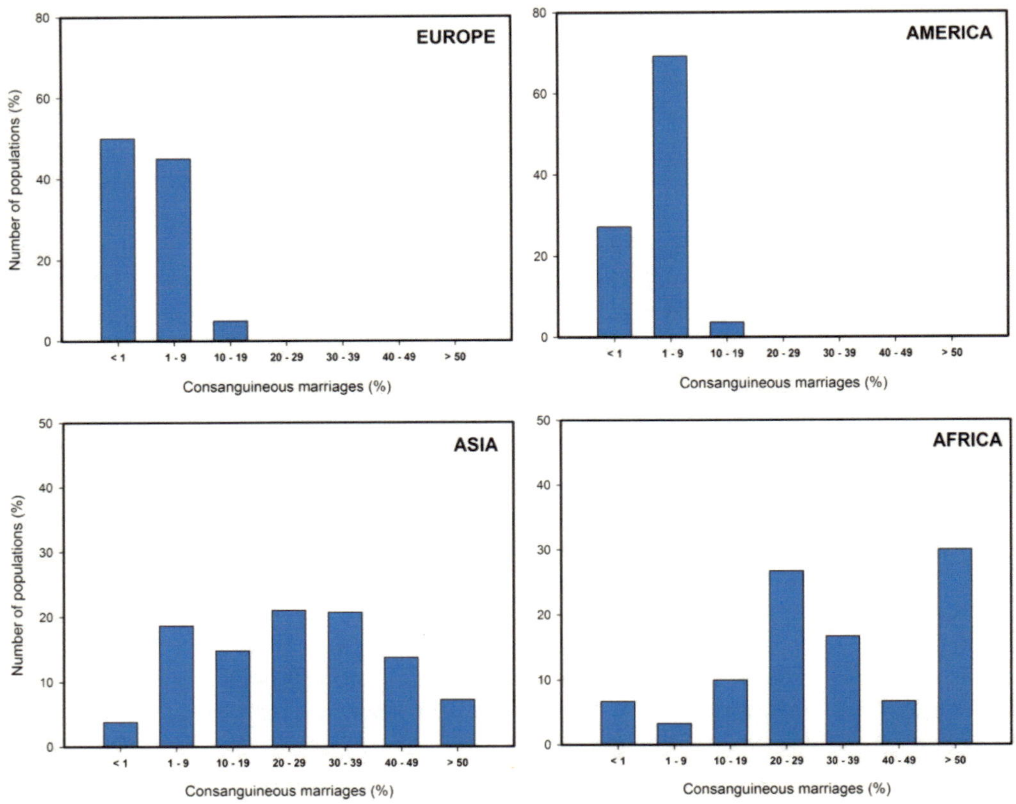

Fig. 1. Percentage of consanguineous marriages in human populations from four continents. (Data from consag.net)

Consanguinity studies in population minorities, isolates and migrants reveal that there is a great heterogeneity between close communities around the world. Figure 2 shows the incidence of consanguineous marriages in population minorities, isolates and migrants for more than 100 populations from 22 countries (data from consang.net). In the nomadic Bedouin Baggara Arabs community that inhabits Nyertiti state in Sudan, for example, 71.7% of their matrimonies are consanguineous marriages, with a clear preference for first-cousin unions. In Japan, where only 8.98% of all marriages are consanguineous, an isolate population as the Arihara community in the Kansai region presented 47.8% of consanguineous marriages. Samaritan isolate community from Israel has a clear preference for first cousin unions. While in Israel other Hebrew communities have on average 7.6% of consanguineous unions, Samaritans have 46.4%. In Europe, some migrant populations maintain their traditions while living abroad. For instance, Pakistani community of Great Britain living in Bradford has 67% of consanguineous marriages with average consanguinity being 0.0377. Pakistani community in Norway also has high incidence of consanguineous unions since 31% of their marriages are consanguineous. In the Unites States, where first cousin marriages are criminal offence in eight states and illegal in a further 31 states, exceptions have been incorporated to permit uncle-niece marriage within the Jewish community of Rhode Island. High incidence of consanguineous marriages has been reported in isolates minorities from USA such as a Gypsy community from Boston with

61.9% of consanguineous unions, and Christian Anabaptists Mennonites from Kansas with 33.0% of their matrimonies being between relatives.

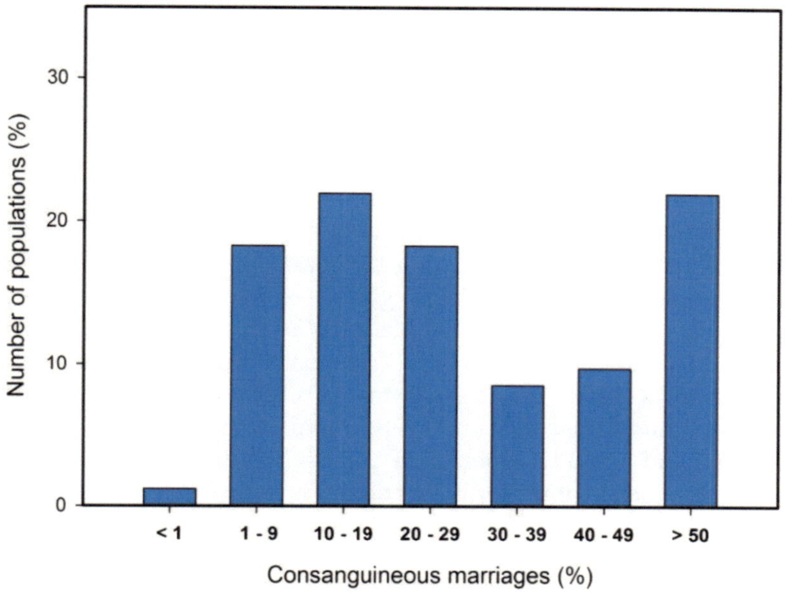

Fig. 2. Percentage of consanguineous marriages in minorities, isolates and migrant populations around the world. (Data from consag.net)

Consanguineous marriage is favored in many societies, especially from Asia and Africa, as a mean of preserving family goods and lands (Bittles, 2006). Social and cultural advantages such as strengthened family ties, enhanced female autonomy, more stable marital relationships, greater compatibility with in-laws, lower domestic violence, lower divorced rates or simplified premarital arrangements along with economic considerations may be the actual motives for the preference of consanguineous unions particularly in rural societies. Furthermore, consanguinity was also common among European royalty and aristocracy up until the middle of 1900s, and nowadays is still present punctually in rich families and aristocracy. Consanguineous marriage cannot be restricted to any specific society or religion, although the attitude of the different societies toward consanguinity is highly influenced by religious beliefs or creeds (Bittles et al., 1991). Marriage regulations in Islam permit first-cousin and double first-cousin unions and the Quran expressly prohibits uncle-nice matrimonies. Unlike Islam, Hinduism attitude over consanguinity is non-uniform. The Aryan Hindus of northern India prohibit marriages between relatives for approximately seven generations. By comparison, Dravidian Hindus of south India strongly favor marriage between first cousin of the type mother's brother's daughter, and particularly in the states of Andhra Pradesh, Karnataka and Tamil Nadu uncle-nice marriages are also widely contracted (Table 1). Buddhism and its two major branches Theravada and Mahayana which are spread through all Asia prohibit any type of consanguineous relationship in marriage. Christianity and Judaism attitude over consanguinity is based in the book of Leviticus, third book of the Hebrew Bible and Torah. Many examples of consanguineous unions are cited in the biblical texts, for example Abraham and Sarah, identified as half siblings (*Genesis* 20:12) or Moses´ parents, related as nephew and aunt (*Exodus* 6:20). However, in the book of Leviticus is expressed that "None of you shall approach any one of his close relatives to uncover nakedness. I am the Lord" (*Leviticus 18:5*). Despite these sentences, the Leviticus has been interpreted in different ways. Judaic lax interpretation of the Leviticus led its followers to permit first-cousin and even uncle-nice unions. Christianity attitude over consanguineous marriage is characterized by its lack of uniformity. Orthodox churches have a strict interpretation of the Leviticus since they prohibit consanguineous marriage of any form. For members of the Latin Church the effect of the rules addressed in the Leviticus was to prohibit marriage with a biological relative usually up to and including third cousin. Dispensation could, however, be granted at Diocesan level for related couples who wished to marry within the prohibited degrees of consanguinity, albeit with payment of an appropriate benefaction to the church. Among the constellation of different churches arose from Reformed Protestant the existing biblical guidelines were generally adopted, although the closest form of approved union usually has been between first cousins. Paradoxically, the highest rates of consanguineous unions historically recorded in Europe, and even nowadays, appear to be in the southern Roman Catholic countries rather than in the northern Protestant European countries. This pattern is followed also by the Catholic countries of South and Central America in comparison with Protestants, Anabaptist, Anglicans and Restorationists from North America.

3. Inbreeding and genetic disease

In his classic study of inborn errors of metabolism, Archibald Garrod noted that an unusual high proportion of patients with alkaptonuria were progeny of consanguineous marriages. After this observation carried out at the early years of the 20th century, a very large number of studies have consistently shown that recessive traits occur with increased frequency in the progeny of consanguineous mates, and this outcome is one of the most important clinical consequences of inbreeding. In Europe and Japan, for example, the frequency of first-cousin marriages among the parents of affected individuals with recessive traits such as albinism, phenylketonuria, ichthyosis congenital and microcephaly is remarkably higher than frequency of first-cousin marriages in the corresponding general population (Bodmer & Cavalli-Sforza, 1976; pp. 372-377). In general, the rarer the disease, the higher the proportion of consanguineous marriage among the parents of affected individuals. Similarly, the closer the inbreeding, the higher the effect. The genetic explanation for these observations is simple and derives from basic principles of population genetics. In a random mating population, the frequency of recessive homozygotes *aa* will be q^2 for an allele *a* that has frequency q, according to the Hardy-Weinberg law. In an inbred population with inbreeding level F, the frequency of recessive homozygotes will be $q^2 + (1 - q)qF$ and therefore the ratio of the frequency of the homozygote *aa* in an inbred population relative to a random mating one will be $1 + F(1 - q)/q$. The ratio is very large for low allele frequencies and increases with the level of inbreeding. For example, when F = 1/16 corresponding to the progeny of a first cousin marriage and q = 0.01, there are more than seven times as many affected individuals in the inbred group as in the non-inbred population. For illustrative purposes, Table 2 shows the risk of recessive disease among progeny of first-cousin marriages and among progeny of unrelated parents for three values of allelic frequency. On this rationale, parental consanguinity can be a useful criterion in clinical diagnosis. Thus, when the parents of a patient suffering from a previously unknown disease are consanguineous the diagnosis of a recessive genetic disease is of serious consideration.

Allele frequency (q)	Offspring of unrelated parents	Offspring of first cousins
0.01	1:10,000	1:1,400
0.005	1:40,000	1:3,000
0.001	1:1,000,000	1:16,000

Table 2. Risk of affected individual for rare recessive disease in offspring of unrelated and first-cousin parents

Several studies have reported the occurrence of a number of detrimental health effects in the progeny of consanguineous marriages. In general, the offspring of consanguineous couples presented increased levels of morbidity and significant medical problems such as major malformations, congenital anomaly and structural birth defects in first few days of life (Bennett et al., 2002; Bittles, 2001, 2006). The estimation of the absolute risk for the offspring of consanguineous unions is often very difficult because an important number of factors such as sociodemographic variables, methods of subject ascertainment and others that are influencing the risk of a given population. Many of these non-genetic variables are hardly controlled in the data analysis. A way to circumvent such problems is to compare the risk in the offspring of consanguineous marriages with that corresponding to non-consanguineous unions. In a compilation based on data from a number of studies, the increased risk for a significant birth defect in progeny of a first cousin marriage varied between 1.7 and 2.8% above that of the non-consanguineous population (Bennett et al., 2002). An important number of abnormalities have also been reported in the offspring of first degree incestuous unions. A compilation from data of several studies shows that 11.7% (25/213) of the incestuous progeny presented known autosomal recessive disorders, 16.0% (34/213) congenital malformations, 11.7% (25/213) nonspecific severe intellectual impairment and 14.6% (31/213) mild intellectual impairment (Bennett et al., 2002).

In contrast with the extensive evidence on the effect of inbreeding for Mendelian diseases the contribution of consanguinity to complex or multifactorial diseases is less known. There is, however, growing evidence for adverse effects of inbreeding on complex human diseases of public health importance. The relationship between inbreeding and blood pressure (BP), and the related late-onset disease, essential hypertension, has been investigated in isolate populations from Dalmatian islands, Croatia (Rudan et al., 2003b). A strong linear relationship between the inbreeding coefficient (F) and both systolic and diastolic BP among 2760 adult individuals from 25 villages within Croatian island isolates was found. The individual inbreeding coefficient was computed for each study participant based on pedigree information from four to five ancestral generations. An increase in F of 0.01 corresponded to an increase of approximately 3 mm Hg in systolic and 2 mm Hg in diastolic BP, and 10-15 % of the total variation in BP in those populations could be explained by recessive or partially recessive quantitative trait locus (QTL) alleles. It was estimated that several hundred (300-600) recessive QTLs could contribute to BP variation. Moreover, it was inferred that inbreeding accounts for 36 % of all hypertension in those populations. Dalmatian island populations have been also used to investigate the relationship between inbreeding and the prevalence of 10 late onset complex diseases: coronary heart disease, stroke, cancer, schizophrenia, epilepsy, uni/bipolar depression, asthma, adult type diabetes, gout and peptic ulcer, which are commonly occurring disorders in those islands (Rudan et al., 2003a). The study was carried out in 14 isolate villages on three neighboring islands in middle Dalmatia which present a wide range of levels of inbreeding and endogamy, and relative uniformity of environment so that the potential effects of inbreeding on those complex diseases may be detected. Disease prevalence was investigated by comparisons between villages grouped by the level of inbreeding as high (average F = 0.036), moderate (average F = 0.013) and low (average F = 0.006). An increase in disease prevalence across villages associated with an increase in average inbreeding coefficient was observed for gout, depression, peptic ulcer, schizophrenia, cancer, epilepsy, coronary heart disease, stroke and asthma (the last three not statistically significant) but not for type 2 diabetes (Table 3). The results indicated that between 23 % and 48 % of the incidence of these disorders in the population sample (other than type 2 diabetes) could be attributed to inbreeding. These findings provide indirect evidence in support of a major polygenic component to disease susceptibility due to many deleterious recessive alleles located throughout the genome. Rudan et al. (2003a) have suggested that the genetic component of late onset diseases may be caused by large number of rare variants in numerous genes maintained at low frequency in populations by mutation-selection balance, according to the common disease/rare variant (CD/RV) hypothesis (Wright et al., 2003). From this point of view, the study of inbred populations could be very useful in the detection of genetic effects on complex disease since inbred individuals will show stronger phenotypic effects compared with outbred individuals, where most alleles are present in heterozygotes (Rudan et al., 2003b).

A number of evidences suggest that inbreeding is also an important risk factor in susceptibility to infectious diseases in humans. Association between inbreeding and susceptibility to infectious disease has been investigated through microsatellite genome scan data for tuberculosis (TB) in The Gambia, leprosy in India and persistent hepatitis B virus infection both in The Gambia and Italy (Lyons et al., 2009b). In this study, inbreeding coefficients were estimated from correlations in heterozygosity among markers because genealogical information was not available for the studied individuals; r^2 values between heterozygosities were calculated from two sets of randomly selected unlinked markers. In The Gambia, where the frequency of first-cousin marriage is approximately 30%, the correlations in heterozygosity among markers were larger in affected individuals than in unaffected ones for both hepatitis and TB. This result suggests that inbred individuals are more common among the infected cases for both hepatitis and TB and, therefore, consanguinity appears significantly to increase the risk of these two major infectious causes of death in humans. Significant differences in r^2 values between affected and unaffected individuals were not found for persistent hepatitis in the Italian genome scan, probably due to the low levels of inbreeding in that population. Correlations in heterozygosity among markers were not different between affected and unaffected individuals for leprosy in India, where the frequency of consanguineous marriages is high, suggesting no effect of inbreeding on this infectious disease. Furthermore, evidence for an association between infectious disease and homozygosity has been also reported. In a case-control study of fatal invasive bacterial diseases in Kenyan children that was performed by using a genome-wide scan with microsatellite markers, homozygosity was significantly increased in 148 children aged <13 years who died of invasive bacterial diseases such as bacteraemia, meningitis and neonatal sepsis compared to the control sample constituted by 137 age-matched, healthy children (Lyons et al., 2009a). Of a total number of 134 microsatellite markers analyzed, homozygosity was strongly associated with mortality at five markers. These results indicate that homozygosity significantly contribute to the risk of childhood death due to invasive bacterial disease.

Disease		High Inbreeding (Mean F=0.036)	Moderate Inbreeding (Mean F=0.013)	Low Inbreeding (Mean F=0.006)
Coronary heart disease		13.28	11.95	11.23
Stroke		2.43	2.79	1.73
Cancer		4.54***	3.44*	1.93
Schizophrenia		1.23***	0.96*	0.14
Uni/bipolar depression		10.26***	7.63**	4.51
Asthma		3.63	2.64	2.60
Tipe II diabetes		6.02	7.35	6.77
Gout		9.25***	7.19***	3.96
Peptic ulcer		6.92***	4.29**	2.18
Epilepsy		1.47***	0.78	0.31

Statistically significance (P values) in highly and moderately inbred groups is calculated against the low inbreeding group: * $P<0.05$; ** $P<0.01$; *** $P<0.001$

Table 3. Prevalence (%) of 10 complex diseases in groups of villages with relatively "high", "moderate" and "low" inbreeding coefficient (F) in Dalmatia islands, Croatia. (From Rudan et al., 2003a)

4. Inbreeding depression

One of the adverse effects of consanguineous mating is the phenomenon of inbreeding depression. In population genetics, inbreeding depression is usually defined as the decreased fitness of offspring from related parents (Charlesworth & Willis, 2009). Inbreeding depression occurs in many species of animal and plants as well as in humans and is caused by increased homozygosity of individuals. There are two major hypotheses to explain how increased homozygosity can lower fitness. The "overdominance hypothesis" suggests that heterozygotes at loci determining fitness are superior to homozygotes for either allele so that heterozygote advantage (overdominance) is responsible for inbreeding depression. The "partial dominance hypothesis" assumes that inbreeding depression is caused by recessive or partially recessive deleterious alleles maintained in the population at low frequencies by mutation-selection balance. A number of studies on the genetics of quantitative fitness traits in *Drosophila* and other species suggest that inbreeding depression is predominantly caused by deleterious alleles generated by mutation and kept at low frequency in the population by natural selection, even though some alleles at higher frequencies maintained by some form of balancing selection such as heterozygote advantage or temporal, spatial or frequency-dependent selection could be also involved (Charlesworth & Charlesworth, 1999; Charlesworth & Willis, 2009).
The first experimental research on the harmful effects of consanguinity including inbreeding depression was performed by Charles Darwin and was published in his book "*The effects of*

cross and self-fertilization in the vegetable kingdom" (Darwin, 1876). Darwin carried out carefully controlled experiments in the Down House greenhouse that involved self-fertilization and outcrossing between unrelated individuals in 57 plant species. In these experiments the offspring of self-fertilized plants were on average shorter, flowered later, weighted less and produced fewer seeds than the progeny of cross-fertilized plants. By these experiments Darwin documented the phenomenon of inbreeding depression for numerous plant species. Darwin´s laborious study on inbreeding had its origin in his interest on plant reproductive systems. In fact, his experiments were performed to explain why numerous plant species have systems that prevent self-fertilization and why reproduction by outcrossing is prevalent in nature. However, it is very likely that Darwin also had a personal interest on this matter. Charles Darwin was married to his first cousin Emma Wedgwood and they had 10 children along their lifetime. Darwin was worried about the health of his children, who were very often ill and three of them died before adulthood. Darwin´s own ill health led him to fear that his children could have inherited his medical problems but he also suspected that his marriage to his first cousin might have caused some of his children´s health problems (Jones, 2008; Moore, 2005). For a long time, it has been commonly accepted that Charles Darwin´s concerns on the harmful effects of first-cousin marriage were unjustified because they were based on the extrapolation from ill-effects of self-fertilization in plants to the outcomes of first-cousin marriage in humans. Nevertheless, recent researches on both survival and fertility in the Darwin/Wedgwood dynasty support the view that inbreeding was effectively involved in a number of health problems of Darwin´s children (Berra et al., 2010; Golubosvky, 2008). First-cousin marriage had a widespread acceptance among the upper middle class of Victorian England in such a way that the first-cousin marriage of Charles and Emma was not unusual in that time. In fact, three of Emma´s brothers were married to relatives: Josiah Wedgwood III married his first cousin Caroline Darwin, who was Charles´s sister, Hensleigh Wedgwood was married to his first cousin Frances MacKintosh and Henry Wedgwood was married to his double first cousin Jessie Wedgwood. All these consanguineous marriages are represented in the pedigree of the Darwin/Wedgwood dynasty shown in Figure 3, which was specifically constructed to compute inbreeding coefficients for Charles Darwin, his progeny and related families combining genealogical information obtained from numerous sources. The inbreeding coefficients computed from the Darwin/Wedgwood pedigree shows that some individuals of the dynasty presented rather high levels of inbreeding. Thus, the children of Henry Wedgwood had a high inbreeding coefficient (F = 0.1255) because their parents were double first cousins. The progeny of both Charles Darwin and Josiah Wedgwood III had a moderate inbreeding coefficient (F = 0.0630), and the progeny of Hensleigh Wedgwood had an inbreeding of 0.0625. Charles Darwin´s mother, Susannah Wedgwood, and her brother, Josiah Wedgwood II, had very low inbreeding values (F = 0.0039). All the remaining individuals in the pedigree depicted in Figure 1 had F = 0, as did Charles Darwin and his father, Robert Darwin. From these data, a statistically significant positive association between child mortality (deaths from birth to 10 years) and inbreeding coefficient was detected in the progeny of 25 marriages belonging to four consecutive generations of the Darwin/Wedgwood dynasty (Berra et al., 2010). Child mortality was clearly higher for those families whose progeny had high inbreeding coefficient (Figure 4). Mean child mortality in progeny of 21 non consanguineous Darwin/Wedgwood marriages was 10.67%, whereas progeny mortality was nearly twice in the consanguineous marriages: 20.00% in those families with F = 0.0625 - 0.0630 and 16.67% in one family with F = 0.1255. Regarding the own Darwin family, the offspring of Charles and Emma had an inbreeding coefficient of 0.0630 and presented one of the highest mortalities (30.0%) among the 25 Darwin/Wedgwood families investigated. Of the three Darwin´s children that died before adulthood (Anne Elizabeth, Mary Eleanor and Charles Waring), the cause of death is known for two of them. Anne Elizabeth (1841-1851), Darwin´s second child and first daughter, probably died of child tuberculosis and Charles Waring (1856-1859), the last Darwin´s child, died of scarlet fever. The recent evidence of inbreeding as an important risk factor in susceptibility to infectious diseases such as hepatitis and tuberculosis as well as the association between homozygosity and childhood mortality resulting from invasive bacterial disease (Lyons et al., 2009a,b) gives a strong support to the hypothesis that inbreeding was directly involved in a number of health problems in Darwin´s children. Furthermore, it has been also suggested that inbreeding might have influenced the fertility of Darwin´s children (Golubovsky, 2008). It is known that three of Charles Darwin´s six children with long-term marriage history suffered from infertility (William Erasmus, Henrietta and Leonard) and a likely cause of that unexplained infertility might be the segregation of some recessive autosomal meiotic mutation manifested in Darwin progeny as a result of inbreeding.

At the present time, there is extensive evidence on the harmful effects of inbreeding on survival before adulthood in humans. Most of this empirical evidence comes from mortality data of the progeny of first cousins as this type of marriage is the most prevalent consanguineous union in human populations. A compilation based on data from 31 studies for various stages of prereproductive mortality showed that the offspring of consanguineous marriages have a higher risk of mortality compared with the offspring of unrelated parents (Khalt & Khoury, 1991; Khoury et al., 1987). The median relative risk for the progeny of first cousin marriages compared with the non consanguineous progeny was 1.41 for prereproductive mortality including all deaths from stillbirths to deaths below 20 years. In other meta-analysis based on data from 38 populations located in eastern and southern Asia, the Middle East, Africa, Europe and South America the progeny of first cousins presented an absolute increase in mortality from birth to a median age of 10 years of 4.4% ± 4.6 (Bittles & Neel, 1994; Figure 5). The most recent compilation on inbreeding depression for survival in humans revealed an absolute increase in mortality from approximately 6 months gestation to an average of 10 years of age of 3.5 % among first-cousin progeny and comprised 69 populations resident in 15 countries located across four continents (Bittles & Black, 2010). It should be emphasized, however, that the above figures represent population averages and they do not reflect the fact that the magnitude of inbreeding depression is highly variable among human populations. Thus, the absolute increase in mortality at first-cousin level varied from nearly zero to approximately 19 % across populations in one of the above mentioned compilations (Bittles & Neel, 1994). Regarding inbreeding depression for high inbreeding levels, the available evidence is at present less abundant than that corresponding to moderate inbreeding from first-cousin marriage. In humans, the most extreme cases of close inbreeding correspond to incestuous unions such as father-daughter, mother-son and brother-sister. Several studies have investigated the adverse effects of inbreeding from children of such incestuous unions, but the results obtained are difficult to interpret because difficulties associated with sample size, unbiased data and suitable controls (Adams & Neel, 1967; Carter, 1967, Seemanová, 1971).

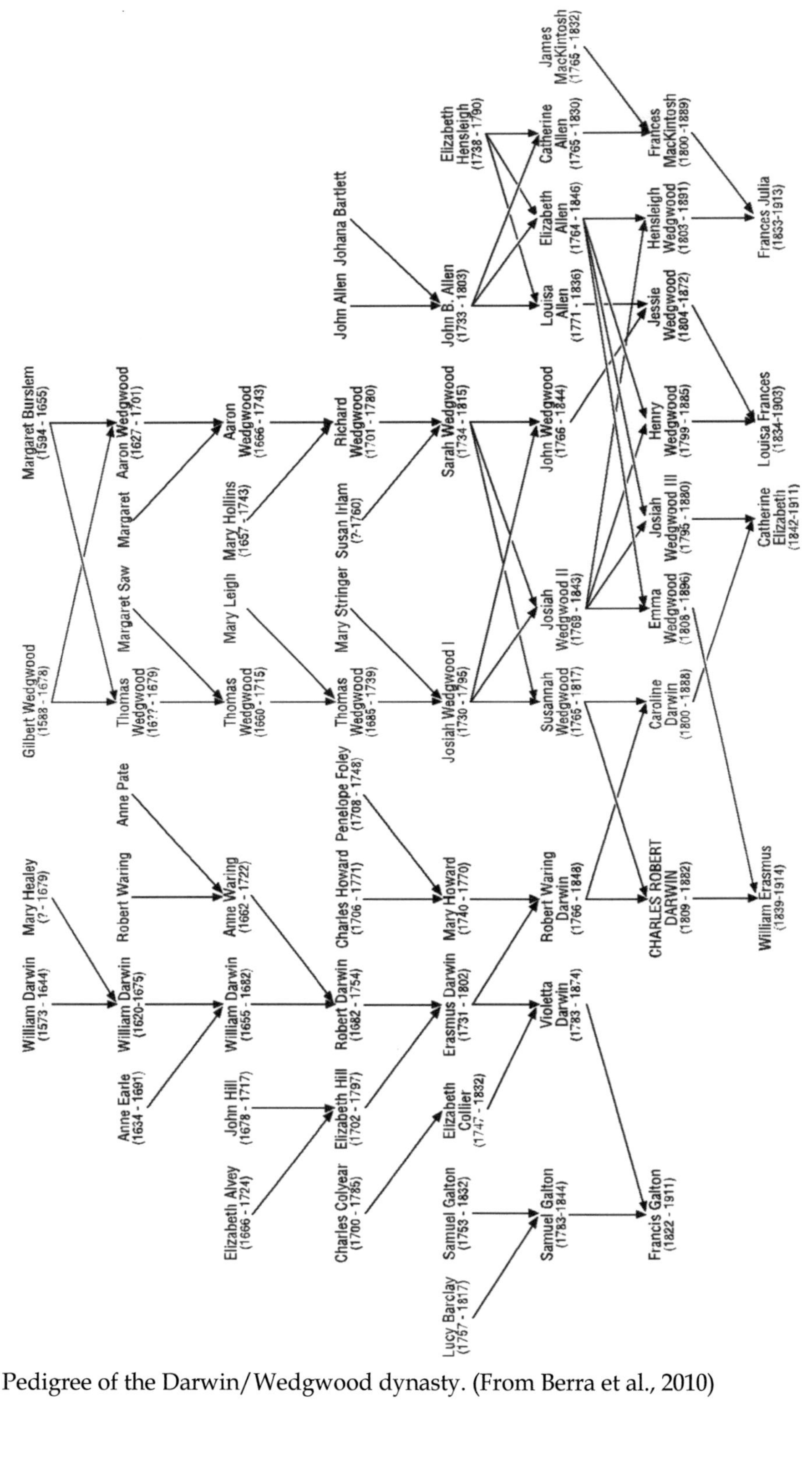

Fig. 3. Pedigree of the Darwin/Wedgwood dynasty. (From Berra et al., 2010)

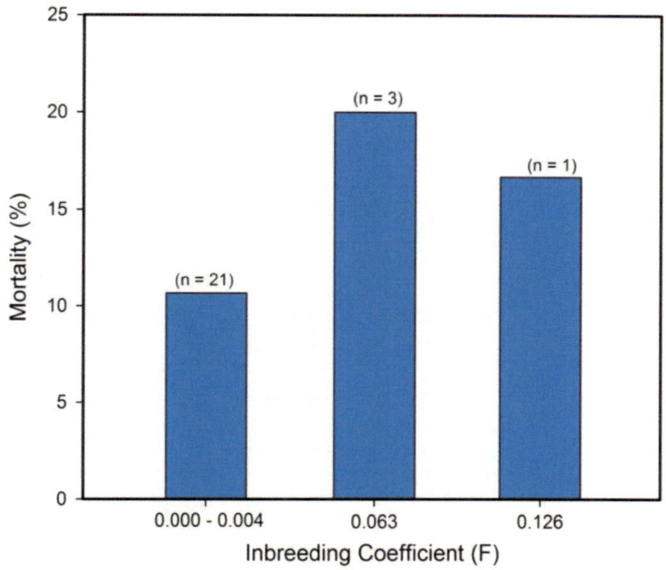

Fig. 4. Mortality from birth to 10 years and inbreeding coefficient (F) in offspring of 25 marriages of the Darwin/Wedgwood dynasty (n = number of marriages) (Data from Berra et al., 2010)

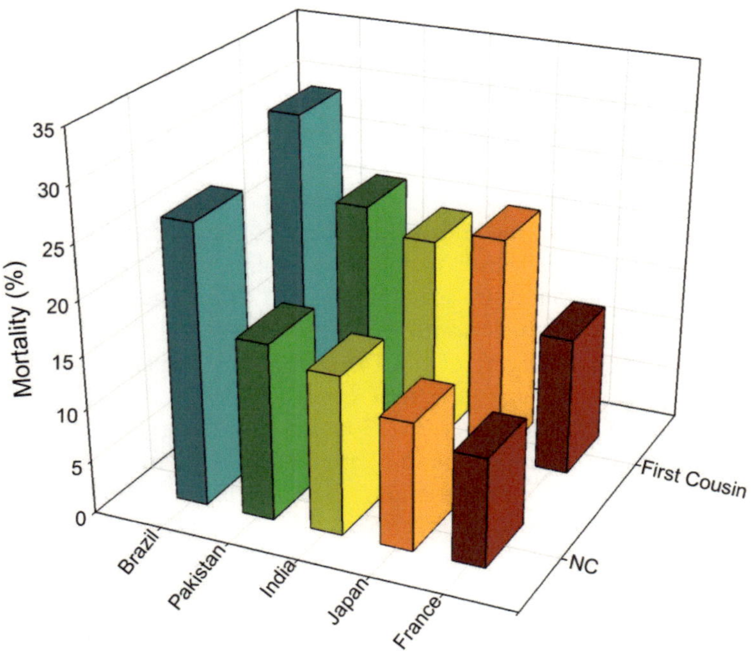

Fig. 5. Mortality in offspring of first cousin and non-consanguineous marriages in Brazil (average of 8 populations), Pakistan (average of 9 populations), India (average of 10 populations), Japan (average of 7 populations) and France (average of 2 populations). (Data from Bittles & Neel, 1994)

King	F		King´s wife	F		Type of consanguineous marriage
Philip I (1478-1506)	0.025		Joanna I of Castile	0.039		Third cousins
Charles I (1500 – 1558)	0.037		Isabella of Portugal	0.101		First cousins
Philip II (1527 – 1598)	0.123		Mary of Portugal	0.123		Double first cousins
			Mary I of England	0.008		First cousins one removed
			Elizabeth of Valois	0.001		Remote kinship
			Anna of Habsburg	0.106		Uncle – niece
Philip III[1] (1578 – 1621)	0.218		Margaret of Habsburg	0.139		First cousins once removed
Philip IV (1605 – 1665)	0.115		Elizabeth of Bourbon	0.007		Third cousins
			Mariana of Habsburg	0.155		Uncle - niece
Charles II[2] (1661 – 1700)	0.254		Maria Luise d'Orleans	0.078		Second cousins
			Maria Anna of Neoburg	0.008		Remote kinship

1. Child of Philip II and Anna of Habsburg
2. Child of Philip IV and Mariana of Habsburg

Table 4. Inbreeding coefficient (F) of the Spanish Habsburg kings and their wives (From Alvarez et al., 2009)

The European royal dynasties of the Modern Age provide very rich materials for the study of the effects of high inbreeding levels in humans (Alvarez et al., 2009). Consanguineous marriages such as uncle-niece, first cousins and other non-incestuous unions were very frequent in those dynasties along prolonged periods of time and the genealogical records available in the historical sources are very extensive and accessible in such a way that inbreeding coefficients can be computed with extreme precision from extended pedigrees. One of the most important European royal dynasties of the Modern Age was the Habsburg dynasty (also known as the House of Austria) and the Spanish branch of this dynasty ruled over the world-wide Spanish Empire since 1517 until 1700. Along this time, the six kings of the Spanish Habsburg branch contracted 11 marriages and 9 (81.8%) of them were consanguineous unions in a degree of third cousins or closer: two uncle-niece marriages, one double first cousin marriage, one first cousin marriage and other consanguineous unions. The inbreeding coefficient of the Spanish Habsburg kings computed from an extended pedigree up to 16 generations in depth that involves more than 3,000 individuals experienced a strong increase along generations from 0.025 for king Philip I, the founder of the dynasty, to 0.254 for Charles II, the last Spanish Habsburg king (Table 4). The progeny of the Spanish Habsburg kings suffered an important inbreeding depression for survival in such a way that inbreeding at the level of first cousins ($F = 0.0625$) exerted an adverse effect on survival to 10 years (miscarriages, stillbirth and neonatal deaths not included) of 17.8% ± 12.3. The relationship between survival and inbreeding coefficient in the progeny of 71 Habsburg marriages belonging to both branches of the dynasty (Spanish and Austrian Habsburgs) is shown in Figure 6 (unpublished results). The evidence of a strong inbreeding depression for survival in the Habsburg dynasty is confirmed from this large data set. The absolute decrease in survival to 10 years for the progeny of a first cousin marriage was

13.54% ± 5.40 and the cost of inbreeding for an F value of 0.254, which is the inbreeding coefficient of Charles II, was 54.99%. Statistically significant deviations of a linear relationship between survival and inbreeding coefficient were not detected by the nonlinearity t test which compares the change in mean survival between two low levels of F and that between two high levels of F (Lynch & Walsh, 1998, p 267-268). Yet, departures from linearity were not detected for log-transformed data. These results must be taken, however, with caution because the statistical power of the test was probably not high enough to conclude that factors potentially promoting deviations of linearity such as epistatic interactions among loci or purging selection can be discarded. In any case, these findings suggest that linearity deviations for inbreeding depression on survival could be not very strong in humans so that, at least as a first approximation, estimates of inbreeding depression obtained from low inbreeding levels could be linearly extrapolated to predict the extent of depression for high inbreeding in a given population.

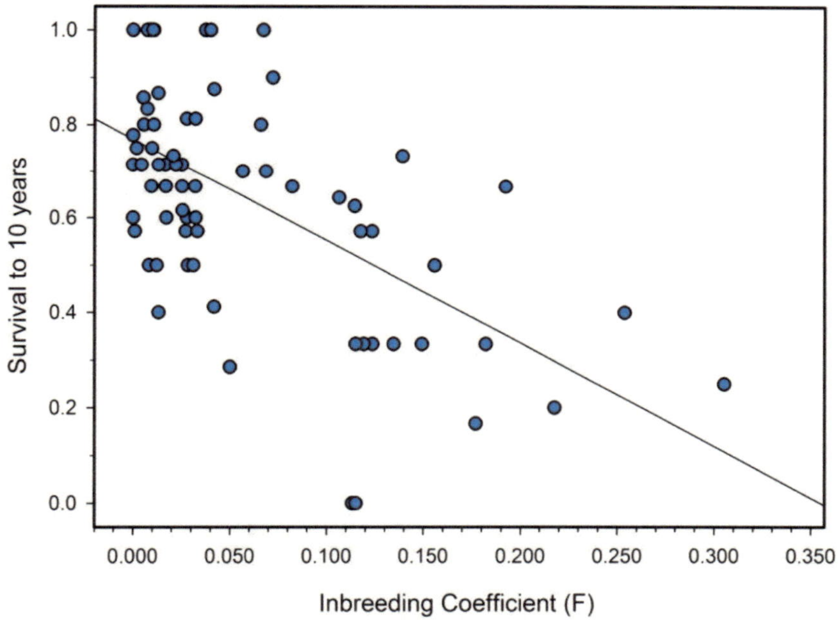

Fig. 6. Survival and inbreeding coefficient (F) of offspring of 71 marriages from the Habsburg royal dynasty

The Spanish Habsburg dynasty died out when Charles II, the last king of the dynasty, died in 1700 since no children were born from his two marriages. Indeed, the inbreeding depression on survival suffered by the dynasty was a relevant factor contributing to its extinction but, in the last instance, an effect of inbreeding on morbidity probably was also involved in the extinction of the Spanish Habsburg lineage. Charles II presented important physical and mental disabilities suffering from a number of different diseases during his life, hence being known in Spanish history as *El Hechizado* ("The Hexed") (Gargantilla, 2005). In the light of the knowledge of the current clinical genetics and taking into account that Charles II had an extremely high inbreeding coefficient (F = 0.254) which means that approximately 25.4% of his autosomal genome was autozygous, a tentative hypothesis based on the simultaneous occurrence in this king of two recessive genetic disorders has been advanced to explain most of his complex clinical profile, including his impotence/infertility which in last instance led to the extinction of the Spanish Habsburg lineage (Alvarez et al., 2009). According to contemporary writings, Charles II was often described as "big headed" and "weak breast-fed baby". He was unable to speak until the age of 4, and could not walk until the age of 8. He was short, weak and quite lean and thin. He was described as a person showing very little interest on his surroundings (abulic personality). He first marries at 18 and later at 29, leaving no descendants. His first wife talks of his premature ejaculation, while his second spouse complaints about his impotency. He suffers from sporadic hematuria and intestinal problems (frequent diarrhoea and vomits). He looked like an old person when he was only 30 years old, suffering from edemas on his feet, legs, abdomen and face. During the last years of his life he barely can stand up, and suffers from hallucinations and convulsive episodes. His health worsens until his premature death when he was 39, after an episode of fever, abdominal pain, hard breathing and comma. From these evidences, two recessive genetic disorders, combined pituitary hormone deficiency (CPHD, OMIM 26260) and distal renal tubular acidosis (dRTA, OMIM 602722), could explain an important part of the complex clinical profile of Charles II. Combined pituitary hormone deficiency leads to a multiple endocrine deficit of pituitary hormones: thyroid stimulating hormone (TSH), growth hormone (GH), prolactin (PRL), gonadotropin and adrenocorticotropic hormone (ACTH) (University of Washington, Genetest.gov). This disease shows a slow progression and is frequently caused by a genetic disorder produced by mutations of some of the transcription factors expressed in the pituitary gland, such as *PROP1* (5q), *POU1F1* (3p), *LHX3* (9q), *LHX4* (1q), *HESX1* (3p), *TBX19* (1q), *SOX2* (3q) and *SOX3* (Xq). Mutations occurring in *PROP1* are the most frequent genetic cause of hereditary CPHD, and they are inherited as autosomal recessives. Mutations in *PROP1* are associated with progressive endocrine deficiencies highly variable in both, intensity and in the first clinic sign manifestation (Kelberman & Dattani, 2007; Reynaud et al., 2005). Charles II showed clinical characteristics of hypothyroidism such as muscular weakness, hypotonia, delayed onset of speech and abulic behaviour, and the lack of GH could account for his short stature. His hypogonadotropic hypogonadism could explain his infertility/impotency, and a PRL deficit has been associated with decreased fertility in males. ACTH deficit usually presents in adults with common gastrointestinal symptoms such as nausea, vomit and diarrhoea. At the same time, the patients are fatigued, with general weakness, asthenia and hypotension. Any additional physical stress will exacerbate these clinical manifestations, often resulting in intense abdominal pain, fever, lethargy followed by hypovolemic vascular collapse (Agarwal et al., 2000; McGraw Hill, Access Medicine). The variety and scope of clinical symptoms afflicting Charles II could have been caused by an additional disease responsible for his muscular weakness at a young age, rickets, hematuria and his big head relative to his body size. These symptoms might have been manifestations of a secondary metabolic alteration originated in a renal disease such as severe hyperchloremic hypokalemic distal renal tubular acidosis (dRTA). This disease presents with alterations of the urine acidification mechanisms leading to severe metabolic hyperchloremic hypokalemic acidosis, prominent renal tract calcification with persistent hematuria and rickets. It may be caused by autosomal recessive mutations in *ATP6V0A4* (7q) or *ATP6V1B1* (2q) genes (Stover et al., 2002; Vargas-Possou et al., 2006). In this way, most of the symptoms showed by Charles II might be caused by these two different recessive genetic disorders. From this perspective, inbreeding effects on both survival and fertility due to prolonged consanguineous marriage led to the fall of the Spanish Habsburg lineage which constitutes one of the most dramatic examples of detrimental effects of inbreeding in humans.

Because most studies of inbreeding depression in humans have focused on prereproductive stages of the life cycle, research on effects of inbreeding on fitness traits such as fertility has received less attention. The analysis of the effects of inbreeding on reproductive success are subject to a number of potential limitations associated with lack of control for important sociodemographic variables such as age at marriage, literacy, use of contraceptives and duration of marriage. A number of studies have compared the fertility in consanguineous unions with that of unrelated couples. In this way, the effect of the degree of relatedness between spouses on fertility is investigated. The relatedness between individuals is usually expressed as their kinship coefficient (θ), which is equal to the inbreeding coefficient (F) of their offspring (Hedrick, 2005, pp. 269; Lynch & Walsh, 1998, pp. 135-140). In several studies, the total number of offspring (completed fertility) produced by related couples has been found to be higher than that corresponding to unrelated ones (Bittles et al., 2002; Helgason, et al., 2008). In a meta-analysis based on data from a wide range of different human populations (30 populations) located in India, Pakistan, Japan, Kuwait and Turkey, the number of live born children produced by non-consanguineous unions were compared with the number of live born children in four categories of consanguineous unions: double first cousin or uncle-niece ($\theta = 0.125$ in the two cases), first cousin ($\theta = 0.0625$), first cousin once removed/double second cousin ($\theta = 0.0313$), and second cousin ($\theta = 0.0156$) (Bittles et al., 2002). A positive association between kinship and fertility was found at all levels of kinship tested, although the differences between consanguineous and non-consanguineous couples were statistically significant only for first cousin couples. Since these positive associations between consanguinity and fertility could largely be due to uncontrolled socio-demographic variables, Bittles et al. (2002) performed an analysis based on data of first cousin marriages from the National Family and Health Survey conducted in India during 1992-1993. Multivariate analysis showed that fertility is importantly influenced by a number of factors such as illiteracy, earlier age at marriage, lower contraceptive use, duration of marriage and reproductive compensation which were, in turn, positively associated with consanguineous marriage. When the effects of these various factors were adjusted at the multivariate analysis, differences in fertility between first cousin and non-consanguineous couples were not detected. In contrast with these results based on a large data set, some studies provide convincing evidence for a positive association between kinship and fertility in some particular human population. Thus, a significant positive association between kinship and fertility was detected in a study performed from all known couples of the Icelandic population born between 1800 and 1965 (Helgason et al., 2008). Iceland is one of the most socioeconomically and culturally homogeneous societies in the world and is characterized by relatively low levels of inbreeding. The kinship of couples was computed on a depth of up to 10 generations from each couple so that differences in fertility across a fine scale of kinship values was assessed. Research on the inbreeding effect on fertility at an individual level has been also performed through the measurement of fertility in inbred males and females. A significant effect of inbreeding on female fecundity has been found in a 15-year study performed in Hutterite colonies in South Dakota (Ober et al. 1999). The socio-economic conditions are relatively uniform within the Hutterite community so that inbreeding effects can be studied without the confounding effects of uncontrolled socio-economic variables. Hutterite women with $F \geq 0.04$ showed significantly reduced fecundity as evidenced by longer interbirth intervals. There were no significant effects of father´s F or of the kinship of couples on the interbirth interval. In contrast, completed family sizes did not differ among the more and the less-inbred Hutterite women who were born after 1920, even though the adverse effect of inbreeding on fecundity was evident in those cohorts. These results suggest that reproductive compensation may be occurring in the more inbred, less-fecund women probably to achieve a culturally defined optimal family size. An adverse effect of inbreeding on female fecundity has been also found in a study performed in a small and isolated village in the Swiss Alps where socio-economic factors are rather homogeneous (Postma et al., 2010). A significant negative effect of the inbreeding level of the mother on completed family size was detected so that inbred women had fewer children. On the contrary, an effect of either the inbreeding coefficient of the fathers or the kinship coefficient of the couples was not detected. Moreover, some empirical evidences suggest that sensitivity of fertility to inbreeding might vary with parental age. The effect of consanguineous marriages on reproduction studied in a cohort of women born in the late 19th century in north-eastern Quebec, Canada, showed that the inbreeding coefficient of the father strongly affects reproduction rates along reproductive period as inbred fathers showed a strong asymmetry in the number of children produced during the first half in comparison with the second half (Robert et al., 2009). These results suggest that temporal aspects of reproduction may be relevant in the study of inbreeding depression for fertility in humans.

5. Conclusion

Inbreeding defined as the mating between relatives is a phenomenon that occurs in many animal and plant species as well as in humans. Genetic effects of inbreeding are basically due to the fact that the inbred individual will frequently inherit the same gene from each parent, who inherited it from a common ancestor. In this way, inbreeding increases the amount of homozygosity so that recessive traits such as many human genetic disorders will occur with increased frequency in the progeny of consanguineous couples. Studies on genome-wide homozygosity through the genome scan technology have opened new possibilities for understanding inbreeding from a genomic perspective. Long homozygous chromosomal segments have been detected through whole-genome scans in human chromosomes. These long homozygous tracts are the result of autozygosity (homozygous by descent) because inbred individuals have segments of their chromosomes that are homozygous as a result of inheriting identical genomic segments through both parents. The distribution of such homozygous tracts throughout the genome has been studied in inbred individuals affected by recessive Mendelian disorders providing valuable information on the genomic architecture underlying human genetic diseases associated with inbreeding. Recent researches have shown that extended tracts of genomic homozygosity are globally widespread in many human populations providing new perspectives in the study of past consanguinity and population isolation. Autozygosity has also practical implications for the identification of human disease genes. Thus, at present, homozygosity mapping is the method of choice for mapping human genes that cause recessive traits from the DNA of affected children from consanguineous marriage. This approach involves the detection of the disease locus on the basis that the adjacent region will be homozygous by descent in such inbred children.

Consanguineous marriage is frequently found in many human populations all over the world. The highest rates of consanguineous marriages occur in north and sub-Saharan Africa, the Middle East, and west, central, and south Asia, where, in some populations, 20 to 60% of all marriages are between relatives. First-cousin marriage is the most common form of consanguineous union in most human populations. There are clear social and economic advantages to consanguinity mainly associated with the maintenance of family structure and property, particularly in rural societies. Consanguineous marriages cannot be linked to any specific religion or religious rules. It is practiced among people of various religions, and the attitudes towards consanguineous marriages vary among followers of the same religion.

Offspring of consanguineous parents are at risk both for monogenic autosomal recessive disorders and for conditions with multifactorial inheritance. Consanguineous marriage increases the chance that both members of a couple will carry any recessive variant that is being transmitted in their family, and that this will manifest in the homozygous state in their children. Thus, a large number of studies have reported this outcome as one of the most important clinical consequences of consanguineous marriage. In general, the offspring of consanguineous couples present increased levels of morbidity and significant medical problems such as major malformations, congenital anomaly and structural birth defects. Furthermore, consanguinity has been implicated in susceptibility to a number of complex diseases such as heart disease, cancer, depression, gout, peptic ulcer, schizophrenia, epilepsy and asthma. Consanguinity has been also proven to be a risk factor for infection by a diverse range of pathogens responsible for a number of human infectious diseases.

The phenomenon of inbreeding depression, that is, the reduced survival and fertility of offspring of related individuals, has been documented in many human populations reflecting the consequences of increased homozygosity for alleles affecting reproductive fitness. Estimates of inbreeding depression in survival have been obtained for a number of human populations comparing the prereproductive mortality in the progeny of first-cousin and non consanguineous marriages. The mean increase in mortality among the offspring of first-cousin marriages ($F = 0.0625$) was 4.4% ± 4.6 from data of 38 worldwide human populations and a more recent estimate obtained from 69 populations was 3.5%, but it is necessary to emphasize that the extent of inbreeding depression on survival presents a large variation among populations. By contrast, there is little information on inbreeding depression in survival for inbreeding levels higher than those corresponding to first-cousin progenies. Recent studies conducted on European royal dynasties of the Modern Age where inbreeding coefficients were much higher than that corresponding to first-cousins are filling this gap of information. It is expected that these studies could provide a deeper understanding of the genetic basis of inbreeding depression in human populations.

6. References

Adams, M.S. & Neel, J.V. (1967). Children of Incest. *Pediatrics*, Vol. 40, No. 1, pp. 55-62

Agarwal, G.; Bhatia, V., Cook, S. & Thomas, P.Q. (2000). Adrenocorticotropin Deficiency in Combined Pituitary Hormone Deficiency Patients Homozygous for a Novel PROP1 Delection. *Journal of Clinical Endocrinology and Metabolism*, Vol. 85, pp. 4556-4561

Alvarez, G.; Ceballos, F.C. & Quinteiro, C. (2009). The Role of Inbreeding in the Extinction of a European Royal Dynasty. *PLoS ONE*, 4(4): e5174.doi:10.1371/journal.pone.0005174

Balloux, F.; Amos, W. & Coulson, T. (2004). Does Heterozygosity Estimate Inbreeding in Real Populations?. *Molecular Ecology*, Vol. 13, pp. 3021-3031

Bennett, R.L.; Motulsky, A.G., Bittles, A., Hudgins, L., Uhrich, S. et al. (2002). Genetic Counseling and Screening of Consanguineous Couples and Their Offspring: Recommendations of the National Society of Genetic Counselors. *Journal of Genetic Counseling*, Vol. 11, No 2, pp. 97-119

Berra, T.M.; Alvarez, G. & Ceballos, F.C. (2010). Was the Darwin/Wedgwood Dynasty Adversely Affected by Consanguinity?. *BioScience*, Vol. 60, No. 5, pp. 376-383

Bittles, A.H. (2001). Consanguinity and Its Relevance to Clinical Genetics. *Clinical Genetics*, Vol. 60, pp. 89-98

Bittles, A.H. (2006). A Background Summary of Consanguineous Marriage. Available from http://www.consang.net

Bittles, A.H. & Black, M.L. (2010). Consanguinity, Human Evolution, and Complex Diseases. *Proceedings of the National Academy of Sciences USA*, Vol. 107, No. Suppl. 1, pp. 1779-1786

Bittles, A.H.; Grant, J.C., Sullivan, S.G. & Hussain, R. (2002). Does Inbreeding Lead to Decreased Human Fertility. *Annals of Human Biology*, Vol. 29, No. 2, pp. 111-130

Bittles, A.H.; Mason, W.M., Greene, J. & Appaji Rao, N. (1991). Reproductive Behavior and Health in Consanguineous Marriages. *Science*, Vol. 252, pp. 789-794

Bittles, A.H. & Neel, J.V. (1994). The Costs of Human Inbreeding and Their Implications for Variations at the DNA Level. *Nature Genetics*, Vol. 8, pp. 117-121

Bodmer, W.F. & Cavalli-Sforza, L.L. (1976). *Genetics, Evolution, and Man*, W.H. Freeman and Company, ISBN 0-7167-0573-7, San Francisco, USA

Botstein, D. & Risch, N. (2003). Discovering Genotypes Underlying Human Phenotypes: Past Successes for Mendelian Disease, Future Approaches for Complex Disease. *Nature Genetics*, Vol. 33, pp. 228-237

Boyce, A.J. (1983). Computation of Inbreeding and Kinship Coefficients on Extended Pedigrees, *Journal of Heredity*, Vol. 74, pp. 400-404

Broman, K.W. & Weber, J.L. (1999). Long Homozygous Chromosomal Segments in Reference Families from the Centre d´Étude du Polymorphisme Humain, *The American Journal of Human Genetics*, Vol. 65, pp. 1493-1500

Carothers, A.D.; Rudan, I., Kolcic, I., Polasek, O. Hayward, C. et al. (2006). Estimating Human Inbreeding Coefficients: Comparison of Genealogical and Marker Heterozygosity Approaches. *Annals of Human Genetics*, Vol. 70, pp. 666-676

Carter, C.O. (1967). Children of Incest. *Lancet*, Vol. i, pp. 436

Cavalli-Sforza, L. L. & Bodmer, W. F. (1971). *The Genetics of Human Populations*, W. H. Freeman and Company, ISBN 0-7167-1018-8, San Francisco, USA

Charlesworth, B. & Charlesworth, D. (1999). The genetic Basis of Inbreeding Depression. *Genetical Research*, Vol. 74, pp. 329-340

Charlesworth, D. & Willis, J.H. (2009). The Genetics of Inbreeding Depression. *Nature Reviews Genetics*, Vol. 10, pp. 783-796

Consanguinity/Endogamy Resource. April 2009. Date of access March 2011. Available from: http://www.consang.net/index.php/Main_Page

Darwin, C.R. (1876). *The Effects of Cross and Self-Fertilization in the Vegetable Kingdom*, John Murray, London, England

Gargantilla, P. (2005). *Enfermedades de los Reyes de España: Los Austrias,* La Esfera de los Libros, ISBN 84-9734-338-7, Madrid, Spain

Gibson, J.; Morton, N.E. & Collins, A. (2006). Extended Tracts of Homozygosity in Outbred Human Populations. *Human Molecular Genetics,* Vol. 15, No. 5, pp. 789-795.

Golubovsky, M. (2008). Unexplained Infertility in Charles Darwin´s Family: Genetic Aspect. *Human Reproduction,* Vol. 23, pp. 1237-1238

Hedrick, P. W. (2005). *Genetics of Populations,* Jones and Bartlett Publishers, ISBN 0-7637-4772-6, Sudbury, Massachusetts, USA

Helgason, A.; Pálsson, S., Gudbjartsson, D., Kristjánsson, P. & Stefánsson, K. (2008). An Association Between the Kinship and Fertility of Human Couples. *Science,* Vol. 319, pp. 813-816

Hildebrandt, F.; Heeringa, S.F., Rüschendorf, F., Attanasio, M.,Nürnberg, G., et al. (2009). A Systematic Approach to Mapping Recessive Disease Genes in Individuals from Outbred Populations. *PLoS Genetics,* 5(1):e1000353.doi:10.1371/journal.pgen.1000353

Jones, S. (2008). *Darwin´s Island. The Galapagos in the Garden of England,* Little, Brown, ISBN 978-1-4087-0000-6, London, England

Kelberman, D. & Dattani, MT. (2007). Hypothalamic and Pituitary Development: Novel Insights Into the Aetiology. *European Journal of Endocrinology,* Vol. 157, pp. S3-S14

Khlat, M. & Khoury, M. (1991). Inbreeding and Diseases: Demographic, Genetic, and Epidemiologic Perspectives. *Epidemiologic Reviews,* Vol. 13, pp. 28-41

Khoury, M.J.; Cohen, B.H., Chase, G.A. & Diamond, E.L. (1987). An Edidemiologic Approach to the Evaluation of the Effect of Inbreeding on Prereproductive Mortality. *American Journal of Epidemiology,* Vol. 125, No. 2, pp. 251-262

Kirin, M.; McQuillan, R., Franklin, C.S., Campbell, H., McKeigue, P.M. & Wilson, J.F. (2010). Genomic Runs of Homozygosity Record Population History and Consanguinity. *PLoS ONE* 5(11):e13996.doi: 10.1371/journal.pone.0013996

Lander, E.S. & Botstein, D. (1987). Homozygosity Mapping: A Way to Map Human Recessive Traits with the DNA of Inbred Children. *Science,* Vol. 236, pp. 1567-1570

Lynch, M. & Walsh, B. (1998). *Genetics and Analysis of Quantitative Traits,* Sinauer Associates, ISBN 0-87893-481-2, Sunderland, Massachusetts, USA

Lyons, E.J.; Amos, W., Berkley, J.A., Mwangi, I., Shafi, M. et al. (2009a). Homozygosity and Risk of Childhood Death Due to Invasive Bacterial Disease. *BMC Medical Genetics,* 10:55,doi:10.1186/1471-2350-10-55

Lyons, E.J.; Frodsham, A.J., Zhang, L., Hill, A.V.S. and Amos, W. (2009b). *Biology Letters,* Vol. 5, pp. 574-576

MacCluer, J.W.; Boyce, A.J., Dyke, B., Weitkamp, L.R., Pfennig, D.W. et al. (1983). Inbreeding and Pedigree Structure in Standardbred Horses. *Journal of Heredity,* Vol. 74, pp. 394-399

McGraw Hill. March 2011. In: Access Medicine. Date of access March 2011. Available from: http://accessmedicine.com/features.aspx

McQuillan, R.; Leutenegger, A.L., Abdel-Rahman, R., Franklin, C.S., Pericic, M. et al. (2008). Runs of Homozygosity in European Populations. *The American Journal of Human Genetics,* Vol. 83, pp. 359-372

Moore, J. (2005). Good Breeding: Darwin Doubted His Own Familiy´s "Fitness". *Natural History,* Vol. 114, pp. 45-46

Nalls, M.A.; Simon-Sanchez, J., Gibbs, J.R., Paisan-Ruiz, C., Bras, J.T. et al. (2009). Measures of Autozygosity in Decline: Globalization, Urbanization, and Its Implications for Medical Genetics. *PLoS Genetics*, 5(3):e1000415.doi:10.1371/journal.pgen.1000415

Ober, C.; Hyslop, T. & Hauck, W.W. (1999). Inbreeding Effects on Fertility in Humans: Evidence for Reproductive Compensation. *The American Journal of Human Genetics*, Vol. 64, pp. 225-231

Postma, E.; Martini, L. & Martini, P. (2010). Inbred Women in a Small Swiss Village Have Fewer Children. *Journal of Evolutionary Biology*, Vol. 23, pp. 1468-1474

Reynaud, R.; Barlier, A., Vallette-Kasis, S., Saveanu, A., Guillet, M-P. et al. (2005). An Uncommon Phenotype with Familial Central with Hypogonadism Caused by a Novel PROP1 Gene Mutant Truncated in the Transactivation Domain. *Journal of Clinical Endocrinology and Metabolism*, Vol. 90, pp. 4880-4887

Robert, A.; Toupance, B., Tremblay, M. & Heyer, E. (2009). Impact of Inbreeding on Fertility in a Pre-Industrial Population. *European Journal of Human Genetics*, Vol. 17, pp. 673-681

Rudan, I.; Rudan, D., Campbell, H., Carothers, Wright, A. et al. (2003a). Inbreeding and Risk of Late Onset Complex Disease. *Journal of Medical Genetics*, Vol. 40, pp. 925-932

Rudan, I; Smolej-Narancic, N., Campbell, H., Carothers, A., Wright, A. et al. (2003b). Inbreeding and the Genetic Complexity of Human Hypertension. *Genetics*, Vol. 163, pp. 1011-1021

Seemanová, E. (1971). A Study of Children of Incestuous Matings. *Human Heredity*, Vol. 21, pp. 108-128

Stover, E.H.; Borthwick, K.J., Bavalia, C., Eady, N. & Fritz, D.M. (2002). Novel ATP6V1B1 and ATP6V0A4 Mutations in Autosomal Recessive Distal Renal Tubular Acidosis with New Evidence for Hearing Loss. *Journal of Medical Genetics*, Vol. 39, pp. 796-803

University of Washington. March 2011. In: Gene Test. Date of access March 2011. Available from: http://ncbi.nlm.nih. gov/sites/GeneTest/?db=GeneTest

Vargas-Poussou, R.; Houillier, P., Le Poittier, N., Strompf, L., Loirat, C. et al. (2006). Genetic Investigation of Autosomal Recessive Distal Renal Tubular Acidosis: Evidence for Early Sensorineural Hearing Loss Associated with Mutations in the ATP6V0A4 gene. *Journal of the American Society of Nephrology*, Vol. 17, pp. 1437-1443

Vogel, F. & Motulsky, A.G. (1997). *Human Genetics*, Springer Verlag, ISBN 3-540-60290-9, Berlin, Germany

Woods, C.G.; Cox, J., Springell, K., Hampshire, D.J., Mohamed, M.D. et al. (2006). Quantification of Homozygosity in Consanguineous Individuals with Autosomal Recessive Disease. *The American Journal of Human Genetics*, Vol. 78, pp. 889-896

Woods, C.G.; Valente, E.M., Bond, J. & Roberts, E. (2004). A New Method for Autozygosity Mapping Using Single Nucleotide Polymorphisms (SNPs) and EXCLUDEAR. *Journal of Medical Genetics* 41:e101

Wright, A.; Charlesworth, B., Rudan, I., Carothers, A. & Campbell, H. (2003). A Polygenic Basis for Late-Onset Disease. *Trends in Genetics*, Vol. 19, No. 2, pp. 97-106

3

Cytogenetic Techniques in Diagnosing Genetic Disorders

Kannan Thirumulu Ponnuraj
Universiti Sains Malaysia
Malaysia

1. Introduction

When the discovery of giant banded, salivary chromosomes in *Drosophila* was made by Painter in 1934, it gave a tremendous impact to the cytological work carried out in *Drosophila.* This made it possible to identify the chromosomes individually and also to discern the specific segments of the chromosome. Followed by this, cytogenetics bloomed with the establishment of chromosome number in man as 46 in the year 1956. Since then, lot of advancements and improvements have taken place over the years and combination of techniques have made cytogenetics as an undisputable source in diagnosing the various genetic disorders and now, human cytogenetics has completed its glorious 50 years after the discovery of chromosome number in normal human cells. This chapter provides an insight into the fundamentals of cytogenetics and its importance in the diagnosis of commonly occurring syndromes and disorders.

2. History of cytogenetics

When the genetic importance of polytene chromosomes of Diptera was rediscovered in the early thirties, almost every *Drosophila* geneticist started studying the salivary glands. Nageli, the Swiss botanist first described thread like structures in the nuclei of plant cells in the 1840s and called them "transitory cytoblasts", which represented what now are called chromosomes. Later, the term "chromosome" was coined by Waldeyer in 1888 after staining techniques had been developed which made them better discernible (*chromos* = Greek for colour; *soma* = Greek for body). In 1909, Johannsen coined the term 'gene'. This triggered the beginning of modern cytogenetics, but yet, the progress was moving at a snail's pace. Still, attempts were going on to find the number of chromosomes, which became a serious issue and a matter of great concern among the various researchers. The quality of chromosomes were poor and the numbers varied each and every time. Even determining the diploid number of a mammalian species was considered a difficult accomplishment. The chromosomes were crowded in metaphase and considerations of biological function of the chromosomes and in particular, of modern genetics were beyond the scope of cytological research in the 19th century. It was quite cumbersome to obtain nice slides with good metaphase spreads for easy counting. However, in 1950s, there were advent of new techniques for chromosome preparations, like addition of colcemid and hypotonic treatment, led to the establishment of the diploid number of chromosomes in man as 46 (Tjio

& Levan, 1956) and the peripheral leucocyte culture method of Moorehead *et al.* (1960) was adopted by many cytogeneticists. Once the correct description of the normal human chromosome number was established, chromosome abnormalities were recognized to be clearly associated with specific congenital defects. It was possible to arrange the chromosomes in different groups based on their size and location of the centromere which enabled easy counting as well as detection of numerical chromosome aberrations like trisomy 21 in Down syndrome (Lejeune *et al.* 1959), 45X in Turner syndrome (Ford *et al.* 1959), 47XXY in Klinefelter syndrome (Jacobs & Strong, 1959), trisomy 13 (Patau *et al.* 1960) and trisomy 18 (Edwards *et al.* 1960), Philadelphia chromosome, a structural aberration involving chromosomes 9 and 22, was recognized in a patient with chronic myeloid leukemia (Nowell & Hungerford, 1960). The metaphase chromosomes were classified into 7 groups based on the Denver classification (1960), with revisions at the London Conference (Hamerton *et al.* 1963) and the Chicago Conference (1966). Karyotype is the normal nomenclature where the chromosomes are arranged in homologous pairs in a systematic manner to describe the normal or abnormal chromosomal complement of an individual, tissue or cell line (ISCN, 2005). Jau-hong Kao *et al.* (2008) described chromosome classification based on the band profile similarity along approximate medial axis. This was soon followed by amniocentesis to determine the chromosomal abnormalities in fetal cells in the amniotic fluid, which formed the core of prenatal genetic diagnosis (Steele & Breg, 1966). After the advent of these protocols and discoveries, the heyday of cytogenetics research appeared to be over (Hans Zellweger and Jane Simpson, 1977), the power of cytogenetics analysis improved with the development of staining protocols by Caspersson *et al.* (1968), that made chromosomes of the same group, which previously could not be distinguished from each other, discernible. This banding pattern was based on a fluorescent staining technique and the fluorescence intensity quickly quenched which made the technique less optimal for routine studies of patients. Hence, several other banding techniques were developed like G-, R-, C- and NOR banding each having their own specific properties and applications (Rooney, 2001). These banding patterns became the barcodes with which cytogeneticists could easily identify chromosomes, detect subtle deletions, inversions, insertions, translocations, fragile sites and other more complex rearrangements and refine breakpoints (Caspersson *et al.* 1970).

3. Cytogenetics

Cytogenetics is the study of the structure and properties of chromosomes, chromosomal behaviour during somatic cell division in growth and development (mitosis) and germ cell division in reproduction (meiosis), chromosomal influence on the phenotype and the factors that cause chromosomal changes (Hare & Singh, 1979). Discovery of new techniques, improvements of existing techniques or new combinations of well established techniques are often followed by progress in the biosciences. This is strikingly exemplified by the development of cytogenetics in the last 100 years.

3.1 Chromosomes and normal chromosome complement

Chromatins are dark staining materials present in the nucleus of a cell and in interphase, these chromatin materials are organised into a number of long, loosely coiled, irregular strands or threads called the chromatin reticulum. At the time of cell division, these chromatin bodies condense into shorter and thicker threads called chromosomes, that carry the genes and functions in the transmission of hereditary information. In a normal diploid cell, there are 46 chromosomes (23 chromosome pairs), where one of each pair is derived from the father and the other from the mother of the individual. The first 22 pairs are called the autosomes (non-sex chromosomes) and the 23rd pair is called the sex-chromosomes. In males, the 23rd pair is XY and in females, it is XX. The X-chromosome is maternally derived and the Y-chromosome is paternally derived. The karyotypes of a normal male (Figure 1) and female (Figure 2) are presented. Except in the case of mosaic individuals (where they have two or more populations of cells which differ in chromosome number), all the cells of an individual have the same chromosome complement in their diploid cells. In the case of gametic cells (sperm and ovum), or otherwise called haploid cells, they have only single chromosome from each pair.

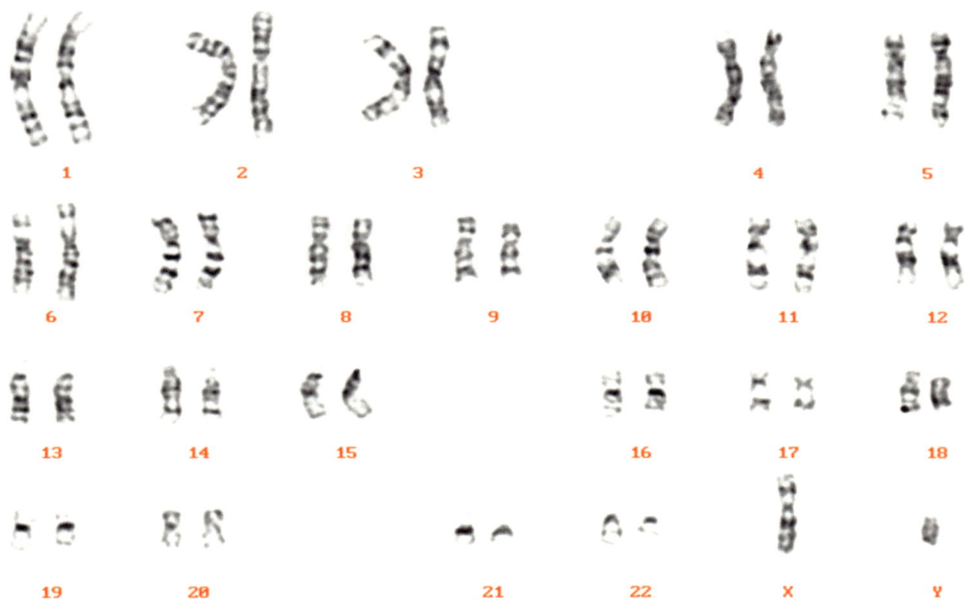

Fig. 1. A karyotype of a normal male (46,XY)
(Reproduced courtesy of Human Genome Centre, Universiti Sains Malaysia, Malaysia)

3.2 Cytogenetic analysis of chromosomes

3.2.1 Whole blood culture

The main advantage of whole blood culture is that blood is one of the most and easily accessible human tissues. Also, it has a very good growth potential after mitogenic stimulation. They have a cell cycle which is well characterized and the results can be obtained after a culture duration of 3 days.

3.2.1.1 Short term culture

The most commonly used technique for preparation of chromosomes is peripheral blood culture. The materials and reagents needed for culture are as below.

1. Sodium heparin - which is used as an anti-coagulant
2. Culture medium (E.g. RPMI 1640, TC 199 etc.) - provides nutrients and amino acids needed for the growth of the cells

3. Fetal bovine serum - contains a rich variety of proteins that enhances the growth of cells
4. Antibiotics - suppreses the growth of contaminants
5. Mitogen - (E.g. Phytohaemagglutinin) - induces the cells to undergo mitosis
6. Colchicine or its synthetic derivative, Colcemid - arrests cell division
7. Potassium chloride solution (hypotonic treatment) - induces swelling of cells through osmosis
8. Methanol: Acetic acid - for fixation of cells

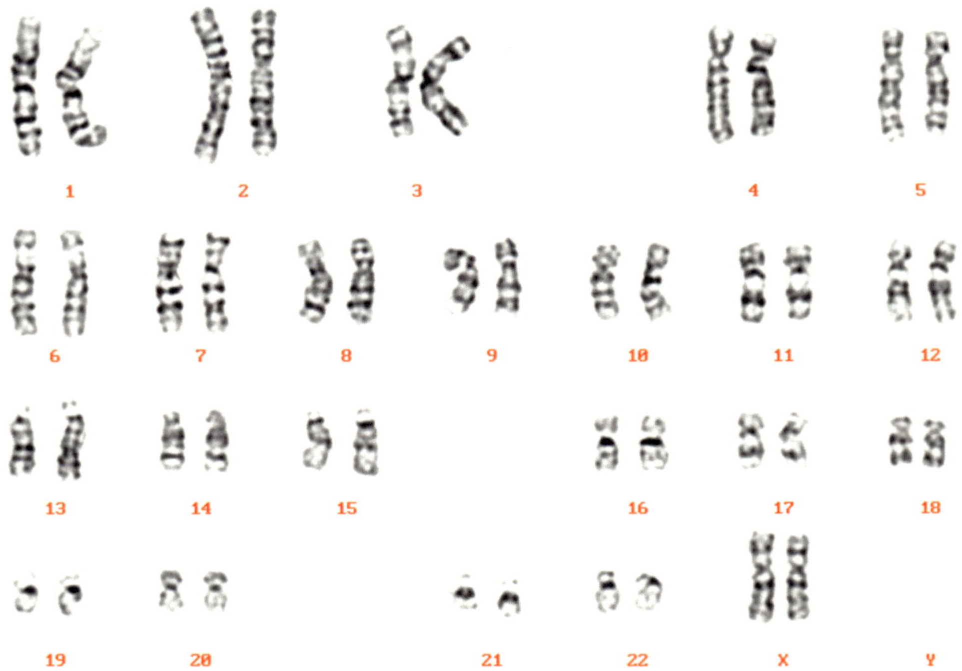

Fig. 2. A karyotype of a normal female (46,XX)
(Reproduced courtesy of Human Genome Centre, Universiti Sains Malaysia, Malaysia)

Blood is collected in sterile tubes containing sodium heparin. Whole blood, leucocytes separated from red blood cells or purified lymphocytes are put in culture medium supplemented with serum and antibiotics. Then, mitogen is added to induce mitosis. Once the cultures are set, they are incubated at 37°C for 72 hours in a CO_2 incubator. The cultures have to be shaken at least twice daily which significantly increases mitosis. Then, colchicine or its synthetic derivative, colcemid is added to the cultures few hours before harvesting (usually 2 to 3 hours) to arrest the cells in metaphase. Colcemid prevents formation of cell spindle and hence prevents cells from progressing to the next phase of the cell cycle, anaphase. Colcemid can also cause contraction of chromosomes if added in larger quantities or if the cells are exposed for a longer duration of time. This varies from laboratory to laboratory and hence needs optimisation to obtain chromosomes of good quality. After incubation for 72 hours, the centrifuge tubes in which the cultures are set is centrifuged at 1000 rpm for 10 minutes. Then, the supernatant is discarded and the cells are gently suspended. To this, freshly prepared potassium chloride solution is added, called the hypotonic treatment. Potassium chloride causes swelling of the cells through the process of osmosis and hence proper dispersion of chromosomes. The hypotonic treatment is achieved by incubating the centrifuge tubes in a CO_2 incubator at 37°C for about 30 minutes. Then, the process of centrifugation is repeated followed by addition of 3:1 methanol:acetic acid, which acts as a fixative. Methanol in the fixative denatures and precipitates the proteins by dehydration under acid conditions and acetic acid coagulates the nucleoproteins and casues swelling of cells thus counteracting the shrinking caused by methanol. The fixative penetrates the cells rapidly, preserves the chromosome structure and to a large extent, strips cytoplasmic proteins from cells. The fixative washes are repeated as many times as necessary until a clear cell button is obtained at the bottom of the tube. Then, the chromosomes are prepared by dropping the cell suspension on a clean, grease free slide, where, the drop spreads out and the chromosomes get fixed on the slides. Once the slides are prepared, suitable staining techniques are carried out as needed for the diagnosis of chromosomal disorders.

3.2.1.2 Bone marrow culture

The bone marrow culture is used to identify chromosome anomalies in hematopoietic cells, especially for hematological disorders like pre-leukemia and leukemia. Bone marrow aspirate of about 0.5 to 2.0 ml is collected in a heparinized syringe. Strict aseptic techniques are a must right from the beginning of collection until the final process is completed. Bone marrow is collected in transport media and mixed thoroughly. Then, the samples are spun at around 900 rpm for 10 minutes followed by pipetting off the supernatant. This is then followed by addition of about 1ml of sample to complete culture media (medium + Fetal bovine serum + L-glutamine + Antibiotics). After about 45 minutes, colcemid is added to this and mixed thoroughly. Then, the cultures are incubated at 37°C in a CO_2 incubator for 24 hours. This is followed by the routine hypotonic and fixative treatments as for the whole blood culture. The chromosomes are prepared on clean grease free slides, stained and examined under microscope for analysis.

3.2.2 Banding techniques

The different banding techniques allow precise identification of each chromosome as well as to detect structural chromosomal rearrangements. A combination of several banding techniques also help in obtaining the information necessary for chromosomal analysis.

3.2.2.1 Q-banding

This banding technique does not require any prior treatment of the chromosomes but requires a fluorescent microscope for analysis. Caspersson *et al.* (1970) discovered one of the first chromosome banding techniques, which involves staining chromosomes with a fluorochrome, such as quinacrine mustard or quinacrine dihydrochloride, and examining them with fluorescence microscopy. The Q-bands appear along each chromosome in alternating bright and dull bands with varying intensity. However, Q-banding does not permit permanent preparations. Certain antibiotics like anthracyclines produce fluorescent bands similar to Q-bands and are more stable than those produced by quinacrine.

3.2.2.2 G-banding

G-bands are produced by staining the chromosomes with a stain, Giemsa. This is done by treating the chromosomes with substances (usually trypsin), that alters the structure of proteins followed by staining with a Giemsa solution (Rowley, 1973). It is the most common method of banding, as it produces the same banding pattern as quinacrine with even greater resolution; it allows permanent preparations and does not necessitate the use of fluorescence microscopy. Thus, G-band patterns can be used to pair and identify each of the human chromosomes accurately.

3.2.2.3 R-banding

R-bands are just the reverse of G-bands, which can be produced by a variety of methods. A modification of method of Dutrillaux and Lejeune (1971) involves thermic denaturation in Earle's balanced salt solution (at 87°C), which is the most common method. Since the staining ability of the chromosomes is somewhat lost due to heating, the use of phase contrast objectives gives a better contrast of the chromosomes for analysis.

3.2.2.4 C-banding

C-bands localize the heterochromatic regions of chromosomes. Pardue & Gall (1970) first reported C-bands in 1970 when they discovered that the centromeric region of mouse chromosomes is rich in repetitive DNA sequences and stains dark with Giemsa. The original method of Arrighi and Hsu (1971) involves treating the slides with 0.2 N hydrochloric acid followed by treatment with RNAse and sodium hydroxide. Many chromosomes have regions that differ among individuals but have no pathological importance. These polymorphic regions can be visualized optimally with C-band methods and are most often seen on acrocentric chromosomes, the centromeric region of chromosomes 1, 9, and 16, and the distal portion of the Y chromosome. C-banding is also useful to show chromosomes with multiple centromeres, to study the origin of diploid molar pregnancies and true hermaphroditism and to distinguish between donor and recipient cells in bone marrow transplantation.

3.2.2.5 T-banding

This method involves staining the telomeric (end) regions of the chromosomes. Dutrillaux (1973) treated the slides with either phosphate buffer or Earle's balanced salt solution and then stained using mixed Giemsa solution to produce the T-bands.

3.2.2.6 CT-banding

Scheres, (1974) developed a method to stain both the centromeric heterochromatin as well as the telomere of chromosomes. He treated the slides with barium hydroxide to produce the CT-bands. Chamla & Ruffie (1976) obtained complete C- and T-bands by incubating the slides in Hank's balanced salt solution.

3.2.2.7 Nucleolar Organizing Region-banding

Nucleolar organizing region (NOR)-banding is a technique that stains NORs of chromosomes (Matsui & Sasaki, 1973). These regions are located in the satellite stalks of acrocentric chromosomes and house genes for ribosomal RNA. NOR-bands may represent structural non-histone proteins that are specifically linked to NOR and bind to ammoniacal silver. Goodpasture *et al.* (1976) developed a simple silver nitrate staining technique that is now used widely. NOR-banding is useful in clinical practice to study certain chromosome polymorphisms, such as double satellites. This method is also helpful to identify satellite stalks that are occasionally seen on non-acrocentric chromosomes.

3.2.2.8 The choice of banding technique

For routine analysis, the banding technique using trypsin and Giemsa became the most accepted worldwide (Seabright, 1971). Since the banding pattern enabled the detection of various structural aberrations like translocations, inversions, deletions, and duplications next to the already well-known numerical aberrations, not only potentially unbalanced cases (patients) could be studied but also healthy individuals as possible carriers of a balanced aberration. For instance, healthy family members of already known carriers and couples suffering from repetitive spontaneous abortions were cytogenetically investigated (Dominique FCM Smeets, 2004).

3.2.2.9 High resolution banding

Despite the above banding patterns, resolution of chromosome studies remained relatively limited with an approximate count of 500 bands per haploid genome (resolution ≈ 6 million base pairs ≈ 50 genes per band) because the total number of bands produced on metaphase chromosomes are less and it is difficult to detect rearrangements involving small portions of chromosomes due to excessive condensation. This was improved by the development of so-called high-resolution banding by Yunis (1976) which was achieved by synchronizing the lymphocyte cultures and obtaining more number of cells in pro-metaphase or even prophase (increasing resolution from 500 to over 1000 bands in a haploid genome). High resolution cytogenetics provides precision in the delineation of chromosomal breakpoints and assignment of gene loci, greater than with earlier techniques, since analysis of late prophase sub-banding reveals more than twice the number of bands seen at metaphase (Sawyer & Hozier, 1986). By applying this technique, several already well-known clinical syndromes like Prader Willi and Angelman syndrome with a deletion at the proximal long arm of chromosome 15, Smith-Magenis and Miller-Dieker syndrome with (different) deletions in the short arm of chromosome 17 and DiGeorge/Velo Cardio Facial (VCF) syndrome with deletions in the long arm of chromosome 22 could be linked to small chromosome aberrations and the concept of the micro-deletion or contiguous gene syndrome was born (Schmickel, 1986).

3.2.2.10 Sex chromatin analysis

The number of sex chromatin bodies is one less than the number of X chromosomes in the chromosome complement. This is obtained by taking buccal smears on a clean slide followed by fixing them in ethanol, air drying, hydrolysing in hydrochloric acid, washing in distilled water to remove the acid and then finally staining using cyrstal violet. The presence of a chromatin mass, called the "Barr body" indicates a chromatin positive cell.

3.3 Specialized techniques to visualize chromosomes

3.3.1 Sister Chromatid Exchange (SCE)

SCE staining is accomplished in cell cultures by incorporating BrdU (bromodeoxyuridine) (in place of thymidine) into replicating cells for 2 cell cycles. As a result of semi-conservative DNA replication, chromosomes have one chromatid with BrdU in one strand of DNA and the other chromatid has BrdU in both strands of DNA. This produces an acridine fluorescence pattern in which one chromatid fluoresces more brightly than the other chromatid. Sister chromatid exchanges appear as an interchange between sister chromatids of brightly and dully fluorescent segments. The biologic importance of SCEs is uncertain, but some mutagens and carcinogens increase their frequency (Perry & Evans, 1975).

3.3.2 Fragile sites and chromosome breakage

Certain uncondensed portions of DNA in chromosome structure can be visualized as gaps in the staining pattern and these gaps are prone to chromosome breakage. Gaps that are consistently seen at the same chromosome locus are called fragile sites. Fragile sites can be induced by modifying the culture media in ways that interfere with DNA synthesis and are best visualized in chromosomes by using non-banding or Q-banding methods. Some fragile sites are associated with specific medical conditions such as fragile X syndrome, (Figure 3), which is associated with a fragile site at Xq27.3 (Lubs, 1969). The symptoms associated with the syndrome include mental retardation, altered speech patterns and other physical attributes. The syndrome is named so because it is related to the tip of the X chromosome that breaks more frequently that other chromosomal regions.

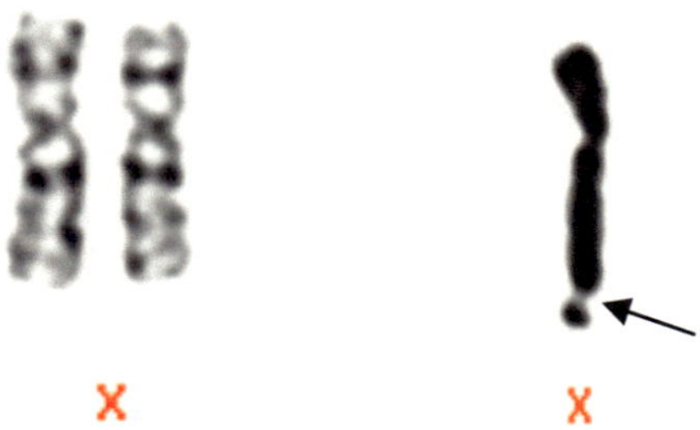

Fig. 3. A micrograph showing normal X-chromosomes (on the left) and an abnormal X-chromosome with a fragile-X site (indicated by arrow)
(Reproduced courtesy of Human Genome Centre, Universiti Sains Malaysia, Malaysia)

3.4 Molecular cytogenetics

3.4.1 Fluorescent in situ Hybridization (FISH)

Even with the technique of high resolution chromosome banding, it was difficult to visualize the aberrations at the cytogenetics level. In 1986, Pinkel *et al.* (1986a) developed a method to visualize chromosomes using fluorescent-labeled probes called FISH. FISH allowed chromosomal and nuclear locations of specific DNA sequences to be seen through the microscope. FISH technology permits the detection of specific nucleic acid sequences in morphologically preserved chromosomes, cells and tissues. FISH can be performed on either metaphase or interphase cells and involves denaturing genomic DNA by using heat and formamide. Slide preparations are flooded with chromosome-specific DNA sequences attached to colored fluorochromes and incubated at 37°C. During this time, probe DNA anneals with complementary DNA sequences in the chromosomes. The presence or absence of FISH signals is observed with a fluorescence microscope. FISH probes are generally classified by where they hybridize in the genome or by the type of chromosome anomaly they detect. These techniques are useful in the work-up of patients with various congenital and malignant neoplastic disorders, especially in conjunction with conventional chromosome studies. Fluorescent tags are safer and simpler to use, can be stored indefinitely, give higher resolution which opened up prospects for simultaneously locating several DNA sequences in the same cell by labelling them with different fluorochromes (Barbara J Trask, 2002). Using FISH, cytogeneticists could detect chromosomal abnormalities that involved small segments of DNA. Even more importantly, FISH opened up the nuclei of non-dividing cells to karyotype analysis. Using FISH and chromosome-specific probes, cytogeneticists could enumerate chromosomes, simply by counting spots in each nucleus (Pinkel *et al.* 1986b).

3.4.2 Spectral Karyotyping (SKY) and Multicolour FISH (M-FISH)

After the advent of FISH, where a single copy gene could fluoresce, a more powerful technology called SKY or M-FISH was developed. M-FISH allows all the 24 human chromosomes to be painted in different colours. By making use of various combinations and concentrations of fluorescent dyes, it is even possible to give every single chromosome a different color (SKY) which can be of particular use when dealing with complex aberrations often associated with various types of solid tumors. SKY or M-FISH enables production of chromosome-specific 'paints': combines fluorochromes to produce 24 colour combinations, one for each chromosome (Ried *et al.* 1992) and hence multicolour analyses. SKY paints the entire chromosome in the same colour, whereas in the case of M-FISH, various fluorescence dyes to represent different painting probes at the same time are used. This offers the simultaneous presentation of all 24 different human chromosomes with a single hybridization. The unequivocal colour signature for each chromosome enables the analysis of hidden or complex chromosome aberrations as well as the composition of marker chromosomes. These imaging systems can be programmed to classify each chromosomal segment automatically and they offer the first real hope of automated karyotype analysis. SKY and M-FISH have proved to be extremely useful in detecting translocations and other complex chromosomal aberrations.

3.4.3 Comparative Genomic Hybridization (CGH)

While FISH investigations have proved to be advantageous in many ways, it also has demerits. Like all probes, it has to be hybridized and later microscopically analyzed. Moreover such procedures were time-consuming and difficult to automate. This led to the development of technique of FISH called CGH (Kallioniemi *et al.* 1992). Later, a further improved technique was developed which was an array based on comparative genomic hybridization (Sabina Solinas-Toldo *et al.* 1997; Albertson & Pinkel, 2003). In contrast to analysis carried out on banded chromosomes, CGH does not require preparation of metaphase chromosomes from the cells. Instead of hybridizing a labeled probe to human chromosomes on a slide, we now have the potential to print thousands of different and well-characterized probes on a glass slide. Subsequently, complete isolated and fragmented DNA from the patient is labeled in a certain color and mixed with exactly the same amount of DNA of a normal control (or a mix of controls) which is labeled in a different color. This DNA mix is then hybridized to the denatured probe DNA on the glass slide. After several washing steps, the fluorescence pattern of each spot can be analyzed and the ratio of test (patient) over reference (control) is measured. The array-CGH is even more promising than the conventional CGH (Pinkel *et al.* 1998). Array-CGH is the equivalent of conducting thousands of FISH experiments at once and provides better quantification of copy number and more precise information on the breakpoints of segments that are lost or gained than does conventional CGH. These techniques will tell us much more about changes and variation within the human genome.

4. Prenatal genetic diagnosis

The term prenatal diagnosis refers broadly to a number of different techniques and procedures that can be performed during a pregnancy to provide information about the health of a developing fetus. Prenatal diagnosis of chromosomal aberrations requires cytogenetic analysis of amniotic fetal cells (Verma *et al.* 1998). Amniocentesis is an invasive, well-established, safe, reliable, and accurate procedure performed during pregnancy to detect chromosomal abnormalities as well as other specific genetic diseases. Fuchs and Riis (1956) reported the first use of amniotic fluid examination in the diagnosis of genetic disease in 1956 in their seminal article in "Nature". The determination of fetal sex led to the prenatal management of patients with Haemophilia in 1960 and Duchenne muscular dystrophy in 1964. Steele and Breg very importantly demonstrated in their seminal paper in the Lancet in 1966 that cultured amniotic fluid cells were suitable for karyotyping (Steele & Breg, 1966). Cytogenetic investigation of spontaneous pregnancy losses provides the basic information for accurate genetic counseling (Neus Baena *et al.* 2001). The prenatal genetic diagnosis is necessary in cases where the sonographic findings leads one to doubt on the chromosomal disorders, especially the syndromes associated with various trisomies. It is also warranted in individuals with a high risk of trisomic pregnancies based on pedigree analysis for chromosomal disorders to know the family history of trisomy, increased maternal age, and increased incidence of meiotic or mitotic non-disjunction and couples who are suspected or known to be carriers of inherited genetic disorders.

4.1 Amniocentesis and amniotic fluid culture

Amniocentesis is an invasive test during pregnancy that removes a small amount of fluid from the sac around the baby to look for birth defects and chromosomal problems. A reliable quality of preparations is important in amniocentesis as repeated removal of amniotic fluid and chorionic villi increases the risk of fetal loss. However, with good ultrasound scanning, samples can be obtained safely and reliably. Since, the cells in amniotic fluid consists of cells derived from skin, kidney, bladder, gut as well as from other fetal tissues, it is better to collect samples from multiple sites. A proper collection of sample along with proper culture technique leads to a proper interpretation of the results. Amniocentesis is done from 12 to 15 weeks of gestation for chromosomal analysis. There are basically two methods of culturing the cells; one is culturing and processing on coverslips, which retains the individual colonies of the cells and the other is culturing in flasks, removing the cells with trypsin, which mixes all the colonies in the flask.

After the amniotic sample is received in the laboratory, the sample is centrifuged at 750 rpm for 10 minutes. The amniotic fluid is then carefully decanted from the cell pellet into a sterile test tube and then the cell pellet is re-suspended in amniotic fluid. Then, suitable medium supplemented with fetal bovine serum, L-glutamine and antibiotics are added and the cultures are incubated at 37°C in 5% CO_2 incubator. The cells are harvested at 8-10 days after culture, subjected to routine hypotonic and fixative treatments as for whole blood culture and the chromosomes are analyzed.

5. Syndromes associated with chromosomal abnormalities

5.1 Down syndrome (Trisomy 21)

Down syndrome represents one of the better-known cytogenetic diseases. In most of the cases, this is due to trisomy of chromosome 21 (where the chromosome 21 appears thrice). Various types of chromosome +21 anomalies can cause this syndrome. The extra chromosome results in abnormalities of the body and brain development. The physical development is slower and may also have delayed mental development. The symptoms of Down syndrome vary from one person to another ranging from mild to severe.

Symptoms

- Nose is flattened
- Small ears and mouth
- Upward slanting of the eyes
- Flat face (hypoplastic maxilla)
- Decreased muscle tone at birth
- Single palmar crease of the hand
- Rounded inner corner of the eyes
- Wide, short hands with short fingers
- Abundant nuchal skin at the nape of the neck
- Head smaller than normal and abnormally shaped
- Separated joints between the sutures of the skull bone
- Brushfield spots (white spots on the coloured part of the eye)

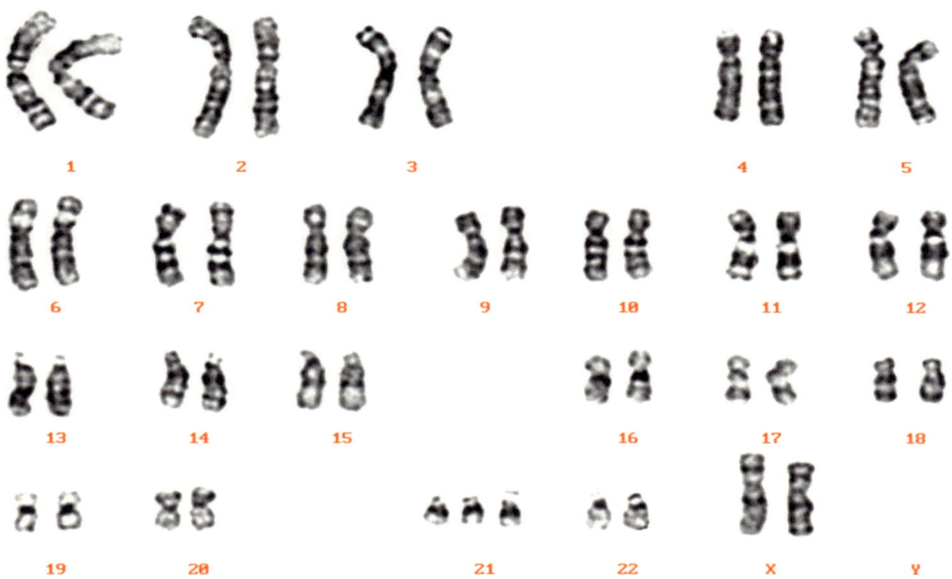

Fig. 4. A karyotype of a Down syndrome patient (47, XX,+21)
(Reproduced courtesy of Human Genome Centre, Universiti Sains Malaysia, Malaysia)

Other medical conditions may also be noticed in Down syndrome people like birth defects of heart (atrial septal defect or ventricular septal defect), dementia, problems related to eye (cataract), hearing problem, dysplastic pelvis, sleep apnea and hypothyroidism. Currently, there is no known treatment for Down syndrome. However, certain defects require surgery like heart problems etc. The risk is higher among women aged 35 years and above and couples having a Down syndrome baby have an increased risk of having another baby with the condition. A typical karyotype of a Down syndrome patient is given in Figure 4.

5.2 Edwards syndrome (Trisomy 18)

Edwards syndrome is a rare genetic chromosomal syndrome where the child has an extra third copy of chromosome 18. Most of the fetuses abort before term and is more severe than Down syndrome. This syndrome results in mental retardation and various physical defects which causes mortality of the infants at an early stage. Delayed psychomotor development as well as pre and post natal growth failure are the most common findings associated with this syndrome. Sometimes, only some of the body cells have an extra copy of chromosome 18. Hence, there is a mixed population of cells in the individual (called mosaicism). If the individual is a mosaic, then the individual exhibits fewer abnormalities compared to the typical Edwards syndrome features.

Symptoms

- Small face
- Low set ears
- Omphalocele
- Upturned nose
- Arthrogryposis
- Cleft lip/palate
- Cryptorchidism
- Ptosis of eyelids
- Prominent occiput
- Overlapping fingers
- Small jaw and mouth
- Limited hip abduction
- Drooping upper eyelids
- Developmental retardation
- Clubfoot or rocker bottom feet
- Malformations of heart and kidney
- Webbing of the second and third toes
- Widely spaced small eyes with narrow eyelid folds

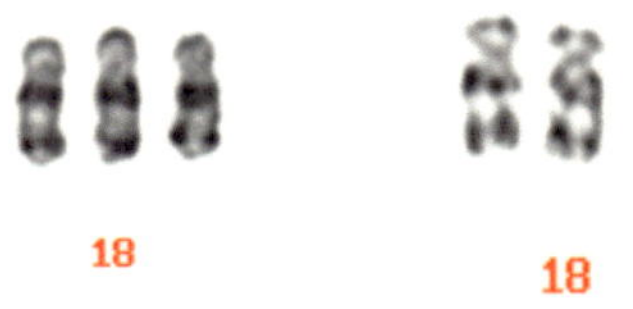

Fig. 5. A micrograph of trisomy 18 (Edwards syndrome) in comparison with its corresponding normal chromosomes
(Reproduced courtesy of Human Genome Centre, Universiti Sains Malaysia, Malaysia)

The Edwards syndrome is untreatable but treatment can be provided for certain symptoms of the disease. Proper attention should be paid on providing proper nutrition as well as to keep them clean as they are more prone to infections. The survival rate is very low in the Edwards syndrome as half of them die while in the womb. Of those born, fifty percent die within two or three months of their birth, while others die by the time they enter their first year. A typical karyotype of an Edwards syndrome patient is given in Figure 5.

5.3 Patau syndrome (Trisomy 13)

Patau syndrome is a genetic disorder in which a person has three copies of chromosome 13, instead of the usual two copies. Rarely, the extra material may be attached to another chromosome (translocation). Trisomy 13 can appear as complete trisomy 13 or as mosaic or as partial trsiomy 13.

Symptoms

- Hernias
- Coloboma
- Small eyes
- Hypotonia
- Polydactyly
- Low set ears
- Micrognathia
- Microcephaly
- Hypertonicity
- Cleft lip/ palate
- Epicanthal folds
- Clenched hands
- Single palmar crease
- Skeletal abnormalities
- Developmental retardation
- Close-set eyes (eyes may actually fuse together into one)

The infants who are born often have congenital heart disease (atrial septal defect, patent ductus arteriosus, ventricular septal defect). Most of the children with trisomy 13 die in the first month of their life. The patients with trisomy 13 also have other complictions like breathing difficulty, deafness, feeding problems, seizures and vision problems. Hence, treatment involves case by case basis. A typical karyotype of a Patau syndrome patient is given in Figure 6.

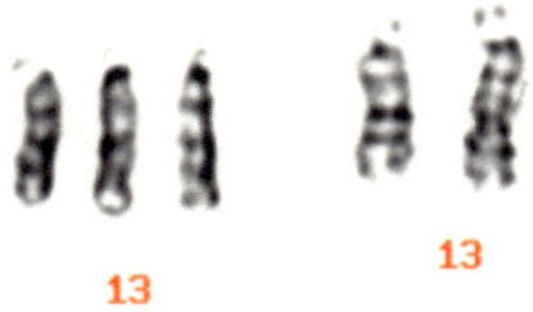

Fig. 6. A micrograph of trisomy 13 (Patau syndrome) in comparison with its corresponding normal chromosomes
(Reproduced courtesy of Human Genome Centre, Universiti Sains Malaysia, Malaysia)

5.4 Trisomy 9 syndrome

Trisomy 9 is one of the rare chromosomal disorders in which the entire 9th chromosome appears three times rather than twice in cells of the body. However, there are other variations, which comprise of trisomy 9 mosaic, trisomy 9p, tetrasomy 9p, trisomy 9q and monosomy 9. This can occur either as a mosaic or non-mosaic pattern and may be caused by errors during the division of a parent's reproductive cells (meiosis) or during the division of body tissue cells (somatic cells) early in the development of the embryo (mitosis). Non-mosaic or complete trisomy 9 is a lethal diagnosis, with most fetuses dying prenatally or during the early postnatal period with most of the cases ending in spontaneous abortion in the first trimester.

Symptoms

- Club foot
- Small face
- Micropenis
- Low set ears
- Clinodactyly
- Webbed neck
- Micrognathia
- Bulbous nose
- Brachydactyly
- Ear anomalies
- Hypertelorism
- Short sternum
- Cyrptorchidism
- Abnormal brain
- Wide fontanelles
- Bilateral club foot
- Prominent occiput
- Mental retardation
- High arched palate
- Rocker bottom feet
- Small, deep set eyes
- Overlapping fingers
- Limited hip abduction
- Abnormal hands and feet
- Developmental retardation
- Upslanting palpebral fissures
- Head - larger and cloverleaf shaped

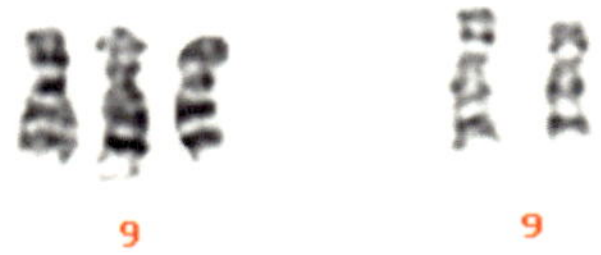

Fig. 7. A micrograph of trisomy 9 in comparison with its corresponding normal chromosomes (Reproduced courtesy of Human Genome Centre, Universiti Sains Malaysia, Malaysia)

The infants who are born have congenital heart defects, kidney anomalies, musculoskeletal, genital and/or additional abnormalities. Most of those individuals that survive to be born at term are mosaics. Infants with non-mosaic trisomy 9 are more severely affected than those with mosaicism. The incidence and severity of malformations and mental deficiency correlate with the percentage of trisomic cells in the different tissues. A typical karyotype of a Trisomy 9 syndrome patient is given in Figure 7.

5.5 Turner syndrome

Turner syndrome, gonadal dysgenesis or gonadal agenesis represents a special variant of hypergonadotrophic hypogonadism, and is due to the lack of the second sex chromosome or parts of it. The wide range of somatic features in Turner syndrome is due to a number of different X-located genes. Though many karyotype abnormalities have been described in association with Turner syndrome, monoclonal monosomy X and its various mosaicisms, each with an X monosomic (XO) cell clone, are the most frequent karyotype anomalies.

Symptoms

- Dry eyes
- Infertility
- Short stature
- Vaginal dryness
- Broad, flat chest
- Drooping eyelids
- Wide carrying angle
- Primary amenorrhea
- Widely spaced nipples
- Swollen hands and feet
- Wide and webbed neck
- Underdeveloped breasts
- Scanty pubic and axillary hair
- Absence of secondary sexual characters
- Rudimentary uterus and bilateral streak ovaries

Fig. 8. A micrograph of Turner (XO) in comparison with its corresponding normal (XY) chromosomes
(Reproduced courtesy of Human Genome Centre, Universiti Sains Malaysia, Malaysia)

The symptoms of this syndrome have been logically deduced to be caused by a single dosage of genes that are normally present and active in two dosages. Growth hormone may be advocated in a child with Turner syndrome to grow taller. The Turner syndrome patients can have a normal life though they are prone to complications like arthritis, cataracts, diabetes, heart defects, high blood pressure, renal problems, ear infections, obesity etc. A typical karyotype of a Tunrner syndrome patient is given in Figure 8.

5.6 Klinefelter syndrome

Klinefelter syndrome is the presence of an extra X chromosome in a male. The XXY karyotype is the most frequent of this syndrome.

Symptoms

- Infertility
- Thinness
- Tall stature
- Gynecomastia
- Cryptorchidism
- Delayed talking
- Speech difficulty
- Sparse facial hair
- Difficulty writing
- Delayed language
- Small firm testicles
- Normal intelligence
- Muscular hypotonia
- Inability to produce sperm
- Sparse pubic and axillary hair
- Abnormal legs, short trunk, shoulder equal to hip size

Hormonal treatment may be advocated which may help the growth of body hair, improve the apperance of muscles, increase libido and strength. Some of the complications include enlarged teeth with a thinning surface (taurodontism), depression, learning disabilities, osteoporosis and breast cancer in men. A typical karyotype of a Klinefelter syndrome patient is given in Figure 9.

Fig. 9. A micrograph of Klinefelter (XXY) in comparison with its corresponding normal (XY) chromosomes
(Reproduced courtesy of Human Genome Centre, Universiti Sains Malaysia, Malaysia)

6. Conclusion

So far, no system can classify banded chromosomes as robustly and accurately as a skilled cytogeneticist, despite the millions of dollars that have been invested in automated karyotype analysis since 1968. Currently cytogenetics is paving its way into the molecular approaches in deciphering the structure, function and evolution of chromosomes. Still, conventional cytogenetics where routine banding techniques are employed remains a simple and popular technique to get an overview of the human genome as a whole (Thirumulu Kannan Ponnuraj & Zilfalil Alwi, 2009). Routine banded karyotype analysis can now be combined with M-FISH and other molecular techniques leading to more precise detection of various syndromes in children. Through the analysis of chromosome banding patterns, thousands of chromosomal abnormalities have been associated with inherited or *de novo* disorders, generating many leads to the underlying molecular causes of these disorders and today, when high resolution genetic linkage analysis can be conducted easily, the discovery of a patient whose disorder is caused by a gross chromosomal abnormality is heralded as a valuable resource for locating the disease gene. Solid tumors also present a myriad of complex chromosomal aberrations and each is a possible clue to tumor initiation and progression. The challenge is to navigate from the visible morphological alteration to the DNA sequence level. In other words, chromosomal abnormalities exist as nature's guide to the molecular basis of many unexplained human disorders. Hence, cytogenetics continue to remain as indispensable tools for the diagnosis of various genetic disorders which gives an overall picture of the whole genome for analysis. This could possibly also pave a way for treatment and management related to chromosomal disorders.

7. References

Albertson, D. & Pinkel, D. (2003). Genomic microarrays in human genetic disease and cancer. *Human Molecular Genetics* 12: 145–152.

Arrighi, F.E. & Hsu, T.C. (1971). Localization of heterochromatin in human chromosomes. *Cytogenetics* 10: 81-86.

Barbara J Trask. (2002). Human cytogenetics: 49 chromosomes, 46 years and counting. *Nature* 3: 769-778.

Caspersson, T., Farber, S., Foley, G.E., Kudynowski, J., Modest, E.J., Simonsson, E., Wagh, U. & Zech, L. (1968). Chemical differentiation along metaphase chromosomes. *Experimental Cell Research* 49: 219-222.

Caspersson, T., Zech, L. & Johansson, C. (1970). Differential binding of alkylating fluorochromes in human chromosomes. *Experimental Cell Research* 60: 315-319.

Chamla, Y. & Ruffie, M. (1976). Production of C and T bands in human mitotic chromosomes after treatment. *Human Genetics* 34: 213-216.

Chicago Conference, (1966). Standardization in Human Cytogenetics. Birth defects: Original Article Series, 11:2, New York, The National Foundation.

Denver Conference. (1960). The identification of individual chromosomes especially in man. *American Journal of Human Genetics* 12: 384–389.

Dominique FCM Smeets. (2004). Historical prospective of human cytogenetics: from microscope to microarray. *Clinical Biochemistry* 37: 439–446.

Dutrillaux, B. & Lejeune, J. (1971). Sur une nouvelle technique d'analyse du caryotype humain. C.R. Acad. Sci. Paris 272: 2638-2640.

Dutrillaux, B. (1973). Noveau susteme de marquage chromosomique: les bandes T. *Chromosoma* 41: 395-402.

Edwards, J.H., Harnden, D.G., Cameron, A.H., Crosse, V.M. & Wolff, O.H. (1960). A new trisomic syndrome. *Lancet* 1: 787–790.

Ford, C.E., Jones, K.W., Polani, P.E., De Almeida, J.C. & Briggs, J.H. (1959). A sex chromosome anomaly in a case of gonadal dysgenesis (Turner's syndrome). *Lancet* 1: 711-713.

Fuchs, F. & Riis, P. (1956). Antenatal sex determination. *Nature* 177: 330.

Goodpasture, C., Bloom, S.E., Hsu, T.C. & Arrighi, F.E. (1976). Human nucleolus organizers: the satellites or the stalks? *American Journal of Human Genetics* 28: 559-566.

Hans Zellweger & Jane Simpson. (1977). Chromosomes of Man. William Heinemann Medical Books Ltd. J.B.Lippincott Co. Philadelphia.

Hamerton, J.L., Klinger, H.P., Mutton, D.E. & Lang, E.M. (1963). The London Conference on the normal human karyotype, 28th-30th August, 1963. *Cytogenetics* 25: 264-268.

Hare, W.C.D. & Singh, E.L. (1979). Cytogenetics in Animal Reproduction. Commonwealth Agricultural Bureaux, UK.

ISCN, 2005. An international system for human cytogenetics nomenclature (2005): recommendations of the International Standing Committee on Human Cytogenetic Nomenclature / editors, Lisa G. Shaffer, Niels Tommerup Basel ; Farmington, CT : Karger.

Jacobs, P.A. & Strong, J.A. (1959). A case of human intersexuality having a possible XXY sex-determining mechanism. *Nature* 183: 302–303.

Jau-hong Kao, Jen-hui Chuang. & TsaipeiWang. (2008). Chromosome classification based on the band profile similarity along approximate medial axis. *Pattern Recognition* 41: 77 - 89.

Johannsen, W. (1909). Elemente der exakten Erblichkeitslehre. Gustav Fischer, Jena.

Kallioniemi, A., Kallioniemi, O.P., Sudar, D., Rutovitz, D., Gray, J.W., Waldman, F. & Pinkel, D. (1992). Comparative genomic hybridization for molecular cytogenetic analysis of solid tumors. *Science* 258: 818–821.

Lejeune, J., gautier, M. & Turpin, R. (1959). Etude des chromosomes somatiques de neuf enfants mongliens. *Comptes Rendus Hebd Seances Acad Sci* 248 (11) : 1721–1722.

Lubs, H.A. (1969). A marker X chromosome. *American Journal of Human Genetics* 21: 231-244.

Matsui, S. & Sasaki, M. (1973). Differential staining of nucleolus organisers in mammalian chromosomes. *Nature* 246: 148-150.

Moorehead, P.S., Nowell, P.C., Mellman, W.J., Battips, D.M. & Hungerford, D.A. (1960). Chromosome preparations of leukocytes cultured from human peripheral blood. *Experimental Cell Research* 20: 613-616.

Neus Baena., Miriam Guitart., Joan Carles Ferreres., Elisabet Gabau., Manuel Corona., Francisco Mellado., Josep Egozcue & Maria Rosa Caballin. (2001). Fetal and placenta chromosome constitution in 237 pregnancies. *Annales de Genetique* 44: 83-88.

Nowell, P.C. & Hungerford, D.A. (1960). A minute chromosome in human chronic granulocytic leukemia. *Science* 132: 1497–1501.

Painter, T.S. (1934). A new method for the study of chromosome aberrations and the plotting of chromosome maps in Drosphila melanogaster. *Genetics,* 19: 175-188.

Pardue, M.L. & Gall, J.G. (1970). Chromosomal localization of mouse satellite DNA. *Science* 168: 1356-1358.

Patau, K., Smith, D.W., Therman, E., Inhorn, S.L. & Wagner, H.P. (1960). Multiple congenital anomaly caused by an extra autosome. *Lancet* 1: 790–793.

Perry, P. & Evans, H.J. (1975). Cytological detection of mutagen-carcinogen exposure by sister chromatid exchange. *Nature* 258: 121-125.

Pinkel, D., Seagraves, R., Sudar D., Clark, S., Poole, I., Kowbel, D., Collins, C., Kuo, W.L., Chen, C., Zhai, Y., Dairkee, S.H., Ljung, B.M., Gray, J.W. & Albertson, D.G. (1998). High resolution analysis of DNA copy number variation using comparative genomic hybridization to microarrays. *Nature Genetics* 20: 207–211.

Pinkel, D., Gray, J.W., Trask, B., van den Engh, G., Fuscoe, J. & van Dekken, H. (1986a). Cytogenetic analysis by in situ hybridization with fluorescently labeled nucleic acid probes. *Cold Spring Harbor Symposia on Quantitative Biology* 51: 151-157.

Pinkel, D., Straumem T. & Gray, J.W. (1986b). Cytogenetic analysis using quantitative, high-sensitivity, fluorescence hybridization. *Proceedings of the National Academy of Sciences USA* 83: 2934-2938.

Ried, T., Landes, G., Dackowski, W., Klinger, K. & Ward, D.C. (1992). Multicolor fluorescence *in situ* hybridization for the simultaneous detection of probe sets for chromosomes 13, 18, 21, X and Y in uncultured amniotic fluid cells. *Human Molecular Genetics* 1: 307–313.

Rooney, D.E. (2001). Human cytogenetics: constitutional analysis. New York: Oxford Univ. Press.

Rowley, J.D. (1973). A new consistent chromosomal abnormality in chronic myelogenous leukaemia identified by quinacrine fluorescence and Giemsa staining. *Nature* 273: 290–293.

Sabina Solinas-Toldo., Stefan Lampel., Stephan Stilgenbauer., Jeremy Nickolenko., Axel Benner., Hartmut Döhner., Thomas Cremer. & Peter Lichter. (1997). Matrix-based comparative genomic hybridization: biochips to screen for genomic imbalances. *Genes Chromosomes Cancer* 20: 399–407.

Sawyer, J.R. & Hozier, J.C. (1986). High resolution of Mouse chromosomes: Banding conservation between man and mouse. *Science* 232: 1632-1639.

Scheres, J.M.J.C. 1974. Production of C and T bands in human chromosomes after heat treatment at high ph and staining with "stains-all". *Human Genetics* 23: 311-314.

Schmickel, R.D. (1986). Contiguous gene syndromes: a component of recognizable syndromes. *Journal of Pediatrics* 109: 231–241.

Seabright, M. (1971). A rapid banding technique for human chromosomes. *Lancet* 2: 971-972.

Steele, M.W. & Breg, W.R. (1966). Chromosome analysis of human amniotic-fluid cells. *Lancet* 1: 383–385.

Thirumulu Ponnuraj Kannan & Zilfalil Alwi. (2009). Cytogenetics: Past, Present and future. *Malaysian Journal of Medical Sciences* 16(2): 4-9.

Tjio, J.H. & Levan, A. (1956). The chromosome number in man. *Hereditas.* 42: 1-6.

Verma, L., MacDonald, F., Leedham, P., McConachie, M., Dhanjal, S. & Hulten, M. (1998). Rapid and simple prenatal DNA diagnosis of Down's syndrome. *The Lancet* 352: 9-12.

Waldeyer, W. (1888). Über Karyokinese und ihre Beziehungen zu den Befruchtungsvorgängen. *Archiv für mikroskopische Anatomie und Entwicklungsmechanik*. 32: 1-122.

Yunis, J.J. (1976). High resolution of human chromosomes. *Science* 191: 1268–1270.

4

Functional Interpretation of Omics Data by Profiling Genes and Diseases Using MeSH–Controlled Vocabulary

Takeru Nakazato, Hidemasa Bono and Toshihisa Takagi
Database Center for Life Science, Research Organization of Information and Systems
Japan

1. Introduction

One of the major aims of molecular biology and medical science is to understand disease mechanisms. A genetic disorder is a disease caused by abnormalities in genes and chromosomes, and researchers often report the identification of disease-relevant genes and correlations between phenotypes and genotypes (Butte & Kohane 2006; Lamb 2007; Perez-Iratxeta *et al.* 2002, 2005, 2007).

Omics analysis using microarray, new generation sequencing (NGS) technology, and mass spectrometry is widely employed for determining genome sequences and profiling gene expression. Changes in gene expression on a genome-wide scale can be detected by omics analysis, which provides various types of huge datasets. These data are often archived in public databases; nucleotide sequences in the DDBJ/EMBL/GenBank International Nucleotide Sequence Database (INSD) (Cochrane *et al.* 2011), gene expression in Gene Expression Omnibus (GEO) (Barrett *et al.* 2011), and journal articles in MEDLINE. Currently, research cannot continue without the use of these databases. In Japan, the Database Center for Life Science (DBCLS) has developed infrastructure for researchers to access and easily reuse these data by providing index sites such as INSD and GEO yellow pages and by constructing a portal site for life science databases and tools. Researchers can easily analyze public data in conjunction with their own omics data.

Here we present an analytical method to clarify the associations between genes and diseases. We characterized genes and diseases by assigning a MeSH-controlled vocabulary (Nakazato *et al.* 2008, 2009). Our objective was to help interpret omics data from molecular and clinical aspects by comparing these feature profiles.

2. Omics databases

2.1 Microarray data and its repository sites

Microarray technology is one of the most widely employed tools for genome-wide analyses of changes in gene expression under various conditions including diseases and drug treatments. This approach is also useful for examining genome copy number variations, methylation status, and transcription factor binding.

Microarray data are archived in public databases such as GEO at the National Center for Biotechnology Information (NCBI) (Barrett *et al.* 2011) and ArrayExpress at the European

Bioinformatics Institute (EBI) (Parkinson *et al.* 2011). GEO is a public functional genomics data repository that accepts array- and sequence-based data. It has been developed and maintained by NCBI since 2000. GEO archives three types of data: datasets derived from research projects, samples such as species and cell lines used, and platforms to produce data (i.e., chipsets and massively parallel sequencers). GEO contains approximately 22,000 series of experiments, approximately 8500 platforms, and approximately 540,000 samples as of March 2011.

GEO data are freely downloadable (http://www.ncbi.nlm.nih.gov/geo/); therefore, researchers can utilize the data to perform further analyses and compare their own data as omics analysis. However, it is extremely difficult to grasp the GEO archived data because experimental conditions referred in each GEO entry are complicated and partially described in plain English.

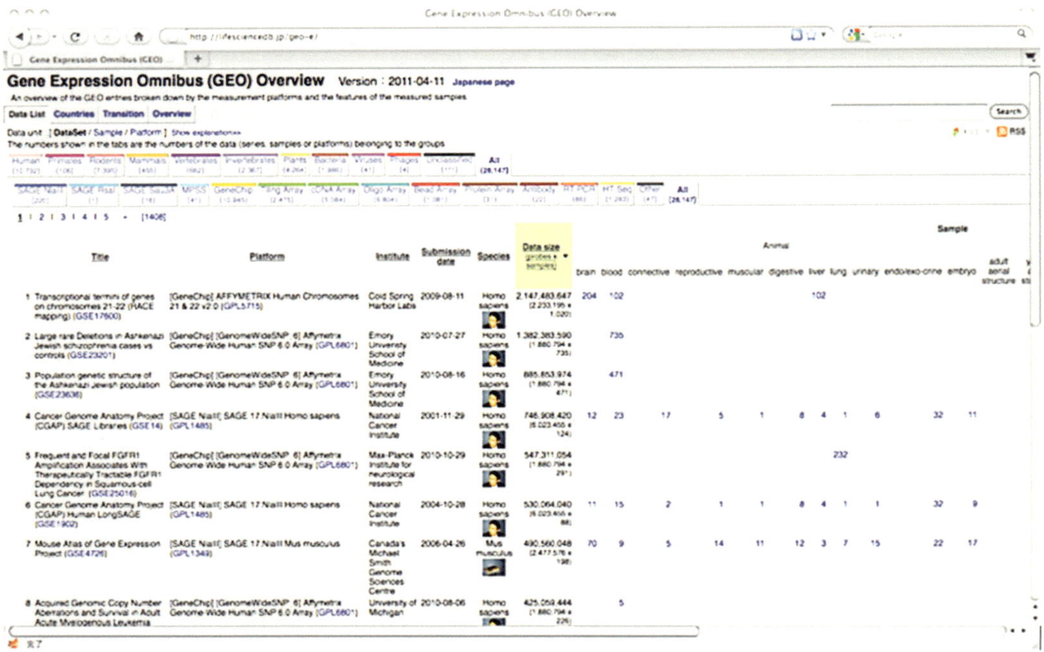

Fig. 1. Snapshot of the GEO Overview

To ease this situation, Dr. Okubo and his colleagues at the National Institute of Genetics (Japan) have developed a web service of an index site as a yellow page called the GEO Overview (http://lifesciencedb.jp/geo/), which is maintained by DBCLS (Fig. 1). It shows a list of project titles with their platforms and data provider names. In the GEO Overview, the datasets archived in GEO are categorized and organized by taxonomy (species type) and platform (methods or instruments). Researchers can easily refine the results by clicking the tabs corresponding to the taxonomy and platform of interest. In addition, the datasets can be searched using the search box at the top of the page. Hit data are categorized by histology with a hyperlink to the original GEO entry, and total data size is also provided. The GEO Overview should be helpful in outlining the abundant amount of gene expression data available from GEO. A tutorial movie for the GEO Overview is available on the TogoTV site (http://togotv.dbcls.jp/20100816.html).

2.2 NGS and its repository sites

Microarray technology has been widely employed to detect genome-wide gene expression. More recently, NGS, also called next-generation sequencing, has been performed for the same purpose. NGS is an ultra-high throughput nucleotide sequencing technology that drastically reduces the cost and time than previously possible (Shendure & Ji 2008). NGS technology has rapidly spread to approach whole-genome sequencing, metagenomics, and transcriptomics, and it also applies to epigenetics and genome-wide association study (GWAS) (Kahvejian *et al.* 2008).

NGS provides a tremendous of captured images and numerous sequence reads (Nat. Biotechnol. Editorial Board 2008), and the in-process files require huge amounts of disk space. However, NGS data are important for researchers and should be shared as well as microarray data in GEO. Thus, the NGS data are also archived in public databases; the Sequence Read Archive (SRA) (Leinonen *et al.* 2011 b) at NCBI, European Nucleotide Archive (ENA) (Leinonen *et al.* 2011 a) at EBI, and DNA Data Bank of Japan (DDBJ) Sequence Read Archive (DRA) (Kaminuma *et al.* 2010) at DDBJ. These databases are an archive databank for raw data from NGS, and the data are collaboratively synchronized. Researchers can search and download the archived data from the DDBJ site (http://trace.ddbj.nig.ac.jp/dra/).

Downloaded data from the SRA/ENA/DRA sites can be used for genome mapping, assembly, and annotation (Kaminuma *et al.* 2010). DBCLS has developed an index site for NGS data, called the Survey of Read Archives (http://sra.dbcls.jp/) as well as the GEO Overview site, to make this data more searchable and usable. The deposited NGS data contain not only sequence reads but also experimental conditions including project titles, species or cell lines, sample names, and sequencing platforms as metadata. The metadata consist of six files in XML format: submission, study, experiment, run, sample, and analysis. However, each submission does not contain all of these metadata because additional experiments or runs to be assigned to a previous project are often performed and archived as a new submission. Therefore, we determined the connections among each type of corresponding metadata and developed a project list as an index site. We attempted to curate the metadata by correcting misspellings and disambiguating spelling variations.

The Survey of Read Archives site provides a list with project titles, sample names, and a hyperlink to corresponding experiments and run data. It categorizes the data by study type including whole genome sequencing, transcriptome analysis, and metagenomics. Furthermore, the archived data are divided by platform and sample taxonomy. Thus, researchers can easily obtain final results with corresponding features of interest. The Survey of Read Archives site provides NGS statistical data such as the number of projects assigned to each study, platforms, and sample taxonomy. Table 1 shows the top ten list of NGS statistical data as of March 2011.

In addition, the Survey of Read Archives site offers a publication list that refers to NGS data. We obtained PubMed IDs (PMIDs) cited in the SRA database as reference articles. We also extracted hyperlinks and descriptions of SRA IDs from PubMed articles. The publication list provides article titles, journals, and project titles. Using this publication list, researchers can retrieve NGS data of sufficiently high quality for analysis. Users can narrow down the publication list by referring to NGS's study types, platforms, and sample species.

Study type	
Study type	The number of projects
Whole genome sequencing	2799
Transcriptome analysis	778
Metagenomics	564
Epigenetics	365
Resequencing	276
Other	259
Population genomics	110
RNASeq	104
Gene regulation study	37
Cancer genomics	18

Platforms	
Platform	The number of projects
Illumina Genome Analyzer II	1628
454 GS FLX	1209
454 Titanium	1121
Illumina Genome Analyzer	753
454 GS FLX Titanium	274
GS FLX	150
GS 20	135
Unspecified	109
Illumina HiSeq 2000	99
454 GS 20	61

Species of samples	
Species	The number of projects
Unidentified	460
Homo sapiens	414
Mus musculus	230
Metagenome sequence	170
Drosophila melanogaster	149
Marine metagenome	87
Caenorhabiditis elegans	75
Escherichia coli str. K-12 substr. MG1655	66
Arabidopsis thaliana	55
Saccharomyces cerevisiae	51

Table 1. List of top ten study types, platforms, and sample species of NGS data archived in SRA databases

3. Disease database

3.1 Online Mendelian Inheritance in Man (OMIM)

OMIM is one of the most widely referred disease databases by biological researchers (Amberger *et al.* 2009; Hamosh *et al.* 2002, 2005). It contains more than 21,000 detailed entries of genetic diseases and disease-relevant human genes as a knowledge bank. Each disease entry provides a full-text overview in some categories including clinical features, diagnoses, and pathogenesis, and gene entry consists of sections such as cloning, gene function, and allelic variants sections.

OMIM was originally created as a printed version called the Mendelian Inheritance in Man (MIM), which has been annotated by Dr. McKusick and his colleagues for over 40 years (McKusick 2007). OMIM, which is the online version of MIM, is accessible through the internet from the NCBI site (http://www.ncbi.nlm.nih.gov/omim/). Its contents are the copyright of Johns Hopkins University. Data are updated daily on this database, and approximately 70 new entries are added per month (http://www.ncbi.nlm.nih.gov/Omim/dispupdates.html). The OMIM content is derived from the peer-reviewed biomedical literature.

3.2 Previous work using OMIM data

OMIM is an excellent resource to obtain information on genetic diseases and disease-relevant genes and for researchers attempting to understand disease features. Using Entrez Gene or Ensembl as a gene database, gene features including gene names, genomic locations, and gene ontology (GO) terms can be obtained. However, OMIM is not completely exploited for omics analysis because of its bibliographic data structure; it is written in plain English (Bajdik *et al.* 2005). To overcome these difficulties, previous studies attempted to extract knowledge described in OMIM and make it easier to use that knowledge for biological research, including omics analysis.

Some groups focused on terms referred in the clinical synopsis (CS) section of OMIM (Cantor & Lussier 2004; Freudenberg & Propping 2002; Hishiki *et al.* 2004; Masseroli *et al.* 2005 a; van Driel *et al.* 2006). The OMIM CS section contains keywords and key phrases for the mode of inheritance, symptoms, and phenotypes such as eye color, pain sensitivity, height, and weight.

Table 2 shows a partial list of terms referred in the CS section for Prader–Willi syndrome (OMIM ID: 176270) as an example.

This section describes clinical features of disorders and their modes of inheritance such as autosomal dominant, body system such as almond-shaped eyes, and endocrine features such as growth hormone deficiency.

As a previous study, categorization of each OMIM disease entry using particular criteria such as episodes, etiology, tissue, onset, and inheritance has been attempted (Freudenberg & Propping 2002). They also calculated correlations between OMIM entries on the basis of profile similarities.

Masseroli *et al.* normalized various descriptions such as Neuro and Neurologic in the CS section and characterized OMIM disease entries (Masseroli *et al.* 2005 a). They developed a web service called GFINDer to analyze phenotypes of inherited disorders (Masseroli *et al.* 2005 b).

Cohen *et al.* also developed a web service to search the OMIM CS section called CSI-OMIM (Cohen *et al.* 2011).

Using CS terms, researchers can retrieve disease information from OMIM without using text-mining techniques. Although the OMIM full-text content includes detailed biological and genetic descriptions, the CS terms are mainly clinical and diagnostic, and therefore, it is difficult to decipher disease information in conjunction with biological process data such as gene expression data. Furthermore, the CS terms such as Cardiac and Cardiovascular are ambiguous because the assigned terms are often defined by the author's original description in the cited articles. We therefore utilized the medical subject headings (MeSH)-controlled vocabulary to characterize OMIM entries.

Headings	Subheadings	Feature
Inheritance	-	Isolated cases
Growth	Height	Mean adult male height, 155 cm
		Mean adult female height, 147 cm
		Steady childhood growth
	Weight	Onset of obesity from 6 months to 6 years
		Central obesity
Respiratory	-	Hypoventilation
		Hypoxia
Skeletal	-	Osteoporosis
		Osteopenia
Endocrine features	-	Hyperinsulinemia
		Growth hormone deficiency
		Hypogonadotropic hypogonadism
Miscellaneous	-	Food related behavioral problems include excessive appetite and obsession with eating
		Temperature instability
		High pain threshold
Molecular basis	-	Microdeletion of 15q11 in 70% of patients confirmed by fluorescent in situ hybridization
		Remainder of cases secondary to maternal disomy
		Rare cases secondary to chromosome translocation

Table 2. Keywords and key phrases referred in the OMIM CS section for Prader–Willi syndrome (partial)

4. Feature profiling of OMIM data using MeSH keywords

Many methods such as noise reduction (Li & Wong 2001 a, 2001 b), hierarchical clustering (Eisen *et al.* 1998), and self-organization maps (Tamayo *et al.* 1999) have been proposed for analyzing omics data including microarray. However, these methods are statistical approaches, and molecular biology and medicine researchers often need to grasp their microarray data from a biological viewpoint.

Researchers often use a controlled vocabulary, called ontology, to annotate biological features including genes. The most popular ontology for biologists is GO (Ashburner *et al.* 2000). GO consists of three categories: biological process, molecular function, and cellular component. For omics analysis, GO terms are often utilized by assigning corresponding terms to genes of interest (Khatri & Draghici 2005; Zeeberg *et al.* 2003, 2005). However, GO cannot be applied to annotate OMIM diseases because it focuses on features at the molecular level, and no term corresponding to specific diseases or chemical substance exists.

Here we introduce MeSH terms to characterize genes and diseases.

4.1 MeSH

MeSH (http://www.nlm.nih.gov/mesh/) is a controlled vocabulary and contains more than 23,000 keywords (Nelson *et al.* 2004). These keywords are hierarchically categorized into 15 concepts such as disease, chemicals and drugs, and anatomy. MeSH was originally curated for indexing MEDLINE articles by the National Library of Medicine (NLM). Researchers can view MeSH keywords assigned to each MEDLINE article in PubMed results. In a PubMed search, some queries are automatically added by corresponding MeSH terms, and PubMed is searched by a converted query. PubMed also accepts MeSH keywords as an input query. MeSH has over 177,000 entry terms that assist in finding the most appropriate MeSH heading. For example, vitamin C is an entry term for ascorbic acid. In addition, another approximately 200,000 terms of chemical compounds and proteins are available as the Substance Names. MeSH is freely on the NLM site in XML and ASCII formats and is updated annually.

4.2 Feature profiling of OMIM data

4.2.1 Data collection

We retrieved OMIM data available as of January 2010 by downloading them from the NCBI FTP site (ftp://ftp.ncbi.nih.gov/repository/OMIM/) and by using the web service with Entrez Programming Utilities (eUtils, http://eutils.ncbi.nlm.nih.gov/). We obtained MeSH terms (2010 release) from the NLM web site (http://www.nlm.nih.gov/mesh/meshhome.html). MEDLINE article data were also obtained from NLM.

4.2.2 Article extraction related to each OMIM entry

As previously described, MeSH is originally used for keywords to index MEDLINE articles and is not directly linked to OMIM entries. Thus, we developed a method to retrieve articles referred in each OMIM entry. A schematic view of the pipeline for generating OMIM-PMID associations is shown in Fig. 2. The pipeline consists of three steps.

First, we retrieved PMIDs cited in the OMIM reference section (Fig. 2 a). Alzheimer Disease, AD (OMIM ID: 104300) was used as an example, and 191 articles were referred in the OMIM reference section as of March 2011. Previous studies also extracted hyperlinks to external databases to utilize MeSH terms for interpreting microarray data (Djebbari *et al.* 2005; Masys *et al.* 2001).

Next, we retrieved OMIM IDs referred in the Secondary Source ID section of MEDLINE articles (Fig. 2 b). We also collected the OMIM ID descriptions from full-text articles by searching PubMed Central. IDs of external databases including GenBank and GEO referred in full-text articles are often assigned to MEDLINE articles as a Secondary Source ID. As of April 2010, 5463 OMIM IDs were assigned to MEDLINE articles as a Secondary Source ID. These Secondary Source IDs are assigned by NLM, but not all IDs are extracted.

In the last step, we obtained PMIDs of articles assigned with MeSH terms corresponding to each OMIM entry (Fig. 2 c). As described above, MeSH contains disease category terms; therefore, there is often a MeSH keyword corresponding to each OMIM entry. For example, the OMIM entry for Alzheimer Disease, AD corresponded to the MeSH term Alzheimer Disease.

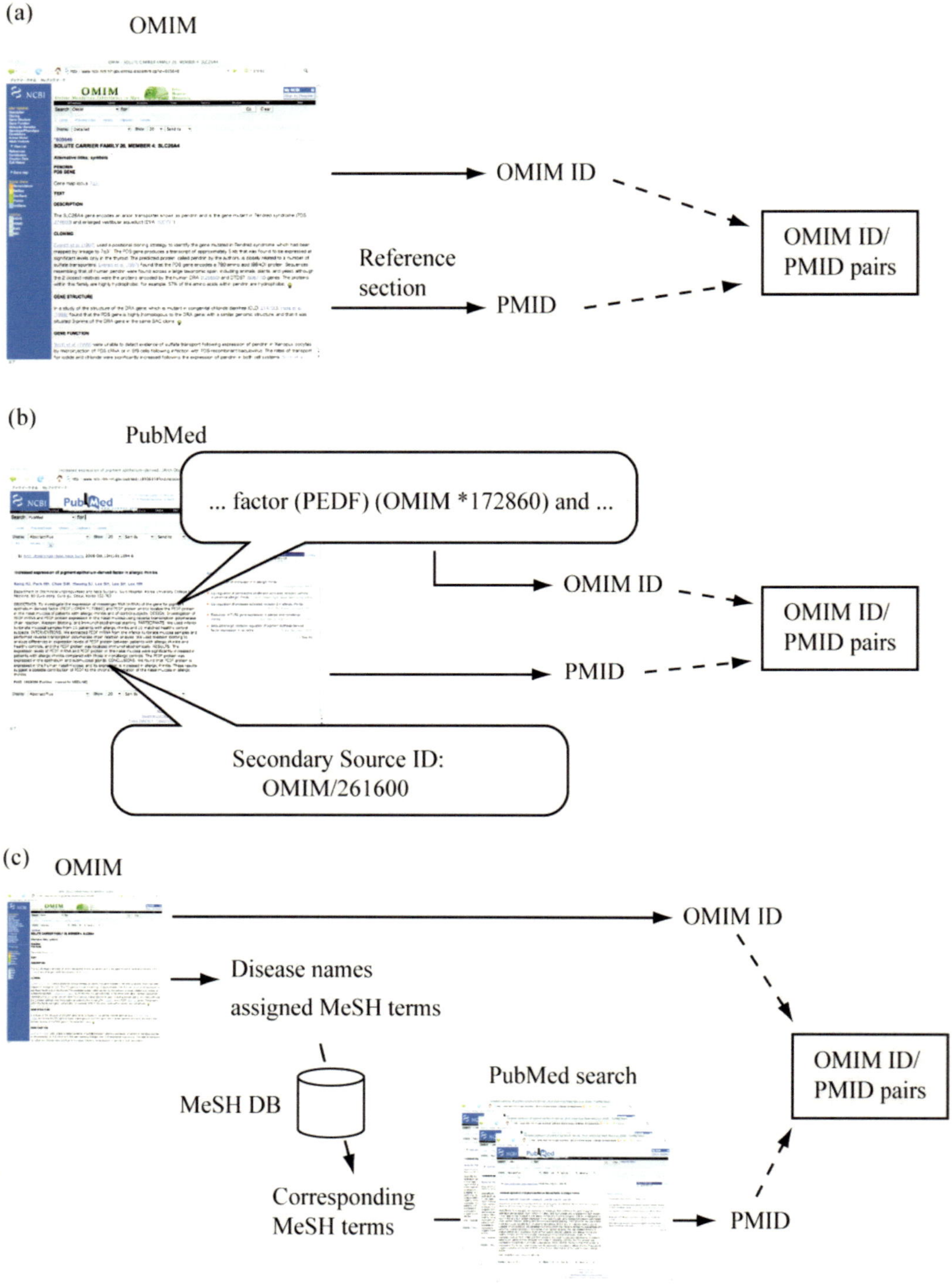

Fig. 2. Schematic view of the pipeline for generating pairs of OMIM entries and relevant PMIDs

We also obtained articles referring to human genes. OMIM contains entries describing not only genetic diseases but also disease-relevant human genes. By obtaining articles related to each OMIM entry using these steps, we also obtained articles on human genes. To complement articles on human genes, we obtained articles using Entrez Gene as a gene database. Using the process described above, we obtained PMIDs referred in Entrez Gene, describing Entrez Gene ID in the abstract, and assigned them to corresponding MeSH terms.

Accordingly, we retrieved approximately 500,000 unique pairs of OMIM IDs and PMIDs and generated approximately 2,000,000 OMIM–MeSH pairs.

In a previous version (Nakazato *et al.* 2008, 2009), we retrieved PMIDs by searching PubMed using disease names. To identify contexts indicating genes and diseases from articles is a major theme, and many approaches using text mining, such as named entity recognition (NER), have been reported (Gaudan *et al.* 2005; Hirschman *et al.* 2005; Jensen *et al.* 2006; Shatkay 2005). One of the difficulties is that a single disease often has many names, e.g., type 2 diabetes, non-insulin dependent diabetes, and NIDDM. Another problem is that the same abbreviation may refer to several diseases, genes, or drugs; e.g., EVA refers to enlarged vestibular aqueduct (disease), epithelial V-like antigen (gene), and ethylene vinyl acetate (chemical). Thus, we attempted to overcome this by creating abbreviations/long-form pairs for disease names, such as PWS and Prader–Willi syndrome, and searched MEDLINE for articles co-occurring with both names. However, this text-mining approach is noisy, and therefore, we discontinued applying this step in this version of data creation.

4.2.3 Scoring associations between OMIM entries and MeSH terms

OMIM contains gene entries as molecular mechanisms and disease entries as their phenotypes (Amberger *et al.* 2009). We calculated the scores of diseases and genes separately. These types are indicated by symbols prefixed to the OMIM ID such as #143100 (Huntington Disease; HD) and *613004 (Huntingtin; HTT). We divided the OMIM entries into three groups according to these types: sequence known (*, +), locus known (%), and phenotype (#, none). We then calculated p values as scores of OMIM–MeSH pairs in each group. The p value is the probability of the actual or a more extreme outcome under the null hypothesis. A lower p value means a larger significance of association. We used R language to calculate the p values.

4.2.4 Data visualization

To visualize retrieved features of OMIM disease entries with relevant MeSH terms, we developed a web-based software application called the gene disease features ontology-based overview system (Gendoo) (Nakazato *et al.* 2008, 2009). Gendoo accepts OMIM IDs, OMIM titles, Entrez Gene IDs, gene names, and MeSH terms as input queries. For disease names, Gendoo currently uses descriptions of title, alternative titles, and symbols referred in OMIM, and therefore, not all synonyms are included in the disease name dictionary. We will increase the number of synonyms by adding the canonical name and synonyms (entry terms) for corresponding MeSH terms and by extracting disease names from MEDLINE and OMIM resources using text mining. Gendoo generates high-scoring lists that display relevant MeSH terms for diseases, drugs, biological phenomena, and anatomy together with their scores. These MeSH terms are sorted according to their scores. The background color of each association indicates its p value. Gendoo also provides a hierarchical tree view of MeSH terms associated with diseases of interest using JavaScript and cascading style sheet (CSS) resources from the Yahoo! User Interface (YUI) library (http://developer.yahoo.com/yui/).

Gendoo can be openly accessed at http://gendoo.dbcls.jp/. Every association file including Entrez Gene/OMIM IDs, MeSH, and their scores is available from the web site. Dictionary files including gene/disease names, synonyms, and IDs are also downloadable. These web services and files are freely available under a Creative Commons Attribution 2.1 Japan license (http://creativecommons.org/licenses/by/2.1/jp/deed.en).

4.3 Obtained feature profiles

4.3.1 Example 1: Positive control

Table 3 shows a list of scores and MeSH terms closely associated with Alzheimer Disease, AD (OMIM ID: 104300) and Amyloid Beta A4 Precursor Protein, APP (OMIM ID: 104760) as a positive control.

Alzheimer Disease; AD		
MeSH terms	Category	p value
Alzheimer Disease	Disease	0
Amyloid Beta Protein	Chemicals and Drugs	0
Brain	Anatomy	0

Amyloid Beta A4 Precursor Protein; APP		
MeSH terms	Category	p value
Alzheimer Disease	Disease	4.20×10^{-231}
Amyloid Beta Protein	Chemicals and drugs	5.12×10^{-214}
Brain	Anatomy	7.32×10^{-35}

Table 3. Lists of scores and keywords related to Alzheimer Disease and the Amyloid Beta A4 Precursor Protein

Alzheimer disease is a neurodegenerative disorder caused by accumulation of amyloid plaques in the brain. Here we used three MeSH terms as keywords to describe features of Alzheimer disease: Alzheimer Disease, Amyloid Beta Protein, and Brain. The scores among the keywords and the OMIM entry of Alzheimer Disease were small; thus, the retrieved associations seemed to properly illustrate features of the disease. The entry of the Amyloid Beta A4 Precursor Protein as an example of a gene was also strongly associated with these keywords.

4.3.2 Example 2: Retrieved profile

Table 4 lists the top three keywords related to Prader–Willi syndrome (OMIM ID: 176270) for the features of the fields, such as Diseases, Chemicals and Drugs, Biological Phenomena, and Anatomy, as examples of retrieved profiles.

Prader–Willi syndrome results from deletion of paternal copies of the imprinted small nuclear ribonucleoprotein polypeptide N (SNRPN) and necdin genes within chromosome 15 (Horsthemke & Wagstaff 2008). The results showed that the keyword clearly reflected the features of Prader–Willi syndrome, including Chromosomes, Human, Pair 15, Genomic Imprinting, and Ribonucleoproteins, Small Nuclear. For the features of Prader–Willi syndrome, the OMIM CS section presents morphologies and clinical and diagnostic fields such as mean height and temperature instability (Table 2). This approach illustrates the disease features from a clinical and biological perspective. To retrieve more clinical and diagnostic features with MeSH, we increased the number of novel associations using terms from the MeSH category Analytical, Diagnostic, and Therapeutic Techniques and Equipment.

MeSH category	MeSH terms	*p* value
Diseases	Prader–Willi syndrome	0
	Angelman syndrome	4.05×10^{-140}
	Obesity	6.94×10^{-128}
Chemicals and Drugs	Human growth hormone	5.86×10^{-68}
	Ribonucleoproteins, small nuclear	4.29×10^{-62}
	Ghrelin	1.58×10^{-50}
Biological Phenomena	Chromosomes, human, pair 15	0
	Genomic imprinting	2.47×10^{-131}
	Obesity	1.69×10^{-121}
Anatomy	Chromosomes, human, pair 15	0
	Chromosomes, human, 13–15	1.25×10^{-30}
	Adipose tissue	3.93×10^{-13}

Table 4. List of top three keywords related to Prader–Willi syndrome

4.3.3 Example 3: Comparison of profiles between diseases

We applied this analysis to types 1 and 2 diabetes mellitus (OMIM IDs 222100 and 125853, respectively). Figure 3 shows a summary of typical features and their scores for type 1 and 2 diabetes mellitus. Each cell color on the heat map reflects the *p* value of the association.

Figure 3 summarizes the feature profiles; only type 1 diabetes mellitus was closely related to Autoimmune Diseases and Spleen (their *p* values were 4.55×10^{-5} and 5.53×10^{-7}, respectively), whereas type 2 diabetes was associated with Obesity (*p* value = 1.18×10^{-15}) and Adipocytes (*p* value = 5.17×10^{-5}). Type 1 diabetes mellitus involves the immune system, whereas type 2 diabetes mellitus is a metabolic disorder (Rother 2007). These retrieved profiles reflect the biological features of the diseases. This result suggests that MeSH profiles can clarify the differences and similarities in features between OMIM entries.

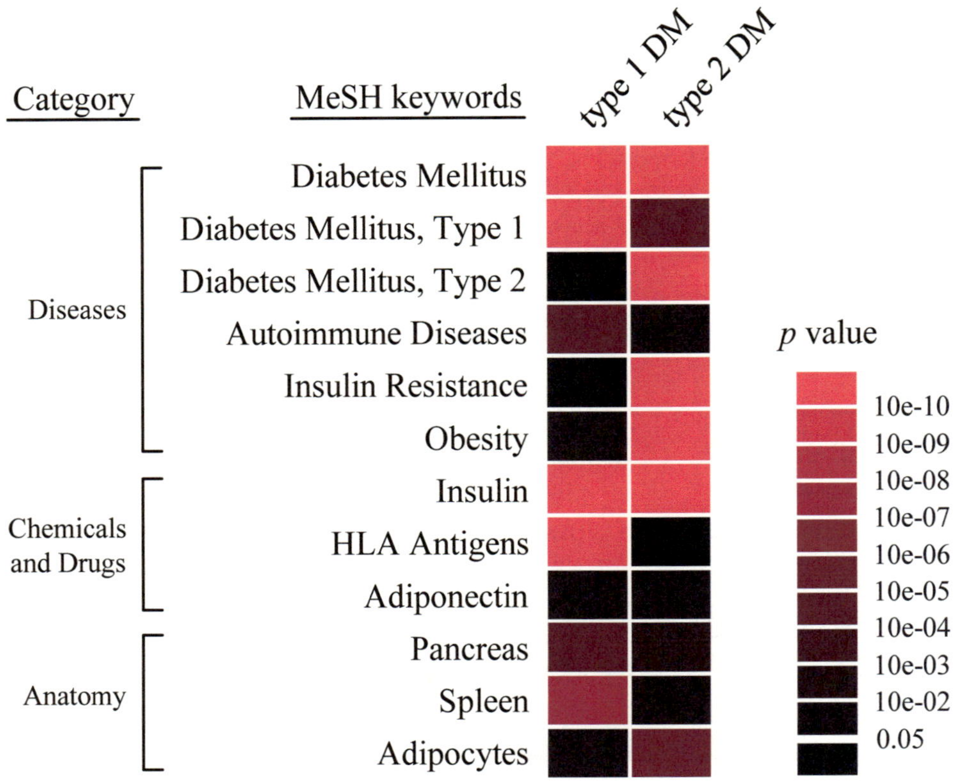

Fig. 3. Differences and similarities between feature profiles of type 1 and 2 diabetes mellitus. DM, diabetes mellitus

5. Discussion

Diverse types of life science data are available including nucleotide sequences at the molecular level and clinical records at the individual level. Omics analysis makes it easy to detect genome-wide upregulation and downregulation of gene expression under various conditions. We analyzed these raw data using several approaches such as statistical clustering and pathway analysis. In addition, to decipher phenotype information in conjunction with molecular data, we often relate genes that drastically change their expression levels to diseases as a result of omics analysis. However, molecular biologists only understand mechanisms for specific diseases. Although OMIM is an excellent knowledge bank for various diseases, it is not completely exploited for omics analysis because of the bibliographic data structure of OMIM. Moreover, drug information is not linked to elements associated with diseases and genes of interest. To alleviate this problem, we comprehensively characterized diseases and genes referred in OMIM with MeSH-controlled vocabulary. MeSH profiles allow disease features to be shared and compared.

Using GO terms, researchers can decipher their omics data from a molecular viewpoint. The developed feature profiles illustrate related diseases and drugs. We could obtain more clinical and medical data using these MeSH profiles.

Furthermore, the profiles can be applied to analyses of disease-relevant genes by comparing the similarities among profiles of OMIM entries and groups of genes such as those found in the gene expression clustering results. Researchers can also obtain overviews of the features of unfamiliar diseases.

Genetic disease subtype entries are available in OMIM. For example, diabetes mellitus, non-insulin dependent, 3 (NIDDM3, OMIM ID: 603694) is a genetic subtype of diabetes mellitus, non-insulin dependent (NIDDM, OMIM ID: 125853, i.e., type 2 diabetes mellitus), which is linked to chromosome 20q12-q13.1. Another genetic type of NIDDM, NIDDM1 (OMIM ID: 601283), is reportedly linked significantly to chromosome 2q37.3. The differences in the clinical features between these two NIDDM genetic types seem to be unclear but the genetic mechanisms are probably different. Omics analysis emphasizes these genetic differences.

The diabetes mellitus entry was missing in OMIM, although the entries diabetes mellitus, insulin-dependent (type 1 diabetes mellitus) and diabetes mellitus, non-insulin dependent (type 2 diabetes mellitus) were present. We plan to create a dictionary of diseases using not only OMIM but also MeSH disease category and ICD-10 terms.

6. Conclusion

We characterized diseases and genes by generating feature profiles for associated drugs, biological phenomena, and anatomy using MeSH keywords. We developed a web service called Gendoo to visualize retrieved profiles. This approach illustrates disease features not only from a clinical but also a biological viewpoint. We also clarified the differences and similarities between disease features by comparing their profiles. Retrieved feature profiles are easy to remix such that Gendoo accelerates the process of omics analysis.

7. Acknowledgment

We thank Prof. Shoko Kawamoto and Prof. Kousaku Okubo for their helpful discussions. This work was supported by Integrated Database Project of the Ministry of Education, Culture, Sports, Science and Technology of Japan.

8. References

Amberger, J., Bocchini, C. A., Scott, A. F., and Hamosh, A. (2009). McKusick's Online Mendelian Inheritance in Man (OMIM). *Nucleic Acids Res*, Vol.37, Database issue, pp. D793-796. ISSN 1362-4962

Ashburner, M., Ball, C. A., Blake, J. A., Botstein, D., Butler, H., Cherry, J. M., Davis, A. P., Dolinski, K., Dwight, S. S., Eppig, J. T., Harris, M. A., Hill, D. P., Issel-Tarver, L., Kasarskis, A., Lewis, S., Matese, J. C., Richardson, J. E., Ringwald, M., Rubin, G. M., and Sherlock, G. (2000). Gene ontology: tool for the unification of biology. The Gene Ontology Consortium. *Nat Genet*, Vol.25, No.1, pp. 25-29. ISSN 1061-4036

Bajdik, C. D., Kuo, B., Rusaw, S., Jones, S., and Brooks-Wilson, A. (2005). CGMIM: automated text-mining of Online Mendelian Inheritance in Man (OMIM) to identify genetically-associated cancers and candidate genes. *BMC Bioinformatics*, Vol.6, pp. 78. ISSN 1471-2105

Barrett, T., Troup, D. B., Wilhite, S. E., Ledoux, P., Evangelista, C., Kim, I. F., Tomashevsky, M., Marshall, K. A., Phillippy, K. H., Sherman, P. M., Muertter, R. N., Holko, M., Ayanbule, O., Yefanov, A., and Soboleva, A. (2011). NCBI GEO: archive for functional genomics data sets--10 years on. *Nucleic Acids Res*, Vol.39, Database issue, pp. D1005-1010. ISSN 1362-4962

Butte, A. J., and Kohane, I. S. (2006). Creation and implications of a phenome-genome network. *Nat Biotechnol*, Vol.24, No.1, pp. 55-62. ISSN 1087-0156

Cantor, M. N., and Lussier, Y. A. (2004). Mining OMIM for insight into complex diseases. *Medinfo*, Vol.11, No.Pt 2, pp. 753-757. ISBN 1-58603-444-8

Cochrane, G., Karsch-Mizrachi, I., and Nakamura, Y. (2011). The International Nucleotide Sequence Database Collaboration. *Nucleic Acids Res*, Vol.39, Database issue, pp. D15-18. ISSN 1362-4962

Cohen, R., Gefen, A., Elhadad, M., and Birk, O. S. (2011). CSI-OMIM - Clinical Synopsis Search in OMIM. *BMC Bioinformatics*, Vol.12, pp. 65. ISSN 1471-2105

Djebbari, A., Karamycheva, S., Howe, E., and Quackenbush, J. (2005). MeSHer: identifying biological concepts in microarray assays based on PubMed references and MeSH terms. *Bioinformatics*, Vol.21, No.15, pp. 3324-3326. ISSN 1367-4803

Eisen, M. B., Spellman, P. T., Brown, P. O., and Botstein, D. (1998). Cluster analysis and display of genome-wide expression patterns. *Proc Natl Acad Sci U S A*, Vol.95, No.25, pp. 14863-14868. ISSN 0027-8424

Freudenberg, J., and Propping, P. (2002). A similarity-based method for genome-wide prediction of disease-relevant human genes. *Bioinformatics*, Vol.18 Suppl 2, pp. S110-115. ISSN 1367-4803

Gaudan, S., Kirsch, H., and Rebholz-Schuhmann, D. (2005). Resolving abbreviations to their senses in Medline. *Bioinformatics*, Vol.21, No.18, pp. 3658-3664. ISSN 1367-4803

Hamosh, A., Scott, A. F., Amberger, J., Bocchini, C., Valle, D., and McKusick, V. A. (2002). Online Mendelian Inheritance in Man (OMIM), a knowledgebase of human genes and genetic disorders. *Nucleic Acids Res*, Vol.30, No.1, pp. 52-55. ISSN 1362-4962

Hamosh, A., Scott, A. F., Amberger, J. S., Bocchini, C. A., and McKusick, V. A. (2005). Online Mendelian Inheritance in Man (OMIM), a knowledgebase of human genes and genetic disorders. *Nucleic Acids Res*, Vol.33, Database issue, pp. D514-517. ISSN 1362-4962

Hirschman, L., Yeh, A., Blaschke, C., and Valencia, A. (2005). Overview of BioCreAtIvE: critical assessment of information extraction for biology. *BMC Bioinformatics*, Vol.6 Suppl 1, pp. S1. ISSN 1471-2105

Hishiki, T., Ogasawara, O., Tsuruoka, Y., and Okubo, K. (2004). Indexing anatomical concepts to OMIM Clinical Synopsis using the UMLS Metathesaurus. *In Silico Biol*, Vol.4, No.1, pp. 31-54. ISSN 1386-6338

Horsthemke, B., and Wagstaff, J. (2008). Mechanisms of imprinting of the Prader-Willi/Angelman region. *Am J Med Genet A*, Vol.146A, No.16, pp. 2041-2052. ISSN 1552-4833

Jensen, L. J., Saric, J., and Bork, P. (2006). Literature mining for the biologist: from information retrieval to biological discovery. *Nat Rev Genet*, Vol.7, No.2, pp. 119-129. ISSN 1471-0056

Kahvejian, A., Quackenbush, J., and Thompson, J. F. (2008). What would you do if you could sequence everything? *Nat Biotechnol*, Vol.26, No.10, pp. 1125-1133. ISSN 1546-1696

Kaminuma, E., Mashima, J., Kodama, Y., Gojobori, T., Ogasawara, O., Okubo, K., Takagi, T., and Nakamura, Y. (2010). DDBJ launches a new archive database with analytical tools for next-generation sequence data. *Nucleic Acids Res*, Vol.38, Database issue, pp. D33-38. ISSN 1362-4962

Khatri, P., and Draghici, S. (2005). Ontological analysis of gene expression data: current tools, limitations, and open problems. *Bioinformatics*, Vol.21, No.18, pp. 3587-3595. ISSN 1367-4803

Lamb, J. (2007). The Connectivity Map: a new tool for biomedical research. *Nat Rev Cancer*, Vol.7, No.1, pp. 54-60. ISSN 1474-175X

Leinonen, R., Akhtar, R., Birney, E., Bower, L., Cerdeno-Tarraga, A., Cheng, Y., Cleland, I., Faruque, N., Goodgame, N., Gibson, R., Hoad, G., Jang, M., Pakseresht, N., Plaister, S., Radhakrishnan, R., Reddy, K., Sobhany, S., Ten Hoopen, P., Vaughan, R., Zalunin, V., and Cochrane, G. (2011). The European Nucleotide Archive. *Nucleic Acids Res*, Vol.39, Database issue, pp. D28-31. ISSN 1362-4962

Leinonen, R., Sugawara, H., and Shumway, M. (2011). The sequence read archive. *Nucleic Acids Res*, Vol.39, Database issue, pp. D19-21. ISSN 1362-4962

Li, C., and Wong, W. H. (2001). Model-based analysis of oligonucleotide arrays: expression index computation and outlier detection. *Proc Natl Acad Sci U S A*, Vol.98, No.1, pp. 31-36. ISSN 0027-8424

Li, C., and Wong, W. H. (2001). Model-based analysis of oligonucleotide arrays: model validation, design issues and standard error application. *Genome Biol*, Vol.2, No.8, pp. RESEARCH0032. ISSN 1465-6914

Masseroli, M., Galati, O., Manzotti, M., Gibert, K., and Pinciroli, F. (2005). Inherited disorder phenotypes: controlled annotation and statistical analysis for knowledge mining from gene lists. *BMC Bioinformatics*, Vol.6 Suppl 4, pp. S18. ISSN 1471-2105

Masseroli, M., Galati, O., and Pinciroli, F. (2005). GFINDer: genetic disease and phenotype location statistical analysis and mining of dynamically annotated gene lists. *Nucleic Acids Res*, Vol.33, Web Server issue, pp. W717-723. ISSN 1362-4962

Masys, D. R., Welsh, J. B., Lynn Fink, J., Gribskov, M., Klacansky, I., and Corbeil, J. (2001). Use of keyword hierarchies to interpret gene expression patterns. *Bioinformatics*, Vol.17, No.4, pp. 319-326. ISSN 1367-4803

McKusick, V. A. (2007). Mendelian Inheritance in Man and its online version, OMIM. *Am J Hum Genet*, Vol.80, No.4, pp. 588-604. ISSN 1432-1203

Nakazato, T., Takinaka, T., Mizuguchi, H., Matsuda, H., Bono, H., and Asogawa, M. (2008). BioCompass: a novel functional inference tool that utilizes MeSH hierarchy to analyze groups of genes. *In Silico Biol*, Vol.8, No.1, pp. 53-61. ISSN 1386-6338

Nakazato, T., Bono, H., Matsuda, H., and Takagi, T. (2009). Gendoo: functional profiling of gene and disease features using MeSH vocabulary. *Nucleic Acids Res*, Vol.37, Web Server issue, pp. W166-169. ISSN 1362-4962

Nat. Biotechnol. Editorial Board, (2008). Prepare for the deluge. *Nat Biotechnol*, Vol.26, No.10, pp. 1099. ISSN 1546-1696

Nelson, S. J., Schopen, M., Savage, A. G., Schulman, J. L., and Arluk, N. (2004). The MeSH translation maintenance system: structure, interface design, and implementation. *Stud Health Technol Inform*, Vol.107, No.Pt 1, pp. 67-69. ISSN 0926-9630

Parkinson, H., Sarkans, U., Kolesnikov, N., Abeygunawardena, N., Burdett, T., Dylag, M., Emam, I., Farne, A., Hastings, E., Holloway, E., Kurbatova, N., Lukk, M., Malone, J., Mani, R., Pilicheva, E., Rustici, G., Sharma, A., Williams, E., Adamusiak, T., Brandizi, M., Sklyar, N., and Brazma, A. (2011). ArrayExpress update--an archive of microarray and high-throughput sequencing-based functional genomics experiments. *Nucleic Acids Res*, Vol.39, Database issue, pp. D1002-1004. ISSN 1362-4962

Perez-Iratxeta, C., Bork, P., and Andrade, M. A. (2002). Association of genes to genetically inherited diseases using data mining. *Nat Genet*, Vol.31, No.3, pp. 316-319. ISSN 1061-4036

Perez-Iratxeta, C., Wjst, M., Bork, P., and Andrade, M. A. (2005). G2D: a tool for mining genes associated with disease. *BMC Genet*, Vol.6, pp. 45. ISSN 1471-2156

Perez-Iratxeta, C., Bork, P., and Andrade-Navarro, M. A. (2007). Update of the G2D tool for prioritization of gene candidates to inherited diseases. *Nucleic Acids Res*, Vol.35, Web Server issue, pp. W212-216. ISSN 1362-4962

Rother, K. I. (2007). Diabetes treatment--bridging the divide. *N Engl J Med*, Vol.356, No.15, pp. 1499-1501. ISSN 1533-4406

Shatkay, H. (2005). Hairpins in bookstacks: information retrieval from biomedical text. *Brief Bioinform*, Vol.6, No.3, pp. 222-238. ISSN 1467-5463

Shendure, J., and Ji, H. (2008). Next-generation DNA sequencing. *Nat Biotechnol*, Vol.26, No.10, pp. 1135-1145. ISSN 1546-1696

Tamayo, P., Slonim, D., Mesirov, J., Zhu, Q., Kitareewan, S., Dmitrovsky, E., Lander, E. S., and Golub, T. R. (1999). Interpreting patterns of gene expression with self-organizing maps: methods and application to hematopoietic differentiation. *Proc Natl Acad Sci U S A*, Vol.96, No.6, pp. 2907-2912. ISSN 0027-8424

van Driel, M. A., Bruggeman, J., Vriend, G., Brunner, H. G., and Leunissen, J. A. (2006). A text-mining analysis of the human phenome. *Eur J Hum Genet*, Vol.14, No.5, pp. 535-542. ISSN 1476-5438

Zeeberg, B. R., Feng, W., Wang, G., Wang, M. D., Fojo, A. T., Sunshine, M., Narasimhan, S., Kane, D. W., Reinhold, W. C., Lababidi, S., Bussey, K. J., Riss, J., Barrett, J. C., and Weinstein, J. N. (2003). GoMiner: a resource for biological interpretation of genomic and proteomic data. *Genome Biol*, Vol.4, No.4, pp. R28. ISSN 1465-6914

Zeeberg, B. R., Qin, H., Narasimhan, S., Sunshine, M., Cao, H., Kane, D. W., Reimers, M., Stephens, R. M., Bryant, D., Burt, S. K., Elnekave, E., Hari, D. M., Wynn, T. A., Cunningham-Rundles, C., Stewart, D. M., Nelson, D., and Weinstein, J. N. (2005). High-Throughput GoMiner, an 'industrial-strength' integrative gene ontology tool for interpretation of multiple-microarray experiments, with application to studies of Common Variable Immune Deficiency (CVID). *BMC Bioinformatics*, Vol.6, pp. 168. ISSN 1471-2105

5

Targeted Metabolomics for Clinical Biomarker Discovery in Multifactorial Diseases

Ulrika Lundin[1], Robert Modre-Osprian[2] and Klaus M. Weinberger[1]
[1]*Biocrates Life Sciences AG, Innsbruck*
[2]*AIT Austrian Institute of Technology GmbH, Graz*
Austria

1. Introduction

The vast majority of this book deals with monogenic disorders which are relatively rare but have just one or a small number of characteristic genotypes and usually very pronounced clinical and biochemical phenotypes. In contrast, this chapter will try to discuss multifactorial diseases which are far more prevalent and pose a completely different kind of challenge both for the socio-economic systems and for biomedical research. As an example we will focus on chronic kidney disease (CKD) and relevant animal models thereof. In fact, together with diabetic retinopathy, myocardial infarction, and stroke, diabetic nephropathy is one of the most severe sequelae of type II diabetes mellitus (T2D) and, considering the obesity-related pandemic of T2D, will represent a major health issue in the decades to come (Mensah et al., 2004; James et al., 2010).

Of course, all of these diseases have an important genetic component as demonstrated by pedigree analyses and a growing number of twin studies (Walder et al., 2003; Vaag & Poulsen, 2007). Still, with rare exceptions, this genetic component is rather seen as a predisposition for than as a cause of the actual disease. In particular, recent genome-wide association studies (GWAS) on large population-based cohorts have revealed a couple of single nucleotide polymorphisms (SNPs) that are significantly associated with T2D but the contribution of single SNPs to the individual's risk of developing T2D are marginal (Groop & Lyssenko, 2009). To fully understand the interaction of the identified genetic loci and to appreciate the meaning of the genetic background in a personalized medicine approach, complex haplotypes would have to be analyzed, and this has not even been achieved in basic diabetes research, let alone in any clinical application.

Yet, genetic research in diabetology has gained a new momentum in the last few years since it became obvious that a combination of GWAS with a more detailed phenotyping than just a generic diagnosis of T2D immediately led to improved statistics and to a much better biochemical plausibility of the findings (Gieger et al., 2008; Illig et al., 2010). Specifically, genome-wide significances could be achieved on much smaller cohorts than in classical GWAS rendering a more cost-efficient tool in biomedical research. The statistical power could be further improved by defining metabolic phenotypes based on the knowledge of the underlying biochemical pathways, e.g., by using groups of metabolites that are synthesized or degraded by the same enzymes or by calculating ratios of the concentrations of products and substrates of enzymatic reactions. This approach clearly reduces the inherent variability of the data set and, thus, offers great potential for robust diagnostic applications. In addition, it turned out that, in contrast to many GWAS results so far, the hits were not predominantly located in intergenic regions. In fact, eight of the nine loci that could be replicated with genome-wide significance in two independent cohorts (KORA and UK Twins) were in or very near a gene encoding for either an enzyme or a transporter. So, for the very first time, a convincing connection between genotype and metabolic phenotype could be demonstrated in a multifactorial disease.

Even so, the field may still be far from a true systems biology view on T2D covering all the different omics levels but the application of GWAS (or next generation sequencing, for that matter) on quantitative metabolic traits clearly paves the way for a better understanding of epidemiology and pathophysiology at the same time, and this approach has already been confirmed in other areas of genetic research (Weikard et al., 2010).

The systematic analysis of these metabolic traits is called metabolomics. Based on spectral methods such as nuclear magnetic resonance (NMR) spectroscopy or mass spectrometry, it is increasingly recognized as the most informative discipline in functional genomics because it is closest to depicting actual biochemical phenotypes, and thus delivers signatures or biomarkers that mirror genetic predisposition and the sum of environmental influences in one data set (Altmaier et al., 2008; Altmaier et al., 2009; Altmaier et al., 2011). In conclusion, metabolomics-based biomarkers are expected to be more predictive and descriptive than their genomic and proteomic counterparts. They may help trigger a paradigm shift from damage-oriented to function-oriented diagnostics, ultimately allowing diseases to be detected at earlier stages and subtyped more accurately contributing to the overarching goal of personalized medicine (Weinberger, 2008; Suhre et al., 2010).

Moreover, one of the most appealing advantages of metabolomics is that the majority of its analytes are not species-specific, i.e. most amino acids, sugars, lipids, etc. are structurally identical in mice, rats, dogs, pigs, monkeys, humans or other mammals, even in many microbes. This makes metabolomics ideally suited as a biomarker platform avoiding the need for redevelopment of the analytical assays for every animal model and for clinical trials.

2. The fundamentals of metabolomics

Metabolomics systematically identifies and quantifies low-molecular weight compounds in biological samples such as body fluids, tissue homogenates or cell culture. Metabolite concentrations allow inferences on the complex interactions between biological processes on a molecular level to be made. As pointed out above, metabolomics is increasingly appreciated as the richest source of information in functional genomics (Nicholson et al., 1999; Weinberger & Graber, 2005). Until recently, systems biology has mainly relied on three other 'omics' technologies, namely genomics, transcriptomics, and proteomics. Important as these areas have been, they fail to provide a real-time phenotype, i.e., a picture of what is actually happening in a dynamic biological system. Recent advances in mass spectrometry have added metabolomics as another powerful and practical tool to the systems biology toolbox (Weckwerth, 2003). The metabolome is the sum of all low molecular weight metabolites in a biological system. By assessing hundreds of metabolites simultaneously, modern mass-spectrometric techniques produce high-resolution biochemical snapshots showing the functional endpoints of genetic predisposition as well as the sum of all environmental influences, including nutrition, exercise, and medication. This snapshot is an almost real-time image of the physiology—or pathophysiology—of a cell or an entire organism (Weckwerth, 2003).

3. Technological advances paved the way into clinical applications

Mass spectrometric assays revolutionized the diagnosis of inherited metabolic disorders, a development co-pioneered in the late 1990s by Adelbert Roscher (Röschinger et al., 2003). This and similar pilot projects around the world taught the diagnostics community some crucial lessons. Quantitation of endogenous metabolites using multiple reaction monitoring (MRM) and stable isotope dilution (SID) for absolute quantitation on tandem mass spectrometers combined with advanced data analysis tools fulfills the most strict quality criteria in terms of precision and accuracy without suffering any of the shortcomings of immunoassays, such as cross-reactivities, which makes this technology an ideal platform for clinical chemistry (Unterwurzacher et al., 2008). What is more, the superior sensitivity of triple quadrupole mass spectrometers combined with MRM and SID enabled the detection of metabolites in biologically relevant sample types, such as plasma or serum, whereas the limited sensitivity in the previous NMR-based workflows restricted their use mainly to urine (urine as a sample type is analytically very convenient but the concentration of metabolites in urine is not regulated in the sense of a strict homeostasis as in blood). Furthermore, it has been proven for many disorders that multiparametric biomarkers reduce biological noise in the data by internal normalization as well as improve diagnostic sensitivity and specificity. Subsequently, it led to a marked reduction of healthcare costs (Röschinger et al., 2003; Weinberger., 2008).

4. Targeted metabolomics or metabolic profiling

There are two approaches to metabolomics usually called targeted metabolomics and metabolic profiling. While both approaches are complementary, targeted metabolomics, i.e., the identification and quantitation of defined sets of structurally known and biochemically annotated metabolites, takes advantage of our functional understanding of many biochemical pathways. In contrast to protein-protein interactions or regulatory relationships at the transcript level, the fact that so many biochemical pathways have been explored in great detail offers an invaluable source of background information that enables evidence-based interpretation of metabolomics data sets. For the majority of these pathways, substrates and products of enzymatic reactions, reaction mechanisms, equilibra, kinetics and energetic of these reactions, as well as cofactors or compartmentalization have been elucidated. This information renders instant functional interpretation of the data set and, thus, phenotyping of the analyzed cell or organism, a straight forward process (Modre-Osprian et al., 2009; Weinberger & Graber, 2005; Weinberger et al., 2005; Weinberger, 2008). One other major advantage of targeted metabolomics is that it generally provides quantitative information. These quantitative data, the molar concentrations of the metabolites involved in a pathway, facilitate the immediate understanding of any alterations between different biological states and allow for comparison and meta-analysis of several independent studies (Enot et al., 2011). Targeted metabolomics enables the systematic quantitation of a wide range of biologically relevant molecule classes in cells, tissues, or clinically relevant fluids. The technology comprises an automated sample preparation workflow integrated with sensitive mass spectrometric methods and a tailor-made software solution. Many hundreds of metabolites can be identified and quantified using this novel platform, which is also well suited for high-throughput and routine applications (Weinberger & Graber, 2005).

5. Proof-of-concept for targeted metabolomics: Neonatal screening

The proof-of-concept for targeted metabolomics was first delivered in clinical diagnostics, namely in neonatal screening for inborn errors of metabolism. As mentioned above, the diagnosis of inherited disorders in amino acid metabolism, such as phenylketonuria, or fatty acid oxidation disorders, such as medium-chain acyl-CoA dehydrogenase (MCAD) deficiency, was revolutionized by the use of mass spectrometric assays (Röschinger et al., 2003). The idea was a logical continuation of Sir Archibald Garrod's (1857–1936) concept of chemical pathology, to quantify specific sets of amino acids and acylcarnitines to diagnose specific metabolic disorders. This laid the foundation for what is now referred to as 'targeted metabolomics'. The introduction of tandem mass spectrometry and the transition from expensive, monoparametric to multiparametric assays has enabled the simultaneous diagnosis of 20–30 monogenic diseases, which is a significant improvement of diagnostic performance, particularly of the specificity and the predictive values for very rare diseases. This improved diagnostic performance was achieved without raising costs. Rather neonatal screening is now reimbursed by health insurance providers in many Western countries and has lead to substantial healthcare savings. These medical and commercial benefits have turned neonatal screening into an impressive success story and led to its introduction in most industrialized countries within less than a decade (Röschinger et al., 2003; Weinberger., 2008).

6. Data exploitation

The whole data-related workflow for targeted metabolomics has recently been summarized (Enot et al., 2011). In the context of this chapter, we only refer to the pathway mapping aspects of this workflow.

The unique level of understanding of metabolomics data that makes them suitable for a key role in functional genomics mainly results from this key step of data handling, namely the biochemical interpretation in the context of pathway and background knowledge. Despite its importance, very few standardized procedures have been developed and/or published for this step, and some experts would probably consider it their proprietary methodology to derive biochemical and pathobiochemical insight from multivariate metabolic datasets.

The last few years have seen multiple efforts to systematically annotate endogenous metabolites and led to databases such as KEGG (Kaneshia & Goto, 2000), Reactome (Vastrik et al., 2007), BioCyc (Karp et al., 2005), HMDB (Wishart et al., 2007) and OMIM (Online mendelian inheritance in man, 2011). Despite suffering from some serious shortcomings in terms of pathway coverage and data curation, these may serve as a more or less accepted framework for future knowledge collection.

These databases also provide the background for various attempts at visualization of metabolic pathways and data mapping on these charts, although most of these projects still follow a static approach of predefined (and predrawn) maps that cannot do justice to the dynamics of biochemical networks. In the following paragraph, we would like to demonstrate a few concepts about how dynamic representation and simulation (Modre-Osprian et al., 2009) of metabolic pathways enable the first steps of generating hypotheses from multivariate datasets.

Firstly, electronic availability of metabolites and metabolic reactions facilitates an almost trivial but nevertheless powerful approach that is analogous to a gene set enrichment analysis (GSEA; Subramanian et al., 2005). Any given set of metabolites which has been identified by statistics as significantly different in two biological states or clinical cohorts can be mapped on the entirety of metabolic pathways, and these pathways can then be ranked by the number of altered metabolites they contain (Fig. 1). This is a way of structuring the data that scientists from transcriptomics and proteomics are familiar with although the definition of metabolic pathways does not follow a similarly strict classification system as the classical gene ontology (GO; Ashburner et al., 2000). Note also that a reliable selection of species-specific enzymatic reactions instead of the generic reference pathways is necessary to reduce the risk of false positive hits.

Pathway		Count
00564	Glycerophospholipid metabolism	15
00590	Arachidonic acid metabolism	7
00591	Linoleic acid metabolism	7
00592	alpha-Linolenic acid metabolism	7
00600	Sphingolipid metabolism	3
00052	Galactose metabolism	2
00051	Fructose and mannose metabolism	1
00310	Lysine degradation	1
00500	Starch and sucrose metabolism	1
00520	Amino sugar and nucleotide sugar metabolism	1

Fig. 1. Ranking of metabolic pathways according to the number of significant differences between a study and control cohort in analogy to a gene set enrichment analysis (MarkerIDQ™ software, Biocrates)

Secondly, starting from a particular metabolite of interest, exploration of the reactions that either synthesize or degrade this metabolite immediately generates a list of enzymes of interest for further investigation. This concept of exploring shells of reactions around a metabolite is exemplarily shown for tryptophan (Trp) metabolism in Fig. 2 and can be expanded stepwise around every metabolite serving as a new seed node. Each of these reactions can then be characterized by a ratio of product and substrate concentrations as a measure of enzymatic activity. Assessment of such ratios reduces biological noise and often dramatically increases the significance of the findings (Altmaier et al., 2008; Gieger et al., 2008; Wang-Sattler et al., 2008).

Lastly, moving even further from a traditional textbook representation of metabolic pathways, one can apply route finding algorithms to find and depict connections between metabolites of interest across the boundaries of (often artificially) predefined pathways. Such algorithms can identify the shortest route, routes up to a defined length, routes that do not share a certain metabolite (termed node-disjoint paths) or enzyme (so-called edge disjoint paths), depending on the respective biological question (Fig. 3). Here, the main prerequisite to avoid a potentially very large number of trivial hits is the exclusion of common cofactors and small inorganic molecules that connect many metabolites to many others, e.g., H_2O, CO_2, ATP, NADP. Using tools like these, and keeping in mind all the caveats discussed above, enzymes and pathways involved in the pathophysiology of a certain disease or in the mode-of-action of a drug can be more efficiently identified. In addition, hypotheses for designing further validation experiments and studies can be formulated.

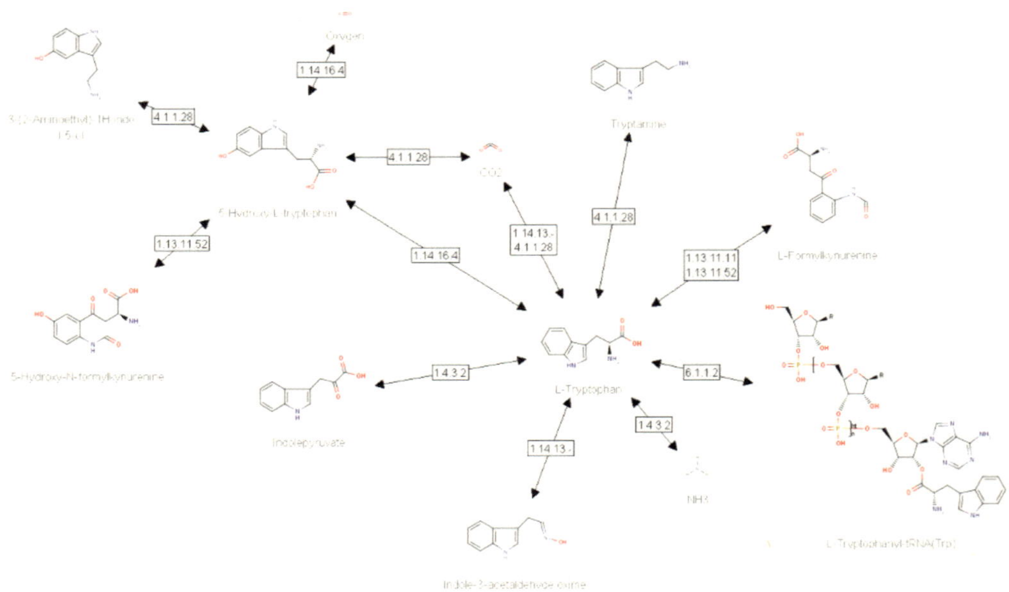

Fig. 2. Shellwise exploration of enzymatic reactions in tryptophan metabolism. L- Trp was used as the first seed node; after expansion of eight synthetic or degrading reactions, 5- hydroxy-tryptophan was used as secondary seed node and further expanded (MarkerIDQ™ software, Biocrates)

Yet, all of this needs to be combined with another plausibility check, which originates from inherent redundancies in metabolism: quite often groups of compounds are metabolized by the same enzyme and should, therefore, be influenced in at least a similar (if not the same) way by regulatory mechanisms, drugs, etc. If this rule of thumb is severely challenged, one should always check for possible analytical or statistical artifacts, or – not uncommon in pharmaceutical R&D – interference by xenobiotics, e.g., a drug or drug metabolite disturbing the signal for an endogenous metabolite.

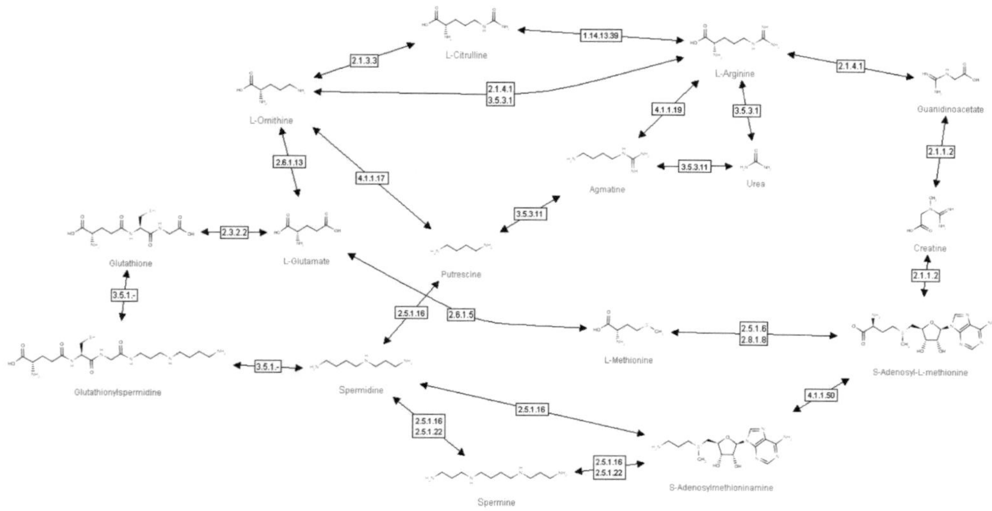

Fig. 3. Route finding across metabolic pathways. Nine paths from arginine to spermine, ranging in length from four to six steps were calculated based on the KEGG dataset, and the settings allowed for joint nodes, e.g., ornithine (MarkerIDQ™ software, Biocrates)

6.1 Quantitative experimental information for computational biology

The quantitative information of targeted metabolomics enables new possibilities in validating computational systems biology approaches using detailed kinetic models to simulate and predict the dynamic response of metabolic networks in the context of human diseases. It also supports the design of tailored kinetic models of human-specific metabolic pathways including detailed knowledge about all metabolic reactions concerned.

Besides statistical model building and data mining-based approaches (Baumgartner et al., 2004; Baumgartner et al., 2005; Baumgartner & Graber, 2008), computational systems biology is essential to combine knowledge of human physiology and pathology starting from genomics, molecular biology and the environment through the levels of cells, tissues, and organs all the way up to integrated systems behaviour. Applying systems biology approaches within the context of human health and disease will definitely gain new insights. Eventually, a new discipline - systems medicine - will emerge at the interface between medicine and systems biology (van der Greef et al., 2006; van der Greef et al., 2007; Lemberger, 2007).

Higher levels of organization are extremely complex, and even models at the cell and subcellular levels are forced to resort to simplifications to minimize modeling and computational complexity (Crampin et al., 2004; Nakayama et al., 2005; Yugi & Tomita, 2004). Additionally, some parameters and constants for kinetics, binding and concentrations of biomolecules are typically not known, thus reducing the model's ability to respond correctly to dynamic changes in external conditions. A high-quality network of human-specific metabolic pathways including detailed knowledge about all metabolic reactions concerned is essential to design tailored kinetic models for better understanding of human physiology and its relationship with diseases. While such large networks are used to analyze the global structure or functional connectivity of the network (Ma et al., 2007), deterministic and stochastic models are mainly used for simulating specific metabolic pathways as well as regulatory and signaling networks (Goel et al., 2006).

Results of *in silico* experiments should be related to quantitative experimental data (e.g. from neonatal screening) in order to reveal better insights into dynamic properties of the complex biochemical networks under the constraints of various disease conditions and finally to obtain a better understanding of pathophysiological aspects of genetic disorders (Modre-Osprian et al., 2009).

7. Use case: Biomarker development in CKD

Chronic kidney disease is a major health problem associated with increased risk of cardiovascular disease, renal failure and other complications (James et al., 2010). The cost for treating these complications puts a disproportionally large part on national health care budgets (Eknoyan et al., 2004; James et al., 2010; Mendelssohn & Wish, 2009). With an aging population and a worldwide epidemic of diabetes, the most common causes of CKD have switched from infection/inflammation and inheritance, to hypertension, other vascular disorders and diabetes as the main triggers.

It is estimated that at least 40 million people in the EU have some degree of CKD. This number is expected to increase every year, even double over the next decade, and the trend is similar all over the world (European Kidney Health Alliance, 2011; James et al., 2010). One of the major reasons for this is the dramatic increase of T2D, accounting for up to 95 % of the total diabetes incidence (American Diabetes Association, 2000; Kurukulasuriya, & Sowers, 2010; Ritz & Stefanski, 1996). Diabetic nephropathy is one of the most severe complications of diabetes and by far the most common cause of end-stage renal disease (ESRD; Susztak & Bottinger, 2006). Most people are unaware of their disease at early stages and do not get the right treatment in time. The classical renal function markers, serum creatinine level and estimated glomerular filtration rate (eGFR) are known to be insensitive and late markers of CKD (National Kidney Foundation, 2002). The gold standard for assessing renal function is measuring the true GFR with test substances like inulin or iothalamate, but this is an invasive and far too tedious procedure for routine application. It is of highest importance to develop markers which have the ability to predict or detect CKD at an earlier stage, making it possible to intervene with therapy to prevent or at least slow down the progression of kidney damage finally leading to ESRD and control related complications. While the classical diagnostic markers are restricted to traditional endpoints for kidney damage, metabolic markers can assess pathophysiological and pathobiochemical changes that play a role in exacerbation of renal damage.

This use case is based on two studies explained in further detail below. In a preclinical study on puromycin-treated Sprague-Dawley rats, several classes of metabolites were quantitated covering the main pathways of metabolism. The absolute concentration of the metabolites was determined by MRM and the application of SID (Jarman et al., 1975). The aim of the preclinical rat study was to evaluate metabolic changes in these rats, focusing on nephrotoxicity.

Cohorts consisted of three dosage groups (10 mg/kg/day, 20 mg/kg/day and 40 mg/kg/day) and one control group where only a vehicle was administered. Samples were taken at day 3, 7, 14 and 22 after start of the experiment, except for the highest dosage group, where all animals had to be sacrificed at day 14 because of complete renal failure. One of the metabolites that was associated with exacerbation of renal damage was symmetric dimethylarginine (SDMA) in plasma (Fig. 4), which has been extensively discussed in the literature as a marker for renal failure (Bode-Böger et al., 2006; Vallance et al., 1992). SDMA is hardly metabolized in the body, but only eliminated by renal excretion and, since no specific tubular resorption has been reported, it could be interpreted as an internal test substance for renal clearance (Bode-Boger et al, 2006; Martens-Lobenhoffer & Bode-Böger, 2006). As seen in figure 4, SDMA was increased in the two highest dosage groups, and there was also an increase over time within these groups.

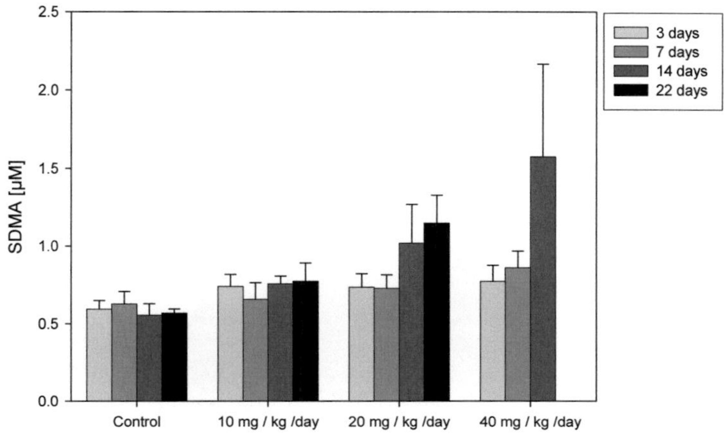

Fig. 4. Time-and dose-dependent increase of SDMA in a nephrotoxicity study in rats. Levels of SDMA increased in a time- ($p=9.9 \cdot 10^{-5}$ in the cohort treated with 20 mg/kg/day, $p=8.4 \cdot 10^{-4}$ in the cohort treated with 40 mg/kg/day) and dose-dependent manner ($p=4.4 \cdot 10^{-6}$, comparing day 14 in all cohorts)

Many of the preclinical findings were confirmed in a clinical biomarker study on progression of CKD that was performed at Montpellier University hospital as part of an EU-funded consortium (ETB Urosysteomics). The participating patients were divided into three cohorts according to severity of kidney disease; no to moderate renal function impairment (eGFR > 30 ml/min/1.73 m^2, corresponding to stages 1 to 3 of CKD as proposed by the National Kidney Foundation, for simplicity referred to as stage 3), severe renal function impairment (30 ml/min/1.73 m^2 > eGFR > 15 ml/min/1.73 m^2, corresponding to stage 4) and renal failure (eGFR < 15 ml/min/1.73 m^2, corresponding to stage 5 treated with dialysis) based on eGFR as proposed by Bauer et al, 2008. The patients in this study were mixed cases from different etiologies of CKD (diabetic and non-diabetic), and several analyses were performed to exclude confounding factors of these diseases and to look at biomarkers influenced by kidney damage, regardless of underlying disease.

Just as in the preclinical study, many of the quantitated metabolites were found to be significantly up- or downregulated with progressing CKD. In a discriminant analysis the data could be separated almost completely which indeed indicates there is information in the data set to distinguish the stages from one another (Fig. 5) and further statistical analyses both identified novel markers (Lundin et al., submitted for publication) and confirmed biomarkers that had already been found in previous studies (e.g., nephrotoxicity of model compounds, early prognostic markers for acute rejection and chronic nephropathy in kidney transplant patients; Boudonck et al., 2009; Lundin & Weinberger, 2009). One of the findings was elevated levels of SDMA, as already observed in the rat model (Fig. 6).

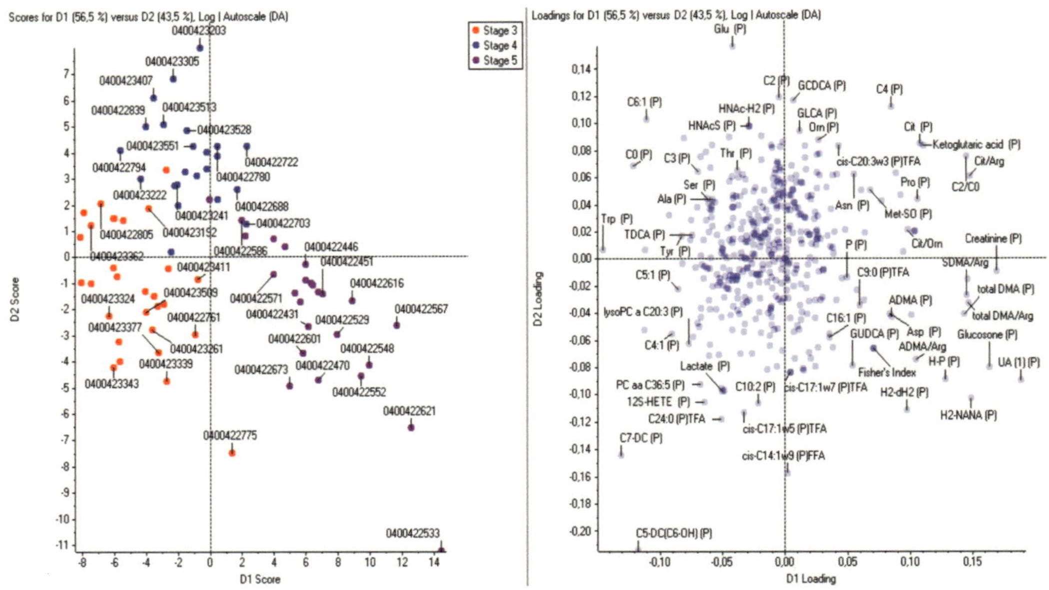

Fig. 5. Discriminant analysis of three stages of CKD. In the scores plot (left) the three stages of CKD are almost perfectly separated. Each point represents one patient and the cohort to which they belong is indicated by colour in the box in the upper right corner. The axes are calculated to minimize variance within the group and maximize it between the groups to get the best separation possible. The loadings plot (right) identifies which metabolites are mostly responsible for the separation, the further away from the origin, the stronger the influence. Since multi-group comparisons are not particularly clear, deeper analysis is required to identify single markers

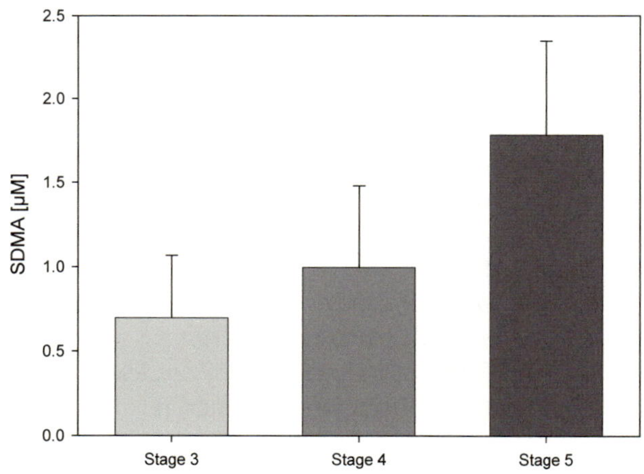

Fig. 6. Increase of plasma SDMA concentrations in progressing CKD. Barplots represent plasma SDMA concentrations in three groups of patients with declining renal function. SDMA shows a highly significant increase in progressing stages of CKD ($p = 1.2 \cdot 10^{-9}$)

Another finding that was reproduced in both studies was changes in concentration of the essential with amino acid Trp. Tryptophan is crucial for protein synthesis and might therefore play an important part in cellular differentiation, development and growth (Badawy, 1988). The drop in concentration of Trp has been associated with impaired kidney function before (Egashira et al., 2006; Saito et al., 2000). In the puromycin-treated rat model of nephrotoxicity, Trp drops to less than a third of its concentration between low- and high dose and at different time points (Fig. 7). The same trend can be observed in the clinical study on progression of CKD (Fig. 8 left) which emphasizes the advantages of being able to use translational research in metabolomics.

This phenomenon could partly be explained by albumin depletion since, in peripheral blood, Trp is bound to albumin to a significant extent (Walser & Hill, 1993). This would result in a drop of Trp when the albumin is being depleted in progressing kidney disease. As seen in figure 8 (right), there is indeed a drop in albumin in the clinical study, but not in the same magnitude as Trp, hence it can be assumed that other mechanisms are also involved here.

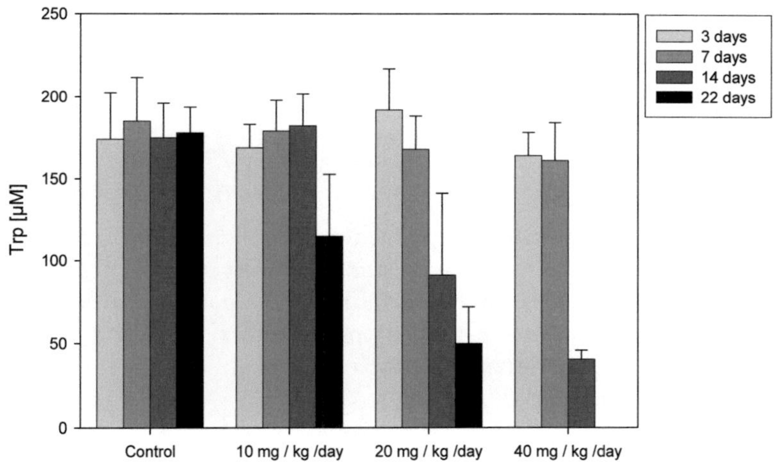

Fig. 7. Tryptophan depletion in puromycin-treated rats. Tryptophan shows both a dose- ($4.9 \cdot 10^{-6}$, comparing day 14 in all cohorts) and time-dependent ($p=1.8 \cdot 10^{-3}$ in the cohort treated with 10 mg/kg/day, $p=1.2 \cdot 10^{-6}$ in the cohort on 20 mg/kg/day, and $p= 2.5 \cdot 10^{-9}$ in the cohort on 40 mg/kg/day) decrease

Another explanation for the drop in concentration of Trp might be in its degrading pathways (see Fig. 9). When analyzing the two main catabolic pathways originating from Trp, both the rat model and the clinical study revealed that actually both pathways (towards serotonin and through kynurenine towards niacin) are upregulated (Fig. 10). The steep increase and high statistical significance of the kynurenine / Trp (product to substrate) ratio in the clinical study suggest there is a markedly increased activity through this pathway, in keeping with the fact that the kynurenine pathway accounts for 95 % of tryptophan catabolism (Walser & Hill, 1993). The Trp degrading indoleamine 2,3-dioxygenase (IDO) enzyme, which catalyzes the initial and rate-limiting step in the niacin pathway, seems to have an increased activity in progressing CKD.

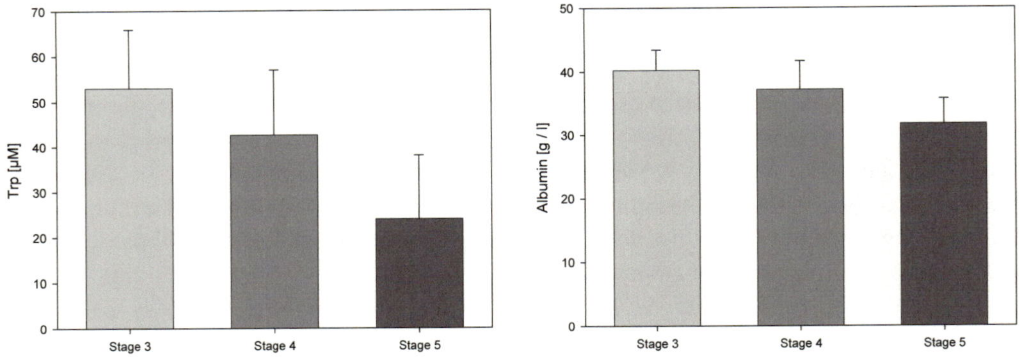

Fig. 8. Changes of Trp and albumin with progression of CKD. Left: Decrease of plasma Trp concentrations in progressing CKD. Barplots represent plasma Trp concentrations in three groups of patients with progressing CKD. Tryptophan shows a highly significant decline in later stages of CKD ($p = 6.2 \cdot 10^{-9}$). Right: This could in part be explained by the fact that it is albumin-bound, but although it is significant ($p=1.56 \cdot 10^{-9}$) the fold-change of the albumin depletion is by far less pronounced than the one for Trp

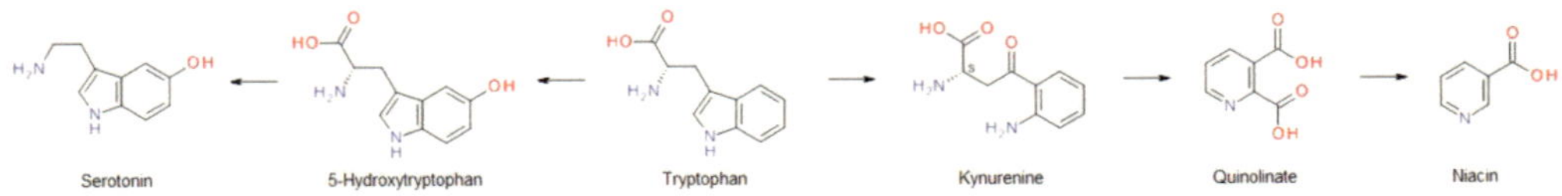

Fig. 9. Simplified scheme of the two main pathways catabolizing Trp. To the right the niacin pathway is illustrated where the rate limiting step is the conversion of Trp to kynurenine catalyzed by IDO (Ball et al., 2009). To the left the serotonin pathway with its two key reactions (tetrahydrobiopterin-dependent tryptophan hydroxylation and pyridoxalphosphate-dependent decarboxylation of 5-hydroxytryptophan) is shown

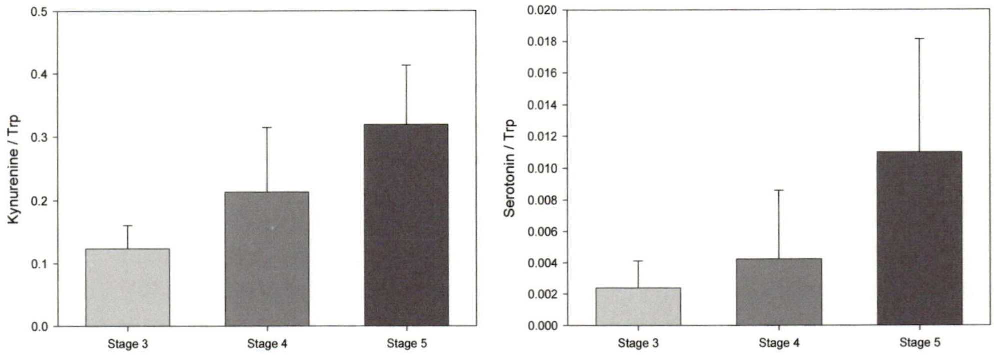

Fig. 10. Upregulation of Trp degrading pathways. There is an upregulation of both the niacin pathway (left, $p=1.44 \cdot 10^{-12}$) and serotonin pathway (right, $p=2.98 \cdot 10^{-6}$) degrading Trp, but the steep increase and high statistical significance of the kynurenine / Trp ratio suggest there is an increased activity of the Trp degrading IDO enzyme

8. Outlook and potential applications

There is a widespread range of potential applications of metabolomics in the areas of biomedical research, pharmaceutical R&D and clinical diagnostics. Besides the well-established procedure of neonatal screening, metabolomics is currently being applied in biomarker and diagnostics research as demonstrated in the example of CKD above. Still, the diagnostic potential of metabolomics is not confined to typical metabolic disorders, but rather extends into fields such as cancer (Osl et al., 2008) and neurologic disorders (Urban et al., 2010). Metabolomics can also be applied in drug development where it is used to uncover new drug targets, prioritize lead compounds and assess drug toxicity, enabling the development of novel, smarter and safer drugs (Weinberger & Graber, 2005). In addition, metabolomics has the possibility to identify individuals likely to benefit from a given therapy, minimizing the risk of side effects and avoiding unnecessary drug use.

9. Conclusion

The most important difference of metabolomics to other -omics approaches is the level of functional understanding that, currently, the metabolome is offering to a much greater extent than the other -omes. The first successful examples of combining GWAS with metabolic phenotypes, so-called metabotypes, have recently been published and show significant promise for a more useful outcome of population based association studies in general. This phenotyping is particularly useful when the disease in question affects metabolically active organs and when large scale transport phenoma are affected. Consequently, metabolomics is very well suited for biomarker discovery in multifactorial diseases like T2D and CKD. It is not only possible to find novel markers but also to explain the pathophysiological effects behind the disease, e.g., inhibition of or upregulation of an enzyme in a specific pathway. Additionally, the fact that there is no need to redevelop the analytic assays, because of the non-species specific properties of the metabolites, makes it cost- and time-saving since there is no need for redevelopment of the analytical assays.

10. Acknowledgment

The authors wish to acknowledge Àngel Argilés and Natalie Gayrard for study design and clinical documentation, Lisa Körner, Stephanie Angeben, Verena Forcher, Doreen Kirchberg, Hai Pham-Tuan, and Ali Alchalabi for excellent lab work, Madhumalar Panneerselvam, Denise Sonntag, Daniel Andres and Torben Friedrich for support with data handling and biostatistics. The studies presented here were in part supported by the EurotransBio Program of the FP6 of the European Comission carried out by the Urosysteomics consortium and the FP7 European Union grant 'SysKid' (HEALTH-F2-2009-241544).

11. References

Altmaier, E., Kastenmuller, G., Romisch-Margl, W., Thorand, B., Weinberger, K.M., Illig, T., Adamski, J., Doring, A. & Suhre, K. (2011). Questionnaire-based self-reported nutrition habits associate with serum metabolism as revealed by quantitative targeted metabolomics. *Eur J Epidemiol*, Vol.26, No.2, pp. 145-156, ISSN 0393-2990

Altmaier, E.; Kastenmuller, G.; Romisch-Margl, W.; Thorand, B.; Weinberger, K.M.; Adamski, J.; Illig, T.; Doring, A. & Suhre, K. (2009). Variation in the human lipidome associated with coffee consumption as revealed by quantitative targeted metabolomics. *Mol Nutr Food Res*, Vol.53, No.11 , pp. 1357-1365, ISSN 1613-4125

Altmaier, E.; Ramsay, S.L.; Graber, A.; Mewes, H.W.; Weinberger, K.M. & Suhre, K. (2008). Bioinformatics analysis of targeted metabolomics--uncovering old and new tales of diabetic mice under medication. *Endocrinology*, Vol.149, No.7, pp. 3478-3489, ISSN 0013-7227

American Diabetes Association. (2000). Type 2 Diabetes in Children and Adolescents. *Diabetes Care*, Vol.23, No.3, pp. 381-389, ISSN 0149-5992

Ashburner, M.; Ball, C.A.; Blake, J.A.; Botstein, D.; Butler, H.; Cherry, J.M.; Davis, A.P.; Dolinski, K.; Dwight, S.S.; Eppig, J.T.; Harris, M.A.; Hill, D.P.; Issel-Tarver, L.; Kasarskis, A.; Lewis, S.; Matese, J.C.; Richardson, J.E.; Ringwald, M.; Rubin, G.M. & Sherlock, G. (2000). Gene ontology: tool for the unification of biology. The Gene Ontology Consortium. *Nat Genet*, Vol.25, No.1, pp. 25-9, ISSN 1061-4036

Badawy, A.A. (1988). Effects of pregnancy on tryptophan metabolism and disposition in the rat. *Biochem J*. Vol.255, No.1, pp. 369-372, ISSN 0264-6021

Ball, H.J.; Yuasa, H.J.; Austin, C.J.; Weiser, S. & Hunt, N.H. (2009). Indoleamine 2,3-dioxygenase-2; a new enzyme in the kynurenine pathway. *Int J Biochem Cell Biol*, Vol.41, No.3, pp. 467-471, ISSN 1357-2725

Bauer, C.; Melamed, M.L. & Hostetter, T.H. (2008) Staging of chronic kidney disease: time for a course correction. *J Am Soc Nephrol*, Vol.19, No.5, pp. 844-846, ISSN 1533-3450

Baumgartner C & Graber A. (2008). Data mining and knowledge discovery in metabolomics, In: Successes and new directions in data mining. Masseglia F.; Poncelet, P. & Teisseire, M. (Ed.), 141-66, ISBN 978-1-59904-645-7, IgI Global, Hershey, PA, USA.

Baumgartner, C.; Böhm, C. & Baumgartner D. (2005). Modelling of classification rules on metabolic patterns including machine learning and expert knowledge. *J Biomed Inf*, Vol.38, No.2 , pp. 89-98, ISSN 1532-0464

Baumgartner, C.; Böhm, C.; Baumgartner, D.; Marini, G.; Weinberger, K.M.; Olgemöller, B.; Liebl, B. & Roscher, A.A. (2004). Supervised machine learning techniques for the classification of metabolic disorders in newborns. *Bioinformatics*, Vol. 20, No.7 , pp. 2985-2996, ISSN 1367-4803

Bode-Böger, S.M.; Scalera, F.; Kielstein, J.T.; Martens-Lobenhoffer, J.; Breithardt, G.; Fobker, M. & Reinecke, H. (2006). Symmetrical dimethylarginine: a new combined parameter for renal function and extent of coronary artery disease. *J Am Soc Nephrol*, Vol.17, No.4, pp. 1128-1134, ISSN 1046-6673

Boudonck, K.J.; Mitchell, M.W.; Nemet, L.; Keresztes, L.; Nyska, A.; Shinar, D. & Rosenstock, M. (2009). Discovery of metabolomics biomarkers for early detection of nephrotoxicity. *Toxicol Pathol*, Vol.37, No.3, pp. 280-292, ISSN 0192-6233

Crampin, E.J.; Halstead, M.; Hunter, P.; Nielsen, P.; Noble, D.; Smith, N. & Tawhai, M. (2004). *Computational physiology and the Physiome Project. Exp Physiol*, Vol.89, No. , pp. 1-26

Egashira, Y.; Nagaki, S. & Sanada, H. (2006). Tryptophan-niacin metabolism in rat with puromycin aminonucleoside-induced nephrosis. *Int J Vitam Nutr Res*, Vol.76, No.1, pp. 28-33, ISSN 0300-9831

Eknoyan, G.; Lameire, N.; Barsoum, R.; Eckardt, K.U.; Levin, A.; Levin, N.; Locatelli, F.; MacLeod, A.; Vanholder, R.; Walker, R. & Wang, H. (2004). The burden of kidney disease: improving global outcomes. *Kidney Int*, Vol. 66, No.4, pp. 1310-1314, ISSN 0085-2538

Enot DP, Haas B, Weinberger KM. Bioinformatics for mass spectrometry-based metabolomics. *Methods Mol Biol.* 2011;719:351-75. (also: Enot, D.; Haas, B. & Weinberger, K.M. (2011). Bioinformatics for mass spectrometry-based metabolomics, In: *Bioinformatics for Omics Data: Methods and Protocols.* B. Mayer (Ed.), 351-75, 978-1-61779-026-3, Humana Press, New York, USA.)

European Kidney Health Alliance (2011). The kidney in health and disease. 2011-03-15, Available from: <http://www.ekha.eu/usr_img/info/factsheet.pdf>

Gieger, C.; Geistlinger, L.; Altmaier, E.; Hrabe de Angelis, M.; Kronenberg, F.; Meitinger, T.; Mewes, H.W.; Wichmann, H.E.; Weinberger, K.M.; Adamski, J.; Illig, T. & Suhre, K.. (2008). Genetics meets metabolomics: a genome-wide association study of metabolite profiles in human serum. *PLoS Genet*, Vol.4, No.11, (Dec), pp. 4:e1000282, ISSN 1553-7404

Goel, G.; Chou, I.C. & Voit, E.O. (2006). Biological systems modeling and analysis: a biomolecular technique of the twenty-first century. *J Biomol Tech*, Vol.17, No.4 , pp. 252-269, ISSN 1524-0215

Greef, J van der.; Martin, S.; Juhasz, P.; Adourian, A.; Plasterer, T.; Verheij, E.R. & McBurney, R.N. (2007). The art and practise of systems biology in medicine: mapping patterns of relationships. *J Proteome Res*, Vol.6, No.4 , pp. 1540-1559, ISSN 1535-3893

Greef,J van der.; Hankemeier, T. & McBurney, R.N. (2006). Metabolomicsbased systems biology and personalized medicine: moving towards n = 1 clinical trials? *Pharmacogenomics*, Vol.7, No.7 , pp. 1087-1094, ISSN 1462-2416

Groop, L. & Lyssenko, V. (2009). Genetics of type 2 diabetes. An overview. *Endocrinol Nutr*, Vol. 56 Suppl 4, pp. 34-7, ISSN 1575-0922

Illig, T.; Gieger, C.; Zhai, G.; Romisch-Margl, W.; Wang-Sattler, R.; Prehn, C.; Altmaier, E.; Kastenmuller, G.; Kato, B.S.; Mewes, H.W.; Meitinger, T.; de Angelis, M.H.; Kronenberg, F.; Soranzo, N.; Wichmann, H.E.; Spector, TD.; Adamski, J. & Suhre, K. (2010). A genome-wide perspective of genetic variation in human metabolism. *Nat Genet*,Vol.42, No.2, (Feb), pp. 137-141, ISSN 1061-4036

James, M.T.; Hemmelgarn, B.R. & Tonelli, M. (2010). Early recognition and prevention of chronic kidney disease. *Lancet*, Vol.375, No.9722, pp. 1296-1309, ISSN 0140-6736

Jarman, M.; Gilby, E.D.; Foster, A.B. & Bondy, P.K. (1975). The quantitation of cyclophosphamide in human blood and urine by mass spectrometry-stable isotope dilution. *Clin Chim Acta*. Vol.58, No.1, pp. 61-9, ISSN 0009-8981

Kanehisa, M. & Goto, S. (2000). KEGG: Kyoto Encyclopedia of Genes and Genomes. *Nucleic Acids Res*, Vol.28, No.1, pp. 27-30, ISSN 0305-1048

Karp, P.D.; Ouzounis, C.A.; Moore-Kochlacs, C.; Goldovsky, L.; Kaipa, P.; Ahrén, D.; Tsoka, S.; Darzentas, N.; Kunin, V.; López-Bigas, N. (2005). Expansion of the BioCyc collection of pathway/genome databases to 160 genomes. *Nucleic Acids Res*, Vol.33, No.19, pp. 6083-9, ISSN 0305-1048

Kurukulasuriya, L.R. & Sowers, J.R. (2010). Therapies for type 2 diabetes: lowering HbA1c and associated cardiovascular risk factors. *Cardiovasc Diabetol*, Vol. 9, pp. 45, ISSN 1475-2840

Lemberger, T. (2007). Systems biology in human health and disease. *Mol Syst Biol*, Vol.3, No.3 , pp. 136, ISSN 1744-4292

Lundin, U. & Weinberger, K.M. (2009) Metabolic Characterization of a rat model of puromycin induced nephrotoxicity. *Proceedings of SOT 48th Annual Meeting & ToxExpoTM*, Baltimore, MD, USA

Ma, H.; Sorokin, A.; Mazein, A.; Selkov, A.; Selkov, E.; Demin, O. & Goryanin, I. (2007). The Edinburgh human metabolic network reconstruction and its functional analysis. *Mol Syst Biol*. Vol. 3, pp. 135, ISSN 1744-4292

Martens-Lobenhoffer, J. & Bode-Boger, S.M. (2006). Fast and efficient determination of arginine, symmetric dimethylarginine, and asymmetric dimethylarginine in biological fluids by hydrophilic-interaction liquid chromatography-electrospray tandem mass spectrometry. *Clin Chem*, Vol.52, No.3, pp. 488-493, ISSN 0009-9147

Mendelssohn, D.C. & Wish, J.B. (2009). Dialysis delivery in Canada and the United States: a view from the trenches. *Am J Kidney Dis*, Vol.54, No.5, pp. 954-964, ISSN 0272-6386

Mensah, G.A.; Mokdad, A.H.; Ford, E.; Narayan, K.M.; Giles, W.H.; Vinicor, F. & Deedwania, P.C. (2004). Obesity, metabolic syndrome, and type 2 diabetes: emerging epidemics and their cardiovascular implications. *Cardiol Clin*. Vol.22, No.4, pp. 485-504, ISSN 0733-8651

Modre-Osprian, R.; Osprian, I.; Tilg, B.; Schreier, G.; Weinberger, K.M. & Graber, A. (2009). Dynamic simulations on the mitochondrial fatty acid beta-oxidation network. *BMC Syst Biol*, Vol.3, pp. 2, ISSN 1752-0509

Nakayama, Y.; Kinoshita, A. &Tomita, M. (2005). Dynamic simulation of red blood cell metabolism and its application to the analysis of a pathological condition. *Theor Biol Med Model*, Vol.2, pp. 18, ISSN 1742-4682

National Kidney Foundation. (2002). K/DOQI clinical practice guidelines for chronic kidney disease: evaluation, classification, and stratification. *Am J Kidney Dis*, Vol.39, No.2Suppl1, pp. S1-266, ISSN 0272-6386

Nicholson, J.K.; Lindon, J.C. & Holmes, E. (1999). 'Metabonomics': understanding the metabolic responses of living systems to pathophysiological stimuli via multivariate statistical analysis of biological NMR spectroscopic data. *Xenobiotica*, Vol.29, No.11, pp. 1181-1189, ISSN 0049-8254

Online Mendelian Inheritance in Man, OMIM®. McKusick-Nathans Institute of Genetic Medicine, Johns Hopkins University (Baltimore, MD), 2011-03-15, Available from: <http://omim.org/>

Osl, M.; Dreiseitl, S.; Pfeifer, B.; Weinberger, K.M.; Klocker, H.; Bartsch, G.; Schafer, G.; Tilg, B.; Graber, A.; & Baumgartner, C. (2008). A new rule-based algorithm for identifying metabolic markers in prostate cancer using tandem mass spectrometry. *Bioinformatics*, Vol.24, No.24 , pp. 2908-2914, ISSN 1367-4803

Ritz, E. & Stefanski, A. (1996). Diabetic nephropathy in type II diabetes. *Am J Kidney Dis*, Vol.27, No.2, pp. 167-194, ISSN 0272-6386

Röschinger, W.; Olgemoller, B.; Fingerhut, R.; Liebl, B. & Roscher, A.A. (2003). Advances in analytical mass spectrometry to improve screening for inherited metabolic diseases. *Eur J Pediatr*, Vol.162 Suppl 1, pp. S67-76, ISSN 0340-6199

Saito, K.; Fujigaki, S.; Heyes, M.P.; Shibata, K.; Takemura, M.; Fujii, H.; Wada, H.; Noma, A. & Seishima, M. (2000). Mechanism of increases in L-kynurenine and quinolinic acid in renal insufficiency. *Am J Physiol Renal Physiol*, Vol.279, No.3, pp. F565-572, ISSN 0363-6127

Subramanian, A.; Tamayo, P.; Mootha, V.K.; Mukherjee, S.; Ebert, B.L.; Gillette, M.A.; Paulovich, A.; Pomeroy, S.L.; Golub, T.R.; Lander, E.S. & Mesirov, J.P. (2005) Gene set enrichment analysis: a knowledge-based approach for interpreting genome-wide expression profiles. *Proc Natl Acad Sci U S A*, Vol.102, No.43, pp. 15545-50, ISSN 0027-8424

Suhre, K., Meisinger, C., Doring, A., Altmaier, E., Belcredi, P., Gieger, C., Chang, D., Milburn, M.V., Gall, W.E., Weinberger, K.M., et al. (2010). Metabolic footprint of diabetes: a multiplatform metabolomics study in an epidemiological setting. *PLoS One*, Vol.5, No.11, pp. e13953, ISSN 1932-6203

Susztak, K. & Bottinger, E.P. (2006). Diabetic nephropathy: a frontier for personalized medicine. *J Am Soc Nephrol*, Vol.17, No.2, pp. 361-367, ISSN 1046-6673

Unterwurzacher, I.; Koal, T.; Bonn, G.K.; Weinberger, K.M. & Ramsay, S.L. (2008). Rapid sample preparation and simultaneous quantitation of prostaglandins and lipoxygenase derived fatty acid metabolites by liquid chromatography-mass spectrometry from small sample volumes. *Clin Chem Lab Med*, Vol.46, No.11, pp. 1589-1597, ISSN 1434-6621

Urban, M.; Enot, D.P.; Dallmann, G.; Körner, L.; Forcher, V.; Enoh, P.; Koal, T.; Keller, M. & Deigner, H.P. (2010). Complexity and pitfalls of mass spectrometry-based targeted metabolomics in brain research. *Anal Biochem*. Vol.496, No.2, pp. 124-31, ISSN 0003-2697

Vaag. A. & Poulsen. P. (2007). Twins in metabolic and diabetes research: what do they tell us? *Curr Opin Clin Nutr Metab Care*. Vol.10, No.5, pp. 591-6, ISSN 1363-1950

Vallance, P.; Leone, A.; Calver, A.; Collier, J. & Moncada, S. (1992). Accumulation of an endogenous inhibitor of nitric oxide synthesis in chronic renal failure. *Lancet*, Vol.339, No.8793, pp. 572-575, ISSN 0140-6736

Vastrik, I.; D'Eustachio, P.; Schmidt, E.; Joshi-Tope, G.; Gopinath, G.; Croft, D.; de Bono, B.; Gillespie, M.; Jassal, B.; Lewis, S.; Matthews, L.; Wu, G.; Birney, E. & Stein, L. (2007). Reactome: a knowledge base of biologic pathways and processes. *Genome Biology*, Vol.8, No.3, pp. R39, ISSN 1465-6906

Walder, K.; Segal, D.; Jowett, J.; Blangero, J. & Collier, G.R. (2003). Obesity and diabetes gene discovery approaches. *Curr Pharm Des*. Vol.9, No.17, pp. 1357-72

Walser, M. & Hill, S.B. (1993). Free and protein-bound tryptophan in serum of untreated patients with chronic renal failure. *Kidney Int*, Vol.44, No.6, pp. 1366-1371, ISSN 0085-2538

Wang-Sattler, R.; Yu, Y.; Mittelstrass, K.; Lattka, E.; Altmaier, E.; Gieger, C.; Ladwig, K.H.; Dahmen, N.; Weinberger, K.M.; Hao, P.; Liu, L.; Li, Y.; Wichmann, H.E.; Adamski, J.; Suhre, K. & Illig, T. (2008). Metabolic profiling reveals distinct variations linked to nicotine consumption in humans - first results from the KORA study. *PLoS ONE*, Vol. 3, No.12, pp. e3863, ISSN 1932-6203

Weckwerth, W. (2003). Metabolomics in systems biology. *Annu Rev Plant Biol.* Vol. 54, pp. 669-689, ISSN 1543-5008

Weikard, R.; Altmaier, E.; Suhre, K.; Weinberger, K.M.; Hammon, H.M.; Albrecht, E.; Setoguchi, K.; Takasuga, A. & Kühn, C. (2010). Metabolomic profiles indicate distinct physiological pathways affected by two loci with major divergent effect on Bos taurus growth and lipid deposition. *Physiol Genomics.* Vol.42A, No.2, ISSN 1094-8341

Weinberger, K.M. & Graber, A. (2005). Using Comprehensive Metabolomics to Identify Novel Biomarkers. *Screening Trends in Drug Discovery*, Vol.6, pp. 42-45

Weinberger, K.M. (2008). Metabolomics in diagnosing metabolic diseases. *Ther Umsch*, Vol.65, No.9, pp. 487-491, ISSN 0040-5930

Weinberger, K.M..; Ramsay, S.L. & Graber, A. (2005). Towards the biochemical fingerprint.*Biosyst Solut,* Vol.12, 36–37

Wishart, D.S.; Tzur, D.; Knox, C. et al. (2007) HMDB: the Human Metabolome Database. *Nucleic Acids Res*, Vol.35, Database issue, pp. D521-6, ISSN 0305-1048

Wolf, G. & Ritz, E. (2003). Diabetic nephropathy in type 2 diabetes prevention and patient management. *J Am Soc Nephrol*, Vol.14, No.5, pp. 1396-1405, ISSN 1046-6673

Yugi, K. & Tomita, M. (2004). A general computational model of mitochondrial metabolism in a whole organelle scale. *Bioinformatics*, Vol. 20, No.11 , pp. 1795-1796, ISSN 1367-4803

Part 2

Unifactorial or Unigenetic Disorder

6

Thalassemia Syndrome

Tangvarasittichai Surapon
Chronic Diseases Research Unit, Department of Medical Technology,
Naresuan University, Phitsanulok
Thailand

1. Introduction

Thalassemia is an inherited disorder of autosomal recessive gene disorder caused by impaired synthesis of one or more globin chains. The impairment alters production of hemoglobin (Hb) (Ridolfi et al., 2002). Thalassemia causes varying degrees of anemia, which can range from significant to life threatening. People of Mediterranean, Middle Eastern, African, and Southeast Asian descent are at higher risk of carrying the genes for thalassemia (Weatherall, 1997). These hereditary anemias are caused by mutations that decrease hemoglobin synthesis and red cell survival. These hereditary anemia caused by decreased or absent production of one type of globin chain either α or β globin chain. These hematologic disorders range from asymptomatic to severe anemia that can cause significant morbidity and mortality. It was first recognized clinically in 1925 by Dr. Thomas Cooley, who described a syndrome of anemia with microcytic erythrocytes. Then it was called Cooley's anemia. Later Wipple and Bradford renamed this disease as "Thalassemia". Because it was found in the region of the Mediterranean Sea (thalasa is an old Greek word for sea) (Cooley, 1946). Thalassemias can cause significant problems because these are inherited disorders, newborn screening and prenatal diagnosis are important in management of patients. This topic will review the clinical features of thalassemia while focusing on pathophysiology, clinical features, complication, management, screening and diagnosis. Formerly the distribution of thalassemia had been mainly limited to the areas from the Mediterranean basin through the Middle East and Indian subcontinent up to Southeast Asia so called "thalassemia belt" (Chernoff, 1959). However, recent migrations of people have spread thalassemia genes throughout the world.

2. Pathophysiology

Hemoglobin (Hb) is the molecule that carries and transports oxygen all through the body. Normal human hemoglobin is a tetramer formed by two pairs of globin chains attached to heme. The hemoglobin type is determined by the combination of tetra-globin chains (α, β, δ, and γ chains). Each globin chain is structurally different and thus has different oxygen affinity, electrical charge, and electrophoretic mobility. Normal adult hemoglobins are expressed as A_2, A and F (fetal). Ninety-five to ninety-eight percent of adult hemoglobin is A the major hemoglobin, which consists of two α- and two β-chains (α_2, β_2). Hemoglobin A_2 (α_2, δ_2), the remainder of hemoglobin in adults is a minor component (less than 3.3%), and 1% or less of F (α_2, γ_2) (Nathan & Oski, 1993.), the gamma hemoglobin (Hb-F) is the predominant hemoglobin found only during fetal development. The equal production of α and non-α (β, δ, γ) globin chains is necessary for normal red blood cell (RBC) function. The failure in hemoglobin synthesis is a main cause of microcytosis and anemia in many population groups around the world. Hb variants are characterized by the gene mutation of the globin chains form hemoglobin (i.e., the replacement of different amino acids at a certain position). Thalassemia occurs when there is decreased or absent production of one of the types of globin chains (most commonly either α or β), that cause insufficeient amount of normal structure globin chains. This results in an imbalance between α- and β-chains and causes the clinical features of thalassemia (Nathan & Gunn, 1966), it can be separated into two major types such as α-thalassemia and β- thalassemia.

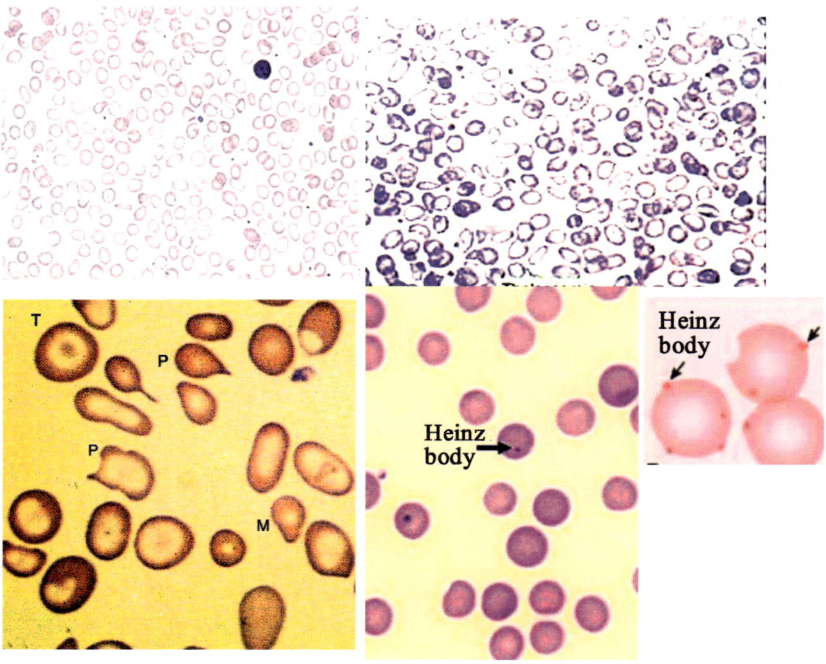

Fig. 1. Red blood cell morphology is altered in patients with all forms of thalassemia. Hypochromic microcytes and target cells are the main features in asymptomatic individuals. Patients with more severe forms of thalassemia have the anisocytosis and poikilocytosis, hypochromic microcytic, target cells, ovalocytes, occasional fragmented red blood cells

The absence or decreased of normal production of α-globin chains results in a relative excess of γ-globin chains in the fetus and newborn, and β-globin chains in children and adults. When globin chains are not produced in equal amounts, any excess chains accumulate and precipitate damaging the RBC and accelerating its destruction. The absence of normal production of α-chains results in a relative excess of γ-globin chains in the fetus and newborn, and β-globin chains in children and adults. Further, the β-globin chains are capable of forming soluble tetramers (β-4, or Hb-H); yet this form of hemoglobin is unstable and tends to precipitate within the cell forming insoluble inclusions (Heinz bodies) that damage the red cell membrane. α-Thalassemia is generally less severe because the excess unpaired β-chains that accumulate are less damaging to RBCs than the unpaired α chains. Furthermore, diminished hemoglobinization of individual red blood cells results in damage to erythrocyte precursors and ineffective erythropoiesis in the bone marrow, as well as hypochromia and microcytosis of circulating red blood cells. (Fig 1)

In β-thalassemia, reduced amount (β^+) or absence (β^0) of β-globin chains excess α-chains accumulate in the RBC and precipitate because they are highly insoluble. These precipitated globin chains occur in both erythroid precursors in the bone marrow and circulating RBCs. The destruction of precursor RBCs results in ineffective erythropoiesis, increased erythropoietin, and proliferation of the bone marrow. This expanded bone marrow (up 25 to 30 times normal) can result in the characteristic bony abnormalities of β-thalassemia if the process is not prevented by transfusion therapy. Prolonged and severe anemia and increased erythropoietic drive also result in hepatosplenomegaly and extramedullary erythropoiesis, leading to their premature death and hence to ineffective erythropoiesis. The degree of globin chain reduction is determined by the nature of the mutation at the β-globin gene located on chromosome 11. Peripheral hemolysis contributing to anemia is more prominent in thalassemia major than in thalassemia intermedia, and occurs when insoluble α-globin chains induce membrane damage to the peripheral erythrocytes.

Genes that regulate both synthesis and structure of different globins are organized into 2 separate clusters. The α-globin genes are encoded on chromosome 16 and the γ, δ, and β-globin genes are encoded on chromosome 11 as demonstrated in Fig 2. Each individual normally carries a linked pair of α-globin genes, 2 from the paternal chromosome, and 2 from the maternal chromosome. Therefore, each diploid human cell has four copies of the α-globin gene. The four α-thalassemia syndromes thus reflect the disease state produced by deletion or no-function of one, two, three, or all four of the α-globin genes (Higgs et al., 1989) (Table 1). The silent carrier state of α-thalassemia represents a mutation of one copy of the α-globin gene and results in no hematologic abnormalities.

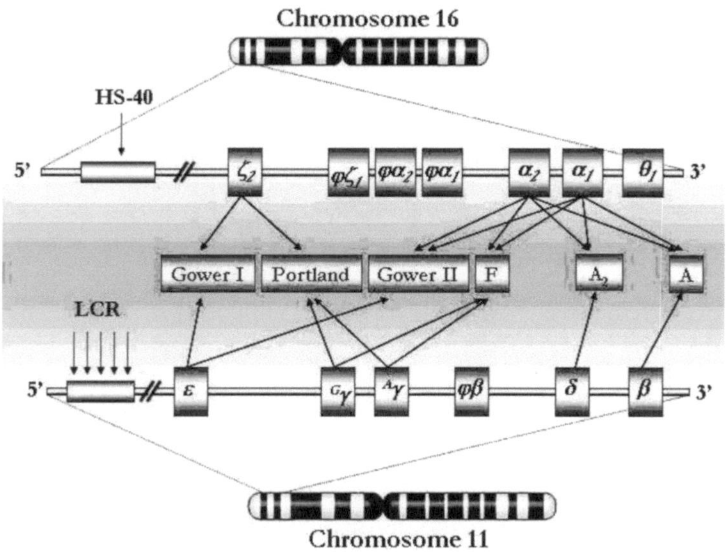

Fig. 2. Schematic represent of the globin gene loci. The upper panel shows the α-globin locus that resides on chromosome 16. Each of the four alpha globin genes contributed to the synthesis of the α-globin protein. The lower panel shows the β-globin locus that resides on chromosome 11. The two γ-globin genes are active during fetal growth and produce hemoglobin F. The "adult" gene, beta, takes over after birth

3. Geographical distribution of thalassemias and the malaria hypothesis

It is a widely accepted conclusion that the high frequency of thalassemias and sickle cell anemia observed in some tropical and subtropical areas of the world (Fig 3). This due to the resistance against malignant malaria (*Plasmodium falciparum*) conferred by these inherited defects to the heterozygous carriers (Allison, 1954). According to the malaria hypothesis, the heterozygous for HbS or a thalassemic (clinically healthy) are resistant to malaria and have a selective advantage over both homozygotes which have a higher chance of dying during the first years of life because of either malaria or anemia. The preferential survival of the heterozygote thus makes possible the persistence at polymorphic frequencies of the abnormal genes in the population, provided that the selective agent (malaria) remains present and active. Because there is a loss of both normal and abnormal genes, an equilibrium between their frequency will be reached in a period of time which depends on the extent of the selective advantage (balanced polymorphism). The malaria hypothesis is supported by the overlapping geographical distribution of these disorders and endemic malaria and by clinical and epidemiological studies showing a positive correlation between malaria endemicity and frequency of abnormal alleles (Siniscalco et al., 1966).

[A]

[B]

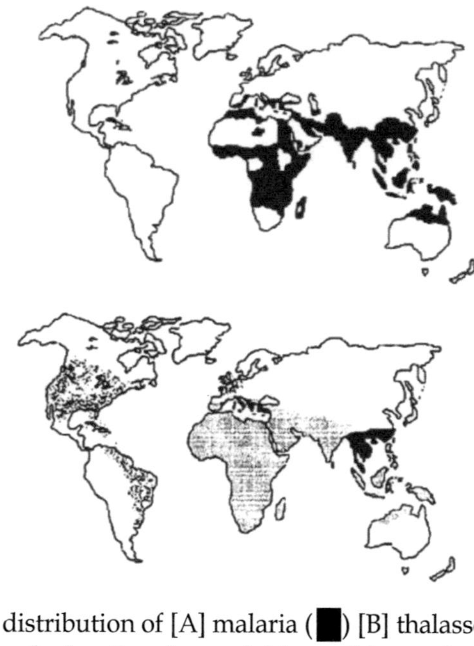

Fig. 3. The geographical distribution of [A] malaria (■) [B] thalassemia (□, α^+- thalassemia α^0- thalassemia). Because of migration, hemoglobinopathies are improved into the area where malaria has never been endemic

The α-thalassemias are most prevalent in Asian and African populations. Persons of Mediterranean and African descent have the highest incidence of β-thalassemia. Thalassemic mutations have maintained a high frequency, particularly in these areas, because the heterozygous state confers some protection against malaria (Weatherall, 1987). Other abnormalities of hemoglobin also occur with increased frequency in these populations: therefore, thalassemia may coexist with other disorders of hemoglobin such as the sickle cell syndromes, hemoglobin E (Hb-E), or hemoglobin C (Hb-C).

Syndrome	Molecular basis	Laboratory values	Clinical Feature
α- Thalassemia			
α- Thalassemia silent carrier	One α- gene deletion (−α/αα) Heterozygous α-thalassemia	No anemia or RBC morphology abnormalities; Asymptomatic may have 1-2 % Hb Bart's at birth	Asymptomatic
α-Thalassemia trait (minor)	Two α-gene deletion (—/αα) Heterozygous α-thalassemia-1 Two α-gene deletion (−α/−α) Homozygous α-thalassemia 2	Mild anemia, microcytosis, and hypochromia; 4-6% Hb Bart's at birth	Asymptomatic
Hb H disease (Hb variants related to mutation in α-globin chain)	Three α-gene deletion (—/−α) α-thalassemia-1/α-thalassemia-2 Hb Constant Spring α-thalassemia-1/Hb Constant Spring	Moderate anemia, microcytosis, hypochromia, RBC fragments; Hb Bart's prominent at birth α- chain has extra 31 amino acids	Jaundice, gallstones, splenomegaly, occasionally need transfusion; antioxidant drugs can precipitate hemolysis
Hb Bart's Hydrops fetalis	Four α-gene deletion (—/—) Homozygous α-thalassemia 1	Severe anemia, nucleated RRCs; only Hb H, Bart's, and Portland present	Death in utero or shortly after birth
β- Thalassemia			
β-Thalassemia trait (minor)	Point mutations Heterozygous β^0-thalassemia Heterozygous β^+-thalassemia	Mild anemia, hypochromia, and microcytosis; RBC morphologic abnormalities; Hb A_2, and F often elevated	Asymptomatic
β-Thalassemia intermedia	Point mutations - β^0-thalassemia/β^+-thalassemia -HbEβ^+-thalassemia	Moderate anemia, microcytosis, and hypochromia; RBC morphologic abnormalities; Hb A, and F increased; Hb A decreased to absent	Maintain Hb of 7 g/dL without transfusion; clinical phenotype between β-thalassemia trait and thalassemia major

Syndrome	Molecular basis	Laboratory values	Clinical Feature
β-Thalassemia major	Point mutations -Homozygous β^0-thalassemia - HbEβ^0-thalassemia (Thalassemia intermediate or thalassemia major)	Severe anemia, microcytosis, and hypochromia; RBC fragments and striking morphologic abnormalities; Hb A_2, and F ncreased; Hb A decreased to absent	Require chronic transfusion; develop iron overload resulting in endocrine abnormalities and chronic organ damage
RBC= red blood cell; Hb H = hemoglobin H			

Table 1. Characteristic of the Thalassemia Syndromes

β-thalassemia is prevalent in Mediterranean countries, the Middle East, Central Asia, India, Southern China, and the Far East as well as countries along the north coast of Africa and in South America. The highest carrier frequency is reported in Cyprus (14%), Sardinia (10.3%), and Southeast Asia (Flint et al., 1998). The high gene frequency of β-thalassemia in these regions is most likely related to the selective pressure from *Plasmodium falciparum* malaria (Flint et al., 1998). Population migration and intermarriage between different ethnic groups has introduced thalassemia in almost every country of the world, including Northern Europe where thalassemia was previously absent. It has been estimated that about 1.5% of the global population (80 to 90 million people) are carriers of β-thalassemia, with about 60,000 symptomatic individuals born annually, the great majority in the developing world. The total annual incidence of symptomatic individuals is estimated at 1 in 100,000 throughout the world and 1 in 10,000 people in the European Union. According to Thalassemia International Federation, only about 200,000 patients with thalassemia major are alive and registered as receiving regular treatment around the world (Thalassemia International Federation: Guidelines for the clinical management of thalassemia 2nd edition. 2008 (http://www.Thalassemia. org. cy)).

4. Molecular basis and classification

The thalassemia syndromes are one of the most thoroughly studied diseases at the molecular level. Consequently, some explanation for the clinical heterogeneity seen in patients can be explained at the molecular level.

4.1 α-Thalassemias

The major clinical syndromes resulting from α-thalassemia were first recognized in the mid 1950s and early 1960s through the association of the abnormal hemoglobins (Hb-H and Hb Bart's) with hypochromic microcytic anemia in the absence of iron deficiency (Minnich et al., 1954, Rigas et al., 1955), Lie-Injo & Jo, 1960). α-Thalassemia is divided into deletional and nondeletional types (Bain 2006). There are at least 40 different deletions. The size of the deletion is important and affects the clinical phenotype of hydrops fetalis. Over 95% of α thalassemia is caused by large deletions involving one or both of the α-globin genes. The α-globin gene cluster occurs on the short arm of chromosome 16, band 16 p 13.3 and includes the α-globin genes as well as the embryonic genes (as two identical α-globin genes (α_1 and α_2) that are aligned one after the other on the chromosome). Common α-thalassemia deletions that spare the embryonic gene allow for the production of functional embryonic hemoglobin early in gestation. In contrast, the large deletions (severe) lack the benefit of embryonic hemoglobin. Non-deletion mutations may have a more severe phenotype than most of the deletional mutations. The most common non-deletional α-thalassemia mutation is Hemoglobin Constant Spring; this mutation of the stop codon results in 31 amino acids being added to α chain. Depending on the production of α-globin chains, α-thalassemia determinants can be classified into two groups: α° and α^{+}. In α°-thalassemia the production of α-chains by the affected chromosome is completely abolished; α^{+}-thalassemia is defined by the variable amounts of α polypeptide chains which can still be expressed in cis to the thalassaemic cluster. This nomenclature, which describes α-thalassemias in terms of α-globin chain expression/haplotype, has replaced the previous classification of these defects into severe (α-thalassaemia-1) and mild (α-thalassaemia-2) forms (Weatherail & Clegg, 1981).

In the passed, genetics of these syndromes were more confusing. This was because the adult carriers of α-thalassemia do not produce large amounts of either Hb-H or Hb Bart's. Although the relatives of the affected individuals do not have a readily defined phenotype, it was eventually shown that the offspring of individuals with Hb-H disease have raised levels of Hb Bart's (γ_4) in the neonatal period (Na-Nakorn et al., 1969), and the parents of individuals with Hb-H disease and the Hb Bart's hydrops fetalis syndrome have mildly hypochromic, microcytic red cell indices (Ali, 1969); sometimes Hb-H inclusions could be demonstrated in occasional red cells (McNiel JR, 1968). By 1969 it had been shown that Hb-H disease results from the inheritance of α-thalassemia-1 x α-thalassemia-2 and the Hb Bart's hydrops fetalis syndrome results from α-thalassemia-1 x α-thalassemia 1) (Na-Nakorn et al., 1969, Pootrakul et al., 1967).

The structural organization of the α-globin genes revealed by blot hybridization analysis (Orkin, 1978), Normal individual have two α-genes on each chromosome 16 or four copies of the α-globin gene (αα/αα) and carriers for α-thalassemia have either three (–α/αα) or two (– –/αα) α genes. Thus, the most frequently encountered genotype of Hb-H disease is – –/– α and Hb Bart's hydrops fetalis is – –/– – (Orkin, 1978, Orkin et al., 1979, Phillips 3d et al., 1980). Thus by 1980 the molecular genetics of α-thalassemia was understood. The four α-thalassemia syndromes thus reflect the disease state produced by deletion or nonfunction of one, two, three, or all four of the α-globin genes (Higgs et at., 1989). α-Thalassemia trait occurs with deletion or nonfunction of two α-globin genes. The two genes are deleted from the same chromosome (cis-deletion) or one gene is lost from each chromosome 16 (trans-deletion). The cis-deletion is most common in Asian and Mediterranean populations, whereas individuals of African descent usually have the trans-deletion (Higgs et al., 1989). Both varieties of α-thalassemia trait produce an asymptomatic, mild anemia associated with microcytosis. Hemoglobin H (Hb-H) disease, a three-gene deletion, usually results from inheritance of the cis α-thalassemia trait from one parent and the one gene deletion from the other parent. Therefore, this abnormality is rare in the black population because the cis-deletion is uncommon. Hydrops fetalis results from deletion of all four α-globin genes and generally causes death in utero because no physiologically useful hemoglobin is produced beyond the embryonic stage. Although the α-thalassemia syndromes also are of varying clinical severity, these differences cannot be explained by the number of deleted or nonfunctional genes. One of the most frequent α-thalassemia mutations is the $--^{SEA}$ deletion, which deletes both α-globin genes but spares the embryonic gene. Homozygosity for this deletion ($--^{SEA}$) is the most common cause of hydrops fetalis (Chui & Waye 1998). The sparing of the embryonic gene allows enough functional embryonic hemoglobin (Hemoglobin Portland 1 and Hemoglobin Portland 2) to allow gestation to continue and the

phenotype of hydrops fetalis to develop. In contrast, other common α-thalassemia mutations ($-- ^{FIL}$, $-- ^{THAI}$) also lack the entire embryonic α-globin cluster, and therefore do not produce the functional embryonic Hemoglobin Portland. These embryos may terminate unnoticed early in gestation (Chui & Waye 1998). Over 5% of individuals in the Philippines are carriers for the $-- ^{SEA}$ or $-- ^{FIL}$ mutation. Hydrops fetalis, while most common in Southeast Asia, is found worldwide among many ethnic groups; $-- ^{MED}$ is a common α^0-thalassemia mutation in Mediterranean regions, particularly Greece and Cyprus. It has resulted in hydrops fetalis.
Non-deletional α-thalassemia is found throughout the world. Up to 8% of Southeast Asians are carriers of Hemoglobin Constant Spring. In the Middle East, Hemoglobin αTSaudiα is a common α-thalassemia non-deletional mutation. It is a mutation of the polyadenylation signal sequence of the α 2 gene, resulting in decreased expression of structurally normal α chains. Hemoglobin Koya Dora, another structural non-deletional mutation, is found in India. Other structural mutations, such as hemoglobin Quong Sze found in Southeast Asia, are highly unstable and result in defects in the hem pocket (Skordis, 2006, Leung et al., 2002).

4.2 α Thalassemia trait

α-Thalassaemia trait is usually caused either by the interaction of the normal haplotype with a α°- or a α^{+}-thalassaemia determinant or by the homozygosity for two α^{+} haplotypes. Much less frequently this phenotype can be the result of compound heterozygosity for a deletional α^{+}- thalassaemia and a α^{+} determinant caused by a point mutation or even homozygosity for the latter kind of determinant. Depending on the nature and localization of the mutation, the phenotype of the trait can thus range from the silent cartier to individuals showing very pronounced haematological abnormalities.
Patients with α-thalassemia trait have microcytosis, hypochromia, and mild anemia. Small amounts of hemoglobin Bart's (a tetramer of γ chains: γ_4) may be noted on a newborn screen. Individuals with this disorder are asymptomatic and do not require transfusions or any other treatment. The diagnosis of α-thalassemia trait is considered when the patient has the appropriate RBC abnormalities, when iron deficiency and β-thalassemia trait have been excluded, and when family studies (CBC, hemoglobin profile, and review of the peripheral smear) are consistent with the diagnosis (Nathan & Oski 1993). To make the diagnosis with complete certainty requires characterization of gene deletions with restriction endonuclease mapping or globin chain synthesis studies showing a decreased (α:β ratio. However, this confirmation rarely is indicated clinically.

4.3 Hemoglobin H disease

Hemoglobin H (Hb-H) disease is the most severe non-fatal form of α-thalassemia syndrome, mostly caused by molecular defects of the α-globin genes in which α-globin expression is decreased, causes a moderate anemia with hypochromia, microcytosis, and red cell fragmentation. Two common genotypes lead to the phenotype of Hb-H disease are α-thalassemia-1/α-thalassemia-2 and Hb Constant Spring/α-thalassemia-1. Both genotypes are equally common but Hb Constant Spring/α-thalassemia-1 is more severe than α-thalassemia-1/α-thalassemia-2 (Fucharoen et al., 1988). Compound heterozygotes for α^0- and α^+-thalassemia (--/-α) with only one functional α-globin gene have a severe imbalance in globin chain synthesis with a two- to five-fold excess of β-globin chains synthesis (Nathan & Oski 1993.). Newborns have large amounts of Bart's Hb. (Higgs et al., 1989). When the switch from γ- to β-globin chain production occurs, Hb Bart's (γ_4) switches to Hb-H (β_4) and the typical picture of Hb-H disease results. The excess β-globin chains precipitate and form a characteristic abnormal hemoglobin; hemoglobin H (Hb-H) or β-globin tetramer ($β_4$). This causes a phenotype of mild to moderate chronic hemolytic anemia named Hb-H disease characterized by readily detectable Hb-H inclusion bodies in the peripheral blood cells. Hb-H is unable to transport oxygen at physiologic conditions; therefore, patients have a more severe deficit in oxygen carrying capacity than would be expected from their measured hemoglobin level (Nathan & Oski 1993). Increased red cell destruction occurs because Hb-H containing cells are sensitive to oxidative stress. Thus the complications of the disease are related to hemolysis and include jaundice, hepatosplenomegaly, gallstones, and leg ulcers. Most affected individuals have a mild disorder with an Hb concentration of 7-10 g/dL and require only symptomatic care with occasional transfusions. Therefore, iron overload is rarely a problem in these patients.

The clinical phenotypes of Hb-H disease found in nondeletional α-thalassemia (--/αTα) are often more severe than those caused by $α^+$-thalassemia resulting from simple deletion (--/-α). Recent molecular analysis of more than 500 thalassemia carriers at the Department of Pediatrics, Siriraj Hospital, Thailand, revealed that the frequency of deletional α-thalassemia is significantly higher compared with non-deletional mutations (mainly Hb CS and Pakse) in Thai population (15%-20% vs 1%-2%, respectively). However, the number of symptomatic patients with Hb-H disease due to non-deletional mutations appeared to be higher than those with deletional Hb-H (60% vs 40% from 350 Hb-H disease patients), as shown in Table 1, suggesting that non-deletional Hb-H patients have more significant clinical symptoms and require more medical attention (Fucharoen & Viprakasit, 2009).

A striking clinical feature of Hb-H disease is the sudden drop in the Hb concentration with associated symptoms of acute anemia during episodes of pyrexia (Chinprasertsuk et al., 1994). It has been postulated that fever either alone or together with oxidative substances released in the process of infection, induces the unstable Hb-H to precipitate in the red cells as inclusion bodies. These red cells then either hemolyze or are rapidly destroyed by the reticuloendothelial cells. Blood transfusions should be given together with treatment for infections. Body temperature should be normalized as quickly as possible in order to reduce induction of Hb-H precipitation within the red cells. Hb Constant Spring is detected in addition to Hb-A and H in patients with Hb Constant Spring α-thalassemia-1. They are slightly more severe than classical Hb-H disease with lower Hb concentrations, larger spleens, higher levels of Hb-H and more red cells containing inclusion bodies (Fucharoen et al., 1988).

4.4 Hemoglobin Bart's Hydrops fetalis syndrome

Hydrops fetalis, the most severe form of α-thalassemia, occurs in infants whose parents both have α-thalassemia syndrome (Higgs et al., 1989). As discussed previously, these infants have deletion of all four α-globin genes and produce only Hb Bart's, Hb-H, and small amounts of embryonic hemoglobins. Therefore, they have very little physiologically useful hemoglobin and are hydropic secondary to severe anemia. These infants are usually stillborn or die shortly after delivery (Chui & Waye, 1998, Leung et al., 2008, Lorey et al., 2001, Michlitsch et al., 2009, Weatherall 2008) Advances in perinatal care and recognition of surviving homozygous thalassemia newborns have precipitated studies of long-term survivors with this disorder. Recently, the Newborn Screening Program of California reported 8 surviving α-thalassemia major newborns along with 500 Hemoglobin H babies (Michlitsch et al., 2009). In southern China, the prevalence of $α^0$-thalassemia trait is 8.5% and 0.23% of births had homozygous α-thalassemia (Chui & Waye, 1998). In addition to China and Southeast Asia, Bart's hydrops fetalis is now being recognized in Greece, Turkey, Cyprus, India, Sardinia, and other parts of the world (Chui & Waye 1998, Yang & Li, 2009, Suwanrath-Kengpol et al., 2005)

Clinical and haematological examinations reveal severely anaemic infants with variable hemoglobin levels (3-10g/dl) and marked anisopoikilocytosis with large hypochromic red cells and with the presence of numerous erythroblasts. The analysis of the hemolysate shows, in the hydrops caused by the deletion of four α genes, about 80% Hb Bart's (γ_4) and 20% Hb Portland 1 ($\zeta_2 \gamma_2$) with very small amounts, if any, of Hb Portland 2 ($\zeta_2 \beta_2$) and HbH (β_4) (Kutlar et al., 1989). Lower levels of Hb Portland 1 have been observed in genetic compounds for the SEA deletion and the large Fil deletion which also eliminates the ζ gene (Kutlar et al., 1989). In the rare cases of Hb-H disease with hydrops fetalis, in addition to Hb Bart's and the embryonic Hb Portland 1 and 2, variable amounts of HbH, HbF and HbA can also be detected (Chan et al., 1997). The lack of hem-hem interaction or Bohr effect and binds oxygen irreversibly tightly and high oxygen affinity of Hb Bart's make this γ tetramer unsuitable for the delivery of oxygen to the tissues. The ensuing hypoxia is the cause of fetal hydrops and intrauterine death caused by massive organomegaly, severe albuminemia, and heart failure. This leads to gross body edema, growth failure.

4.5 β-Thalassemias

The β-thalassemias are widespread throughout the Mediterranean region, Africa, the Middle East, the Indian subcontinent and Burma, Southeast Asia including southern China, the Malay Peninsula, and Indonesia. Estimates of gene frequencies range from 3 to 10 percent in some areas. (Weatherall, 1994) Within each population at risk for β-thalassemia a small number of common mutations are found, as well as rarer ones; each mutation is in strong linkage disequilibrium with specific arrangements of restriction-fragment length polymorphisms, or haplotypes, within the β-globin cluster. A limited number of haplotypes are found in each population, so that 80 percent of the mutations are associated with only 20 different haplotypes. This observation has helped demonstrate the independent origin of β-thalassemia in several populations (Flint et al., 1993). There is evidence that the high frequency of β-thalassemia throughout the tropics reflects an advantage of heterozygotes against. *Plasmodium falciparum* malaria, (Weatherall, 1987) as has already been demonstrated in α-thalassemia (Allen et al., 1997).

The β-globin gene cluster is located on chromosome 11 and is not duplicated like the α-globin genes. Therefore, each diploid cell contains only two β-globin genes. Mutations are described that affect every step in the process of gene expression from transcription and translation to post-translational stability of the β-globin chain (Kazazian Jr., 1990) The variable clinical severity of the β-thalassemia syndromes depends on how significantly these different mutations affect β-globin synthesis. Although over ninety such mutations are known, a given mutation generally is found in one ethnic group and not another. Nearly 200 different mutations have been described in patients with β-thalassemia and related disorders. Although most are small nucleotide substitutions within the cluster, deletions may also cause β-thalassemia (Weatherall 1994). All the mutations result in either the absence of the synthesis of β-globin chains (β^0-thalassemia) or a reduction in synthesis (β^+-thalassemia) (Fig. 2). Mutations in or close to the conserved promoter sequences and in the 5' untranslated region down-regulate transcription, usually resulting in mild β^+ -thalassemia. Transcription is also affected by deletions in the 5' region, which completely inactivate transcription and result in β^0 -thalassemia. Both splicing of the messenger RNA (mRNA) precursor and ineffective cleavage of the mRNA transcript are result in β-thalassemia. In some mutations, no normal message is produced, whereas other mutations only slightly reduce the amount of normally spliced mRNA. Mutations within invariant dinucleotides at intron–exon junctions, critical to the removal of intervening sequences and the splicing of exons to produce functional mRNA, result in β^0 -thalassemia. Mutations in highly conserved nucleotides flanking these sequences, or in "cryptic" splice sites, which resemble a donor or acceptor splice site, result in severe as well as mild β^+-thalassemia. Substitutions or small deletions affecting the conserved AATAAA sequence in the 3' untranslated region result in ineffective cleavage of the mRNA transcript and cause mild β^+-thalassemia. Mutations that interfere with translation involve the initiation, elongation, or termination of globin-chain production and result in β^0 -thalassemia. Approximately half of all β-thalassemia mutations interfere with translation; these include frame-shift or nonsense mutations, which introduce premature termination codons and result in β^0-thalassemia. A more recently identified family of mutations, usually involving exon 3, results in the production of unstable globin chains of varying lengths that, together with a relative excess of α-globin chains, precipitate in red-cell precursors and lead to ineffective erythropoiesis, even in the heterozygous state. This is the molecular basis for dominantly inherited (β^+) thalassemia. In addition, missense mutations, resulting in the synthesis of unstable β-globin chains, cause β-thalassemia. β-thalassemia includes three main forms: Thalassemia Major, variably referred to as Cooley's Anemia and Mediterranean Anemia, Thalassemia Intermedia and Thalassemia Minor also called " β-thalassemia carrier", "β-thalassemia trait" or "heterozygous β-thalassemia". According to Thalassemia International Federation, only about 200,000 patients with thalassemia major are alive and registered as receiving regular treatment around the world (Thalassemia International Federation: Guidelines for the clinical management of thalassemia 2nd edition. 2008 [http://www.thalassemia. org.cy]). The most common combination of β-thalassemia with abnormal Hb or structural Hb variant with thalassemic properties is β-thalassemia/Hb-E which is most prevalent in Southeast Asia where the carrier frequency is around 50%.

4.6 β-Thalassemia trait

Carriers of thalassemia, individuals with this disorder are heterozygous for a mutation that affects β-globin synthesis (Kazazian Jr., 1990). They are mildly anemic with hypochromic, microcytic RBCs. Targeting and elliptocytosis are often seen. As with α-thalassemia trait, one must exclude iron deficiency to make the diagnosis. In general, patients with β-thalassemia trait have a lower mean corpuscular volume (MCV) and a higher red cell count for the degree of anemia than seen in iron deficiency. Thus, the Mentzer index (MCV/RBC) is useful as a screening test to differentiate thalassemia from iron deficiency. If the Mentzer index is < 13, thalassemia is more likely; if > 13, iron deficiency is more common. Hb electrophoresis is normal with iron deficiency, but with β-thalassemia trait the hemoglobin A_2, (Hb A_2) is often elevated. Globin chain synthesis studies show an excess of α-chains (Nathan & Oski 1993). These patients need no treatment, but should receive genetic counseling regarding the potential for having a child with β-thalassemia major or a combination of β-thalassemia trait and sickle hemoglobin (Sβ-thal). When both parents are carriers there is a 25% risk at each pregnancy of having children with homozygous thalassemia. Within the first months of life, adult hemoglobin containing 2 pairs of α and β-chain (Hb-A: $\alpha_2\beta_2$) physiologically replaces fetal hemoglobin (HbF: $\alpha_2\gamma_2$). In β–thalassemia, deficient of production structurally normal β–chain lead to anemia, largely as a consequence of ineffective hemopoiesis (Olivieri 1999, Nathan & Gunn, 1966).

4.7 Thalassemia intermedia

These β-thalassemia patients who clinically are between the extremes of thalassemia trait and thalassemia major (Nathan & Oski 1993), have milder anemia and by definition do not require or only occasionally require transfusion. The regular transfusion therapy is not required initially. These patients usually maintain a hemoglobin level of 7 g/dL without transfusions. At the severe end of the clinical spectrum, patients present between the ages of 2 and 6 years and although they are capable of surviving without regular blood transfusion, growth and development are retarded. At the other end of the spectrum are patients who are completely asymptomatic until adult life with only mild anemia. Therefore, pregnant or older patients are less able to tolerate the anemia and may need transfusion support. Hypertrophy of erythroid marrow with the possibility of extramedullary erythropoiesis, a compensatory mechanism of bone marrow to overcome chronic anemia, is common. Its consequences are characteristic deformities of the bone and face, osteoporosis with pathologic fractures of long bones and formation of erythropoietic masses that primarily affect the spleen, liver, lymph nodes, chest and spine. Enlargement of the spleen is also a consequence of its major role in clearing damaged red cells from the bloodstream.

4.8 β-Thalassemia major (Cooley's anemia)

A Detroit pediatrician, Thomas Cooley, first described this disorder in 1925 after noticing similarities in the appearance and clinical findings in several anemic children of Greek and Italian immigrants (Cooley et al., 1927). Prior to the advent of routine transfusion therapy, β-thalassemia major patients did not survive beyond the first few years of life. Survival is now improved with hypertransfusion regimens, iron chelation therapy, and bone marrow transplantation. Serious thalassemia is associated with iron overload, tissue damage, and increased risk of cardiovascular complications. β-Thalassemias are the most important among the thalassemia syndromes with an average trait prevalence of 7% in Greece, 15% among Cypriots, and 4.8% in Thailand (Weatherall, 1998, Weatherall & Clegg, 2001).

Clinical presentation of thalassemia major occurs between 6 and 24 months. Affected infants fail to thrive and become progressively pale. Feeding problems, diarrhea, irritability, recurrent bouts of fever, and progressive enlargement of the abdomen caused by spleen and liver enlargement may occur. In some developing countries, where due to the lack of resources patients are untreated or poorly transfused, the clinical picture of thalassemia major is characterized by growth retardation, pallor, jaundice, poor musculature, genu valgum, hepatosplenomegaly, leg ulcers, development of masses from extramedullary hematopoiesis, and skeletal changes resulting from expansion of the bone marrow. Skeletal changes include deformities in the long bones of the legs and typical craniofacial changes (bossing of the skull, prominent malar eminence, depression of the bridge of the nose, tendency to a mongoloid slant of the eye, and hypertrophy of the maxillae, which tends to expose the upper teeth).

In β-thalassemia major, severity of anemia requires initiation of blood tranfusions during infancy. If a regular transfusion program that maintains a minimum Hb concentration of 9.5 to 10.5 g/dL is initiated, growth and development tends to be normal up to 10 to12 years (Thalassemia International Federation: Guidelines for the clinical management of thalassemia 2nd edition. 2008 (http://www.thalassemia.org.cy)). Transfused patients may develop complications related to iron overload. Complications of iron overload in children include growth retardation and failure or delay of sexual maturation. Later iron overloadrelated complications include involvement of the heart (dilated myocardiopathy or rarely arrythmias), liver (fibrosis and cirrhosis), and endocrine glands (diabetes mellitus, hypogonadism and insufficiency of the parathyroid, thyroid, pituitary, and, less commonly, adrenal glands) (Borgna-Pignatti & Galanello, 2004).

4.9 Hemoglobin E (Hb-E)

The most common combination of β-thalassemia with abnormal Hb or structural Hb variant with thalassemic properties is Hb-E/β-thalassemia which is most prevalent in an area stretching from northern India and Bangladesh, through Laos, Carmbodia, Thailand, Vietnam, Malaysia, the Philippines, and Indonesia where the carrier frequency is around 50%. Hb-E is caused by a mutation of the 26th amino acid of a normal β-chain, glutamine, is replace by lysine. This mutation also activates a cryptic synthesis of the β-globin chain and leads to a thalassemic phenotype. Furthermore, the hemoglobin E gene, which can interact with β-thalassemic alleles and cause a broad phenotypic spectrum, reaches a frequency of up to 50% in Thailand (Weatherall 1998). These Hb-E/beta-thalassemias may be identified to three categories depending on the severity of symptoms:

4.10 Mild Hb-E/β-thalassemia

It is observed in about 15% of all cases in Southeast Asia. This group of patients maintains Hb levels between 9 and 12 g/dl and usually does not develop clinically significant problems. No treatment is required.

4.11 Moderately severe Hb-E/β-thalassemia

The majority of Hb-E/β-thalassemia cases fall into this category. The Hb levels remain at 6-7 g/dl and the clinical symptoms are similar to thalassemia intermedia. Transfusions are not required unless infections precipitate further anemia. Iron overload may occur.

4.12 Severe Hb-E/β-thalassemia

The Hb level can be as low as 4-5 g/dl. Patients in this group manifest symptoms similar to thalassemia major and are treated as thalassemia major patients.

Hb-E/β-thalassemia is more frequent than homozygous β-thalassemia in Thailand because of the high frequency of Hb-E (Fucharoen & Winichagoon, 2000) It is the most common severe thalassemia syndrome in adults. There are two types of Hb-E/β-thalassemia, classified based on the presence or absence of Hb-A, Hb-E/β^{+}-thalassemia and Hb-E/β^{0}-thalassemia. In patients with Hb- E/β^{0}-thalassemia, only Hb-E and Hb-F are present without detectable Hb-A. Hb-E constitutes between 40-60% of the hemoglobin with the rest Hb-F. Hb-A is present in Hb-E/β^{+}-thalassemia, resulting in a milder clinical picture than Hb-E/β^{0}-thalassemia. Since Hb-E/β-thalassemia is unique to Southeast Asia in general and to Thailand in particular, details of clinical manifestations as well as variability in disease severity will be discussed. In addition, as population migrations have caused the demography of the disease to shift worldwide, this thalassemia syndrome currently has more global implications.

5. Management of β-thalassemia major

5.1 Transfusions

Goals of transfusion therapy are the primary means of treatment for patients with severe β-thalassemia (Fosburg & Nathan 1990) for correction of anemia, suppression of erythropoiesis and inhibition of gastrointestinal iron absorption, which occurs in non transfused patients as a consequence of an increased ineffective erythropoiesis. The decision to start transfusion in patients with confirmed diagnosis of thalassemia should be based on the presence of severe anemia (Hb < 7 g/dl for more than two weeks, excluding other contributory causes such as infections). However, also in patients with Hb > 7 g/dl, other factors should be considered, including facial changes, poor growth, evidence of bony expansion and increasing splenomegaly. Post-transfusion Hb level of 9 to 10 g/dl - 13 to 14 g/dl prevents growth impairment, organ damage and bone deformities, allowing normal activity and quality of life (Thalassemia International Federation: Guidelines for the clinical management of thalassemia 2nd edition. 2008 [http://www.thalassemia.org.cy], Borgna-Pignatti & Galanello, 2004). The frequency of transfusion is usually every two to four weeks. Shorter intervals might further reduce the overall blood requirement, but are incompatible with an acceptable quality of life. The amount of blood to be transfused depends on several factors including weight of the patient, target increase in Hb level and hematocrit of blood unit. Appropriate graphs and formulae to calculate the amount of blood to be transfused are available (Thalassemia International Federation: Guidelines for the clinical management of thalassemia 2nd edition. 2008 [http://www.thalassemia. org.cy]). In general, the amount of transfused RBC should not exceed 15 to 20 ml/kg/day, infused at a maximum rate of 5 ml/kg/hour, to avoid a fast increase in blood volume. To monitor the effectiveness of transfusion therapy, some indices should be recorded at each transfusion, such as pre- and posttransfusion Hb, amount and hematocrit of the blood unit, daily Hb fall and transfusional interval. These measurements enable two important parameters to be calculated: red cell requirement and iron intake. Hypertransfusion and iron chelation is the standard therapy for thalassemia major. These transfusion regimens will provide a marked improvement in survival, growth and sexual development, prevent disfiguring bony abnormalities, decrease cardiac effort, and limit the development of hepatosplenomegaly. The red blood cell transfusions are lifesavers for patients with thalassemi. They are responsible for a series of inevitable complications and expose the patients to a variety of risks of long term transfusion therapy is iron overload.

6. Complications

In developed countries, patients are now given routine transfusion therapy, which has lengthened survival and altered the clinical course of the disease. Assessment and treatment of iron overload patients maintained on a regular transfusion regimen progressively develop clinical manifestations of iron overload. Iron overload of tissue is fatal with or without transfusion if not prevented or adequately treated. It is the most important complication of β-thalassemia and is a major focus of management (Olivieri & Brittenham 1997). Iron status should be accurately assessed in order to evaluate its clinical relevance, the need for treatment, and the timing and monitoring of chelation therapy. The iron status of multitransfused patients can be assessed by several methods. Serum ferritin has in general been found to correlate with body iron stores (Brittenham et al., 1993). After approximately one year of transfusions, iron begins to be deposited in parenchymal tissues (Risdon et al., 1973), where it may cause substantial toxicity as compared with that within reticuloendothelial cells (Hershko &Weatherall 1988, Hershko et al., 1998) Morbidity and mortality are now the result of chronic transfusion induced iron overload and most patients die of heart dysfunction of iron deposition (Zurlo et al., 1989). Iron accumulation in the liver causes fibrosis and cirrhosis (Fosburg & Nathan, 1990). Endocrine abnormalities related to iron overload include diabetes mellitus and impaired glucose tolerance, adrenal insufficiency, hypothyroidism, osteoporosis, hypoparathyroidism and hypogonadism (Fosburg & Nathan, 1990).

In the presence of excess metal iron can generate reactive oxygen species (ROS) (Stohs & Bagchi, 1995) that can modify oxidant-mediated intracellular signaling and cause oxidative damage to lipids, protein, and DNA. A well-studied physiologic biochemical iron reacts with O_2 species through the Fenton and Haber-Weiss reactions to form cytotoxic hydroxyl radicals. In this reaction, ferrous (Fe^{2+}) iron reacts with hydrogen peroxide to produce ferric (Fe^{3+}) iron and highly reactive hydroxyl radicals. This reaction is of particular importance in the liver because this organ, like the heart, has high steady-state production of O_2 and H_2O_2 from abundant mitochondrial activity (Eaton & Qian 2002). In addition to reacting with H_2O_2, ferrous iron may react with O_2 to produce ferric iron and a superoxide radical. The superoxide radical may engage in a series of reactions to generate hydrogen peroxide, which may serve as a substrate in the Fenton reaction to further result in the production of hydroxyl radicals. The hydroxyl radical can non-selectively attack proteins, nucleic acids, polysaccharides and lipids. Indeed, the production of hydroxyl radicals has been demonstrated in rats exhibiting iron overload (Kadiiska et al., 1995).

As indicate iron $$Fe^{3+} + O_2^{\bullet-} \rightarrow Fe^{2+} + O_2$$

$$Fe^{2+} + H_2O_2 \rightarrow Fe^{3+} + OH^- + \bullet OHOO$$

Net reaction: $$O_2^{\bullet-} + H_2O_2 \rightarrow \bullet OHOO + OH^- + O_2$$

These free radicals cause oxidative damage via lipid peroxidation, DNA hydroxylation, and protein oxidation (Schaible & Kaufmann 2004). Oxidative stress is another prominent mechanism of vasculopathy. In hemolytic disorders, the erythrocyte may be a major determinant of the global redox environment. The thalassemias have increased concentrations of ROS compared with normal red blood cells (Aslan & Freeman, 2004, Hebbel et al., 1982, Chakraborty & Bhattacharyya, 2001). Overproduction of ROS, such as superoxide, by both enzymatic (Xanthine oxidase, NADPH oxidase, uncoupled eNOS) and nonenzymatic pathways (Fenton chemistry), promotes intravascular oxidant stress that can likewise disrupt NO homeostasis and produce the highly oxidative peroxynitrite (Wood et al., 2008). Alters cell membrane lipids and abnormal erythrocyte phosphatidylserine (PS) exposure triggered in part by oxidative stress may also contribute to the early demise of the red blood cell in circulation, making them more vulnerable to enzymatic breakdown by secretory phospholipase A2, an important lipid mediator in inflammation. PS exposure also induces binding of red cells to endothelial cells, leading to sequestration of PS-exposing cells in peripheral blood vessels. This process can contribute to vascular dysfunction, hemolysis, and a pro-thrombotic state (Neidlinger et al., 2006). In the alterations in glutathione buffering system common to these hemoglobinopathies (Chakraborty & Bhattacharyya, 2001, Chakraborty & Bhattacharyya, 2001, Reid et al., 2006) may render erythrocytes incapable of handing the increased oxidant burden, thereby predisposing them to hemolysis. Hydroxyl radical formed by iron catalyzed reactions reacts with a polyunsaturated fatty acid of a membrane lipid caused lipid peroxidation. The resulting lipid hydroperoxides can affect membrane fluidity and membrane protein function. A large number of lipid breakdown products are generated including malondialdehyde (MDA) and 4-hydroxy-2-nonenal (4-HNE). In rat models of iron overload, lipid peroxidation has been found in whole liver and also in isolated cellular fractions including mitochondria, microsomes and lysosomes (Bacon et al., 1983, Britton et al., 1987). The reactive aldehydes

(MDA and HNE) can react with proteins to form adducts. The MDA and HNE-lysine adducts have been found in hepatocytes and plasma from rats fed a diet containing carbonyl iron for 13 weeks (Houglum et al., 1990).

Iron overload causes vitamin C to be oxidized at an increased rate, leading to vitamin C deficiency in these patients. Vitamin C in children <10 years and 100 mg >10 years at the time of DFO infusion may increase the chelatable iron available in the body, thus increasing the efficacy of chelation. However there is currently no evidence supporting the use of vitamin C supplements in patients on DFP, DFX or combination treatment. Vitamin C may increase iron absorption from the gut, labile iron and hence iron toxicity and may therefore be particularly harmful to patients who are not receiving DFO, as iron mobilized by the vitamin C will remain unbound, causing tissue damage. The effectiveness and safety of vitamin E supplementation in thalassemia major has not been formally assessed and it is not possible to give recommendations about its use at this time.

7. Assessment of iron overload

Patients maintained on a regular transfusion regimen progressively develop clinical manifestations of iron overload: hypogonadism (35-55% of the patients), hypothyroidism (9-11%), hypoparathyroidism (4%), diabetes (6-10%), liver fibrosis, and heart dysfunction (33%) (Cunningham et al., 2004, Borgna-Pignatti et al., 2004). Iron status should be accurately assessed in order to evaluate its clinical relevance, the need for treatment, and the timing and monitoring of chelation therapy. The iron status of multitransfused patients can be assessed by several methods. Serum ferritin has in general been found to correlate with body iron stores (Brittenham et al 1993). However, as a single value it is not always reliable because, being an acute phase reactant, it is influenced by other factors such as inflammatory disorders, liver disease, malignant. Despite this, serial measurements of serum ferritin remain a reliable and the easiest method to evaluate iron overload and efficacy of chelation therapy. Determination of liver iron concentration in a liver biopsy specimen shows a high correlation with total body iron accumulation and is considered the gold standard for the evaluation of iron overload (Angelucci et al., 2000). However, liver biopsy is an invasive technique with the possibility (though low) of complications. Moreover, we should consider that the presence of hepatic fibrosis, which commonly occurs in individuals with iron overload and HCV infection, and heterogeneous liver iron distribution can lead to possible false negative results (Villeneuve et al., 1996). In recent years, nuclear magnetic resonance imaging (MRI) techniques for assessing iron loading in the liver and heart have been introduced (Wood et al., 2004, Tanner et al., 2006). R2 and T2* parameters have been validated for liver iron concentration. Cardiac T2* is reproducible, transferable between different scanners, correlates with cardiac function, and relates to tissue iron concentration.

As the body has no effective means for removing iron, the only way to remove excess iron is to use iron binders (chelators), which allow iron excretion through the urine and/or stool. As a general rule, patients should start iron chelation treatment once they have had 10-20 transfusions or when ferritin levels rise above 1000 ng/ml (Thalassemia International Federation: Guidelines for the clinical management of thalassemia 2nd edition. 2008 [http://www.thalassemia.org.cy]). Chelation of iron with desferoxamine is effective in reducing iron load and extending life expectancy. However, to be effective, this drug must be given by subcutaneous continuous infusion each day and is not without side effects including hearing and visual loss (Fosburg & Nathan, 1990). Several oral agents for chelation are in various stages of testing and, if effective, will improve the quality of life for

chronically transfused patients (Nathan & Piomelli 1990). Other therapies such as splenectomy and vitamin and folic acid supplements are also of benefit.
The first drug available for treatment of iron overload was deferoxamine (DFO), an exadentate iron chelator that is not orally absorbed and usually as a subcutaneous 8- to 12-hour nightly infusion, 5-7 nights a week. Average dosage is 20-40 mg/kg body weight for children and 30-50 mg/kg body weight for adults (Thalassemia International Federation: Guidelines for the clinical management of thalassemia 2nd edition. 2008 [http://www.thalassemia.org.cy], Borgna-Pignatti & Galanello, 2004). In high risk cases, continuous administration of DFO via an implanted delivery system (Port-acath) or subcutaneously, at doses between 50 and 60 mg/ kg per day, were the only options to intensify the chelation treatment before the advent of the combined therapy with DFO and deferiprone (Anderson et al., 2004). Implanted delivery systems are associated with risk of thrombosis and infection. With DFO, iron is excreted both in faeces (about 40%) and in urine. The most frequent adverse effects of DFO are local reactions at the site of infusion, such as pain, swelling, induration, erythema, burning, pruritus, wheals and rash, occasionally accompanied by fever, chills and malaise.

7.1 Iron overload-related complications

Iron overload of tissue with or without transfusion is fatal, which is the most important complication of β-thalassemia if not prevented or adequately treated, which is a major focus of management (Olivieri & Brittenham, 1997). In patients who are not receiving transfusions, abnormally regulated iron absorption results in increases in body iron burden, depending on the severity of erythroid expansion (Pippard et al., 1979, Pootrakul et al., 1988). Regular transfusions may double this rate of iron accumulation. Most clinical manifestations of iron loading do not appear until the second decade of life in patients with inadequate chelation. After approximately one year of transfusions, iron begins to be deposited in parenchymal tissues, (Risdon et al., 1973) where it may cause substantial toxicity as compared with that within retic-uloendothelial cells (Hershko & Weatherall 1988, Hershko et al., 1998). As iron loading progresses, the capacity of serum transferrin, the main transport protein of iron, to bind and detoxify iron may be exceeded and a non-transferrin-bound fraction of plasma iron may promote the generation of free hydroxyl radicals, propagators of oxygen-related damage (Hershko & Weatherall 1988, Hershkoet al., 1998). The advances in free-radical chemistry have clarified the toxic properties of these and other oxygen-derived species generated by iron, which may cause widespread tissue damage (Hershkoet al., 1998). Although the body maintains a number of antioxidant mechanisms against damage induced by free radicals, including superoxide dismutases, catalase, and glutathione peroxidase, in patients with large iron burdens these may not prevent oxidative damage (Hershko & Weatherall 1988, Hershkoet al., 1998). In the absence of chelating therapy the accumulation of iron results in progressive dysfunction of the heart, liver, and endocrine glands (Olivieri & Brittenham 1997). Extensive iron deposits are associated with cardiac hypertrophy and dilatation, degeneration of myocardial fibers, and in rare cases fibrosis (Buja & Roberts 1971). In patients who are receiving transfusions but not chelating therapy, symptomatic cardiac disease has been reported within 10 years after the start of transfusion (Wolfe et al., 1985) and may be aggravated by myocarditis (Kremastinos et al., 1995) and pulmonary hypertension (Aessopos et al., 1995, Duet al., 1997). Iron-induced liver disease is a common cause of death in older patients (Zurlo et al., 1989) and is often aggravated by infection with hepatitis C virus. Within two years after the start of transfusions, collagen formation (Iancu et al., 1977) and portal fibrosis (Thakerngpol et al., 1996) have been reported; in the absence of chelating therapy, cirrhosis may develop in the first decade of life (Risdon et al., 1973, Witzleben & Wyatt 1961, Jean et al., 1984). The striking increases in survival in patients with β-thalassemia over the past decade have focused attention on abnormal endocrine function (delayed puberty, hypogonadism and assisted reproduction), now the most prevalent iron-induced complication in older patients. Iron loading within the anterior pituitary is the primary cause of disturbed sexual maturation, reported in 50 percent of both boys and girls with the condition (Italian Working Group on Endocrine Complications, 1995) and also cause growth deficiency, which therapeutic used of GH to thalassemia patients proven to have GH deficiency, who may have a satisfactory response to treatment (Karydis et al., 2004, Wu et al., 2003). Furthermore, early secondary amenorrhea occurs in approximately one quarter of female patients over the age of 15 years (Italian Working Group on Endocrine Complications, 1995).

Even in the modern era of iron-chelating therapy, diabetes mellitus is observed in about 5 percent of adults (Italian Working Group on Endocrine Complications, 1995). As the iron burden increases and iron-related liver dysfunction progresses, hyperinsulinemia occurs as a result of reduced extraction of insulin by the liver, leading to exhaustion of beta cells and reduced circulating insulin concentrations (cause diabetes and impaired glucose tolerance) (Cavallo-Perin et al., 1995). Studie reporting reduced serum concentrations of trypsin and lipase (Gullo et al., 1993) suggest that the exocrine pancreas is also damaged by iron loading. Over the long term, iron deposition also damages the thyroid (hypothyroidism), parathyroid (hypoparathyroidism), and adrenal glands (Magro et al., 1990, Sklar et al., 1987) and may provoke pulmonary hypertension, right ventricular dilatation, and restrictive lung disease (Du et al., 1997, Factor et al., 1994, Tai et al., 1996).

In most studies, bone density is markedly reduced (cause osteoporosis) in patients with β-thalassemia, particularly those with hypogonadism. Osteopenia may be related to marrow expansion, even in patients who receive transfusions, (Pootrakul et al., 1988) or to iron-induced osteoblast dysfunction, diabetes, hypoparathyroidism, or hypogonadism (Anapliotou et al., 1995).

7.2 Splenectomy

If the annual red cell requirement exceeds 180-200 ml/Kg of RBC (assuming that the Hct of the unit of red cells is about 75%), splenectomy should be considered, provided that other reasons for increased consumption, such as hemolytic reactions, have been excluded. Other indications for splenectomy are symptoms of splenic enlargement, leukopenia and/or thrombocytopenia and increasing iron overload despite good chelation (Weatherall & Clegg 2001).

8. Bone marrow and cord blood transplantation

Successful allogeneic bone marrow transplant for severe β-thalassemia was first reported in 1982 (Thomas et al., 1982). Since that time, numerous transplants have been performed with the best outcome for well chelated patients with no liver disease (Lucarelli et al., 1990). Bone marrow transplantation (BMT) from HLA-identical donors has been successfully performed worldwide. BMT remains the only definitive cure currently available for patients with thalassemia. The outcome of BMT is related to the pretransplantation clinical conditions, specifically the presence of hepatomegaly, extent of liver fibrosis, history of regular chelation and hence severity of iron accumulation. In patients without the above risk factors, stem cell transplantation from an HLA identical sibling has a disease free survival rate over 90% (Gaziev & Lucarelli, 2003). The major limitation of allogenic BMT is the lack of an HLA-identical sibling donor for the majority of affected patients. In fact, approximately 25-30% of thalassemic patients could have a matched sibling donor. BMT from unrelated donors has been carried out on a limited number of individuals with β-thalassemia. Provided that selection of the donor is based on stringent criteria of HLA compatibility and that individuals have limited iron overload, results are comparable to those obtained when the donor is a compatible sib (La Nasa et al., 2005). However, because of the limited number of individuals enrolled, further studies are needed to confirm these preliminary findings. If BMT is successful, iron overload may be reduced by repeated phlebotomy, thus eliminating the need for iron chelation. Complications include a rate of Chronic graft versus-host disease (GVHD) of variable severity may occur in 2-8% of individuals and a variable incidence of mixed chi-merism (Angelucci et al., 1997). Post-transplantation management of preexisting hepatic iron overload, iron-induced cardiac dysfunction, and viral hepatitis may prevent progression of these processes (Angelucci et al., 1997). Cord-blood transplantation, the use of unrelated phenotypically matched donors, and in utero transplantation (Westgren et al., 1996), offers a good probability of a successful cure and is associated with a low risk of GVHD (Locatelli et al., 2003, Pinto & Roberts, 2008). By this mean, for couples who have already had a child with thalassemia and who undertake prenatal diagnosis in a subsequent pregnancy, prenatal identification of HLA compatibility between the affected child and an unaffected fetus allows collection of placental blood at delivery and the option of cord blood transplantation to cure the affected child (Orofino et al., 2003). On the other hand, in cases with an affected fetus and a previous normal child, the couple may decide to continue the pregnancy and pursue BMT later, using the normal child as the donor. At present this therapy is of limited applicability because only a small number of patients have a related, human leukocyte antigen matched donor. Improvements in transplantation from unrelated donors may expand the use of this treatment in the future.

9. Genetic counseling and prenatal diagnosis

Prevention of β-thalassemia is based on carrier identification, genetic counseling and prenatal diagnosis (Cao et al., 1998). Carrier detection has been previously described. Genetic counseling provides information for individuals and at risk couples (i.e. both carriers) regarding the mode of inheritance, the genetic risk of having affected children and the natural history of the disease including the available treatment and therapies under investigation. Prenatal diagnosis for pregnancies at increased risk is possible by analysis of DNA extracted from fetal cells obtained by amniocentesis, usually performed at approximately 15-18 weeks gestation or chorionic villi sampling (CVS) at 10-11 weeks gestation. Both disease-causing alleles must be identified before prenatal testing can be performed. Analysis of fetal cells in maternal blood and analysis of fetal DNA in maternal plasma for the presence of the father's mutation are currently under investigation (Mavrou et al., 2007, Lo 2005). Pre-implantation genetic diagnosis may be available for families in which the disease-causing mutations have been identified.

10. Screening and diagnosis for hemoglobin variants and thalassemia

There are many techniques that have been used to screen and diagnose for hemoglobin variants and thalassemia, mostly done in combinations. These techniques were ranging from screening to extensive analysis, including a few indirect studies. Screening techniques can indicate a defect in hemoglobin synthesis. Positive results from these tests need confirmation by a more extensive analysis technique. Negative results normally help in cutting down the number of subjects that need to be further diagnosed by a more advanced and complicated testing. Extensive analysis techniques can give more precise information in types of thalassemia or types of Hb variants. They normally perform with higher instruments and technologies, and therefore are more expensive than screening techniques. The flow chart shown in Fig 4 summarizes the techniques for diagnosis of thalassemia and hemoglobinopathies that are commonly used in most laboratories.

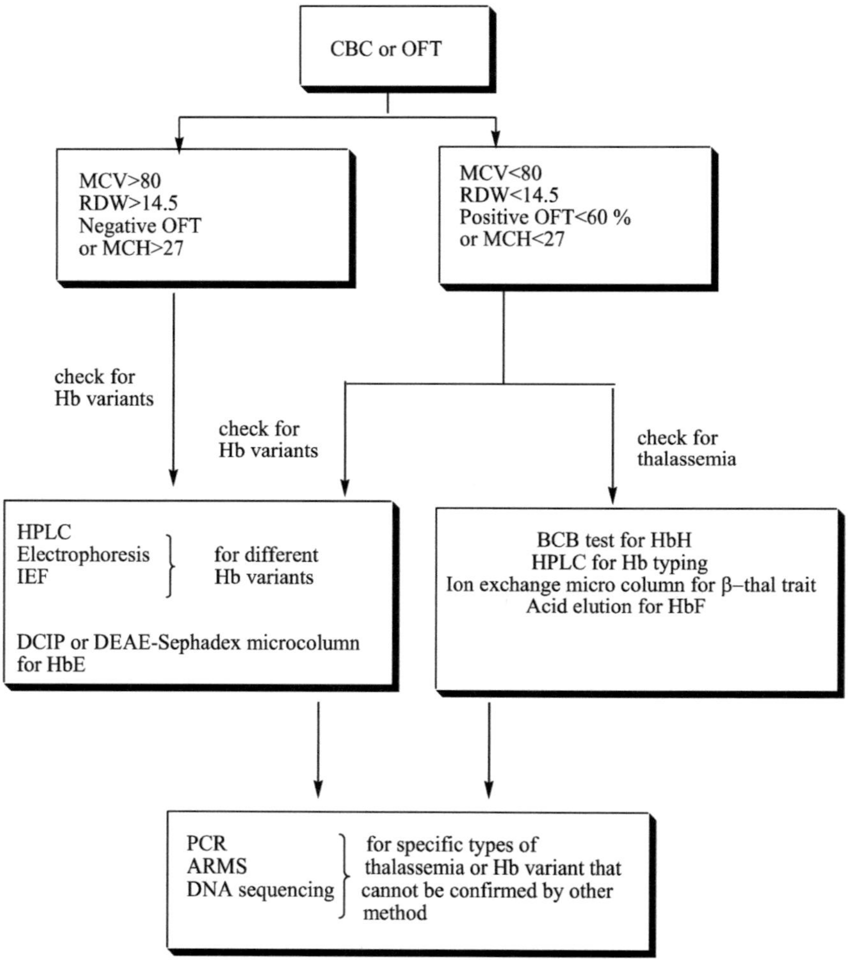

Fig. 4. The summerised chart of normal process of hemoglobin variants and thalassemia

10.1 Screening techniques for thalassemia

Screening techniques are defined as simple techniques and low cost which can indicate the possibility of having thalassemia. These techniques should involve the least sample pretreatment and be rapid, and may not need special instrumentation. These techniques could be used in any primary health care setting. This would lead to low cost and high sample throughput analysis. Positive samples need further confirmatory test while negative samples can be eliminated from further complicated and expensive testing. These screening techniques cannot provide the information on the exact type of hemoglobinopathies, but can help in cutting down the number of samples from unnecessary complicated and expensive testing.

10.1.1 Complete blood count (CBC)

Complete blood count, a primary screening for thalassemia used an electronic blood-cell counter to provide accurate erythrocyte indices as the characteristics of the blood (Hillman & Ault, 1980). The main features of the blood tested in the CBC are the total white blood cell count (WBC), red blood cell count (RBC), hematocrit (Hct), hemoglobin (Hb), red cell distribution width (RDW), peripheral blood smear and other important erythrocyte indices (EI), included mean corpuscular volume (MCV), mean corpuscular hemoglobin (MCH), and mean corpuscular hemoglobin concentration (MCHC) (Klee et al., 2000). Among these parameters, MCV and MCH are the most important indicies that can indicate the existence of thalassemia trait, i.e., when individuals who have hypochromic microcytosis with MCV< 80 fL and MCH< 27 pg should be investigated further.

Parameter	Normal range
RBCs (x10^{12}/L)	3.8 - 5.8
Hb (g/dL)	11.5 - 16.5
Hct (%)	37.0 - 47.0
MCV (fL)	76 - 96
MCH (pg)	27 - 32
MCHC (g/dL)	30.0 - 35.0
RDW (%)	11.5 - 14.5

Table 2. The normal ranges of each parameter

In table 2 summarizes the tests performed in the CBC, the calculation needed for each parameters and the approximate normal cutoff level. However, due to the similar lowed blood cell count between the patients with thalassemia and the ones with iron deficiency, it has been suggested that in the geographic regions where iron deficiency rate is high, the cutoffs for thalassemia interpretation should be adjusted to more suitable values by using a receiver operator char acteristic (ROC) curve (Kotwal et al., 1999), which in this case should better differentiate thalassemic microcytosis from non-thalassemic ones (i.e., iron deficiency patients). As the study in Thailand, they used the combination of MCH (25) pg, RDW (14.5%) and OFT (<55%) with the lower cutoff to increase the screening specificity in those area (Tangvarasittichai et al., 2004). Many laboratories use a CBC autoanalyzer which can provide many blood parameters (such as MCH, MCV, RDW) also be added along with osmotic fragility test an alternative screening test for specific thalassemia testing.

Combined red blood cells indices for α-Thalassemia-1 Screening

1. Red blood cells (RBC) indices included hemoglobin (Hb), hematocrit (Hct), mean corpuscular volume (MCV), mean corpuscular hemoglobin (MCH), MCHC, and RDW from the automated blood cell analyzer
2. In the study of Tangvarasittichai et al. (2004) used the ROC curve and the AUC of each parameters showed the % specificity of each parameter and their combination for screening the α-thalassemia-1 elute as in the table below.

Parameters (Cut-off point)	% Specificity
MCH/OFT/RDW (25 pg/55%/14.5%)	92.4
MCH/OFT/MCV (25 pg/55%/75 fL)	91.9
MCH/OFT (25 pg/55%)	91.7
MCH/RDW/MCV (25 pg/14.5%/75 fL)	90.0
MCH/RDW (25 pg/14.5%)	89.6
MCH/MCV (25 pg/75 fL)	88.5

Table 3. The combined red blood cells indices to increase the specificity for screening α-thalassemia 1

10.1.2 Osmotic fragility test (OFT)

The main purpose of this technique is used as a diagnostic test for the hereditary spherocytosis and it is also useful for screening of thalassemia. This simple technique utilizes osmosis, the movement of water from lower to higher salt concentration region, to test for the osmotic resistance of the red blood cell (Fernandez-Alberti et al., 2000). A single hypotonic saline solution can be prepared from dilution of a Tyrode's solution, which is composed of NaCl, KCl, $CaCl_2 \cdot 6H_2O$, $MgCl_2 \cdot 6H_2O$, $NaHCO_3$, NaH_2PO_4, glucose and distilled water (Electron Microscope Sciences Catalog, Available: http://www.emsdiasum. com/ems/chemicals/ salt. html (October 16, 2003). Different laboratories may be using slightly different recipes for preparation of hypotonic salt solution, but all are normally based on the same concept of kinetic osmotic fragility. The most simple of a single hypotonic saline solution can be prepared which is composed of 0.45% glycerine and 0.36% sodium chlorine in phosphate buffer (pH7.4) (Sirichotiyakul et al., 2004). Whole blood is thoroughly mixed with this solution. In a hypotonic condition, the concentration of salt on the outside of a cell is lower than that on the inside, resulting in net water movement into cells. Normal red blood cells are broken within 1–2 min and the mixture then turns clear and reddish. Abnormal red blood cells have deviated osmotic resistances as compared to normal red cells. Spherocytes and erythrocytes with various membrane defects may show decreased osmotic resistance. However, red blood cells of thalassemia have higher osmotic resistance and thus have slower rupture rate, therefore the mixture remains turbid even after 1-2 h (Silvestroni & Bianco 1983). The OFT is a quick preliminary and very economic test before performing further studies of the blood cells.

The percent hemolysis of more than 60% was considered normal (no α-thalassmia-1 or β-thalassemia trait). The screening test (OFT) was considered abnormal or positive test when the percent hemolysis is of 60% or less [β-thalassemia trait= 30.5±1.4%; α-thalassmia 1 = 30.8±1.2%] and the positive test of gold standard or final diagnosis was considered either when HbA2 levels of 4.1–9% or positive PCR (SEA type).

10.2 Conventional confirmatory tests for thalassemia and Hb variants

These are useful tests to confirm the existence of certain Hb variants or abnormal level of some Hb types. Confirmatory tests for Hb variants include deoxyhemoglobin solubility test (DST) for detection of HbS and dichlorophenol indophenol precipitation test (DCIP) for detection of HbE. HbH disease which relates to α-thalassemia can be detected by DCIP and brilliant cresyl blue test (BCB). Alkaline resistant hemoglobin test (ART) and acid elution stain (AES) are used for detection of abnormal levels of HbF, which can help identify some types of thalassemia. The ion exchange microcolumn technique is used to quantify the amount of HbA2 and HbF to identify β-thal trait, E-trait and EE homozygotes. These conventional techniques are relatively low cost and do not require complicated instrumentation. However, some of these techniques may need a highly experienced operator to translate the results. Therefore, availability of more modern instrumentation that can provide more precise information with little requirement of an experienced operator and less usage of toxic chemicals diminishes the use of some of these conventional techniques such as DST and ART.

10.2.1 Deoxyhemoglobin solubility test

Deoxyhemoglobin solubility test for HbS based on its insolubility in a potassium phosphate saponin buffer solution (composed of K_2HPO_4, KH_2PO_4, saponin and distilled water). Turbidity would be observed within 5 min if the whole blood containing HbS were mixed with sodium hyposulfite and saponin buffer. This test can discriminate samples with HbS from samples with almost all other hemoglobins except Hb Bart's and some rare sickle Hb, if a positive test result is shown (i.e., high enough turbidity that newsprint cannot be seen through the test mixture when placed behind the tube), then a follow-up test by electrophoresis is recommended. A false-negative result may be from a high anemic condition (Fairbanks, 1980, Nalbandian et al., 1971, Greenberg et al., 1972).

10.2.2 Hemoglobin precipitation test

Some hemoglobin variants such as HbH (β4 with α- thalassemia) and Hb Koln ($\beta^{98Val \rightarrow Met}$) are classified as unstable hemoglobins which can be precipitated by heating or adding a chemical such as isopropanol or dichlorophenol indophenol (Dispenzieri, 2001, Winichagoon et al., 2002).

10.2.2.1 The heat instability test

Test can be carried out at either medium temperature (50°C) for 1-2 h or at high temperature (68°C) with chemical reaction aids for 1 min. Although taking longer time, the medium temperature stability test is very simple. The clear supernatant of erythrocyte hemolysate in Tris buffer medium, obtained after removing plasma, hemolyzing with distilled water and removing stroma, is placed in the 50 ◦C water bath for 1 h. Normal hemolysates remain completely clear, while unstable hemoglobins cause flocculation of various turbidities. The test can be done much faster by using chemicals, i.e., KCN and $K_3Fe(CN)_6$, to form hemolysate cyanmethemoglobin. In a phosphate buffer medium, this hemolysate cyanmethemoglobin is agitated rapidly in the 68 ◦C hot water bath. After 1 min, normal hemolysate may show slight cloudiness and therefore this high temperature method, even though very fast, may need high experience in interpretation in order to avoid a false-positive interpretation (Klee, 1980, Dacie et al., 1964).

Hemolysate preparation (For heat, isopropanol precipitation)

Reagent: (i) 0.9% NaCl, (ii) Transformation solution (TS): consist with 0.2 g $K_3Fe(CN)_6$ and 0.2 g KCN in 1000 ml distill water (DW) (iii) Carbon tetrachloride (CCl_4) solution
Sample: EDTA whole blood. **Reagent**: 0.15 M Tris-HCl buffer.

Type	%Hb instability
Normal	2.3±1.2
HbH	9.7±2.4
α-Thalassemia trait	4.3±1.7
Homozygous β-thalassemia	5.4±1.6
β-Thalassemia trait	4.3±2.3
β-Thalassemia/HbE	6.4±2.2

Table 4. % Hb instability value by Heat Precipitation

10.2.2.2 Isopropanol precipitation test

Another way to demonstrate the Hb instability is with isopropanol precipitation. Packed erythrocytes, cold deionized water and CCl_4 (1:1:1.5 ratio) are placed in a closed tube and vortexed for a few minutes, followed by centrifugation. The clear supernatant is then mixed with isopropanol–Tris buffer at a control temperature of about 37 ◦C. Unstable hemoglobins cause more turbidity over time, while normal hemoglobins remain clear for at least 30 min. The isopropanol test is reported to have some limitations on the subjects that contain ≥5% HbF, and those that are inappropriately preserved (i.e., unrefrigerated or too old samples) may give false positive results. Adding anticoagulating reagent can help reduce the false reading but it is suggested that the samples with high HbF should be tested by heat stability, as it is not interfered by HbF (Klee, 1980, Brosious et al., 1976, Carrell & Kay, 1972).
Reagent: 0.1 M Tris-HCl buffer pH 7.4; Isopropanol buffer: as a mixture of 17 ml isopropanol with 83 ml of Tris-HCl buffer

Type	%Hb instability
Normal	1.2±1.1
HbH	16.1±5.2
α-Thalassemia trait	3.5±1.9
Homozygous β-thalassemia	4.2±3.0
β-Thalassemia trait	3.2±2.1
β-Thalassemia/HbE trait	2.9±1.7

Table 5. % Hb instability value by Isopropanol Precipitation

10.2.2.3 Dichlorophenol indophenol (DCIP) precipitation test

The dichlorophenol indophenol (DCIP) precipitation test is also used widely to screen for HbE and HbH. DCIP can oxidize HbE and HbH faster than any other type of hemoglobin, and therefore it can be used to screen for HbE and HbH. Interpretation of results can be difficult since it involves observing the cloudiness in a deep blue color of DPIC solution. However, a reducing agent may be added to overcome this problem. For example, in the AOAC standard titration method for ascorbic acid, the color of an oxidant DCIP is changed from dark blue to light blue on the way to the end point pink (Helrich, 1995). Therefore, if a small amount of ascorbic acid were added to the DCIP thalassemia test, then the observation could be made more accurately under the light blue condition.
Reagents: DCIP reagent: Tris base 4.36 g, EDTA $Na_2.2H_2O$ 2.68 g, DCIP (Sigma) 0.0276 g, Saponin 0.05 g dissolve in DW adjusted pH 7.5 by 6M HCl , then DW to 500 ml store at 4°C.
Interpretation results: Negative = Clear; Positive = cloudiness in a deep blue color of DCIP solution. Hemoglobin precipitation tests can be used to screen for some hemoglobin variants but they may not be able to speciate the types of hemoglobins (i.e., HbE and HbH show similar results). Further tests are needed to pinpoint the exact type.

10.2.3 Brilliant cresyl blue test or new methylene blue test

Both simple colorimetric tests are based on the same procedures with different reagents, specifically performed for HbH diagnosis. HbH is unstable and it precipitates in the red cells, giving the appearance of many small golf balls inside the cells that can be observed when staining the blood film with brilliant cresyl blue ($C_{17}H_2OClN_3O$) or new methylene blue ($C_{18}H_{22}ClN_3S{:}SClZnCl_2$) (Brilliant cresyl blue MSDS sheet, Available: http://www.proscitech. com/ catalogue/ msds/ c085.pdf (April 14, 2003), New Methylene,

Blue MSDS Sheet. Available: http://www.jtbaker. com/ msds/ englishhtml/n2700.htm (April 20, 2003)). The incubation time of blood and the reagents (brilliant cresyl blue in sodium citrate media) takes about 1 h in a controlled temperature setting of about 37 °C (Rigas et al., 1961). This test is very useful to confirm for α-thalassemia involving HbH inclusion body. However, the technique yields low sensitivity for α-thal trait and therefore it should only be used as a confirmatory test, but not for screening of α-thalassemia.

10.2.4 Alkaline resistant hemoglobin test

This is a test for abnormal level of fetal hemoglobin (HbF). Normally hemoglobins are denatured at alkaline pH such as in NaOH solution and they can be precipitated readily with saturated ammonium sulfate ($(NH_4)_2SO_4$) solution. However, HbF is not denatured as easily and remains soluble. Differences in alkaline resistance of the normal Hb and fetal Hb allow for rapid testing for the amount of HbF in blood. The procedure consists of a few experimental and calculation steps (Klee, 1980, Singer et al., 1951, Betke et al., 1959). A suspended mixture of Hb-cyanide-ferricyanide (or cyanmethemoglobin) is prepared by adding packed red cells, obtained from centrifugation of whole blood in isotonic saline solution, into a cyanide-ferricyanide solution (KCN and $K_3Fe(CN)_6$ in distilled water). Then NaOH is added and the solution is mixed for a few minutes before adding the saturated $(NH_4)_2SO_4$ solution. Coagulated protein can be removed by filtering the mixture until a clear filtrate is obtained. The percent of alkaline resistant hemoglobin is calculated based on the absorbance of the filtrate (Df) and the absorbance of the 1:10 dilution of the original cyanmethemoglobin without NaOH and $(NH_4)_2SO_4$ added (Db) at 540 nm, using the following equation: (100 Df)/(10 Db).

In a normal person more than 1 year old, the percentage of HbF should be expressed as being less than 1-2% by using this method. Higher levels of HbF will be suspected of having a hemoglobin disorder of some kind. Although the method was found to mistakenly yield lower results for a subject with HbF higher than 30% of total hemoglobin, such as in umbilical cord blood of newborns, this method was sufficiently sensitive and reproducible for measuring 1-10% HbF, providing that final cyanmethemoglobin concentration is higher than 480 mg/100 ml (Pembrey et al., 1972). In the cases where high amount of HbF is present, an alternative method such as immunological determination of HbF, e.g., by the gel precipitation or immuno-diffusion, involving the use of monoclonal antibody against HbF, may be used (Weatherall & Clegg, 2001, Yuregir 1976, Dover et al., 1979).

Reagent: (i) TS as 0.2 g $K_3(FeCN)_6$ and 0.2 g KCN in 100 ml DW (ii) 1.2 N NaOH (iii) saturated (sat) $(NH_4)2SO_4$

Type	%HbF
Normal	<1
β-Thalassemia trait	1- 10 %
β-Thalassemia major	>50%

Table 6.

10.2.5 Acid elution stain (modified Kleihauer–Betke test)

This is a simple test for HbF and Hb Bart's. After smearing a blood sample on the slide and letting it dry, the slide is immersed in an 80% alcohol solution (ethyl, methyl or propyl alcohol) for 2-3 min. After that, the slide is immersed in a staining solution of Amido Black 10B ($C_{22}H_{14}N_6O_9S_2Na_2$) prepared in alcohol with pH adjusted to 2.0. After 3 min, the slide is washed under running water for 1 min. In the acidic condition, HbA, HbA_2, HbE, and HbH will be eluted out of the blood cells, leaving the cells empty (ghost cells) and showing no color. HbF and Hb Bart's can tolerate acid and are stained by the Amido Black 10B, showing dark blue color of the cells which can be observed under the microscope. There are a few precautions that need to be taken when working with this technique. If the slide is left dry for too long, HbA will not be eluted out. The concentration of alcohol is also important because alcohol higher than 85% will cause HbA to stay in the cell, while lower than 65% will cause vacuolization of HbF. In addition, if the pH of the solution is higher than 2.5, HbA will not be eluted. All these cases will show false results (Research Organics. Available: http://www.resorg.com/(October 17, 2003), Betke & Sanguansermsri, 1972). The drawbacks of this technique are time consuming and subjected to human error. Another possible way of detection of HbF is flow cytometry which is more precise as described later.

10.2.6 Ion exchange micro-column

In the regions where economic restriction does not allow for the use of a relatively higher cost instrument such as HPLC, a cheaper method such as this ion exchange microcolumn along with other inexpensive tests can be used in combination to diagnose the type of thalassemia. This technique is based on ion exchange chromatography as a simplified version of high performance liquid chromatography. The use of diethylaminoethyl DEAE anion exchanger, packed in a relatively cheap and small syringe, and Tris-HCl mobile phase can be adapted to separate HbA2 and HbF effectively. The relative amounts of these Hbs can be estimated by calculating the peak areas of the absorbance, measured at 415 nm, of fractions eluted from the column. It has been shown that the results obtained from the batchwise micro-column are in agreement with those from HPLC, though the method lacks automation and yields lower precision (Dozy et al., 1968, Brosious et al., 1978, Srisawang et al., 2003). However, the result from ion exchange micro-column technique is acceptably accurate and precise and can be used to confirm some types of thalassemias such as β-thalassemia trait. In addition, with its simplicity and low cost, some laboratories perform this technique together with the OF tests as regular screening techniques, especially where thalassemia cases related to abnormal ratio of HbA2 and HbF is commonly found such as in Thailand. It has been estimated that the cost for chemicals and materials per test of the micro-column technique is approximately five times less than that of HPLC. Even though the total analysis time per run is longer than automated HPLC (4 h versus 20 min), many ion exchange micro-columns can be set up and run at the same time. Therefore, the total analysis time of, e.g., 50 tests using multiple micro-columns at one time is less than performing 50 continuous HPLC runs (16 h using HPLC and 4 h using ion exchange micro-columns). In addition, an attempt to reduce the analysis time per run and to make the micro-column technique more automated has been carried out. A flow injection analysis system was joined together with a much smaller ion exchange column to improve the analysis time for hemoglobin typing as compared to the batch process (Srisawang et al., 2003). More work needs to be done, but the preliminary results have suggested that the flow based and reduced volume ion exchange column system has the potential to improve the analysis time per run and to greatly reduce the amount of blood sample needed for the analysis.

Hemoglobin E detection: DEAE Sepharose Microcolumn (GE Healthcare BioSciences, Uppsala, Sweden)

Sufficient DEAE Sepharose was added to columns of 10x1.5 cm to produce a 2 cm Sepharose layer (Figure 5), was saturated with buffer A (0.05 M Tris, pH 8.5). Hemolysate was loaded in the column (40µl of EDTA blood sample to 10 ml 0.05 M, pH 8.0 Tris buffer B. Hb E, which is a weak anion, eluted first from the microcolumn by using buffer B as the elution buffer. The Hb E positive blood samples produced an orange eluted. Hb E negative sample produced a colorless. This Hb E microcolumn testing was approximately 10-15 minutes.

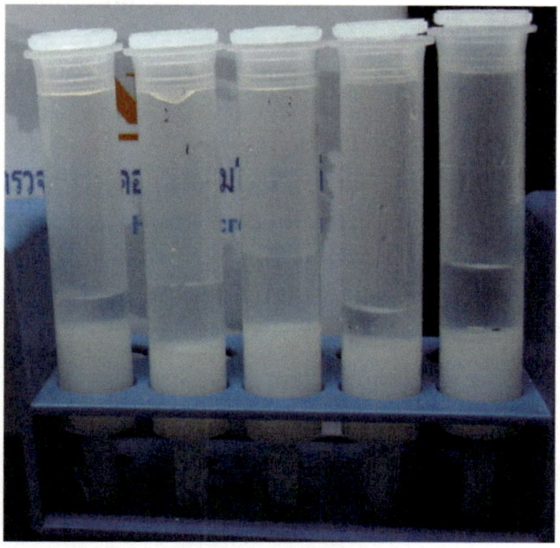

Fig. 5. DEAE Sepharose Microcolumn after preparation for hemoglobin E detection

10.3 Instrumental techniques for determination of thalassemia and Hb variants

These techniques involve modern technologies of complicated instrumentation. They can be automated and are usually faster and more reliable but more expensive than the conventional techniques. Even though these techniques can provide detailed information and can help in diagnosis of many types of Hb variants, there are a few exceptional Hb variant cases that cannot be identified with these techniques, and more extensive confirmatory tests are needed. Most instrumental techniques can perform qualitative and quantitative analysis, but with limited ways to accurately quantitate the signals, such as in gel electrophoresis, these techniques have be used mainly for diagnosis of Hb variants rather than for detection of abnormal level of Hbs in thalassemia diagnosis, as shown in the flow chart in Fig. 4.

10.3.1 High performance liquid chromatography

High-performance liquid chromatographic (HPLC) methods with high sensitivity and specificity have been developed for both screening and confirmation of hemoglobinopathies and thalassemia in newborns. The HPLC technique requires a very small amount of blood samples (µl), therefore, it is very suitable for prenatal diagnosis of thalassemia (Maiavacca et al., 1992, Sanguansermsri et al., 2001, Rao et al., 1997), where sample may be limited and difficult to obtain. In HPLC, particle size of the stationary phase packed in the column is quite small (about 2-5µm). The degree of interactions determines the degree of migration and separation of the components (Skoog & Leary, 1992, Christian, 2004). However, in most laboratories, HPLC has been used for diagnosis of Hb variants rather than for quantification of normal Hb or thalassemia diagnosis. There are many reports showing the agreement of results obtained from HPLC and those obtained from other techniques such as the globin synthesis technique, isoelectrofocusing, carboxymethylcellulose chromatography and DNA sequencing (Sanguansermsri et al., 2001, Rao et al, 1997, Fucharoen et al., 1998).

Cation exchangers, such as CM-cellulose (CMC) and silica supported with carboxylic acid residues with bis-Tris–KCN developer, can also be used for the same purpose (Rouyer-Fessard et al, 1989, Papadea & Cate, 1996, Wilson et al., 1983). The ratio of different globin chains (e.g., β:γ for β- thalassemia diagnosis) can also be determined with HPLC using a reverse phase C18 column and shows similar results to those obtained from CMC which is normally employed for this purpose (Congote, 1981). HPLC was become the preferred method for thalassemia screening because of its speed and reliability. An automated HPLC system has been developed primarily detection of β-thalassemia carriers, HbS, and HbC. In the study of Fucharoen et al. (1998), they used automatic HPLC system (VARIANT ™, Bio-Rad) set up with the α-thalassemia short (ATS) program and β-thalassemia shot (BTS) program to detect various types of thalassemias in both prenatal and postnatal specimens. HPLC has an overall performance better than electrophoresis.

Analyses were performed with a HPLC machine interfaced with a computer program, with an autoinjector or manual injector, and a UV detector at 415 nm. A 3.5 x 0.46 cm cation exchanger column packed with porous (100-nm pore size) 5-gm microparticulate polyaspartic acid-silica (Poly CAT Atm) or Poly LC (Columbia, MD).

Sample preparation by using 100 µl of EDTA whole blood was washed with isotonic saline (NaC1 9 g/L). The cells were then lysed by adding two to three volumes of water, vortex-mixed, and centrifuged at 3000 x g for 5 min. Added 50 µl of hemolysate to 1 mL of mobile phase A, of which 20 µl was injected onto the column. The column effluent was monitored at 415 nm and the peak areas were used for the individual quantitative hemoglobin peaks.

The gradient programwas made up of a mobile phase A (10 mmol/L Bis-Tris, 1 mmol/L KCN, pH 6.87) and mobile phase B (10 mmoIIL Bis-Tris, 1 mmolJL KCN, 200 mmol/L NaCl, pH 6.57). With a flow rate of 1.5 ml/min (a new column should be rinsed with water for 10 mm and with mobile phase B for at least 20 min, and should then be equilibrated with 12% B for another 20 min before sample application). Elution of hemoglobins was performed by increasing the mobile phase B to 40% and to 100% at 8 and 12 min, respectively, and then decreasing to 12% at 13 min. The column was re-equilibrated with 12% mobile phase B for at least 7 min before application of next sample.

Anion exchange resin DEAE and gradient Tris–HCl buffer solution, pH 8.5–6.0, is a widely used stationary-mobile phase system for HbA_2 and HbF quantification to effectively diagnose β-thalassemia and Hb Bart's hydrop fatalis that occur frequently in Southeast Asia (Sanguansermsri et al., 2001, Sanguansermsri et al., 2001). The system can also separate other Hb variants such as HbS, HbC and HbJ (Huisman & Dozy, 1962, Huisman & Dozy, 1965). In the study of Tangvarasittichai et al. (2009), they modified the fast protein liquid chromatography (FPLC) method from microcolumn chromatographic techniques for HbA_2 determination. The FPLC, a general system was used for protein purification and separation. However, they used the method for FPLC application for separation HbA_2, as the diagnosis of β-thalassemia (Tangvarasittichai et al., 2009).

10.3.2 Fast protein liquid chromatography (FPLC) technique for the diagnosis of β-Thalassemia (as demonstrated by Tangvarasittichai et al. (2009)

Hemolysate was prepared by mixing 50 µl of EDTA blood sample with 10.0 ml of Tris buffer A. 0.5 ml of hemolysate was passsed through a 5 x 0.5 cm (1ml) column of diethylaminoethyl (DEAE) sepharose, Hi Trap ™ (GE Healthcare, Sweden) connected to the FPLC (AKTA prime, Amersham Biosciences, USA) with flow rate 2 ml/min. Elluent from column was monitored by a single path ultraviolet monitor at 280 nm in a 10 min path-length high resolution flow cell, and the histogram was saved in the computer. The reagents for FPLC were as linear gradient of buffer A [50 ml of stock Tris buffer (as Tris 60.57 g mixed with 500 ml distilled water, adjusted pH 9.0 with 4 M HCl) was diluted in distilled water 1,000 ml, added 0.1 g KCN (adjusted pH 8.1 with 4 M HCl)], and buffer B (diluted 500 ml of buffer A with 500 ml 1M NaCl). The gradient profile to achieve the separation as in the table

Linear gradient profile of buffer A and B	
Buffer A, volume (ml)	**Buffer b, %**
10.0	0
11.0	10
12.0	30
13.0	50
14.0	70
15.0	90
15.5	100
20.0	0

Table 7. The gradient profile of FPLC technique
The fractions were then separated to HbA_2 or HbE (in the same fraction, HaA_2/E), HbA and HbF

The cut-off values of FPLC for HbA2/E diagnosiswere as follows: Normal (<6%), β-thalassemia (7-10%), He-trait (>10-40%), homozygous HbE (>60%), and β-thalassemia/He (40-60%)

10.3.3 Electrophoresis

Electrophoresis is one of the widely used techniques for analyzing hemoglobin variants based on the movement of different Hb or different globin chains, containing different charges, in the electric field. At an alkaline pH, Hb is negatively charged and will move toward the anode (positively charged) terminal. Electrophoresis of total Hb is different from electrophoresis of separated globin chains. Electrophoresis of hemolysates on cellulose acetate membrane is mainly used in alkaline pH electrophoresis, is a simple, reliable method for detecting abnormal hemoglobin, and capable of separating common hemoglobin variants such as S, f, a, and C. Normal operating voltage is about 250mV and the approximate run time is about 90 min. After that, the membrane needs to be stained, de-stained and air dried before separation of globin chains can be observed. The main limitation of electrophoresis at alkaline pH is a inability to differentiate HbA_2, HbC, HbO and HbE from one another, nor can HbD, HbG and Hb Lepore be differentiated from HbS (Fairbanks, 1980, Rich et al., 1979, Salmon et al., 1978). Therefore, it is normally used to screen for some types of Hb variants. The confirmatory test can be done using electrophoresis in acidic media. At a lower pH of about 6.0, a better separation of different hemoglobins is obtained. Those Hbs that co-migrate in alkaline pH electrophoresis can be separated in acidic media. Nevertheless, the main technique for Hb quantification by densitometric scanning of the gel is still somewhat difficult and unreliable (Fairbanks, 1980) and therefore electrophoresis technique has been used mainly for detection of Hb variants rather than measuring level of Hb in thalassemia diagnosis. It is highly specific in the detection of certain Hb disorders such as sickle cell disease. Even though the electrophoresis in acidic media is quite a powerful technique in separation of many types of Hbs, please keep in mind that not all Hb variants can be separated by electrophoresis in acidic media. For example, Hb Okayama cannot be separated using electrophoresis, but can be done so in HPLC (Frers et al., 2000). Capillary electrophoresis is the new format of electrophoresis where separation takes place in a small fused silica capillary. It is rapid, easily automated and consumes low amounts of reagents, as compared to conventional gel electrophoresis. It also offers much higher throughput as compared to HPLC (Doelman et al., 1997). However, some researchers found that CE has higher instrumentation cost and is less accurate as compared to automated HPLC (Jenkins & Ratnaike, 2003). To perform electrophoresis of globin chains, a few steps need to be done in order to obtain free globin chains. First, heme is removed from hemoglobin by treating with mercaptoethanol. Then the four globin chains are split apart without denaturing them using 8 M urea.

10.3.4 Electrophoresis of hemolysates on cellulose acetate (alkaline buffers)

In this method, erythrocyte hemolysate is electrophoresed on cellulose acetate in urea-2-mercaptoethanol buffers in the presence of additional 2-mercaptoethanol. The latter severs heme from globin, while the urea severs the a- and non-a-globin chains, which migrate on the cellulose acetate according to their electrical charge. The method requires very small amounts of hemolysate, yet it provides excellent resolution of globin chains in alkaline (Ueda & Schneider, 1969).

The electrophoresis apparatus and sample plate, aligning base, applicator, dispenser, and cellulose acetate. Some prepared reagents-such as the pH 8.5 buffer (Supreheme),

Solutions: De-ionized water is used throughout. Concentrated citric acid: 300 g/liter. **Hemolyzing reagent** was 1.0 g of tetrasodium ethylenediaminetetraacetate per liter of water containing 0.2 g of KCN per liter. Staining solution was 5 g of Ponceau S per liter of tri-chloroacetic acid solution (50 g/liter). Dilute acetic acid was 3 ml of glacial acetic acid plus 97 ml of water. Buffer solutions, All pH measurements are made at room temperature.

Alkaline-urea-mercaptoethanol-buffer solutions:

(i) Barbital buffer, pH 8.6, (ii) Tris-EDTA-boric acid buffer, pH 8.5, containing 10.2 g of Tris (about 80 mmol/liter), 0.6 g of EDTA, and 3.2 g of boric acid/liter, (iii) Tris-EDTA-boric acid buffer, pH 8.6, containing 18 g of Tris (about 150 mmol/liter), 2.3 g of EDTA, and 3 g of boric acid/liter.

To about 70 ml of each of these buffers, add 36 g of urea and stir on a mechanical stirrer until the urea dissolves. Adjust the volume (now about 98 ml) to 100 ml with additional buffer. In each case the final pH is about 8.9. These urea-containing buffers are used to dilute the hemolysate and soak the Titan III cellulose acetate. Just before placing buffers into the electrophoresis chambers, add 5 ml of 2-mercaptoethanol per liter.

Collect blood samples by venipuncture into a syringe with anticoagulant, or by finger stick into heparinized hematocrit tubes. Prepare hemolysates by adding one volume of water and 0.4 volume of toluene to one volume of saline-washed, packed erythrocytes. A more rapid alternative is to add three volumes of hemolyzing reagent to one volume of unwashed and sedimented or centrifuged cells (Titan III cellulose acetate plates). In most cases, however, erythrocyte hemolysates (5-10 g of hemoglobin per 100 ml) were electrophoresed directly. Add one volume of the appropriate urea buffer and one-half to one volume of undiluted 2-mercaptoethanol to one volume of hemolysate. (The additional mercaptoethanol is needed for removal of heme from globin.) Convenient volumes are 20 µl each of hemolysate and urea-buffer, and 10 to 20 µl of 2 mercaptoethanol. About 2 µl of this mixture, after it has stood at room temperature for about 0.5 h but not longer than 4 h, are placed into the sample wells.

Electrophoresis

Preparation of cellulose acetate: Mercaptoethanol may soften the Mylar backing of cellulose acetate gels, so soak the Titan III plates for several hours (or longer) in the appropriate urea-buffer without mercaptoethanol. Drain and soak for about 1 h in the corresponding urea-mercaptoethanol buffer, and finally drain and blot before applying samples. Soak Titan II sheets overnight (or longer) in the desired urea-mercaptoethanol buffer. Drain and blot. Application of samples and electrophoresis: Depress the tips of the sample applicators into the wells containing the hemolysate-urea-buffer-mercaptoethanol mixtures and wipe them off, then depress again. Make several trial applications on paper towels, until the lines formed are sufficiently thin. Then hold the applicator down for about 20 s on the Titan III plate positioned in the aligning base. When acid buffers are being used, apply samples about 1 cm from the anodal end of the plate; apply those in alkaline buffers centrally. Always include at least one control sample, usually Hb AS. In the electrophoresis chamber, rest the plates on wicks of filter paper; two or three plates may be analyzed simultaneously (200 to 350 V for 1 to 1.5 h), with a glass plate on each to weight it down.

10.3.5 Isoelectric focusing (IEF)

This technique is based on the electrophoresis technique but with a higher degree of separation. Different Hbs migrate in a pH gradient to the point where their net charges are zero. The order of migration is the same as in alkaline electrophoresis but the narrower bands obtained from this method (IEF) allow for the resolution of HbC, HbE, HbO, HbS, HbD and HbG (Laosombat et al., 2001, Gwendolyn et al., 2000). Two different formats of IEF, thin layer gel and capillary, have been reported (Hempe & Craver, 1994, Hempe et al., 1997). Cossu et al. (1982) applied the immobilized pH gradient method (IPG) with a thin layer gel that has a pH range of 6.7–7.6 to differentiate heterozygous from homozygous β-thalassemia in newborns. The group suggested the use of umbilical cord blood because it contains only HbF, HbA and acetylated HbF (HbFac) and the ratio of HbA:HbFac or HbF:HbA is used instead of the conventional β:α ratio in the IEF of globin chains.
Isoelectric focusing ((IEF) Hicks & Hughes, 1975)

Preparation of hemolysates for isoelectro focusing

The blood used for isoelectrofocusing was collected in vacutainers (Becton-Dickinson, Rutherford, N.J. 07070) with disodium ethylenediaminetetraacetate as anticoagulant. The erythrocytes were washed three times with NaC1 solution (154 mmol/liter) and lysed with an equal volume of distilled water and 0.4 ml of toluene per milliliter of erythrocytes. The mixture was shaken for 5 mm and the hemoglobin solution was cleared of cellular debris by centrifugation (20 mm, 4586 x g). Isoelectric focusing was used to obtain purified hemoglobin biopolymers for our sensitivity studies, the procedure being essentially that recommended by Svensson (1962) and Ui (1971), performed at 4°C with use of carrier ampholytes (Ampholine, 10 g/liter; LKB-Produkter AB, Stockholm, Sweden) and an electrofocusing column (Model 8101, LKB-Produkter AB) of 440-ml capacity. Solutions and linear density gradients in the column were prepared manually. The dense solution used was a sucrose solution (670 g/liter) containing carrier ampholytes (20 g/liter); less-dense solution contained 4 g of carrier ampholytes per liter, with no sucrose. (i)The protein load applied varied from 60 to 80 mg, and the sample was introduced onto the column between the dense solution and the less-dense solution. (ii) The initial voltage was 200 V, the final voltage 750 V. The voltage was increased at 2-h intervals by 200-V increments to the final voltage. (iii) Equilibrium was usually reached in 48 h. (iv) pH range from 6 to 8 was used, this range was used for isoelectrofocusing hemoglobins S, C, F, A, and D or G. (v) Fractions of 2 to 2.5 ml were collected and the absorbance of each fraction was read at 280 nm to identify the various isolated hemoglobin peaks. (vi) The pH of each fraction was determined at 25 °C with a pH meter. (vii) The separated hemoglobins were quantitated by measuring the absorbance at 415 nm with a spectrophotometer.

10.3.6 Capillaries Isoelectric focusing (cIEF)

Capillary IEF showed very promising performance both in qualitative and quantitative aspects. A single IEF run can replace the main tests that normally have to be carried out in combination for qualitative and quantitative analysis of Hbs, for instance, alkaline and acid electrophoresis for major Hb variants, ion exchange chromatography for HbA2 quantification and alkaline resistant test for HbF (Hempe et al., 1997). It has been proven to have a comparable performance to chromatography or radioactive globin chain methods (Dubart et al., 1980) and can be used for analysis of hemoglobin variants in adult and newborn (Mario et al., 1998).

10.3.7 Flow cytometry

Even though acid elution stain test seems to be simple, it is rather time consuming and subject to human error. The more precise and sensitive quantification of HbF can be done using the instrumental based flowcytometric technique (Mundee et al., 2000). The interested component of the cell is bound to a fluorescence label. Light scattering can identify the cell population of interest. Fluorescence intensity is measured to quantify the component of interest. The discovery of monoclonal antibody production has extended the use of flow cytometry. Antibody against HbF tagged with fluorescent dye can be used to specifically determine the amount of HbF. It has been demonstrated that detection of both a fetal cell surface antigen and HbF using two different monoclonal antibodies and two colored dyes is a precise way to identify the fetal cells (van Weeghel et al., 2000, Presented by Purdue University Cytometry Laboratories, Available: http://www. wiley. com/legacy/products/subject/life/cytometry/isac2000/6730.htm). The technique called gradient centrifugation has been proved to enrich the fetal cells from the adult blood and can extend the sensitivity of the flow cytometric analysis of HbF (Chen & Davis, 1997).

10.4 Advanced techniques for thalassemia and Hb variants

These are advanced techniques used to detect thalassemia and Hb variants. They are complicated and expensive techniques which are used in the cases for which there are no other ways to accurately identify or confirm the types of thalassemia or Hb variants. They involve DNA technology that can provide in-depth detailed information of gene mutation.

10.4.1 Polymerase chain reaction (PCR)

PCR selectively amplifies mutant or normal alleles using specific oligonucleotide primers. PCR is a technique that allows a small amount of DNA to be amplified in vitro. The process is composed of cycles of the three following steps: (i) perform heat denaturing to separate the DNA sequence target into two strands, (ii) anneal each strand to the specific primers and (iii) then extend the polymerase chain from the primer termini (Mathews & Holde, 1996). Once there are enough of the DNA target sequences produced for further analysis. DNA fragments can be separated by gel electrophoresis. That is commonly done following the

PCR to different DNA fragments. Many additional methods can be coupled with gel electrophoresis and PCR to obtain better information. Direct DNA sequencing of PCR products is quite a straight forward method to indicate the mutation site (Chern & Chen, 2000). Methods for the detection of point mutations were based on restriction fragment length polymorphism (RFLP) analysis (Saiki et al., 1985), and the effects of base-pair changes on DNA fragment melting temperature (denaturing gradient gel electrophoresis) (Fischer & Lerman, 1983). The RFLP technique can differentiate between different DNA sequences based on the length of fragments yielded by a particular enzyme restriction and can indicate the mutation point of a gene in thalassemia patients (Lee et al., 2002). The detection techniques have utilized allele-specific oligonucleotide (ASO) (Saiki et al., 1986, Conner et al., 1983) hybridization, the single-stranded conformational polymorphism (SSCP) (Orita et al 1989), amplification refractory mutation system (ARMS) (Newton et al., 1989), Primer-guided nucleotide incorporation assays (Hargrove et al., 1990, Takatsu et al., 2004), oligonucleotide ligation assaya (Li et al., 2005), real time PCR (Cheng et al., 2004, Johnson et al., 2004), and DNA microarray technology (Wong et al., 2004, Meaburn et al., 2006). The ARMS-PCR, also known as allele specific PCR, is another technique that has been introduced to be used for thalassemia diagnosis. This technique utilizes two PCR reactions: one contains a primer specific for the normal allele and the other contains one for the mutant allele. Gel electrophoresis is then employed to separate specific DNA bands. The PCR products were separated in 2% agarose gel. The samples were mixed with gel loading buffer and then were slowly loaded into the slots of the agarose gel, which pre-stained with ethidium bromide. The gel then electrophoresed at 150 volts, 15 min for α-thalassemia-1 (SEA type, THAI type), HbCS and HbPS and 150 volts, 25 min for α-thalassemia-2 (3.7 and 4.2 kb deletion) to check the size of PCR product. The size of DNA fragment was checked by comparing the 100 bp or 1 Kb DNA size standard (New England BioLabs) at the same gel. The images were captured using gel documentation (Bio-Rad) under ultraviolet light. Diagnosis of genotyping is based on whether there is amplification in one or both reactions (i.e., the band in normal reaction only indicates normal allele, the band in mutant reaction only indicates mutant allele, and bands in both reactions indicate a heterozygote) (Kanavakis et al., 1997, Old et al., 2000, Simsek et al., 1999). ARMS-PCR is more accurate as compared to RFLP. Single stranded conformation polymorphism (SSCP) is the technique that was developed based on the fact that the mobility in gel electrophoresis of single strands of DNA drastically depends on nucleotide sequence. Single strandedDNA is produced by adding one primer at a concentration higher than another primer in the PCR step. After the primer with lower amount is used up, the reaction will continue producing only the product of the excess primer. The mobilities of single strands are then compared (Takahashi-Fujii et al., 1994). Single stranded DNA may also be produced by denaturing double stranded DNA, as in the technique called denaturing gradient gel electrophoresis (DGGE) (Kanavakis et al., 1997, Vrettou et al., 1999, Losekoot et al., 1990). Table 8 showed some examples of PCR primers for used in thalassemia diagnosis and table 9 summarized of common genotype in thalassemia syndrome in Thailand.

10.4.2 DNA sequencing analysis for β-thalassemia mutation

DNA polymerase amplifies single-stranded DNA templates, by adding nucleotides to a growing chain (extension product). Chain elongation occurs at the 3′ end of a primer, an oligonucleotide that anneals to the template. The deoxynucleotide added to the extension product is selected by base-pair matching to the template. When a dideoxynucleotide is incorporated at the 3′ end of the growing chain, chain elongation is terminated selectively at A, C, G or T because the chain lacks a 3′-hydroxyl group. With 3′-dye labeled dideoxynucleotide (dye terminators), DNA sequencers detect fluorescence from four different dyes that are used to identify the A,C,G and T extension reactions. All four colors and therefore all four bases can be detected and distinguished in a single gel lane and displaed vary in color peak of bases.

Primers	Diagnosis	Reference
P1 (sense): 5′-GCGATCTGGGCTCTGTGTTCT-3′ **P2 (antisense):** 5′-GTTCCCTGAGCCCCGACATG-3′ **P3 (antisense):** 5′-GCCTTGAACTCCTGGACTTAA-3′	α^0-thalassemia (SEA type), (--SEA)	2008; 54:281
P1 (sense): 5′-CCTCCTGGGATTACATCTGG-3′ **P2 (antisense):** 5′-GCACCTCTGGGTAGGTTCTG-3′ **P3 (sense):** 5′-CCCCTGACAATCTCATCATCT-3′	α^0-thalassemia (THAI type), (--THAI)	2005; 8(3): 241
P1 (sense): 5′-AAGTCCACCCCTTCCTTCCTCACC-3′ **P2 (antisense):** 5′-ATGAGAGAAATGTTCTGGCACCTGCACTTG-3′ **P3 (antisense):** 5′-TCCATCCCCTCCTCCCGCCCCTGCCTTTTC-3′	α^+-thalassemia (3.7 kb deletion), (-α3.7)	2005; 8(3): 241
P1 (sense): 5′-TCCTGATCTTTGAATGAAGTCCGAGTAGGC-3′ **P2 (antisense):** 5′-TGGGGGTGGGTGTGAGGAGACAGGAAAGAGAGA-3′ **P3 (antisense):** 5′-ATCACTGATAAGTCATTTCCTGGGGGTCTG-3′	α^+-thalassemia (4.2 kb deletion), (-α4.2)	2005; 8(3): 241
P1 (sense): 5′-GCTGACCTCCAAATACCGTC-3′ **P2 (antisense):** 5′-GTAAACACCTCCATTGTTGG-3′	ARMS for HbCS	2005; 8(3): 241
P1 (sense): 5′-GCTGACCTCCAAATACCGTTAT-3′ **P2 (antisense):** 5′-GTAAACACCTCCATTGTTGG-3′	ARMS for HbPS	2005; 8(3): 241

Table 8. Some examples of PCR primers for used in thalassemia diagnosis

10.4.3 DNA technology: DNA probe/DNA microchip

Analysis of nucleic acids has led to the understanding of the gene expression that controls Hbs formation. This information is more detailed as compared to information obtained from protein analysis that normally only suggests type and amount of different Hbs production. The advance of DNA studies and fabrication technology together has led to the development of methods for diagnosis using a DNA microchip. Normally the segment of a gene of interest first has to be amplified by PCR to obtain a sufficient amount prior to hybridization with allele specific oligonucleotide probes that are immobilized on the solid phase or chip (Bianchi et al., 1997, Saiki et al., 1988, Fotin et al., 1998). The bound target gene can be detected using either labels such as fluorescent substances (Kurg et al., 2000, Kobayashi et al., 1995) or electronic transducers such as piezoelectronic and ion sensitive field effect transistors (ISFETs) (Cailloux, Novel DNA Chips. Patent No. WO/ 2001/064945 (2001)). One example of devices that has been used commonly is a cytometer. Cytometry is a laser based technique that allows for analysis of physical properties and fluorescence intensity of an individual cell in a heterogeneous environment. The image can differentiate different types of cells or DNA sequences that are labeled with different colors by comparing the ratios of fluorescence of different targets. With the aid of a computer, detection and visualization of many different probes can be done simultaneously (Osterhout et al., 1996, Janssen & Hoffmann, 2002).

Phenotype	Common genotype	
α-Thalassemia		
Thalassemia minor	$--/\alpha\alpha$	Heterozygous α-thalassemia-1
Silent Carrier	$-\alpha/\alpha\alpha$	Heterozygous α-thalassemia-2
Hb Bart's hydrops fetalis	$--/--$	Homozygous α-thalassemia-1
Thalassemia minor	$-\alpha/-\alpha$	Homozygous α-thalassemia-2
Hb H disease	$--/-\alpha$	α-thalassemia 1/ α-thalassemia-2
Hb H disease	$--/\alpha^{CS}\alpha$	α-thalassemia 1/Hb Constant spring
β-Thalassemia		
Thalassemia minor		Heterozygous β^0-thalassemia
Thalassemia minor		Heterozygous β^+-thalassemia
Thalassemia major		Homozygous β^0-thalassemia
Thalassemia intermedia		β^0-thalassemia/ β^+-thalassemia
Thalassemia intermedia or Thalassemia major		Hb E-β^0-thalassemia
Thalassemia intermedia		Hb E-β^+-thalassemia

Table 9. Summarized of common genotype in thalassemia syndromes in Thailand

10.5 Indirect thalassemia indication and treatment follow-up

These studies are not to be used for thalassemia diagnosis. However, the relevance of the variable of interest and the existence of thalassemia may help treatment follow-up or a new way to economically test for thalassemia.

10.5.1 Ferritin

Ferritin is the iron storage protein serves to store iron in a non-toxic form, to deposit it in a safe form, and to transport it to areas where it is required. Ferritin level in serum directly relates to the amount of iron stored in the body, which is important for red blood cell production. If ferritin is high, there is iron in excess. Ferritin is also used as a marker for iron overload disorders. Normal ranges of ferritin are 12-300 and 12-150 ng ml−1 for male and female, respectively (Medlineplus, Medical Encyclopedia, The US National Library of Medicine and the National Institutes of Health. Available: http://www.nlm.nih.gov/medlineplus/ency/article/003490.htm (October 16, 2003). The technique commonly used to quantify ferritin is immunoassay (Konjin et al., 1981). A significantly high level of ferritin is found in patients with iron overload and this may help differentiate thalassemia patients from those with iron deficiency, both of which will have a low red blood cell count (Arosio et al., 1981). In addition, any inflammatory disorder can cause a high level of ferritin, act as an acute phase protein. Therefore, long term monitoring of ferritin would be necessary, to gain any additional information for thalassemia diagnosis or treatment follow-up (Telfer et al., 2000).

10.5.2 Nuclear magnetic resonance spectroscopy

The nuclear magnetic resonance technique is the determination of the transverse relaxation time of hepatic water. That is based on the magnetic properties of some nuclei that when placed in the magnetic field, would take up radio frequency energy that matches the magnetic field strength and later re-emit that energy (Gunzler & Williams, 2001). The phenomenon is known as nuclear magnetic resonance (NMR) because it involves the nucleus in a magnetic field that has its strength in resonance with the applied radio frequency. NMR spectroscopy was used for the study of composition of chemical compounds. Later, the technique was developed into the imaging technology, magnetic resonance imaging (MRI), that became a major breakthrough in medical fields because it can reveal the image of the parts of the body and seems to be the most sensitive means at present.. NMR has been widely applied to study body iron overload (Jensen et al., 1994, Mazza et al., 1995, Dixon et al., 1994). NMR spectroscopy has been employed mainly for study of iron level in the fraction of tissue in vitro such as liver, spleen, heart, while NMR imaging has been used mainly for determination of iron in vivo, it is an accurate method of measuring liver iron content, especially when the iron content is below 3% (Dixon et al., 1994). So far, there has been no report on health hazards directly related or side effects to NMR and therefore the NMR technique is considered a safe and non-invasive way to study body iron content with an excellent means of assessing the effectiveness of the various therapeutic strategies used in the management of patients with iron overload.

10.5.3 Whatman 3 MM dried blood spots for identifying α-Thalassemia-1 (as demonstrated by Tangvarasittichai et al., (2008)

This method using small samples spotted onto Whatman 3 MM paper (Whatman chromatography paper, Whatman International Ltd, UK) for measurement of α-Thalassemia-1 by polymerase chain reaction (PCR) method. Forty-microliters of whole blood were multiple spotted onto Whatman 3 MM paper, and let dry at room temperature for a minimum of 3 hours, stored in sealed plastic bag at room temperature until the day of assay everymonth for 6 months. DNA extraction was extraced by Chelex method. The dried blood spot was cut into 3 pieces while for the whole blood test 40 μl of whole EDTA blood was used. Added 1 ml of lysis buffer (1% triton X-100) in a 1.5 ml tube, vortexed and centrifuged at 10,000 g for 1 min, dischared the supernatant and washed the pellets by using 1 ml distilled water and the resuspended in 100 μl of distilled water with the addition of 1 drop of Chelex ® solution. Mixtures were incubated at 56°C for at least 2 hr befor being boiled for 5-10 minutes, Samples were spun down by brief centrifugation. Extracted DNA was stored at 4°C until used. PCR reaction had a volume of 10 μl and contained 1 μl of 10x Tris buffer, 1 μl of 25 mmol/l KCl, 1 μl of glycerol, 1 μl of 2 mmol/l of each dATP, dCTP, dGTP, dTTP, 1 μl of 5 μmol/l of 3 primers, 5 μl of DNA solution and 0.1 μl of 5 U/μl *Tag* polymerase. The composition of the 3 primers is

P1: 5′-GCGATCTGGGCTCTGTGTTCT-3′,

P2: 5′-GTTCCCTGAGCCCCGACACG-3′,

P3: 5′-GCCTTGAACTCCTGGATTAA-3′

The cycling conditions 94 °C for 5 min followed by 40 cycles of amplification, denaturing at 94°C for 40 sec, annealing at 56°C for 40 sec and extension at 72°C for 40 sec. The last cycle extension time was 5 min. The PCR was analyzed by electrophoresis on 2% agarose gel and DNA bands were detected with ethirium bromide by UV transluminator. α-Thalassemia-1 trait (SEA-type) showed a specific 188 bp fragment in addition to a 314 bp fragment obtained from the normal DNA sequence.

11. Conclusion

The rapid increase in understanding of the pathophysiology of thalassemia, diseases of the globin gene have served as a model for the understanding of gene expression and regulation at the molecular level and this knowledge forms the basis for therapeutic interventions, such as gene therapy and augmentation of abnormal hemoglobin levels. Clinical interventions for the treatment of thalassemia patients have also progressed. We have a better knowledge of the optimal amount and method of treatment to provide (such as transfusions and desferrioxamine), as well as of the side-effects of these treatments. Then, the early or prenatal diagnosis of thalassemia is very important, it may base on hematologic and molecular genetic testing. There are many different techniques available for thalassemia diagnosis, but used alone they may not be able to ensure the diagnostic result. Therefore, it is quite common to utilize more than one technique for thalassemia diagnosis. In Fig. 4 summarizes techniques commonly used for diagnosis of Hb variants and thalassemia in most laboratories. If MCV, MCH or OFT screening test reveals a normal result, the possibility of having thalassemia can be eliminated, but analysis of Hb variants should be done. If an abnormal result is obtained from the screening test, there is a possibility of having either Hb variants or thalassemia case. If Hb variants tests do not show any abnormal results, thalassemia tests should still be performed. Choices of techniques depend mainly on budget and equipment available. It should be pointed out that even in laboratories equipped with high technology and many years of experience, quite a few false diagnoses were reported, which resulted in the births of thalassemia children or to have genetic counseling for abortions the unaffected fetuses. It is very important to take precaution in every step of the diagnostic procedures to ensure the most accurate diagnosis. Developments in chemical analysis methodologies are still very useful to this field.

12. References

Aessopos, A, Stamatelos, G, Skoumas, V, Vassilopoulos G, Mantzourani M, et al. (1995). Pulmonary hypertension and right heart failure in patients with β-thalassemia intermedia. *Chest*, 107, p.p.50-53.

Ali, SA. (1969). Hemoglobin H disease in Arabs in Kuwait. *J Clin Pathol*, 22, p.p. 226 - 228.

Allen, S. J., O'Donnell, A., Alexander, N. D. E., Alpers, M. P., Peto, T. E. A., et al. (1997). α^+-Thalassemia protects children against disease caused by other infections as well as malaria. *PNAS*, 94, p.p.14736 - 14741.

Allison, A.C. (1954). Protection Afforded by Sickle-cell Trait Against Subtertian Malarial Infection. *Br Med J*, 1, p.p. 290 - 294.

Anapliotou, M.L.G., Kastanias, I.T., Psara, P., Evangelou, E.A., Liparaki, M., et al. (1995). The contribution of hypogonadism to the development of osteoporosis in thalassaemia major: new therapeutic approaches. *Clin Endocrinol (Oxf)*, 42, p.p. 279-287.

Anderson, L.J., Westwood, M.A., Holden, S., Davis, B., Prescott, E.,et al. (2004). Myocardial iron clearance during reversal of siderotic cardiomyopathy with intravenous desferrioxamine: a prospective study using T2* cardiovascular magnetic resonance. *Br J Haematol*, 127(3), p.p. 348-355.

Angelucci, E., Giovagnoni, A., Valeri, G., Paci, E., Ripalti, M., et al. (1997). Limitations of Magnetic Resonance Imaging in Measurement of Hepatic Iron. *Blood*, 90, p.p. 4736-4742.

Angelucci, E., Brittenham, G.M., McLaren, C.E., Ripalti, M., Baronciani, D., et al. (2000). Hepatic iron concentration and total body iron stores in thalassemia major. *N Engl J Med*, 343(5), p.p. 327-331.

Arosio, P., Iacobello, C., Montesoro, E., & Albertini, A. (1981). Serum ferritin evaluation with radioimmunoassays specific for HeLa and liver ferritin types. *Immunol Lett*, 3(5), p.p. 309-313.

Aslan, M. & Freeman, B.A. (2004). Oxidant-mediated impairment of nitric oxide signaling in sickle cell disease-mechanisms and consequences. *Cell Mol Biol*, 50(1), p.p. 95-105.

Bacon, B.R., Tavill, A.S., Brittenham, G.M., Park, C.H., & Recknagel, R.O. (1983). Hepatic lipid peroxidation in vivo in rats with chronic iron overload. *J Clin Invest*, 71(3), p.p. 429-439.

Bain, B.J. (2006). *Hemoglobinopathy Diagnosis.* 2nd ed. Malden, Mass.: Blackwell Publishing, p. 66.

Betke, K. & Sanguansermsri, T. (1972). Cytological differentiation of blood pigments. Possibilities, results and practical application. *Munch Med Wochenschr*, 114(23), p.p. 1099-1104.

Betke, K., Marti, H.R., & Schlicht, I. (1959). Estimation of small percentages of foetal hemoglobin. *Nature*, 184(Suppl 24), p.p. 1877-1878.

Bianchi, D.W., Williams, J.M., Sullivan, L.M., Hanson, F.W., Klinger, K.W., et al. (1997). PCR quantitation of fetal cells in maternal blood in normal and aneuploid pregnancies. *Am J Hum Genet*, 61(4), p.p.822-829.

Borgna-Pignatti, C. & Galanello, R. (2004). *Thalassemias and related disorders: quantitative disorders of hemoglobin synthesis.* In Wintrobe's Clinical Hematology Volume 42. 11th edition. Lippincott Williams & Wilkins. Philadelphia, p.p. 1319-1365.

Borgna-Pignatti, C., Rugolotto, S., De Stefano, P., Zhao, H., Cappellini, M.D., et al. (2004). Survival and complications in patients with thalassemia major treated with transfusion and deferoxamine. *Haematologica*, 89, p.p. 1187 - 1193.

Brilliant cresyl blue MSDS sheet, Available: http://www.proscitech.com/ catalogue/ msds/c085.pdf (April 14, 2003).

Brittenham, G.M., Cohen, A.R., McLaren, C.E., Martin, M.B., Griffith, P.M., et al. (1993). Hepatic iron stores and plasma ferritin concentration in patients with sickle cell anemia and thalassemia major. *Am J Hematol*, 42(1), p.p. 81-85.

Britton, R.S.; Bacon, B.R. & Recknagel, R.O. (1987). Lipid peroxidation and associated hepatic organelle dysfunction in iron overload. *Chem Phys Lipids*, 45(2-4), p.p. 207-239.

Brosious, E.M., Wright, J.M., Baine, R.M., & Schmidt, R.M. (1978). Micro-chromatographic methods for hemoglobin A2 quantitation compared. *Clin. Chem*, 24, p.p. 2196 - 2199.

Brosious, E.M., Morrison, B.Y., & Schmidt, R.M. (1976). Effects of hemoglobin F levels, KCN, and storage on the isopropanol precipitation test for unstable hemoglobins. *Am J Clin Pathol*, 66(5), p.p. 878-882.

Buja, L.M. & Roberts, W. (1971). Iron in the heart: etiology and clinical significance. *Am J Med*, 51, p.p.209-221.

Cailloux, F. *Novel DNA Chips*. Patent No. WO/ 2001/064945 (2001).
Cao, A.; Galanello, R. & Rosatelli, M.C. (1998). Prenatal diagnosis and screening of the hemoglobinopathies. *Baillieres Clin Haematol*, 11(1), p.p. 215-238.
Carrell, R.W. & Kay, R. (1972). A simple method for the detection of unstable hemoglobins. *Br J Haematol*, 23(5), p.p. 615-619.
Cavallo-Perin, P., Pacini, G., Cerutti, F., et al. (1995). Insulin resistance and hyperinsulinemia in homozygous β-thalassemia. *Metabolism*, 44, p.p. 281-286.
Chakraborty, D. & Bhattacharyya, M. (2001). Antioxidant defense status of red blood cells of patients with beta-thalassemia and Ebeta-thalassemia. *Clin Chim Acta*, 305(1-2), p.p. 123-129.
Chan, V., Chan, V.W., Tang, M., Lau, K., Todd, D.,et al. (1997). Molecular defects in Hb H hydrops fetalis. *Br J Haematol*, 96(2), p.p. 224-228.
Chen, J.C. & Davis, B.H. (1997). Characterization of fetal hemoglobin containing cells by density gradient centrifugation and flow cytometric analysis. *Clinical Immunology Newsletter*, 17(6), p. 88.
Cheng, J.; Zhang, Y. & Li, Q. (2004). Real-time PCR genotyping using displacing probes. *Nucleic Acids Res*, 32, p. e61.
Chern, S.R. & Chen, C.P. (2000). Molecular prenatal diagnosis of thalassemia in Taiwan. *Int J Gynaecol Obstet*, 69(2), p.p. 103-106.
Chernoff, AI. (1959). The Distribution of the Thalassemia Gene: A Historical Review. *Blood*, 14, p.p. 899 - 912.
Chinprasertsuk, S., Wanachiwanawin, W. & Piankijagum, A. (1994). Effect of pyrexia in the formation of intraerythrocytic inclusion bodies and vacuoles in haemolytic crisis of hemoglobin H disease. *Eur J Haematol*, 52, p.p.87-91.
Christian, G.D. (2004). *Analytical Chemistry*, 6th ed., Wiley, New York.
Chui, D.H.K. & Waye, J.S. (1998). Hydrops Fetalis Caused by α-Thalassemia: An Emerging Health Care Problem. *Blood*, 91, p.p. 2213 - 2222.
Congote, L.F. (1981). Rapid procedure for globin chain analysis in blood samples of normal and beta-thalassemic fetuses. *Blood*, 57, p.p. 353 – 360.
Conner, B.J., Reyes, A.A., Morin, C., Itakura, K., Teplitz, R.L., et al. (1983). Detection of Sickle Cell ß S-globin Allele by Hybridization with Synthetic Oligonucleotides. *PNAS*, 80, p.p. 278 - 282.
Cooley, T.B.; Witwer, E. R. & Lee, P. (1927). Anemia in children: With splenomegaly and peculiar changes in the bones report of cases. *Am J Dis Child*, 34, p.p. 347 - 363.
Cooley, TB. (1946), M.D. 1871-1945. *Am J Dis Child*, 71, p.p. 77 - 79.
Cossu, G., Manca, M., Pirastru, M.G., Bullitta, R., Bosisio, A.B., et al. (1982). Neonatal screening of beta-thalassemias by thin layer isoelectric focusing. *Am J Hematol*, 13(2), p.p. 149-157.
Cunningham, M.J., Macklin, EA., Neufeld, E.J., Cohen, A.R., & the Thalassemia Clinical Research Network. (2004). Complications of β-thalassemia major in North America. *Blood*, 104, p.p. 34 - 39.
Dacie, J.V, Grimes, A.J., Meisler, A., Stiengold, L., Hemsted, E.H., et al. (1964). Hereditary heinz-body znaemia. A report of studies on five patients with mild anaemia. *Br J Haematol*, 10, p.p. 388-402.
Dispenzieri, A. (2001). *Primary Hematology*, Humana Press, NJ.
Dixon, R.M., Styles, P., al-Refaie, F.N., Kemp, G.J., Donohue, S.M., et al. (1994). Assessment of hepatic iron overload in thalassemic patients by magnetic resonance spectroscopy. *Hepatology*, 19(4), p.p. 904-910.

Doelman, C.J.A, Siebelder, C.W.M., Nijhof, W.A., Weykamp, C.W., Janssens, J., et al. (1997). Capillary electrophoresis system for hemoglobin A1c determinations evaluated. *Clin Chem*, 43, p.p. 644 – 648.

Dover, G.J., Boyer, S.H., & Zinkham, W.H. (1979). Production of erythrocytes that contain fetal hemoglobin in anemia. Transient in vivo changes. *J Clin Invest*, 63(2), p.p. 173-176.

Dozy, A.M., Kleihauer, E.F., & Huisman, T.H. (1968). Studies on the heterogeneity of hemoglobin. 13. Chromatography of various human and animal hemoglobin types on DEAE-Sephadex. J Chromatogr, 32(4), p.p. 723-727.

Du, Z.D., Roguin, N., Milgram, E., Saab, K., & Koren, A. (1997). Pulmonary hypertension in patients with thalassemia major. *Am Heart J*, 134, p.p.532-537.

Dubart, A., Goossens, M., Beuzard, Y., Monplaisir, N., Testa, U., et al. (1980). Prenatal diagnosis of hemoglobinopathies: comparison of the results obtained by isoelectric focusing of hemoglobins and by chromatography of radioactive globin chains. *Blood*, 56: p.p. 1092 - 1099.

Eaton, J.W. & Qian, M. (2002). Molecular bases of cellular iron toxicity. *Free Radic Biol Med*, 32(9), p.p. 833-840.

Electron Microscope Sciences Catalog, Available: http://www.emsdiasum. com/ems/ chemicals/salt.html (October 16, 2003).

Factor, J.M., Pottipati, S.R., Rappaport, I., Rosner, I.K., Lesser M.L., et al. (1994). Pulmonary function abnormalities in thalassemia major and the role of iron overload. *Am J Respir Crit Care Med*, 149, p.p.1570-1574.

Fairbanks, V.J. (1980). *Hemoglobinopathies and Thalassemia Laboratory Methods and Clinical Cases*, Brian C. Decker, New York.

Fernandez-Alberti A. & Fink, N.E. (2000). Red blood cell osmotic fragility confidence intervals: a definition by application of a mathematical model. *Clin Chem Lab Med*, 38(5), p.p. 433-436.

Fischer, S.G. & Lerman, L.S. (1983). DNA Fragments Differing by Single Base-Pair Substitutions are Separated in Denaturing Gradient Gels: Correspondence with Melting Theory. *PNAS*, 80, p.p. 1579 - 1583.

Flint, J, Harding, R.M, Boyce, A.J. & Clegg, J.B. (1998). The population genetics of the hemoglobinopathies. *Baillieres Clin Haematol*, 11(1), p.p. 1-51.

Fosburg, M.T. & Nathan, D.G. (1990). Treatment of Cooley's anemia. *Blood*, 76, p.p. 435 - 444.

Fotin, A.V, Drobyshev, A.L., Proudnikov, D.Y., Perov, A.N., & Mirzabekov, A.D. (1998). Parallel thermodynamic analysis of duplexes on oligodeoxyribo- nucleotide microchips. *Nucleic Acids Res*, 26, p.p. 1515 - 1521.

Frers, C.R., Dorn, S., Schmidt, W., Kochhan, L., Simon-Schultz, J., et al. (2000). Falsely increased HbA1c values by HPLC and falsely decreased values by immunoassay lead to identification of Hb Okayama and help in the management of a diabetic patient. *Clin Lab*, 46(11-12), p.p. 569-573.

Fucharoen, S. & Winichagoon, P. (2000). Clinical and hematologic aspects of hemoglobin E beta-thalassemia. *Curr Opin Hematol*, 7(2), p.p. 106-112.

Fucharoen, S., Winichagoon, P., Wisedpanichkij, R., Sae-Ngow, B., Sriphanich, R.,et al. (19980. Prenatal and postnatal diagnoses of thalassemias and hemoglo-binopathies by HPLC. *Clin Chem*, 44: p.p.740 - 748.

Fucharoen, S., Winichagoon, P., Pootrakul, P., Piankijagum, A., & Wasi, P. (1988). Difference between two types of Hb H disease, α-thalassemia 1/α-thalassemia 2 and α-thalassemia 1/Hb Constant Spring. *Birth Defect.* ;23 (5A), p.p. 309-315.

Fucharoen, S. & Viprakasit, V. (2009) Hb H disease: clinical course and disease modifiers *Hematology*, 2009, p.p. 26 - 34.

Gaziev, J. & Lucarelli G. (2003). Stem cell transplantation for hemoglobino-pathies. *Curr Opin Pediatr*, 15(1), p.p. 24-31.

Greenberg, M.S., Harvey, H.A. & Morgan, C. (19720. A simple and inexpensive screening test for sickle hemoglobin. *N Engl J Med*, 286(21), p.p. 1143-1144.

GU¨ nzler, H. & Williams A. (2001). *Handbook of Analytical Techniques*, vol.1, Wiley VCH, Germany, p. 509.

Gullo, L., Corcioni, E., Brancati, C., Bria, M., Pezzilli, R., et al. (1993). Morphologic and functional evaluation of the exocrine pancreas in β-thalassemia major. *Pancreas*, 8, p.p.176-80.

Gwendolyn, M.C, Clarke, G.M. & Higgins, T.N. (2000). Laboratory Investigation of Hemoglobinopathies and Thalassemias: Review and Update. *Clin Chem*, 46, p.p. 1284 - 1290.

Hargrove, J.L., Hulsey, M.G., Schmidt, F.H., and Beale, E.G. (1990). A computer program for modeling the kinetics of gene expression. *Biotechniques*, 8(6), p.p. 654-659.

Hebbel, R.P., Eaton, J.W., Balasingam, M., & Steinberg, M.H. (1982). Spontaneous oxygen radical generation by sickle erythrocytes. *J Clin Invest*, 70(6), p.p. 1253-1259.

Helrich, K. (1995). Association of Official Analytical Chemists, AOAC Inc., Virginia.

Hempe, J.M. & Craver R.D. (1994). Quantification of hemoglobin variants by capillary isoelectric focusing. *Clin Chem*, 40, p.p. 2288 - 2295.

Hempe, J.M., Granger, J.N., & Craver, R.D. (1997). Capillary isoelectric focusing of hemoglobin variants in the pediatric clinical laboratory. *Electrophoresis*, 18(10), p.p. 1785-95.

Hershko, C, Konijn, A.M. & Link, G. (1998). Iron chelators for thalassaemia. *Br J Haematol*, 101, p.p.399-406.

Hershko C, Weatherall DJ. (1988). Iron-chelating therapy. *Crit Rev Clin Lab Sci*, 26, p.p.303-345.

Hicks, E.J. & Hughes, B.J. (1975). Comparison of electrophoresis on citrate Agar, cellulose acetate, or starch for hemoglobin identification. *Clin Chem*, 21(8), p.p. 1072-1076

Higgs, D.R., Vickers, M.A., Wilkie, A.O., Pretorius, I.M., Jarman, A.P., et al. (1989). A review of the molecular genetics of the human alpha-globin gene cluster. *Blood*, 73, p.p. 1081 - 1104.

Hillman, R.S. & Ault, K.A. 1995). Hematology in Practical Practice, a Guide to Diagnosis and Management, McGraw-Hill, New York,

Houglum, K, Filip, M., Witztum, J.L., & Chojkier, M. (1990). Malondialdehyde and 4-hydroxynonenal protein adducts in plasma and liver of rats with iron overload. J Clin Invest, 86(6), p.p. 1991-1998.

Huisman, T.H.J. & Dozy, A.M. (1965). Studies on the heterogeneity of hemoglobin: IX. The use of tris(hydroxymethyl)aminomethane—HCl buffers in the anion-exchange chromatography of hemoglobins. *J Chromatography A*, 19, p.p. 160-169

Iancu, T.C, Neustein, H.B. & Landing, B.H. (1977). *The liver in thalassaemia major: ultrastructural observations*. In: Iron metabolism: Ciba Symposium 51. Amsterdam: Elsevier, p.p. 293-309.

Italian Working Group on Endocrine Complications in Non-endocrine Diseases. (1995). Multicentre study on prevalence of endocrine complications in thalassaemia major. *Clin Endocrinol (Oxf)*, 42, p.p.581-586.

Janssen, W.C. & Hoffmann, J.J. (2002). Evaluation of flow cytometric enumeration of foetal erythrocytes in maternal blood. *Clin Lab Haematol*, 24(2), 89-92.

Jean, G., Terzoli, S., Mauri, R., et al. (1984). Cirrhosis associated with multiple transfusions in thalassaemia. *Arch Dis Child*, 59, p.p. 67-70.

Jenkins, M. & Ratnaike, S. (2003). Capillary electrophoresis of hemoglobin. *Clin Chem Lab Med*, 41(6), p.p. 747-54.

Jensen, P.D., Jensen, F.T., Christensen, T., & Ellegaard, J. (1994). Non-invasive assessment of tissue iron overload in the liver by magnetic resonance imaging. *Br J Haematol*, 87(1), p.p. 171-184.

Johnson, M.P., Haupt, LM. & Griffiths, L.R. (2004). Locked nucleic acid (LNA) single nucleotide polymorphism (SNP) genotype analysis and validation using real-time PCR. Nucleic Acids Res, 32, p. e55.

Kadiiska, M.B., Burkitt, M.J., Xiang, Q.H., & Mason, R.P. (1995). Iron supplementation generates hydroxyl radical in vivo. An ESR spin-trapping investigation. *J Clin Invest*, 96(3), p.p. 1653-1657.

Kanavakis, E., Traeger-Synodinos, J., Vrettou, C., Maragoudaki, E., Tzetis, M., et al. (1997). Prenatal diagnosis of the thalassaemia syndromes by rapid DNA analytical methods. *Mol Hum Reprod*, 3: p.p. 523 - 528.,

Karydis, I., Karagiorga-Lagana, M., Nounopoulos, C., & Tolis, G. (2004). Basal and stimulated levels of growth hormone, insulin-like growth factor-I (IGF-I), IGF-I binding and IGF-binding proteins in beta-thalassemia major. *J Pediatr Endocrinol Metab*, 17(1), p.p. 17-25.

Kazazian, Jr. H.H. (1990). The thalassemia syndromes: molecular basis and prenatal diagnosis in 1990. *Semin Hematol*, 27(3), p.p. 209-228.

Klee, G.G., Behrman, R.E.,. Kliegman, R. & Jenson, H.B. (2000). *Nelson Textbook of Pediatrics*, W.B. Saunders.

Klee, G.G. (1980). *Role of Morphology and Erythrocyte Indices in Screening and Diagnosis*, Brian C. Decker, a Division of Thieme-Stratton Inc, New York.

Kobayashi, M., Rappaport, E., Blasband, A., Semeraro, A., Sartore, M., et al. (1995). Fluorescence-based DNA minisequence analysis for detection of known single-base changes in genomic DNA. *Mol Cell Probes*, 9(3), p.p. 175-182.

Konjin, A.M., Levy, R., Link, G. & Hershko C. (1982). A rapid and sensitive ELISA for serum ferritin employing a fluorogenic substrate. *J Immunol Methods*, 54(3), p.p. 297-307.

Kremastinos, D.T., Tiniakos, G., Theodorakis, G.N., Katritsis, D.G. & Toutouzas, P.K. (1995). Myocarditis in β-thalassemia major: a cause of heart failure. *Circulation*, 91, p.p. 66-71.

Kurg, A., Tonisson, N., Georgiou, I., Shumaker, J., Tollett, J., et al. (2000). Arrayed primer extension: solid-phase four-color DNA resequencing and mutation detection technology. Genet Test, 4(1), p.p. 1-7.

Kutlar, F, Reese, A.L., Hsia, Y.E., Kleman, K.M.& Huisman, T.H. (1989). The types of hemoglobins and globin chains in hydrops fetalis. Hemoglobin, 13(7-8), p.p. 671-183.

La-Nasa, G., Argiolu, F., Giardini, C., Pession, A., Fagioli, F., et al. (2005). Unrelated bone marrow transplantation for beta-thalassemia patients: The experience of the Italian Bone Marrow Transplant Group. *Ann NY Acad Sci*, 1054, p.p. 186-195.

Laosombat, V, Wongchanchailert, M., Sattayasevana, B., Wiriyasateinkul, A. & Fucharoen, S. (2001). Clinical and hematologic features of beta^0-thalassemia (frameshift 41/42 mutation) in Thai patients. *Haematologica*, 86, p.p. 138 - 141.

Lee, Y.J., Park, S.S., Kim, J.Y. & Cho, H.I. (2002). RFLP haplotypes of beta-globin gene complex of beta-thalassemic chromosomes in Koreans. *J Korean Med Sci*, 17(4), p.p. 475-478.

Leung, W.C., Leung, K.Y., Lau, E.T., Tang M.H. & Chan, V. (2008). Alpha-thalassaemia. *Semin Fetal Neonatal Med*, 13(4), p.p. 215-222.,

Leung, W.C., Oepkes, D., Seaward, G. & Ryan, G. (2002) Serial sonographic findings of four fetuses with homozygous alpha-thalassemia-1 from 21 weeks onwards. *Ultrasound Obstet Gynecol*, 19(1), p.p. 56-59.

Li, J., Chu, X., Liu, Y., Jiang, J.H., He, Z., et al. (2005). A colorimetric method for point mutation detection using high-fidelity DNA ligase. *Nucleic Acids Res*, 33, p. e168.

Lie-Injo, L & Jo, B.H. (1960) A fast-moving hemoglobin in hydrops foetalis. *Nature*, 185, p. 698.

Lo, Y.M.D. (2005). Recent Advances in Fetal Nucleic Acids in Maternal Plasma. *Journal of Histochemistry & Cytochemistry*, 53, p.p. 293 - 296.

Locatelli, F., Rocha, V., Reed, W., Bernaudin, F., Ertem, M., et al. (2003). Related umbilical cord blood transplantation in patients with thalassemia and sickle cell disease. *Blood*, 101, p.p. 2137 - 2143.

Lorey, F., Cunningham, G., Vichinsky, E.P., Lubin, B.H.,Witkowska H.E. et al. (2001). Universal newborn screening for Hb H disease in California. *Genet Test*, 5(2), p.p. 93-100.

Losekoot, M., Fodde, R., Harteveld, C.L., van Heeren, H., Giordano, P.C., et al. (1990). Denaturing gradient gel electrophoresis and direct sequencing of PCR amplified genomic DNA: a rapid and reliable diagnostic approach to beta thalassaemia. *Br J Haematol*, 76(2), p.p. 269-274.

Lucarelli, G., Galimberti, M., Polchi, P., Angelucci, E., Baronciani, D., et al. (1990). Bone marrow transplantation in patients with thalassemia. *N Engl J Med*, 322(7), p.p. 417-21.

Magro, S., Puzzonia, P., Consarino C., et al. (1990). Hypothyroidism in patients with thalassemia syndromes. *Acta Haematol*, 84, p.p.72-76.

Maiavacca, R., Tedeschi, S., Mosca, A., Calmi, S., De Leonardis, P., et al. (1992). Nonradioactive quantification of low concentrations of hemoglobin A by HPLC for midtrimester prenatal diagnosis of beta-thalassemia. *Clin Chem*, 8, p.p. 1906 - 1908.

Mario, N, Baudin, B. & Giboudeau, J. (1998). Qualitative and quantitative analysis of hemoglobin variants by capillary isoelectric focusing. *J Chromatogr B Biomed Sci Appl*, 706(1), p.p. 123-129.

Mathews, C.K. & Holde, K.E.V. (1996). *Biochemistry, The Benjamin/Cummings*. Publishing Company, New York.

Mavrou, A., Kouvidi, E., Antsaklis, A., Souka, A., Kitsiou Tzeli, S., et al. (2007). Identification of nucleated red blood cells in maternal circulation: a second step in screening for fetal aneuploidies and pregnancy complications. Prenat Diagn, 27(2), p.p. 150-153.

Mazza, P., Giua, R., De Marco, S., Bonetti, M.G., Amurri, B., al et. (1995). Iron overload in thalassemia: comparative analysis of magnetic resonance imaging, serum ferritin and iron content of the liver. *Haematologica*, 80, p.p. 398 - 404.,

McNiel, J.R. (1968). *The inheritance of hemoglobin H disease* (abstr). XII Congress of the International Society of Hematology, p. 52.

Meaburn, E, Butcher, L.M., Schalkwyk, L.C. & Plomin, R. (2006). Genotyping pooled DNA using 100K SNP microarrays: a step towards genomewide association scans. *Nucleic Acids Res*, 34, p. e28.

Medlineplus, Medical Encyclopedia, The US National Library of Medicine and the National Institutes of Health. Available: *http://www.nlm.nih.gov/medlineplus/ency/article/003490.htm* (October 16, 2003).

Michlitsch, J., Azimi, M., Hoppe, C., Walters, M.C., Lubin, B., et al. (2009). Newborn screening for hemoglobinopathies in California. *Pediatr Blood Cancer*, 52(4), p.p. 486-490.

Minnich, V., Na-nakorn, S., Chongchareonsuk, S., & Kochaseni, S. (1954).
Mediterranean Anemia: A Study of Thirty-two Cases in Thailand. *Blood*, 9, p.p.1 - 23.

Mundee, Y, Bigelow, N.C., Davis, B.H.& Porter, J.B. (2000). Simplified flow cytometric method for fetal hemoglobin containing red blood cells. Cytometry, 42(6), p.p. 389-393.

Nalbandian, R.M., Nichols, B.M., Camp, Jr. F.R., Lusher, J.M., Conte, N.F., et al. (1971). Dithionite Tube Test-A Rapid, Inexpensive Technique for the Detection of Hemoglobin S and Non-S Sickling Hemoglobin. Clin Chem, 17, p.p.1028 - 1032.

Na-Nakorn, S., Wasi, P., Pornpatkul, M. & Pootrakul, S.N. (1969). Further evidence for a genetic basis of hemoglobin H disease from newborn offspring of patients. *Nature*, 223(5201), p.p. 59-60.

Nathan, D.G. & Gunn, R.B. (1966). Thalassemia: the consequences of unbalanced hemoglobin synthesis. *Am J Med*, 41(5), p.p. 815-830.

Nathan, D.G. & Piomelli, S. (1990). Oral iron chelators. *Semin Hematol*, 27(2), p.p. 83-5.

Nathan, D.G. & Oski, F.A. (1993). *Hematology of infancy and childhood*, 4th ed. Philadelphia: W B Saunders Co.

Neidlinger, N.A., Larkin, S.K., Bhagat, A., Victorino, G.P. & Kuypers, FA. (2006). Hydrolysis of Phosphatidylserine-exposing Red Blood Cells by Secretory Phospholipase A2 Generates Lysophosphatidic Acid and Results in Vascular Dysfunction. J. Biol. Chem., 281, p.p. 775 – 781.

New Methylene, Blue MSDS Sheet. Available: *http://www.jtbaker.com/msds/englishhtml/n2700.htm* (April 20, 2003)

Newton, C.R., Graham, A., Heptinstall, L.E., Powell S.J., Summers, C.,et al. (1989). Analysis of any point mutation in DNA. The amplification refractory mutation system (ARMS). *Nucleic Acids Res*, 17, p.p. 2503 - 2516.)

Old, J., Petrou, M., Varnavides, L., Layton, M., & Modell, B. (2000). Accuracy of prenatal diagnosis for hemoglobin disorders in the UK: 25 years' experience. *Prenat Diagn*, 20(12), p.p. 986-991.

Olivieri, N.F. & Brittenham, G.M. (1997). Iron-chelating therapy and the treatment of thalassemia. *Blood*, 89, p.p. 739-761.

Olivieri, N.F. (1999). Correction: The (beta)-Thalassemias. N Engl J Med 1999; 341: 99-109 July 8, 1999. *N Engl J Med*, 341(18), p. 1407.

Orita, M., Iwahana, H., Kanazawa, H., Hayashi, K. & Sekiya, T. (1989). Detection of Polymorphisms of Human DNA by Gel Electrophoresis as Single-Strand Conformation Polymorphisms. *PNAS*, 86, p.p. 2766 - 2770.

Orkin, S.H. (1978). The duplicated human globin genes lie close together in cellular DNA. *PNAS*, 75, p.p. 5950 – 5954.

Orkin, S.H., Old, J., Lazarus, H., Altay, C., Gurgey, A., et al. (1979). The molecular basis of alpha-thalassemias: frequent occurrence of dysfunctional alpha loci among non-Asians with Hb H disease. *Cell*, 17(1), p.p. 33-42.

Orofino, M.G., Argiolu, F., Sanna, M.A., Rosatelli, M.C., Tuveri, T., et al. (2003). Fetal HLA typing in beta thalassaemia: implications for haemopoietic stem-cell transplantation. *Lancet*, 362(9377), p.p. 41-42.

Osterhout, M.L., Ohene-Frempong, K. & Horiuchi, K. (1996). Identification of F-reticulocytes by two-stage fluorescence image cytometry. *J Histochem Cytochem*, 44, p.p. 393 – 397.

Papadea, C. & Cate, J.C. (1996). Identification and quantification of hemoglobins A, F, S, and C by automated chromatography. *Clin Chem*, 42, p.p. 57 – 63.

Pembrey, M.E., McWade, P. & Weatherall, D.J. (1972). Reliable routine estimation of small amounts of foetal hemoglobin by alkali denaturation. *J Clin Pathol*, 25, p.p. 738 - 740

Phillips, 3d J.A., Vik, T.A., Scott, A.F.,Young, K.E., Kazazian, Jr H.H., et al. (1980). Unequal crossing-over: a common basis of single alpha-globin genes in Asians and American blacks with hemoglobin-H disease. *Blood*, 55, p.p. 1066 - 1069.

Pinto, F.O. & Roberts, I. (2008). Cord blood stem cell transplantation for hemoglobinopathies. *Br J Haematol*, 141(3), p.p. 309-324.

Pippard, M.J., Callender, S.T., Warner, G.T. & Weatherall, D.J. (1979). Iron absorption and loading in beta-thalassaemia intermedia. *Lancet*, 2, p.p. 819-821.

Pootrakul, P., Kitcharoen, K., Yansukon, P., et al. (1988). The effect of erythroid hyperplasia on iron balance. *Blood*,71, p.p.1124-1129.

Pootrakul, S, Wasi, P, & Na-Nakorn, S. (1967). Hemoglobin Bart's hydrops foetalis in Thailand. *Ann Hum Genet*, 30(4), p.p. 293-311.

Rao, V.B., Natrajan, P.G., Lulla, C.P. & Bandodkar, S.B. (1997). Rapid mid-trimester prenatal diagnosis of beta-thalassaemia and other hemoglobinopathies using a non-radioactive anion exchange HPLC technique-an Indian experience. *Prenat Diagn*, 17(8), p.p. 725-731.

Reid, M., Badaloo, A., Forrester, T. & Jahoor, F. (2006). In vivo rates of erythrocyte glutathione synthesis in adults with sickle cell disease. *Am J Physiol Endocrinol Metab*, 291, p.p. E73 - E79.

Research Organics. Available: *http://www.resorg.com/* (October 17, 2003).

Rich, S.A., Ziegler, F.D., & Grimley, P.M. (2002). Prevention of homozygous beta thalassemia by carrier screening in pregnancy. *Haema*, 5 (3), p.p. 242-245.

Rigas, D.A., Koler, R.D., Cummings, G., Duerst, M.L., Malm, D.R., et al. (1961). Decreased Erythrocyte Survival in Hemoglobin H Disease As a Result of the Abnormal Properties of Hemoglobin H: The Benefit of Splenectomy. *Blood*, 18, p.p. 1 – 17.

Rigas, D.A., Koler, R.D. & Osgood, E.E. (1955). New Hemoglobin Possessing a Higher Electrophoretic Mobility than Normal Adult Hemoglobin. *Science*, 121, p. 372

Risdon, R.A., Flynn, D.M. & Barry, M. (1973). The relation between liver iron concentration and liver damage in transfusional iron overload in thalassaemia and the effect of chelation therapy. *Gut*, 14, p. 421.

Rouyer-Fessard, P., Plassa, F., Blouquit, Y., Vidaud, M., Varnavides, L., et al. (1989). Prenatal diagnosis of hemoglobinopathies by ion exchange HPLC of hemoglobins. *Prenat Diagn*, 9(1), p.p. 19-26.

Saiki, R.K., Chang, C.A., Levenson, C.H., Warren, T.C., Boehm, C.D., et al. (1988). Diagnosis of sickle cell anemia and beta-thalassemia with enzymatically amplified DNA and nonradioactive allele-specific oligonucleotide probes. *N Engl J Med*, 319(9), p.p. 537-541.

Saiki, R.K., Scharf, S., Faloona, F., Mullis, K.B., Horn, G.T., et al.(1985). Enzymatic amplification of beta-globin genomic sequences and restriction site analysis for diagnosis of sickle cell anemia. *Science*, 230, p.p. 1350 - 1354.

Saiki, R.K., Bugawan, T.L., Horn, G.T., Mullis, K.B. & Erlich, H.A. (1986). Analysis of enzymatically amplified beta-globin and HLA-DQ alpha DNA with allele-specific oligonucleotide probes. *Nature*, 324(6093), p.p. 163-166.

Salmon, J.E., Nudel, U., Schiliro, G., Natta, C.L., & Bank, A. (1978). Quantitation of human globin chain synthesis by cellulose acetate electrophoresis. *Anal Biochem*, 91(1), p.p. 146-157.

Sanguansermsri, T., Thanaratanakorn, P., Steger, H.F., Tongsong, T., Sirivatanapa, P.,et al. (2001). Prenatal diagnosis of hemoglobin Bart's hydrops fetalis by HPLC analysis of hemoglobin in fetal blood samples. *Southeast Asian J Trop Med Public Health*, 32(1), p.p. 180-185.

Sanguansermsri, T., Thanarattanakorn, P., Steger, H.F., Tongsong T, Chanprapaph, P., et al. (2001). Prenatal diagnosis of beta-thalassemia major by high-performance liquid chromatography analysis of hemoglobins in fetal blood samples. *Hemoglobin*, 25(1), p.p. 19-27.

Schaible, U.E. & Kaufmann, S.H. (2004). Iron and microbial infection. *Nat Rev Microbiol*, 2(12), p.p. 946-53.

Silvestroni, E. & Bianco, I. (1983). A highly cost effective method of mass screening for thalassaemia. *Br Med J (Clin Res Ed)*, 286, p.p. 1007 - 1009.

Simsek, M., Daar, S., Ojeli, H. & Bayoumi, R. (1999). Improved diagnosis of sickle cell mutation by a robust amplification refractory polymerase chain reaction. *Clin Biochem*, 32(8), p.p. 677-680.

Singer, K., Chernoff, A.I. & Singer, L. (1951). Studies on Abnormal Hemoglobins: I. Their Demonstration in Sickle Cell Anemia and Other Hematologic Disorders by Means of Alkali Denaturation. *Blood*, 6, p.p. 413 - 428.,

Siniscalco, M., Bernini, L., Filippi, G., Latte, B., Khan, M., et al. (1966). Population genetics of hemoglobin variants, thalassaemia and glucose-6-phosphate dehydrogenase deficiency, with particular reference to the malaria hypothesis. *Bull World Health Organ*, 34(3), p.p. 379-393.

Sirichotiyakul, S., Tantipalakorn, C., Sanguansermsri, T., Wanapirak, C. & Tongsong, T. (2004). Erythrocyte osmotic fragility test for screening of alpha-thalassemia-1 and beta-thalassemia trait in pregnancy. *Int J Gynaecol Obstet*, 86(3), p.p. 347-350.

Sklar, C.A., Lew, L.Q., Yoon, D.J., David, R. (1987). Adrenal function in thalassemia major following long-term treatment with multiple transfusions and chelation therapy: evidence for dissociation of cortisol and adrenal androgen secretion. *Am J Dis Child*, 141, p.p. 327-330.

Skoog, D.A. & Leary, J.J. (1992). *Principles of Instrumental Analysis*, Saunders College Publication, New York.

Skordis, N. (2006). The growing child with thalassaemia. *J Pediatr Endocrinol Metab*, 19(4), p.p. 467-469.

Srisawang, B., Kongtawelert, P., Hartwell, S.K., Jakmunee, J. & Grudpan, K. (2003). A simple flow injection-reduced volume column system for hemoglobin typing. *Talanta*, 60(6), p.p. 1163-1170.

Stohs, S.J. & Bagchi, D. (1995). Oxidative mechanisms in the toxicity of metal ions. *Free Radic Biol Med*, 18(2), p.p. 321-336.

Suwanrath-Kengpol, C., Kor-anantakul, O., Suntharasaj, T. & Leetanaporn, R. (2005). Etiology and outcome of non-immune hydrops fetalis in southern Thailand. *Gynecol Obstet Invest*, 59(3), p.p. 134-137.

Svensson, H. (1962). Isoelectric fractionation, analysis and characterization of ampholytes in natural pH gradients. III, Description of apparatus for electrophoresis in columns stabilized by density gradients and direct determination of isoelectric points. *Arch Biochem*, Suppl.I, p. 132.

Tai, D.Y.H., Wang, Y.T., Lou, J., Wang, W.Y., Mak KH., et al. (1996). Lungs in thalassaemia major patients receiving regular transfusion. *Eur Respir J*, 9, p.p. 1389-1394.

Takahashi-Fujii, A., Ishino, Y., Kato, I. & Fukumaki, Y. (1994). Rapid and practical detection of beta-globin mutations causing beta-thalassemia by fluorescence-based PCR-single-stranded conformation polymorphism analysis. *Mol Cell Probes*, 8(5), p.p. 385-393.

Takatsu, K., Yokomaku, T., Kurata, S. & Kanagawa, T. (2004). A new approach to SNP genotyping with fluorescently labeled mononucleotides. *Nucleic Acids Res*, 32, p. e60.

Tangvarasittichai, O., Jongjitwimol, J. & Tangvarasittichai, S. (2008). Whatman 3 MM dried blood spots for identifying alpha-thalassemia-1. *Clin Lab*, 54(7-8), p.p. 281-283.

Tangvarasittichai, O., Jeenapongsa, R., Sitthiworanan, C.& Sanguansermsri, T. (2004). Diagnostic value of combined parameters for α-thalassemia 1 screening in pregnant women. *Naresuan University Journal*, 12, p.p. 19-24.

Tangvarasittichai, S., Tangvarasittichai, O. & Jermnim, N. (2009). Comparison of fast protein liquid chromatography (FPLC) with HPLC, electrophoresis & microcolumn chromatography techniques for the diagnosis of α-thalassemia. *Indian J Med Res*, 129, p.p. 242-248

Tanner, M.A., He, T., Westwood, M.A., Firmin, D.N., Pennell, D.J. & Thalassemia International Federation Heart T2* Investigators. (2006). Multi-center validation of the transferability of the magnetic resonance T2* technique for the quantification of tissue iron. *Haematologica*, 91, p.p. 1388 - 1391.

Telfer, P.T., Prestcott, E., Holden, S., Walker, M., Hoffbrand A.V., et al. (2000). Hepatic iron concentration combined with long-term monitoring of serum ferritin to predict complications of iron overload in thalassaemia major. *Br J Haematol*, 110(4), 971-977.

Thakerngpol, K., Fucharoen, S., Boonyaphipat, P., et al. (1996). Liver injury due to iron overload in thalassemia: histopathologic and ultrastructural studies. *Biometals*, 9, p.p. 177-183.

Thalassemia International Federation. (2008). Guidelines for the clinical management of thalassemia 2nd edition. [*http://www .thalassemia.org.cy*]

Thomas, E.D., Buckner, C.D., Sanders, J.E., Papayannopoulou, T., Borgna-Pignatti, C., et al. (1982). Marrow transplantation for thalassaemia. *Lancet*, 2(8292), p.p. 227-229.

Ueda, S. & Schneider, R.G. (1969). Rapid identification of polypeptide chains of hemoglobin by cellulose acetate electrophoresis of hemolysates. *Blood*, 34, p. 230.

Ui, N. (1971). Isoelectric points and conformation of proteins. I. Effect of urea on the behavior of some proteins in isoelectric focusing. *Biochim Biophys Acta*, 229, p.567.

van Weeghel, R., Steunebrink, G. & Suk, R., (2000). Proceedings of the International Society for Analytical Cytology ISAC2000 International Congress, Poster abstract No. 6730, May 19–35, Presented by Purdue University Cytometry Laboratories,Available: *http://www.wiley.com/legacy/products/ subject/life/cytometry/isac2000/6730.htm.*

Villeneuve, J.P., Bilodeau, M., Lepage, R., Cote, J. & Lefebvre, M. (1996).Variability in hepatic iron concentration measurement from needle-biopsy specimens. *J Hepatol*, 25(2): 172-177.

Vrettou, C., Palmer, G., Kanavakis, E., Tzetis, M., Antoniadi, T., et al. (1999). A widely applicable strategy for single cell genotyping of beta-thalassaemia mutations using DGGE analysis: application to preimplantation genetic diagnosis. *Prenat Diagn*, 19(13): 1209-1216.

Weatherall, D.J. (1987). Common genetic disorders of the red cell and the malaria hypothesis. *Ann Trop Med Parasitol*, 81(5), p.p. 539-548.

Weatherall, D.J. (1994). *The thalassemias*. In: Stamatoyannopoulos, G., Nienhuis, A.W., Majerus, P.H., Varmus, H. eds. The molecular basis of blood diseases. 2nd ed. Philadelphia: W.B. Saunders, p.p. 157-205.

Weatherall, D.J. (1997). Fortnightly review: The thalassaemias *BMJ*, 314, p. 1675.
Weatherall, D.J. (1998). Thalassemia in the next millennium. *Ann N Y Acad Sci*, 850, p.p. 1-9.
Weatherall, D.J. (2008). Hemoglobinopathies worldwide: present and future. *Curr Mol Med*, 8(7), p.p. 592-599.
Weatherail, D.J. & Clegg, J.B. (1981). *The Thalassaemia Syndromes*, 3rd edn. Oxford: Blackwell
Weatherall, D.J. & Clegg, J.B., (2001). *The Thalassemia Syndromes*, 4th ed., Blackwell Science, USA, ,
Weatherall, D.J. & Clegg, J.B. (2001). *The β and $\delta\beta$ thalassemia association with structural hemoglobin variants*. In: Weatherall DJ, Clegg JB. Eds. The Thalassemia syndromes. 4th ed. Oxford, UK: Blackwell scientific Publications, p.p.393-449.
Westgren, M., Ringden, O., Eik-Nes, S., Ek, S., Anvret, M., et al. (1996). Lack of evidence of permanent engraftment after in utero fetal stem cell transplantation in congenital hemoglobinopathies. *Transplantation*, 61(8), p.p. 1176-1179.
Wilson, J.B., Headlee, M.E., & Huisman, T.H. (1983). A new high-performance liquid chromatographic procedure for the separation and quantitation of various hemoglobin variants in adults and newborn babies. *J Lab Clin Med*, 102(2), p.p. 174-86.
Winichagoon, P., Thitivichianlert, A., Lebnak, T., Piankijagum, A. & Fucharoen, S. (2002). Screening for the carriers of thalassemias and abnormal hemoglobins at the community level. *Southeast Asian J Trop Med Public Health*, 33 Suppl 2,p.p. 145-150.
Witzleben, C.L. & Wyatt, J.P. (1961). The effect of long survival on the pathology of thalassaemia major. *J Pathol Bacteriol*, 82, p.p.1-12.
Wolfe, L., Olivieri, N., Sallan, D, et al. (1985). Prevention of cardiac disease by subcutaneous deferoxamine in patients with thalassemia major. *N Engl J Med*, 312, p.p. 1600-1603.
Wong, K.K., Tsang, Y.T.M., Shen, J., Cheng, R.S., Chang, Y.M., et al. (2004).Allelic imbalance analysis by high-density single-nucleotide polymorphic allele (SNP) array with whole genome amplified DNA. *Nucleic Acids Res*, 32, p. e69.
Wood, K.C., Hsu, L.L. & Gladwin, M.T. (2008). Sickle cell disease vasculopathy: a state of nitric oxide resistance. *Free Radic Biol Med*, 44(8), p.p. 1506-1528.
Wood, J.C., Tyszka, J.M., Carson, S., Nelson, M.D. & Coates, T.D. (2004). Myocardial iron loading in transfusion-dependent thalassemia and sickle cell disease. *Blood*, 103, p.p. 1934 - 1936.
Wu, K.H., Tsai, F.J. & Peng, C.T. (2003). Growth hormone (GH) deficiency in patients with beta-thalassemia major and the efficacy of recombinant GH treatment. *Ann Hematol*, 82(10), p.p. 637-640.
Yang, Y. & Li, D.Z. (2009). A survey of pregnancies with Hb Bart's disease in Mainland China. *Hemoglobin*, 33(2), p.p. 132-136.
Yuregir G.T. (1976). Determination of fetal hemoglobin in various age groups by the immunological method of Kohn and Payne. *Clin Chim Acta*, 72(2), p.p. 181-185.
Zurlo, M.G., De Stefano, P., Borgna-Pignatti, C., Di Palma, A., Piga, A., et al. (1989). Survival and causes of death in thalassaemia major. *Lancet*, 2(8653), p.p. 27-30.

Genomic Study in β-Thalassemia

Saovaros Svasti, Orapan Sripichai, Manit Nuinoon,
Pranee Winichagoon and Suthat Fucharoen
*Thalassemia Research Center, Institute of Molecular Biosciences, Mahidol University,
Phutthamonthon, Nakhonpathom
Thailand*

1. Introduction

β-Thalassemia is characterized by the reduced or absent production of β-globin chains in the hemoglobin molecule leading to an excess of α-globin chains. The clinical findings of thalassemia caused by the imbalanced α/non α-globin chains synthesis include many pathological changes of various organs and a lower-than-average life expectancy. Most β-thalassemia major patients who are homozygous or compound heterozygous for β^0-thalassemia mutations have a severe phenotype of β-thalassemia disease and suffer from chronic anemia and requiring regular blood transfusions. In contrast, β^0-thalassemia/HbE disease is a very heterogeneous disorder and patients who carry identical β-thalassemia genotypes may present with a remarkable variability in disease severity. Their hemoglobin levels range from 3 to 13 g/dL with an average level of 7.7 g/dL (Fucharoen et al., 1987). Patients with mild to moderate clinical symptoms usually have normal growth development and survive without regular blood transfusions. Whereas severely affected patients have marked anemia, growth retardation, severe bone changes, hepatosplenomegaly and heavy iron overload similar to that of β-thalassemia major patients.

However, the reasons for this extraordinary clinical heterogeneity are not fully understood. It has been proposed that there are three levels of genetic control of clinical phenotypes in β-thalassemia: 1) primary modifiers due to heterogeneity of the β-thalassemia alleles, 2) secondary modifiers related to the reduced free α-globin pool or increased γ-globin production in adulthood and 3) tertiary modifiers based on candidate genes that may be involved in several pathological alterations, for example, genes that are related to iron absorption, jaundice, cardiac failure and bone defects. However, the fact that many β-thalassemia/HbE patients who have the same β- and α-globin genotypes still have variable clinical symptoms, suggests that there are still some additional factors which influence the severity of the disease. Recently, genome-wide association studies (GWAS) were performed in order to search for other genetic modifying factors. In the first GWAS, approximately 110,000 gene-based single nucleotide polymorphism (SNPs) were initially screened in pooled DNA and then validated in individual samples (Sherva et al., 2010). The second GWAS was conducted using high density SNP arrays to evaluate approximately 600,000 SNPs in individual samples (Nuinoon et al., 2010). The two SNPs association analyses identified highly significant SNPs located in 3 genes/regions (*P-value* of 1.00×10^{-7} to $1.00\times10^{-}$

13): the β-globin gene cluster and olfactory receptor genes upstream of β-globin gene cluster on chromosome 11p15.5, the *HBS1L-MYB* intergenic region on chromosome 6q23 and *BCL11A* on chromosome 2p15 (Nuinoon et al., 2010; Sherva et al., 2010). The three regions have been shown to be associated with fetal hemoglobin (HbF) level by genetic linkage and association studies. Moreover, 101 SNPs on 69 genes also showed association with disease severity with *P-values* of 1.00×10^{-5} to 1.00×10^{-6}. These genes have been shown to have less effect on disease severity as compared to the three mentioned regions. However, their roles in modification of disease severity need further investigation.

2. Hemoglobinopathies

Hemoglobin (Hb) is the protein of the red blood cells that transports oxygen from the lungs to tissues, and carbon dioxide from the tissues back to the lungs. It is composed of four globin chains, two α-like and two β-like globin chains, and each globin contains iron-coordinated heme moieties. The hemoglobinopathies fall into two distinct groups, the structural hemoglobin variants and the thalassemias. Hemoglobin variants result from structural alterations in the globin chain, which are mostly due to single amino acid substitutions, thereby altering the function of the hemoglobin tetramer. The thalassemias are characterized by the absence or reduced synthesis of one of the globin chains. Some mutations also lead to both phenotypes. Hemoglobinopathies are the most common monogenic disorders and it has been estimated that approximately 5.2% of the world population are carriers. Around 1.1% of couples worldwide are at risk for having children with a hemoglobin disorder and 2.7 per 1000 conceptions are affected (Modell & Darlison, 2008).

Thalassemias can be divided according to the globin gene(s) defect into α-thalassemia, β-thalassemia, δβ-thalassemia, γ-thalassemia, δ-thalassemia and εγδβ-thalassemia. However, the major groups of this inherited disorder are α-thalassemia and β-thalassemia.

2.1 α-Thalassemia

The α-like globin locus is located on the short arm of chromosome 16 in band p13.3. It includes an embryonic gene (ζ2), two fetal/adult genes (α2 and α1), three pseudogenes (ψζ1, ψα2, ψα1) and a gene (θ) of unidentified function. α-Thalassemia is classified by a reduction or absence in synthesis of α-globin chains. Molecular defects of α-thalassemia are mainly associated with deletions or mutations of one or more of the α-globin genes, of which now more than 35 known deletional mutations have been discovered (Hardison et al., 1998). α-Thalassemia 1 (--/αα) occurs from a deletion of the duplicated α-globin genes, while deletion or mutation of one copy of the duplicated α-globin genes, which produces a reduced amount of α-globin leads to α-thalassemia 2 (-α/αα). The clinical pathology of the patients is heterogeneous depending mainly on the number of defective genes.

2.2 β-Thalassemia

The β-globin locus is located on the short arm of chromosome 11 in band p15.5. It includes an embryonic gene (ε), two fetal genes ($^{G}\gamma$ and $^{A}\gamma$), two adult genes (δ and β) and a pseudogene (ψβ). β-Thalassemia occurs as a consequence of a quantitative reduction of β-globin chain production. More than 200 point mutations and, rarely deletions, have been reported (Hardison et al., 1998). These genetic defects lead to a variable reduction in β-globin output ranging from a minimal deficit, mild β^+-thalassemia alleles, to the complete absence, β^0-thalassemia.

2.3 Hemoglobin E

HbE, the most common Hb variant among Southeast Asian populations, results from a G to A substitution at codon 26 (GAG to AAG) in exon 1 of the β-globin gene, which substitutes an amino acid residue from Glu to Lys. This abnormal gene produces a structurally abnormal hemoglobin which consists of $\alpha_2\beta^E{}_2$-globin chains. Moreover, the abnormal gene also activates a cryptic 5′ splice site that causes abnormal pre-mRNA splicing. The aberrant splicing leads to a 16 nucleotide deletion of the 3′ end in exon 1 and creates a new inframe stop codon (Orkin et al., 1982). This new cryptic splice site competes with the normal doner splice site, consequently the level of correctly spliced β^E-globin mRNA is decreased. As a result, HbE is synthesized at a reduced rate and thus the β^E-globin gene behaves like a mild form of β^+-thalassemia.

3. β-Thalassemia/HbE disease

β-Thalassemia/HbE disease is the most common form of β-thalassemia in many Asian countries. In Thailand, approximately 3,000 children are born with this condition each year, and there are some 100,000 patients in the population (Fucharoen & Winichagoon, 2000). It accounts for over 50% of cases of severe β-thalassemia in Indonesia and Bangladesh and is also very common in Vietnam, Cambodia, Laos, and Malaysia. It also occurs frequently in the eastern side of Indian subcontinent, including Sri Lanka and Maldives (Fucharoen & Winichagoon, 1997).

The major mechanism underlying the pathophysiology of β-thalassemia/HbE is due to the absence or inadequate β-globin chain production, and can be related to the deleterious effects of imbalanced globin chain synthesis. The excess α-globin chains in β-thalassemia, which are highly unstable, precipitate and lead to oxidative damage in developing (causing dyserythropoiesis) and mature red cells (causing shortened red blood cell survival). Hemolysis and ineffective erythropoiesis cause anemia in β-thalassemia (Rund & Rachmilewitz, 2005). Ineffective erythropoiesis leads to the expansion of marrow cavities and the massive medullar cell proliferation, resulting in skeletal deformities. The erythroid hyperplasia and ineffective erythropoiesis are responsible for the increased iron absorption, which together with regular blood transfusions, results in chronic iron overload and death in these patients.

3.1 Clinical Heterogeneity of β-Thalassemia/HbE disease

β-Thalassemia/HbE is generally classified as thalassemia intermedia. The patients have inherited a β-thalassemia allele and hemoglobin E, which acts as a mild β^+-thalassemia. However, despite seemingly identical genotypes, β-thalassemia/HbE patients have a remarkably wide spectrum of clinical phenotypes. Notable are variations in anemia, growth development, hepatosplenomegaly, and transfusion requirements. The clinical features range from asymptomatic or mild clinical symptoms with normal growth development and survival without transfusions, to transfusion-dependent thalassemia major who have marked anemia, growth retardation, severe bone changes, hepatosplenomegaly and heavy iron overload. A study of 802 β-thalassemia/HbE patients showed that hemoglobin levels in the steady state range from 3 to 13 g/dL with an average level of 7.7 g/dL (Fucharoen et al., 1987). Interestingly, the discordant severity of anemia ranged from 0 to 8.6 g/dL, while the distribution of differences of hemoglobin levels in 216 sib pairs from 98 families showed a remarkable skewness toward the lower values with a mode at 0-0.5 g/dL. This suggests that multiple genetic factors must be involved in determining the clinical variability (Fucharoen et al., 1984). The reasons for this extraordinary clinical heterogeneity are not fully understood.

3.2 β-Thalassemia/HbE disease modifiers

The pathophysiologic change in homozygous β-thalassemia patients is predominantly determined by the amount of excess α-globin chains. *In vitro* globin chain synthesis techniques available in the 1960s revealed that the central mechanism underlying the pathophysiology of β-thalassemia was related to the excess α-globin chains and the degree of chain imbalance (Weatherall et al., 1965). Similar to homozygous β-thalassemia, the effect of imbalanced globin chain synthesis to disease severity of β-thalassemia/HbE patients has been demonstrated. The *in vitro* globin chain synthesis showed a significant difference between α/non α-globin chains ratio of 2.08±0.42 and 2.55±0.34 in mild and severe groups (*P-value*<0.005), respectively (Fucharoen et al., 1987). Interestingly, there were overlaps in the range of α/non α-globin chains ratio of 1.34-2.90 in the mild group and 2.23-3.30 in the severe group. This suggested that other factors also contributed to the clinical symptoms of these patients.

The well-characterized or possible genetic modifiers which influence the severity of β-thalassemia have been classified. As the amount of excess α-globin chains determined the pathophysiologic change in β-thalassaemia, the factors affecting the excess α-globin pools, which may lead to variable clinical phenotype of the patients are classified as primary and secondary modifying factors. While the tertiary modifying factors are genetic factors that do not affect globin imbalance directly but modify complications of the disease in several different ways (Thein, 2008).

Recently in order to explore disease modifying factors we recruited about 1,300 Thai β^0-thalassemia/HbE patients and classified them into three groups, mild, moderate and severe using a scoring system based on criteria of 6 representative parameters; hemoglobin level, age onset, age at the first blood transfusion, requirement of blood transfusion, spleen size or splenectomy, and growth development (Sripichai et al., 2008a). The analysis of known genetic modifiers and genome-wide SNPs association studies (GWAS) were performed using MassARRAY platform (Sequenom, Inc., San Diego, CA, USA) and Illumina Human 610-Quad BeadChips array (Illumina, San Diego, CA, USA) (Nuinoon et al., 2010; Sherva et al., 2010).

3.2.1 Primary modifying factors

The primary modifying factor is described by expression of the β-globin alleles due to the nature of the underlying β-thalassemia mutation itself. β-Thalassemia mutations range from null mutations (β^0-thalassaemia) that cause a complete absence of β-globin production, to those that cause a minimal deficit (β^+-thalassemia). Generally, interaction of two β^+-

thalassemia alleles, in which there is some β-globin production such as the mutations at -28 ATA box (A→G), codon 19 (A→G), results in a milder disease. A recent study in a Thai β-thalassemia/HbE cohort showed that all β^+-thalassemia/HbE patients had mild clinical symptoms (Table 1). On the contrary, co-inheritance of a β^0-thalassaemia mutation, which causes a complete absence of β-globin production from the allele, and HbE results in a wide spectrum of phenotypes.

Since mutation of the β^E-globin gene leads to the alternative splicing of β^E-globin pre-mRNA, the amount of alternative spliced β^E-globin mRNA may play a role in the variability of disease severity. Analysis of *in vitro* globin chain synthesis showed α/β^E-globin chains ratio of 2.69±0.58 and 3.18±0.36 in mild and severe groups respectively (Fucharoen et al., 1987). A study in the 1990s by the RT-PCR technique showed that aberrantly spliced β^E-globin mRNA in patients with severe clinical phenotype was higher than those of mild cases and the level of aberrantly spliced β^E-globin mRNA was correlated with the degree of anemia in the patients (Winichagoon et al., 1995). A recent study using allele specific RT-qPCR confirmed that there were differences in the alternative splicing of the β^E-globin mRNA among the patients and the correctly/aberrantly spliced β^E-globin mRNA ratio in the mild group was higher than that of the severe group (Tubsuwan et al., 2011). Excluding factors correlated to high HbF production, *Xmn*I -158 $^G\gamma$-globin, *HBS1L-MYB* intergenic region and *BCL11A*, the alternative splicing of the β^E-globin mRNA contributed to at least 7.8% of the mild group.

3.2.2 Secondary modifying factors

The severity of anemia in β-thalassemia reflects the degree of α- to non-α-globin chain imbalance and the excess of unmatched α-globin chains with all their deleterious effects on the erythroid precursor cells. Therefore secondary modifying factors are described as factors that affect the degree of globin chain imbalance and the size of the free α-globin chain pool, either via the co-inheritance of α-globin gene mutations or through genetic determinants which increase the level of HbF production.

β-Thalassemia patients who co-inherit α-thalassemia will have less excess α-globin chains and tend to have less severe symptoms (Sripichai et al., 2008b; Wainscoat et al., 1983). The different types of α-thalassemia mutations that predominate in different racial groups display a wide range of severity. The degree of amelioration depends on the number of functional α-globin genes. None of the patients carrying α-thalassemia were in the severe group. After exclusion of β^+-thalassemia mutations, all patients who co-inherited with α-thalassemia 1 heterozygote or α-thalassemia 2 homozygote, who have only 2 functional α-globin genes had mild clinical symptoms. About 90% of the patients who have only one defecteive α-globin gene were in the mild group and 10% were in the moderate group (Table 2). Co-inheritance of α-thalassemia appears to be a major genetic factor underlying the mild clinical phenotype of β-thalassemia/HbE. Moreover, a considerable number of patients, especially those who have co-inheritance of α-thalassemia 1, may have not yet been diagnosed or not presented to hospitals. The prevalence of 0.5% α-thalassemia 1 and 6.9% α-thalassemia 2 in the patients was lower as compared to 4% α-thalassemia 1 and 16% α-thalassemia 2 in Thai population. We suggest that the presence of α-thalassemia genes should always be considered in apparently mild cases of β^0-thalassemia/HbE in Southeast Asia and probably in other countries where α-thalassemia is also prevalent.

	Disease severity				
	Mild			Moderate	severe
β-globin genotype	β^+/β^E	β^0/β^E	β^0/β^E	β^0/β^E	β^0/β^E
α-globin genotype	αα/αα	α-thal	αα/αα	αα/αα	αα/αα
No. of patient*	36 (2.8)	104 (8.1)	278 (21.7)	373 (29.2)	489 (38.2)
Hemoglobin (g/dL)**	7.56±1.05	8.22±1.11	7.53±1.25	5.57±1.51	4.55±1.141
Hemoglobin F (g/dL)**	1.47±0.71	1.94±0.91	3.28±1.20	2.02±0.92	1.50±0.81
Age at first presentation*					
<3 yr	5 (13.9)	18 (17.3)	62 (22.3)	133 (35.7)	377 (77.1)
3-10 yr	10 (27.8)	52 (50.0)	175 (62.9)	220 (59.0)	112 (22.9)
>10 yr	21 (58.3)	34 (32.7)	41 (14.8)	20 (5.3)	0
Age at first transfusion*					
< 5 yr	0	2 (1.92)	11 (3.96)	121 (32.44)	403 (82.41)
5-10 yr	1 (2.78)	12 (11.54)	50 (17.99)	174 (46.65)	83 (16.97)
> 10 yr	35 (97.22)	90 (86.54)	217 (78.06)	78 (20.91)	3 (0.61)
Requirement for transfusions*					
regular	0	2 (1.92)	4 (1.44)	162 (43.43)	421 (86.09)
occasional	0	5 (4.81)	14 (5.04)	129 (34.58)	66 (13.50)
none	36 (100.00)	97 (93.27)	260 (93.53)	82 (21.98)	2 (0.41)
Spleen size*					
size <3 cm	32 (88.89)	71 (68.27)	115 (41.37)	76 (20.38)	12 (2.45)
3-10 cm	4 (11.11)	32 (30.77)	143 (51.44)	130 (34.85)	153 (31.29)
>10 cm or splenectomy	0	1 (0.96)	20 (7.19)	167 (44.77)	324 (66.26)
Height development*					
<3rd percentide	3 (8.33)	17 (16.35)	27 (9.71)	78 (20.91)	220 (44.99)
Weight development*					
<3rd percentide	2 (5.56)	5 (4.81)	19 (6.83)	73 (19.57)	156 (31.90)

* Number of cases (%) ** mean±SD

Table 1. Clinical and hematologic parameters among the different severity groups of β-thalassemia/HbE disease

α-Thalassemias	α-Globin genotype	Mild	Moderate	Severe	Total
		Number (%)	Number (%)	Number (%)	Number (%)
Normal	αα/αα	321	378	501	1200 (90.2)
Triplicated α-globin	$\alpha\alpha\alpha^{anti3.7}/\alpha\alpha$	0 (0.0)	0 (0.0)	6 (0.5)	6 (0.5)
α-thalassemias all genotypes		113 (91.1)	11 (8.9)	0 (0.0)	124 (9.3)
Two α-globin genes defect					
α-thalassemia 1 heterozygote	$--^{SEA}/\alpha\alpha$	7 (100.0)	0 (0.0)	0 (0.0)	7 (0.5)
α-thalassemia 2 homozygote	$-\alpha^{3.7}/-\alpha^{3.7}$	2 (100.0)	0 (0.0)	0 (0.0)	2 (0.2)
One α-globin gene defect					
α-thalassemia 2 (3.7 kb deletion) heterozygote	$-\alpha^{3.7}/\alpha\alpha$	73 (90.1)	8 (9.9)	0 (0.0)	81 (6.1)
α-thalassemia 2 (4.2 kb deletion) heterozygote	$-\alpha^{4.2}/\alpha\alpha$	6 (75.0)	2 (25.0)	0 (0.0)	8 (0.6)
HbCS heterozygote	$\alpha^{CS}\alpha/\alpha\alpha$	23 (95.8)	1 (4.2)	0 (0.0)	24 (1.8)
HbPS heterozygote	$\alpha^{PS}\alpha/\alpha\alpha$	2 (100.0)	0 (0.0)	0 (0.0)	2 (0.2)
Total		434 (32.6)	389 (29.3)	507 (38.1)	1330 (100.0)

Table 2. The effect of α-globin genotype on β-thalassemia/HbE disease phenotypes

Increased α-globin chains are also synthesized from the α-globin triplicated allele (Higgs et al., 1980). The excess α-globin chains lead to a greater globin chain imbalance in β-thalassemia, and hence, the clinical severity of patients is expected to be worsened. The effect of increased α-globin chains by two extra α-globin genes in homozygous triplicated α-globin genes (ααα/ααα) or heterozygous quadruplicated α-globin genes (αααα/αα) was clearly demonstrated in β-thalassemia heterozygotes, which resulted in thalassemia intermedia (Galanello et al., 1983; Thompson et al., 1989). However, the effect of one extra α-globin gene on heterozygous triplicated α-globin genes (ααα/αα) in heterozygous β-thalassemia is more variable and depends on the severity of the β-thalassemia allele (Camaschella et al., 1997; Traeger-Synodinos et al., 1996). Co-inheritance of triplicated α-globin genes (ααα/αα) resulting in severe anemia in β-thalassemia patients has been observed (Camaschella et al., 1995; Galanello et al., 1983; Sripichai et al., 2008a). In this β-thalassemia/HbE cohort, all patients carrying triplicated α-genes (0.5 % of patients) showed a severe clinical phenotype (Table 2). However, the triplicated and quadruplicated α-globin genes occur at a low frequency in most populations. The frequency of triplicated α-globin genes in Cambodian and Chinese cohorts was about 0.5% of patients (Carnley et al., 2006;

Ma et al., 2001). A higher frequency (1–3%) was observed in other countries such as Argentina and Mexico (Bragos et al., 2003; Nava et al., 2006). The quadruplicated α-globin genes were found at an even lower frequency than the triplicated α-globin genes. In Sri Lanka the triplicated and quadruplicated α-globin genes frequencies in the patients were 2.0% and 0.2 %, respectively (Fisher et al., 2003).

The HbF level, which is high at birth and decreases thereafter, is an extremely complex process and still poorly understood. However, the high production of HbF during the neonatal period protects the newborn from the clinical manifestations of β-thalassemia. The role of increased HbF as an ameliorating factor was shown in the group of homozygous β-thalassemia patients who are unable to produce any HbA but showed a mild disease with a reasonable level of HbF (Thein et al., 1988). Studies in β-thalassemia patients have shown that increased Hb F production can reduce the ratio of α- to non-α-globins and ameliorate the severity of the anemia (Rees et al., 1999). The absolute HbF level in mild patients who do not carry the two known modifying factors (β^+-thalassemia or α-thalassemia) was 3.28±1.20 g/dL. This level is significantly higher than that of severe patients, 1.50±0.81 g/dL or mild patients carrying β^+-thalassemia or α-thalassemia, 1.47±0.71 and 1.94±0.91 g/dL, respectively (Table 1).

The broad distribution of HbF levels in normal adults, in which HbF levels decrease steadily with age, and in which females have higher levels than males, suggests that more than one genetic factor may control HbF production. A twin study composed of 264 monozygotic and 511 dizygotic twins showed that approximately 90% of the variations in the level of HbF and F-cells (HbF containing erythrocytes) production in adult life is genetically controlled by some factor located near the γ-globin gene, while other factors are present on different chromosomes (Garner et al., 2000).

It is known that the genetic variant (C→T) at position -158 upstream of $^{G}\gamma$-globin gene, *Xmn*I $^{G}\gamma$-globin polymorphism, is associated with high HbF production (Labie et al., 1985a; Thein et al., 1987). In addition, more than 50% of the genetic variances in levels of F-cells are caused by factors that are not linked to the β-globin gene cluster (Garner et al., 2000). Intensive linkage studies have mapped *trans*-acting quantitative trait loci (QTLs) controlling F-cell levels to three regions of the genome: chromosome 6q23, Xp22 and 8q11 (Craig et al., 1996; Dover et al., 1992; Garner et al., 2002). The genetic factors regulating HbF production are discussed in more detail below.

3.2.3 Tertiary modifying factors

Tertiary modifying factors, while not being involved in hemoglobin synthesis, cause variation in the progression of the disease. For example, the glucuronosyltransferase 1 (*UGT1A*) gene was found to be associated with the levels of bilirubin in response to hemolysis, ineffective erythropoiesis and the incidence of gallstones (Premawardhena et al., 2001). Similarly, the hemochromatosis (Venter et al.) gene has been identified as influencing the degree of iron loading (Longo et al., 1999; Rees et al., 1997) and the apolipoprotein E (*APOE*) ε4 allele is associated with organ damage and cardiac failure (Economou-Petersen et al., 1998). Variability of at least three different loci; vitamin D receptor (*VDR*), type 1 collagen (*COLIA1*) and transforming growth factor beta 1 (*TGFB1*), has the potential to modify the severity of the bone disease, which is particularly common in patients with severe β-thalassemia (Perrotta et al., 2000).

4. General genomic study

Completion of the human genome project (Frazer et al., 2004; Lander et al., 2001; Venter et al., 2001), dramatically accelerated biomedical research. In parallel, characterization of the inherited variation in human populations, focusing mainly on DNA variants that are common in the general population and that confer increases in diseases risk, has led to exploration of disease susceptibility.

4.1 Genomic variation

Genetic and environmental factors are the two keys that cause human phenotypic variation. Although more than 99% of human DNA sequences are the same across the population there is substantial variation in the sequence at many points throughout the genome. DNA sequence variations are described as mutations and polymorphisms. A mutation is defined as any change in a DNA sequence to a rare and abnormal variant in comparison to the normal allele that is prevalent in the population. In contrast, a polymorphism is a DNA sequence variation that is common in the population. The arbitrary cut-off point between a mutation and a polymorphism is 1% (Brookes, 1999). Genetic variations are responsible for individual phenotypic characteristics and impact on how humans respond to diseases, bacterias, viruses, toxins, chemicals, drugs and other therapies.

Since the early 1980s, humans were known to carry a heterozygous site roughly every 1,300 bases. Genetic maps containing a few thousand markers, which are adequate for rudimentary linkage mapping of Mendelian diseases, were constructed in the late 1980s and early 1990s (Lander, 2011; Lander et al., 2001). A map of 1.42 million single nucleotide polymorphisms (SNPs) distributed throughout the human genome was reported in a companion to the human genome project (Sachidanandam et al., 2001). Today, the vast majority of human variants with frequency >5% have been discovered and 95% of heterozygous SNPs in an individual are represented in current databases. The combination of marker alleles on a single chromosome is called a haplotype (*Haplo*id Geno*type*). Haplotype includes markers that tightly linked with each other and these markers often display statistical dependence, called linkage disequilibrium (LD). The International Haplotype Map Project defined the SNPs patterns across the entire genome by genotyping 3 million SNPs (Frazer et al., 2005).

The presence of a specific allele variation can be implicated as a causative factor in human genetic disorders and a genetic modifying factor in disease phenotypes. Therefore, screening for such an allele in an individual might enable detection of a genetic predisposition to disease or particular phenotype. The importance of finding genetic contribution to disease, therefore, has led to collection of DNA samples from a large number of patients with particular disorders. Two major approaches have been used to map genetic variants that influence disease or phenotype: linkage analysis and association studies.

4.2 Linkage studies

Linkage analysis (family-based studies) is based on the principle that a disease locus in a family will segregate as part of an undisturbed chromosomal region. Genetic markers that tag a chromosomal region that includes the disease gene will co-segregate with the disease. In practice, highly variable markers, such as microsatellites that can be distinguished between most mating couples, have been used to tag regions of the chromosomes (Hauser et al., 2004). Families in which sibling pairs are affected with the disorder are typed with genetic markers to find a polymorphism that is co-inherited with the disease. If the polymorphic allele is found in a large number of affected sibling pairs, the polymorphism is probably linked to a gene that confers susceptibility to that disease. The genetic markers and the disease allele must generally be inherited together within the one or two generations spanned by the family. To find polymorphisms that are linked to a specific disease requires the typing of 200–300 families with multiple affected relatives using a set of a few hundred or a few thousand markers, spaced millions of bases apart along the human genome. However, the linkages reported by one group have often not been replicated by others. Failure to replicate the linkages may result from a lack of statistical power or false positive results in the original study. Furthermore, there might also be different sets of susceptibility genes operating in different populations. Linkage analysis has been less successful for polygenic diseases and quantitative traits, perhaps in part because of a limited power to detect the effect of common alleles with modest effects on disease.

4.3 Association studies

Association studies rely on the retention of adjacent polymorphisms over several generations across the population. The prevalences of a particular genetic marker or a set of markers, in affected and unaffected individuals, are compared instead of analysis of large family pedigrees (population-based studies) (Cardon & Bell, 2001; Hirschhorn & Daly, 2005). The "common disease–common variant" hypothesis posited that common genetic variants could have a role in the etiology of common diseases (Reich & Lander, 2001). The vast majority of genetic variance in the population is due to common variants. The susceptibility alleles for a trait will include many common variants unless the alleles have had a large deleterious effect on reproductive fitness over long periods. For common diseases or traits, many susceptibility alleles may have been only mildly deleterious, neutral or even advantageous. By testing all common variants, one could pinpoint key genes and shed light on underlying mechanisms.

Genome-wide association studies (GWAS) are association studies that survey most of the genome for causal genetic variants. In GWAS, hundreds of thousand SNPs tested for association with a disease in hundreds or thousands of persons have revolutionized the search for genetic influences on complex traits (Manolio, 2010). Such conditions, in contrast with single-gene disorders, are caused by many genetic and environmental factors working together, each of which has a relatively small effect and few if any being absolutely required for the disease to occur. Rapid advances in technology and quality control now permit affordable, reliable genotyping of up to 1 million SNPs in a single scan of a person's DNA. In 2010, nearly 600 genome-wide association studies covering 150 distinct diseases and traits were published, with nearly 800 SNP–trait associations being reported as significant (*P-value* $<5\times10^{-8}$).

5. Genomic study in thalassemias

Even after exclusion of known genetic modifying factors, the phenotypic severity in the majority of β-thalassemia/HbE patients still can not be predicted. As mention above, family studies indicated that multiple genetic factors are involved in determining the clinical variability and additional genetic modifying factors remain to be discovered. In order to identify these variants, two GWAS were performed in Thai β-thalassemia/HbE patient cohorts, from which β- or α-globin mutations that are known to affect disease severity were excluded.

The first GWAS was carried out using a two-stage study design, which allowed cost effective identification of a targeted set of SNPs for individual genotyping. Initially pooled DNA of 197 mild and 198 severe cases was examined (Sherva et al., 2010). Then the SNPs with allele frequency differences between the pooled DNA (*P-value* < 0.02) were further genotyped in individual samples of 198 mild and 305 severe cases. The assay panel corresponded to 119,811 gene-based SNPs with a median spacing of 10.4 kilobases, covering approximately 99% of all known and predicted human genes. The pooled genotyping was conducted using the MassARRAY platform (Sequenom, Inc., San Diego, CA, USA). The results showed that 50 SNPs were significantly associated with disease severity (*P-value* $<$ 0.05). Forty-one SNPs in a large linkage disequilibrium (LD) block within the β-globin gene cluster were associated with severe disease, of which the most significant was bthal_bg200 (odds ratio (OR) = 5.56, *P-value* $= 2.6 \times 10^{-13}$).

The second GWAS was conducted using the Illumina Human 610-Quad BeadChips array (Illumina, San Diego, CA, USA) with DNAs from 235 mild and 383 severe cases of Thai β^0-thalassemia/HbE patients (Nuinoon et al., 2010). The result identified 27 SNPs located in three genes/regions, having *P-value* of 1.00×10^{-7} or lower to be associated with the disease severity. The quantile–quantile plot of the observed *P-value* for association to the disease severity and Manhattan plot are shown in Figure 1. The strongest SNPs associated with the disease severity were located in the β-globin gene cluster on chromosome 11p15.5 and olfactory receptor genes upstream of β-globin gene cluster. The 9 most significant disease severity associated SNPs (*P-value* $<1.00 \times 10^{-10}$) were located in a large LD spanning over 62 kb containing the locus control region (LCR) of the β-globin gene cluster, 4 functional β-globin-like genes (ε-, $^G\gamma$-, $^A\gamma$- and δ-globin) and 1 pseudogene (ψβ-globin). The most significantly-associated SNP, rs2071348, was in the ψβ-globin gene (*P-value* $= 2.96 \times 10^{-13}$, OR = 4.33 with 95% CI; 2.74-6.84). The second most significant region was mapped to the *HBS1L-MYB* intergenic region on chromosome 6q23. Five SNPs of this region showed strong association with disease severity (*P-value* $< 1.00 \times 10^{-7}$) and rs9376092 revealed the most significant association with *P-value* $= 2.36 \times 10^{-10}$ (OR = 3.07 with 95% CI; 2.16-4.38). The third significant gene is the *BCL11A* on chromosome 2p15. Four SNPs were significantly associated with the disease severity, with the most significant SNP rs766432 located in intron 2 (*P-value* $= 5.87 \times 10^{-10}$, OR = 3.06 with 95% CI; 2.15-4.37). In addition, 101 SNPs on 69 genes also showed association with disease severity with *P-value*s of 1.00×10^{-5} to 1.00×10^{-6}. These SNPs are located on several genes/regions and can be classified into various biological functions such as cell cycle, cell growth, structural proteins, enzymes, hormones, signaling molecules, genes involved in gene expression, protein degradation, inflammatory response and hypothetical proteins with unknown functions. These genes may have less effect on disease severity compared to the three regions. However, they may play some roles in modification of disease severity and need further investigation.

No SNPs in the *BCL11A* region were typed in the first GWAS, suggested that the pooled genotyping was done on a marker panel that was less dense than the second GWAS and did not have the same level of genome coverage as the high density SNP arrays. However, the low marker density can identify two of the three SNPs highly associated with disease severity identified by the second GWAS, the β-globin gene cluster and *HBS1L-MYB* region.

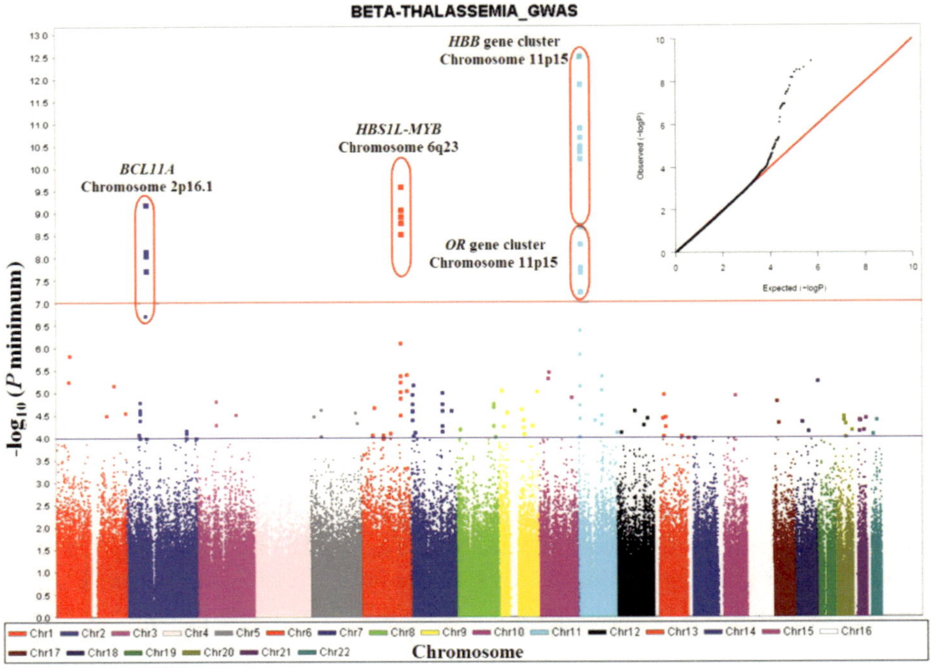

Fig. 1. Genome-wide association study scatter plots of *P-values* (analyzed with disease severity) with chromosome location. The red line denoted the significance threshold (*P-value* = 1.00 x 10^{-7}), and the blue line denoted the suggestive *P-value* (P = 1.00 x 10^{-4}). Inset shows the quantile–quantile plot of the *P-values* (allelic association) (Nuinoon et al., 2010). With kind permission from Springer Science+Business Media

Interestingly, the absolute HbF level among mild β^0-thalassemia/HbE patients without α-thalassemia co-inheritance was significantly higher than those of the mild cases who were β^+-thalassemia/HbE or having co-inheritance of α-thalassemia and the severe cases (Table 1). The three most significant regions associated with disease severity were also reported to be quantitative trait loci (QTLs) associated with HbF level in the previous genetic linkage and association studies.

6. HbF quantitative trait loci

It is clear from isolated family, linkage and GWAS studies that there are several QTLs for HbF and F-cells. Moreover, in many family studies, the high HbF phenotype segregates independently of the β-globin gene cluster, implicating the presence of *trans*-acting factors. The major QTLs for HbF and F-cells that have been extensively studied are located in three loci, one is *in-cis* with the β-globin gene cluster and two are *in-trans* with the β-globin gene cluster, the *HBS1L-MYB* intergenic region and *BCL11A* gene.

6.1 β-globin cluster

It has been recognized since the 1980s that the C→T single base substitution at position -158 in the promoter of the $^{G}\gamma$-globin gene is associated with high HbF levels (Gilman &

Huisman, 1985; Labie et al., 1985a). Evidence for the influence of a genetic variant within the β-globin gene cluster came from families with β-thalassemia or sickle cell anemia which showed a tendency for co-segregation of higher or lower HbF levels with the disease mutation. The HbS mutation is found on four major β-globin cluster haplotypes (HbS-Senegal, -Benin, -Bantu, and –Arab/Indian). Carriers for the β^S gene on the HbS-Senegal or HbS-Arab/Indian β^S haplotype (including the T allele of *Xmn*I -158 $^G\gamma$-globin) have high HbF levels, and a mild clinical course, whereas carriers of the β^S gene on a HbS-Bantu haplotype (including the C allele of *Xmn*I -158 $^G\gamma$-globin) have low HbF levels (Labie et al., 1985b). Despite the long time since the identification of this locus as a major QTL for HbF expression, functional studies have been inconclusive. Identification of the pinpoint causative variant is still unknown, in part because the QTL is located in a large LD block spanning over 62 kb. A plausible explanation of the genetic variant in β-globin cluster and olfactory receptor genes upstream function is the regulation of globin genes expression and hemoglobin switching. In erythroblasts, the β-globin locus forms an erythroid-specific spatial structure called the active chromatin hub (ACH). The ACH composed of the HS sites of the LCR, active β-globin genes, remote 5′ HS sites (HS-110 in human) and 3′ HS-1 (Fang et al., 2007). A chromatin hub is formed by looping 3′ HS-1, 5′ HS-110, and the 5′ part of the LCR together. The β-globin gene locus is surrounded by the genes encoding olfactory receptors that are expressed in olfactory epithelium, but not in erythroid cells (Bulger et al., 1999). The HS-110 and 3′ HS-1 site are located in the olfactory receptor genes (ORGs) cluster. An RNA FISH study in erythroid cells indicated that intergenic transcription of the β-globin locus occurs over a region of more than 250 kb including several genes in the nearby olfactory receptor gene cluster (Miles et al., 2007).

6.2 *HBS1L-MYB* intergenic region

Extensive studies over the years of Thein and colleages showed that a quantitative trait locus (QTL) for HbF expression in adults is located in the *HBS1L-MYB* intergenic region, the so called HBS1L-MYB intergenic polymorphisms (HMIP). A genome-wide linkage analysis study covered seven generations of 210 family members of an Asian-Indian kindred with heterocellular HPFH, β-thalassemia and α-thalassemia identified QTLs for HbF expression on chromosome 6q23-q24 (Lod score = 12.4) (Craig et al., 1996; Garner et al., 1998). Fine mapping of the 1.5 Mb region of human chromosome 6q23 encompassing the area showed five genes, *ALDH8A1, HBS1L, MYB, AHI1* and *PDE7B* (Close et al., 2004). To narrow down the candidate region, a high-resolution association study was performed in twin pairs of North European origin. Three LD blocks within the 79 kb long *HBS1L-MYB* intergenic region showed very strong associations with F-cell levels (*P-value*= 10^{-75}), with the strongest effect in the second block (24 kb) (Thein et al., 2007). The HMIP accounts for about 19% of the North European population trait variance. In Thai β-thalassemia/HbE, a GWAS study also showed that the most significantly-associated SNP with the HbF level in the *HBS1L-MYB* region, rs9399137, is also located within the HMIP second block. The HbF expression QTL at HMIP is also reported in healthy individuals of African descent (Creary et al., 2009), sickle cell patients from Tanzania, Brazil, African American (Creary et al., 2009; Lettre et al., 2008; Makani et al., 2011), β-thalassemia heterozygotes (So et al., 2008) and β-thalassemia patients (Galanello et al., 2009; Nuinoon et al., 2010).

The HMIP has been reported to contain distal regulatory elements that generate a key part of the overall control of the *MYB* expression (Wahlberg et al., 2009). In *MYB* expressing primary human erythroid cells, the core *HBS1L-MYB* intergenic region harbors several potential cis-regulatory elements for GATA-1 signals that coincided with DNase I hypersensitive sites. HbF expression is linked to the kinetics of erythrocyte maturation and differentiation. *MYB* plays role in erythroid proliferation and differentiation, and in turn, the control of HbF levels (Jiang et al., 2006). The HMIP was associated not only with the HbF levels but also with the cell numbers of platelets and monocytes in the peripheral blood (Menzel et al., 2007). Recently, a 3-bp deletion, between 135,460,326 and 135,460,328 bp on chromosome 6q23 in HMIP was identified as the functional motif (Farrell et al., 2011).

6.3 BCL11A gene

The association of *BCL11A* and HbF expression was first identified by two GWAS studies (Menzel et al., 2007; Uda et al., 2008). The first GWAS with the F-cell trait was performed in a European twin cohort, targeting 179 individuals with contrasting extreme F-cell values. Association analysis identified not only the *Xmn*I -158 $^{G}\gamma$-globin and the chromosome 6 locus but also a new F-cell locus in intron 2 of the oncogene *BCL11A* on chromosome 2p15 (Menzel et al., 2007). The second GWAS based on HbF of 4,000 individuals from Sardinia also showed association to the same three loci, the β-globin locus, HMIP and *BCL11A*, which was the first replication of the *BCL11A* locus in patients with SCA and β-thalassemia (Uda et al., 2008). This locus was subsequently replicated in additional SCA patients from the USA and Brazil (Lettre et al., 2008; Sedgewick et al., 2008), and β-thalassemia heterozygotes from Hong Kong and the parents of β-thalassemia/HbE patients from Thailand (Nuinoon et al., 2010; Sedgewick et al., 2008).

The *BCL11A* gene encodes several isoforms of a zinc finger transcription factor, the shorter isoforms appeared to be restricted to primitive erythroblasts, and the full-length isoforms to adult-stage erythroblasts (Sankaran et al., 2008). Down-regulation of BCL11A expression in adult human erythroid precursors results in induction of HbF (Sankaran et al., 2008; Wilber et al., 2011). High-resolution chromatin immunoprecipitation (ChIP)–chip analysis and chromosome conformation capture (3C) assay showed that BCL11A binds the upstream locus control region (LCR), ε-globin and the intergenic regions between γ-globin and δ-globin genes cooperating with SOX6 that reconfigures the β-globin cluster by modulating chromosomal loop formation, which finally leads to transcriptional silencing of the γ-globin genes (Xu et al., 2010).

7. Conclusion

Thalassemias are the most common genetic disease in the world resulting from the defective globin chain synthesis. The main pathophysiologic feature of thalassemia is the accumulation of unpaired globin chains in erythrocyte precursors and red blood cells (β-globin in α-thalassemia and α-globin in β-thalassemia). The unmatched globin chains precipitated in the erythroid precursors in the bone marrow as well as in peripheral erythrocyte membranes contribute to ineffective erythropoiesis and shortened peripheral RBC survival resulting in chronic anemia in these patients. As a monogenic disorder, thalassemia is a very heterogeneous disorder. Patients with identical β-thalassemia genotypes show a remarkable variability in disease severity, ranging from nearly asymptomatic (mild disease) to transfusion-dependent anemia with additional complications (severe disease). Thus, thalassemias are good example of the Mendelian genetic disease that demonstrate phenotypic variations due to the result of multigene interactions. Understanding the roles played by genetic factors in diseases will revolutionize diagnosis, treatment, and prevention, in addition to increase understanding of the environmental contributions. Three levels of genetic modifiers which influence the severity of β-thalassemia have been classified into primary, secondary and tertiary modifiers. The primary modifying factor is described by expression of the β-globin alleles due to the heterogeneity of the molecular lesions of the underlying the β-thalassemia mutation itself. Secondary modifying factors are factors that can affect the degree of globin chain imbalance, which are α-globin genotype and variation in fetal hemoglobin production. Tertiary modifiers are candidate genes which may be involved in several pathological alterations in patients. Our recent GWAS in Thai β-thalassemia/HbE patient cohorts suggests that a number of additional genetic modifier genes may account for the variability in clinical expression. The three genes/regions that are most significant in β-thalassemia/HbE disease severity are also associated with HbF expression, namely the β-globin gene cluster and olfactory receptor genes upstream of β-globin gene cluster on chromosome 11p15.5, the HBS1L-MYB intergenic region on chromosome 6q23 and the *BCL11A* gene on chromosome 2p15. It is noteworthy that the HbF expression QTL in the β-globin cluster was discovered by family and population studies in the 1980s and subsequently validated by genetic studies. The second QTL, the *HBS1L-MYB* intergenic region, was discovered by linkage analysis in extensive kindred in 1990s, and subsequently validated by genetic association studies. The third QTL, the *BCL11A*, was discovered in 2000s by GWAS. This shows the significant development of genomic technologies and knowledge of the human genome. The rapid development of next-generation sequencing technologies seems likely to accelerate further genomic studies. The many less significant variants may be identified in near future. There are several less significant genes compared to the three above mentioned regions, which may play roles in modification of disease severity. More studies are also needed to address the effect of these modifying factors.

8. Acknowledgment

This study was supported in part by the Office of the Higher Education Commission and Mahidol University under the National Research University Initiative, Thailand Research Fund and National Science and Technology Development Agency, Thailand.

9. References

Bragos, I. M.; Noguera, N. I., et al. (2003). Triplication ($/\alpha\alpha\alpha^{anti3.7}$) or deletion ($-\alpha^{3.7}/$) association in Argentinian β-thalassemic carriers. *Ann Hematol,* Vol. 82, No. 11, (Nov), pp. 696-698, ISSN 0939-5555

Brookes, A. J. (1999). The essence of SNPs. *Gene,* Vol. 234, No. 2, (Jul 8), pp. 177-186, ISSN 0378-1119

Bulger, M.; van Doorninck, J. H., et al. (1999). Conservation of sequence and structure flanking the mouse and human β-globin loci: the β-globin genes are embedded within an array of odorant receptor genes. *Proc Natl Acad Sci USA,* Vol. 96, No. 9, (Apr 27), pp. 5129-5134, ISSN 0027-8424

Camaschella, C.; Kattamis, A. C., et al. (1997). Different hematological phenotypes caused by the interaction of triplicated α-globin genes and heterozygous β-thalassemia. *Am J Hematol,* Vol. 55, No. 2, (Jun), pp. 83-88, ISSN 0361-8609

Camaschella, C.; Mazza, U., et al. (1995). Genetic interactions in thalassemia intermedia: analysis of β-mutations, α-genotype, gamma-promoters, and β-LCR hypersensitive sites 2 and 4 in Italian patients. *Am J Hematol,* Vol. 48, No. 2, (Feb), pp. 82-87, ISSN 0361-8609

Cardon, L. R.&Bell, J. I. (2001). Association study designs for complex diseases. *Nat Rev Genet,* Vol. 2, No. 2, (Feb), pp. 91-99, ISSN 1061-4036

Carnley, B. P.; Prior, J. F., et al. (2006). The prevalence and molecular basis of hemoglobinopathies in Cambodia. *Hemoglobin,* Vol. 30, No. 4, pp. 463-470, ISSN 0363-0269

Close, J.; Game, L., et al. (2004). Genome annotation of a 1.5 Mb region of human chromosome 6q23 encompassing a quantitative trait locus for fetal hemoglobin expression in adults. *BMC Genomics,* Vol. 5, No. 1, (May 31), pp. 33, ISSN 1471-2164

Craig, J. E.; Rochette, J., et al. (1996). Dissecting the loci controlling fetal haemoglobin production on chromosomes 11p and 6q by the regressive approach. *Nat Genet,* Vol. 12, No. 1, (Jan), pp. 58-64, ISSN 1061-4036

Creary, L. E.; Ulug, P., et al. (2009). Genetic variation on chromosome 6 influences F cell levels in healthy individuals of African descent and HbF levels in sickle cell patients. *PLoS One,* Vol. 4, No. 1, pp. e4218, ISSN 1932-6203

Dover, G. J.; Smith, K. D., et al. (1992). Fetal hemoglobin levels in sickle cell disease and normal individuals are partially controlled by an X-linked gene located at Xp22.2. *Blood,* Vol. 80, No. 3, (Aug 1), pp. 816-824, ISSN 0006-4971

Economou-Petersen, E.; Aessopos, A., et al. (1998). Apolipoprotein E epsilon4 allele as a genetic risk factor for left ventricular failure in homozygous β-thalassemia. *Blood,* Vol. 92, No. 9, (Nov 1), pp. 3455-3459, ISSN 0006-4971

Fang, X.; Xiang, P., et al. (2007). Cooperativeness of the higher chromatin structure of the β-globin locus revealed by the deletion mutations of DNase I hypersensitive site 3 of the LCR. *J Mol Biol,* Vol. 365, No. 1, (Jan 5), pp. 31-37, ISSN 0946-2716

Farrell, J. J.; Sherva, R. M., et al. (2011). A 3-bp deletion in the HBS1L-MYB intergenic region on chromosome 6q23 is associated with HbF expression. *Blood,* Vol 117, No 18, (May 5), pp. 4935-4945, ISSN 0006-4971

Fisher, C. A.; Premawardhena, A., et al. (2003). The molecular basis for the thalassaemias in Sri Lanka. *Br J Haematol,* Vol. 121, No. 4, (May), pp. 662-671, ISSN 0007-1048

Frazer, K. A.; Ballinger, D. G., et al. (2004). Finishing the euchromatic sequence of the human genome, *Nature,* Vol 431, No 7011, (Oct 21), pp. 931-945, ISSN 0028-0836.

Frazer, K. A.; Ballinger, D. G., et al. (2005). A haplotype map of the human genome. *Nature,* Vol. 437, No. 7063, (Oct 27), pp. 1299-1320, ISSN 0028-0836

Fucharoen, S.&Winichagoon, P. (1997). Hemoglobinopathies in Southeast Asia: molecular biology and clinical medicine. *Hemoglobin,* Vol. 21, No. 4, (Jul), pp. 299-319, ISSN 0363-0269

Fucharoen, S.&Winichagoon, P. (2000). Clinical and hematologic aspects of hemoglobin E β-thalassemia. *Curr Opin Hematol,* Vol. 7, No. 2, (Mar), pp. 106-112, ISSN 1065-6251

Fucharoen, S.; Winichagoon, P., et al. (1984). Determination for different severity of anemia in thalassemia: concordance and discordance among sib pairs. *Am J Med Genet,* Vol. 19, No. 1, (Sep), pp. 39-44, ISSN 1552-4825

Fucharoen, S.; Winichagoon, P., et al. (1987). Variable severity of Southeast Asian β^0-thalassemia/Hb E disease. *Birth Defects Orig Artic Ser,* Vol. 23, No. 5A, pp. 241-248, ISSN 1542-0752

Galanello, R.; Ruggeri, R., et al. (1983). A family with segregating triplicated α globin loci and β-thalassemia. *Blood,* Vol. 62, No. 5, (Nov), pp. 1035-1040, ISSN 0006-4971

Galanello, R.; Sanna, S., et al. (2009). Amelioration of Sardinian β^0-thalassemia by genetic modifiers. *Blood,* Vol. 114, No. 18, (Oct 29), pp. 3935-3937, ISSN 0006-4971

Garner, C. P.; Tatu, T., et al. (2002). Evidence of genetic interaction between the β-globin complex and chromosome 8q in the expression of fetal hemoglobin. *Am J Hum Genet,* Vol. 70, No. 3, (Mar), pp. 793-799, ISSN 0002-9297

Garner, C.; Mitchell, J., et al. (1998). Haplotype mapping of a major quantitative-trait locus for fetal hemoglobin production, on chromosome 6q23. *Am J Hum Genet,* Vol. 62, No. 6, (Jun), pp. 1468-1474, ISSN 0002-9297

Garner, C.; Tatu, T., et al. (2000). Genetic influences on F cells and other hematologic variables: a twin heritability study. *Blood,* Vol. 95, No. 1, (Jan 1), pp. 342-346, ISSN 0006-4971

Gilman, J. G.&Huisman, T. H. (1985). DNA sequence variation associated with elevated fetal $^G\gamma$ globin production. *Blood,* Vol. 66, No. 4, (Oct), pp. 783-787, ISSN 0006-4971

Hardison, R. C.; Chui, D. H., et al. (1998). Access to a syllabus of human hemoglobin variants (1996) via the World Wide Web. *Hemoglobin,* Vol. 22, No. 2, (Mar), pp. 113-127, ISSN 0363-0269

Hauser, E. R.; Watanabe, R. M., et al. (2004). Ordered subset analysis in genetic linkage mapping of complex traits. *Genet Epidemiol,* Vol. 27, No. 1, (Jul), pp. 53-63, ISSN 0741-0395

Higgs, D. R.; Old, J. M., et al. (1980). A novel α-globin gene arrangement in man. *Nature,* Vol. 284, No. 5757, (Apr 17), pp. 632-635, ISSN 0028-0836

Hirschhorn, J. N.&Daly, M. J. (2005). Genome-wide association studies for common diseases and complex traits. *Nat Rev Genet,* Vol. 6, No. 2, (Feb), pp. 95-108, ISSN 1061-4036

Jiang, J.; Best, S., et al. (2006). cMYB is involved in the regulation of fetal hemoglobin production in adults. *Blood,* Vol. 108, No. 3, (Aug 1), pp. 1077-1083, ISSN 0006-4971

Labie, D.; Dunda-Belkhodja, O., et al. (1985a). The -158 site 5' to the $^G\gamma$ gene and $^G\gamma$ expression. *Blood,* Vol. 66, No. 6, (Dec), pp. 1463-1465, ISSN 0006-4971

Labie, D.; Pagnier, J., et al. (1985b). Common haplotype dependency of high Gγ-globin gene expression and high Hb F levels in β-thalassemia and sickle cell anemia patients. *Proc Natl Acad Sci USA,* Vol. 82, No. 7, (Apr), pp. 2111-2114, ISSN 0027-8424

Lander, E. S. (2011). Initial impact of the sequencing of the human genome. *Nature,* Vol. 470, No. 7333, (Feb 10), pp. 187-197, ISSN 0028-0836

Lander, E. S.; Linton, L. M., et al. (2001). Initial sequencing and analysis of the human genome. *Nature,* Vol. 409, No. 6822, (Feb 15), pp. 860-921, ISSN 0028-0836

Lettre, G.; Sankaran, V. G., et al. (2008). DNA polymorphisms at the BCL11A, HBS1L-MYB, and β-globin loci associate with fetal hemoglobin levels and pain crises in sickle cell disease. *Proc Natl Acad Sci U S A,* Vol. 105, No. 33, (Aug 19), pp. 11869-11874, ISSN 0027-8424

Longo, F.; Zecchina, G., et al. (1999). The influence of hemochromatosis mutations on iron overload of thalassemia major. *Haematologica,* Vol. 84, No. 9, (Sep), pp. 799-803, ISSN 0390-6078

Ma, S. K.; Au, W. Y., et al. (2001). Clinical phenotype of triplicated α-globin genes and heterozygosity for β^0-thalassemia in Chinese subjects. *Int J Mol Med,* Vol. 8, No. 2, (Aug), pp. 171-175, ISSN 1107-3756

Makani, J.; Menzel, S., et al. (2011). Genetics of fetal hemoglobin in Tanzanian and British patients with sickle cell anemia. *Blood,* Vol. 117, No. 4, (Jan 27), pp. 1390-1392, ISSN 0006-4971

Manolio, T. A. (2010). Genomewide association studies and assessment of the risk of disease. *N Engl J Med,* Vol. 363, No. 2, (Jul 8), pp. 166-176, ISSN 0028-4793

Menzel, S.; Jiang, J., et al. (2007). The HBS1L-MYB intergenic region on chromosome 6q23.3 influences erythrocyte, platelet, and monocyte counts in humans. *Blood,* Vol. 110, No. 10, (Nov 15), pp. 3624-3626, ISSN 0006-4971

Miles, J.; Mitchell, J. A., et al. (2007). Intergenic transcription, cell-cycle and the developmentally regulated epigenetic profile of the human β-globin locus. *PLoS One,* Vol. 2, No. 7, pp. e630, ISSN 1932-6203

Modell, B.&Darlison, M. (2008). Global epidemiology of haemoglobin disorders and derived service indicators. *Bull World Health Organ,* Vol. 86, No. 6, (Jun), pp. 480-487,

Nava, M. P.; Ibarra, B., et al. (2006). Prevalence of $-\alpha^{(3.7)}$ and $\alpha\alpha\alpha^{(anti3.7)}$ alleles in sickle cell trait and β-thalassemia patients in Mexico. *Blood Cells Mol Dis,* Vol. 36, No. 2, (Mar-Apr), pp. 255-258, ISSN 1079-9796

Nuinoon, M.; Makarasara, W., et al. (2010). A genome-wide association identified the common genetic variants influence disease severity in β^0-thalassemia/hemoglobin E. *Hum Genet,* Vol. 127, No. 3, (Mar), pp. 303-314, ISSN 0340-6717

Orkin, S. H.; Kazazian, H. H., Jr., et al. (1982). Abnormal RNA processing due to the exon mutation of β^E-globin gene. *Nature,* Vol. 300, No. 5894, (Dec 23), pp. 768-769, ISSN 0028-0836

Perrotta, S.; Cappellini, M. D., et al. (2000). Osteoporosis in β-thalassaemia major patients: analysis of the genetic background. *Br J Haematol,* Vol. 111, No. 2, (Nov), pp. 461-466, ISSN 0007-1048

Premawardhena, A.; Fisher, C. A., et al. (2001). Genetic determinants of jaundice and gallstones in haemoglobin E β-thalassaemia. *Lancet,* Vol. 357, No. 9272, (Jun 16), pp. 1945-1946, ISSN 0140-6736

Rees, D. C.; Luo, L. Y., et al. (1997). Nontransfusional iron overload in thalassemia: association with hereditary hemochromatosis. *Blood,* Vol. 90, No. 8, (Oct 15), pp. 3234-3236, ISSN 0006-4971

Rees, D. C.; Porter, J. B., et al. (1999). Why are hemoglobin F levels increased in HbE/β thalassemia? *Blood,* Vol. 94, No. 9, (Nov 1), pp. 3199-3204, ISSN 0006-4971

Reich, D. E.&Lander, E. S. (2001). On the allelic spectrum of human disease. *Trends Genet,* Vol. 17, No. 9, (Sep), pp. 502-510, ISSN 0168-9525

Rund, D.&Rachmilewitz, E. (2005). β-Thalassemia. *N Engl J Med,* Vol. 353, No. 11, (Sep 15), pp. 1135-1146, ISSN 0028-4793

Sachidanandam, R.; Weissman, D., et al. (2001). A map of human genome sequence variation containing 1.42 million single nucleotide polymorphisms. *Nature,* Vol. 409, No. 6822, (Feb 15), pp. 928-933, ISSN 0028-0836

Sankaran, V. G.; Menne, T. F., et al. (2008). Human fetal hemoglobin expression is regulated by the developmental stage-specific repressor BCL11A. *Science,* Vol. 322, No. 5909, (Dec 19), pp. 1839-1842, ISSN 0036-8075

Sedgewick, A. E.; Timofeev, N., et al. (2008). BCL11A is a major HbF quantitative trait locus in three different populations with β-hemoglobinopathies. *Blood Cells Mol Dis,* Vol. 41, No. 3, (Nov-Dec), pp. 255-258, ISSN 1079-9796

Sherva, R.; Sripichai, O., et al. (2010). Genetic modifiers of Hb E/β^0-thalassemia identified by a two-stage genome-wide association study. *BMC Med Genet,* Vol. 11, No. pp. 51, ISSN 1471-2350

So, C. C.; Song, Y. Q., et al. (2008). The HBS1L-MYB intergenic region on chromosome 6q23 is a quantitative trait locus controlling fetal haemoglobin level in carriers of β-thalassaemia. *J Med Genet,* Vol. 45, No. 11, (Nov), pp. 745-751, ISSN 0022-2593

Sripichai, O.; Makarasara, W., et al. (2008a). A scoring system for the classification of β-thalassemia/Hb E disease severity. *Am J Hematol,* Vol. 83, No. 6, (Jun), pp. 482-484, ISSN 0361-8609

Sripichai, O.; Munkongdee, T., et al. (2008b). Coinheritance of the different copy numbers of α-globin gene modifies severity of β-thalassemia/HbE disease. *Ann Hematol,* Vol. 87, No. 5, (May), pp. 375-379, ISSN 0939-5555

Thein, S. L. (2008). Genetic modifiers of the β-haemoglobinopathies. *Br J Haematol,* Vol. 141, No. 3, (May), pp. 357-366, ISSN 0007-1048

Thein, S. L.; Hesketh, C., et al. (1988). The molecular basis of thalassaemia major and thalassaemia intermedia in Asian Indians: application to prenatal diagnosis. *Br J Haematol,* Vol. 70, No. 2, (Oct), pp. 225-231, ISSN 0007-1048

Thein, S. L.; Menzel, S., et al. (2007). Intergenic variants of HBS1L-MYB are responsible for a major quantitative trait locus on chromosome 6q23 influencing fetal hemoglobin levels in adults. *Proc Natl Acad Sci U S A,* Vol. 104, No. 27, (Jul 3), pp. 11346-11351, ISSN 0027-8424

Thein, S. L.; Wainscoat, J. S., et al. (1987). Association of thalassaemia intermedia with a β-globin gene haplotype. *Br J Haematol,* Vol. 65, No. 3, (Mar), pp. 367-373, ISSN 0007-1048

Thompson, C. C.; Ali, M. A., et al. (1989). The interaction of anti 3.7 type quadruplicated α-globin genes and heterozygous β-thalassemia. *Hemoglobin,* Vol. 13, No. 2, pp. 125-135, ISSN 0363-0269

Traeger-Synodinos, J.; Kanavakis, E., et al. (1996). The triplicated α-globin gene locus in β-thalassaemia heterozygotes: clinical, haematological, biosynthetic and molecular studies. *Br J Haematol,* Vol. 95, No. 3, (Dec), pp. 467-471, ISSN 0007-1048

Tubsuwan, A.; Munkongdee, T., et al. (2011) Molecular analysis of globin genes expression in different thalassaemia disorders individual variation of β^E pre-mRNA splicing determine disease severity. *Br J Haematol.* Vol. 154, No. 5, (Sep), pp. 635-643, ISSN 0007-1048

Uda, M.; Galanello, R., et al. (2008). Genome-wide association study shows BCL11A associated with persistent fetal hemoglobin and amelioration of the phenotype of β-thalassemia. *Proc Natl Acad Sci U S A,* Vol. 105, No. 5, (Feb 5), pp. 1620-1625, ISSN 0027-8424

Venter, J. C.; Adams, M. D., et al. (2001). The sequence of the human genome. *Science,* Vol. 291, No. 5507, (Feb 16), pp. 1304-1351, ISSN 0036-8075

Wahlberg, K.; Jiang, J., et al. (2009). The HBS1L-MYB intergenic interval associated with elevated HbF levels shows characteristics of a distal regulatory region in erythroid cells. *Blood,* Vol. 114, No. 6, (Aug 6), pp. 1254-1262, ISSN 0006-4971

Wainscoat, J. S.; Kanavakis, E., et al. (1983). Thalassaemia intermedia in Cyprus: the interaction of α and β thalassaemia. *Br J Haematol,* Vol. 53, No. 3, (Mar), pp. 411-416, ISSN 0007-1048

Weatherall, D. J.; Clegg, J. B., et al. (1965). Globin synthesis in thalassaemia: an in vitro study. *Nature,* Vol. 208, No. 5015, (Dec 11), pp. 1061-1065, ISSN 0028-0836

Wilber, A.; Hargrove, P. W., et al. (2011). Therapeutic levels of fetal hemoglobin in erythroid progeny of β-thalassemic CD34+ cells after lentiviral vector-mediated gene transfer. *Blood,* Vol. 117, No. 10, (Mar 10), pp. 2817-2826, ISSN 0006-4971

Winichagoon, P.; Fucharoen, S., et al. (1995). Role of alternatively spliced β^E-globin mRNA on clinical severity of β-thalassemia/hemoglobin E disease. *Southeast Asian J Trop Med Public Health,* Vol. 26 Suppl 1, No. pp. 241-245,

Xu, J.; Sankaran, V. G., et al. (2010). Transcriptional silencing of γ-globin by BCL11A involves long-range interactions and cooperation with SOX6. *Genes Dev,* Vol. 24, No. 8, (Apr 15), pp. 783-798, ISSN 0890-9369

8

HMG–CoA Lyase Deficiency

Beatriz Puisac, María Arnedo, Mª Concepción Gil-Rodríguez,
Esperanza Teresa, Angeles Pié, Gloria Bueno, Feliciano J. Ramos,
Paulino Goméz-Puertas and Juan Pié
Unit of Clinical Genetics and Functional Genomics
School of Medicine, University of Zaragoza
Spain

1. Introduction

The HMG-CoA lyase (HL) deficiency or 3-hydroxy-3-methylglutaric aciduria (MIM 246450) is an inborn error of intermediary metabolism that was first described in 1976 by Faull et al (Faull et al., 1976). Because its clinical manifestations, it has been included within the Sudden Infant Death Syndrome (Wilson et al., 1984). At present, it is considered a rare disease (<1/100,000 live neonates) that should be diagnosed at early age because there is a simple and effective treatment (Watson et al., 2006).

HL is a mitochondrial enzyme that catalyzes the cleavage of HMG-CoA to acetyl-CoA and acetoacetate, which is the common final step of ketogenesis and leucine catabolism (Figure 1). Patients with this disease suffer on the one hand, the absence of ketone bodies as alternative energy source of glucose and on the other hand, the accumulation of toxic metabolites of leucine catabolism. The most frequently affected organs are the liver and the brain, but the pancreas and the heart can also be involved. This chapter discusses a recent study of differential expression of human HL in liver, pancreas, testis, heart, skeletal muscle and brain that can help us to understand the consequences of this deficiency (Puisac et al., 2010).

It is an autosomal recessive disease caused by mutations in the *HMGCL* gene. The study of these mutations and patients´ origin helps to draw a map of incidence in which three countries stand out for their high frequency: Saudi Arabia (Ozand et al., 1992), Spain and Portugal (Menao et al., 2009).

At present, the functional study of missense mutations is possible thanks to the knowledge of the structure (Fu et al., 2006) and mechanism of the enzyme (Fu et al., 2010) and also by the development of a method of simple and efficient expression of the protein (Menao et al., 2009). Finally, despite the current knowledge of the disease, genotype-phenotype correlations are difficult to establish.

2. HL enzyme

HL is a 325-aminoacid enzyme that has been purified from a variety of organisms and tissues, including pig heart (Bachawat et al., 1955), chicken liver (Kramer et al., 1980) and *Pseudomonas mevalonii* (Scher et al., 1989). In addition to the isoform located in the mitochondrial matrix, it has been described another in peroxisomes (Ashmarina et al., 1994). The native mitochondrial isoform contains a leader peptide of 27 aminoacids at the N-terminal end, which guides HL towards the mitochondrial matrix, where the leader peptide is removed. This final isoform has a molecular mass of 31.5 kDa and an isoelectric point of 6.2.

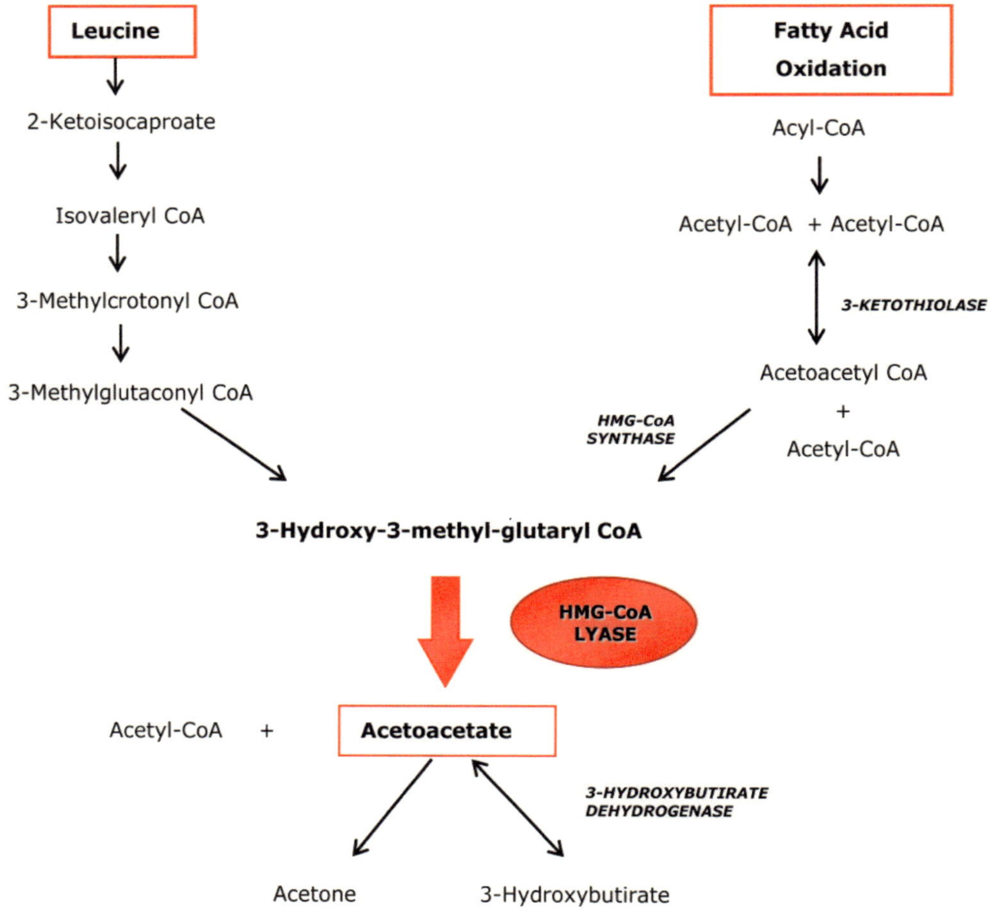

Fig. 1. Metabolic interrelationships of HL

Human HL has 87% simmilarity with its mouse homologue, 82% with its chicken homologue, and 52% with *P. mevalonii*, and the sequence has been highly conserved throughout evolution (Pié et al., 2007). The cathalytic active form is a homodimer of two identical monomers bound by a disulphide bridge (Roberts, 1994). The human enzyme is very sensitive to oxidation, showing higher activity in reductive conditions. It is also sensitive to the conditions of pH, showing an optimum activity at alkaline pH (pH=9). HL activity requires the presence of a divalent cation, such as Mg^{+2} or Mn^{+2}. The Mg^{+2} ion has an octahedral coordination with two water molecules, the imidazole nitrogens of catalitic residues His^{233} and His^{235}, the carboxylate group of Asp^{42} and the amide oxygen of Asn^{275}. Other catalytic residues in the vicinity include Arg^{41} and Cys^{266}.

2.1 Protein structure

The first attempt to build a 3D structural model of human 3-hydroxy-3-methylglutaryl-CoA lyase was based on a threading procedure using the crystallized structure of the TIM-barrel hisA gene from *Thermotoga maritima* as a template (Casals et al., 2003). The proposed model correspond to a $(\alpha\beta)_8$ barrel with short loops on the NH_2 terminal face and, in contrast, long and probably non-structured loops on the COOH-terminal face of the β-barrel. This model showed, for the first time, the structural proximity of the residues involved in the cathalytic activity of the protein: Arg^{41}, Asp^{42}, Glu^{72}, His^{233} and His^{235}, located near the cavity opened in the COOH-terminal face of the protein model (Figure 2).

This model was confirmed when the cristal structure of human HL was obtained (Fu et al., 2006). In addition to the basic TIM barrel structure, the monomer of human HL includes an additional polypeptide region made of residues 290-323 containing β-strand 9, and α-helices 11 and 12. The active site is accessible only from the C-terminal side of the TIM barrel and the N-terminal barrel end is occluded. Crystal structures of the wild-type enzyme complex and inhibitor hydroxyglutaryl-CoA has demostrated the interaction of Arg^{41} and acyl-CoA´s C1 carbonyl oxygen of sustrate and explains why Arg^{41} mutations cause drastic enzyme deficiency (Fu et al., 2010).

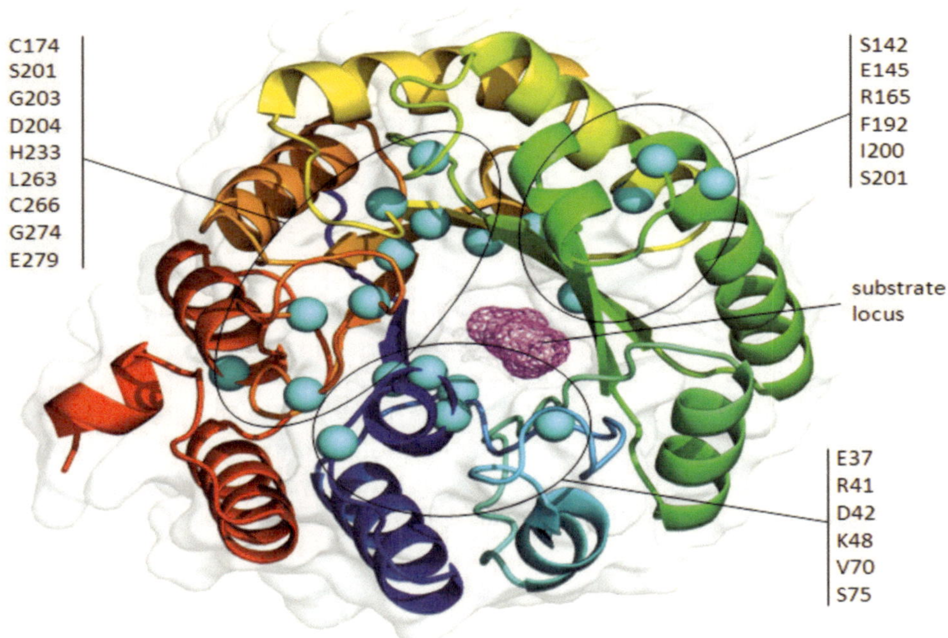

Fig. 2. Structural location of missense mutations in human HL. Blue spheres represent mutated residues

The native enzyme is a dimer in solution (Tuinstra et al., 2002) that was confirmed when the protein was crystallized. The area of contact between monomers is formed by additional secondary elements that are not part of the core TIM barrel structure, β-strand 9, and α-helices 11 and 12. Recently it was suggested that multiple cysteine residues influence covalent adduct formation in HMG-CoA lyase as well as the dependence of enzyme activity on reducing agent (Montgomery & Miziorko, 2011).

2.2 Enzymatic reaction

The cleavage of HMG-CoA, catalyzed by the HL enzyme is the final step of ketogenesis, in which acetyl-CoA, mainly from the β-oxidation of fatty acids, is converted to acetoacetate, β-hydroxybutyrate and acetone (Figure 1). From a chemical point of view, the enzyme reaction is a retro-Claisen condensation, which requires an acid and a base for catalysis (Roberts et al., 1996). The base abstracts a proton from the C3 hydroxyl of HMG-CoA, which leads to the formation of a ketone (acetoacetate) and C2–C3 bond cleavage (Figure 3). In addition, a transient carbanion form of acetyl-CoA, is regenerated by the acid proton. However, the exact identity of molecules or residues that act as base or as acid was not precised. Recently a water molecule, positioned between D42 and the C3 hydroxyl of bound sustrate has been proposed as a proton shuttle (Fu et al., 2010).

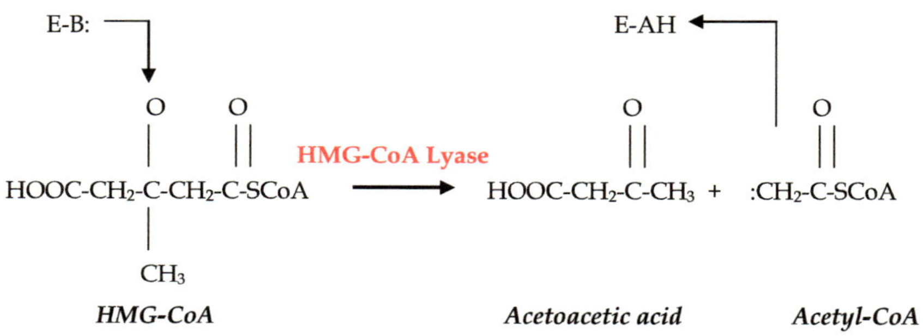

Fig. 3. Chemical reaction catalyzed by the enzyme HMG-CoA lyase. E-B: base, E-AH acid

2.3 Enzyme expression

HL is widely expressed in most tissues (Clikenbeard et al., 1975) mainly because it is necessary not only in tissues that synthesize ketone bodies, but for the catabolism of leucine as well. Activity levels of this enzyme have been reported in different eucaryotes organism tissues: pig heart (Bachawat et al., 1955), bovine liver (Stegink & Coon, 1968) and chicken liver, kidney, heart, brain, ileum and muscle (Clikenbeard et al., 1975). However, its distribution and activity in human tissues have been limited to enzyme assay in fibroblast (Wanders et al., 1988b) lymphoblast (Wysocki et al, 1976b) liver biopsy (Robinson et al,1980) amniocytes and chorionic villi (Wanders et al., 1988b) or pancreatic islets (MacDonald et al., 2007).

Recently, it has been reported the first study of mRNA levels, protein expression and enzyme activity of human HMG-CoA lyase in kidney, pancreas, testis, heart, skeletal muscle and brain (Puisac et al., 2010). The highest HL activity was found in liver and pancreas was the second with more activity (Figure 4c). This finding indicates that the pancreas has a high ketogenic capacity and suggests that if ketone bodies regulate the release of insulin (Biden & Taylor, 1983; Malaisse et al., 1990; Rhodes et al., 1985) some of them could be produced in the pancreas. HL activity in kidney was high and moderately high in testis and skeletal muscle. Surprisingly in muscle, although the mRNA levels were very low (Figure 4a), moderate HL activity was measured. Similar cases are reported in the literature (Lewin et al., 2001), which suggests that certain tissues may have a lower turnover of the HL protein versus an unstable mRNA. In testis, the low activity levels of HL compared with the high enzyme expression (Figure 4b), suggest that HL activity could be regulated after translation in this tissue. However, very little HL is found in heart tissue and it is not present in the mitochondria from human brain.

2.4 Isoforms

Two different protein isoforms of HL have been found, which are codified by a single gene located in chromosome 1. While most HL is found in mitochondria, about 16-20% is located in peroxisomes (Ashmarina et al., 1999). To date, no satisfactory explanation has been found to explain this distribution. The protein found in peroxisomes is guided by the signal CKL tripeptide in the C-terminal end and it has 325 aminoacids, a molecular mass of 34.1 kDa and an isoelectric point of 7.6, which is much more basic than the mitochondrial protein (Ashmarina et al., 1994). As the mitochondrial isoform, it is a dimeric form and has lyase activity; however its role inside peroxisomes is still unknown. Probably, this is related to cholesterol synthesis or long chain fat acids degradation (Krisans et al., 1996).

3. HL deficiency

HMG-CoA lyase deficiency or 3-Hydroxy-3-methylglutaric aciduria (OMIM 246450) is a rare autosomal recessive genetic disorder that affects ketogenesis and L-leucine catabolism. For this reason, it is included within alterations of fatty acid metabolism and also within organic acidemias. This deficiency was first described by Faull et al in 1976 in a 7 month-old male with acidosis and hypoglycemia (Faull et al., 1976). Later, Wysocki et al showed that HL activity in the leukocytes of this patient was null (Wysocky et al., 1976). The gene knock-out in mice results in embryonic lethality (Wang et al., 1998) reflecting the physiological importance of this enzyme.

3.1 Clinical features

3-Hydroxy-3-methylglutaric aciduria is a severe condition in children, in fasting or in high glucose consumption, when ketone bodies are essential as alternative energy substrate. In approximately 30% of the cases the first symptoms appear between the second and fifth days of life or between 3 and 11 months. However, four patients with late onset (puberty and adult) have been reported (Sweetman et al., 1995; Vargas et al., 2007; Bischof et al., 2004; Reimao et al., 2009).

3.1.1 Acute crisis

Acute crises tend to occur when there is no exogenous intake of glucose (starving cases) or when there is an excessive glucose metabolization (conditions of metabolic stress, febrile stress and exercise). Initial symptoms may include poor feeding, vomiting, diarrhea, followed by further complication as hypotonia, hypothermia, lethargy, cyanosis and apnea. (Schutgens et al., 1979; Gibson et al., 1988a; Gibson et al., 1988b). In some cases the progresive lowered state of consciousness leads to coma and subsequent death (Wysocki et al., 1986). Laboratory data that stand out are the metabolic acidosis and non-ketotic hypoglycemia (Table 1). Hypoglycemia can be explained by fasting or other intercurrent illness, while the hipoketonemia shows the inability of patients to synthesize ketone bodies. Metabolic acidosis and aciduria can be explained by the accumulation of acids metabolites from leucine catabolism: 3-hydroxy-isovaleric acid, 3-methylglutaconic acid, 3-methylglutaric acid and 3-hydroxy-3-methylglutaric acid. Occasionally, patients present with increased bilirubin, liver transaminases and prothrombin time. It is also reported the appearance of hyperammonemia associated with increased proteolysis by deficiency of ketone bodies.

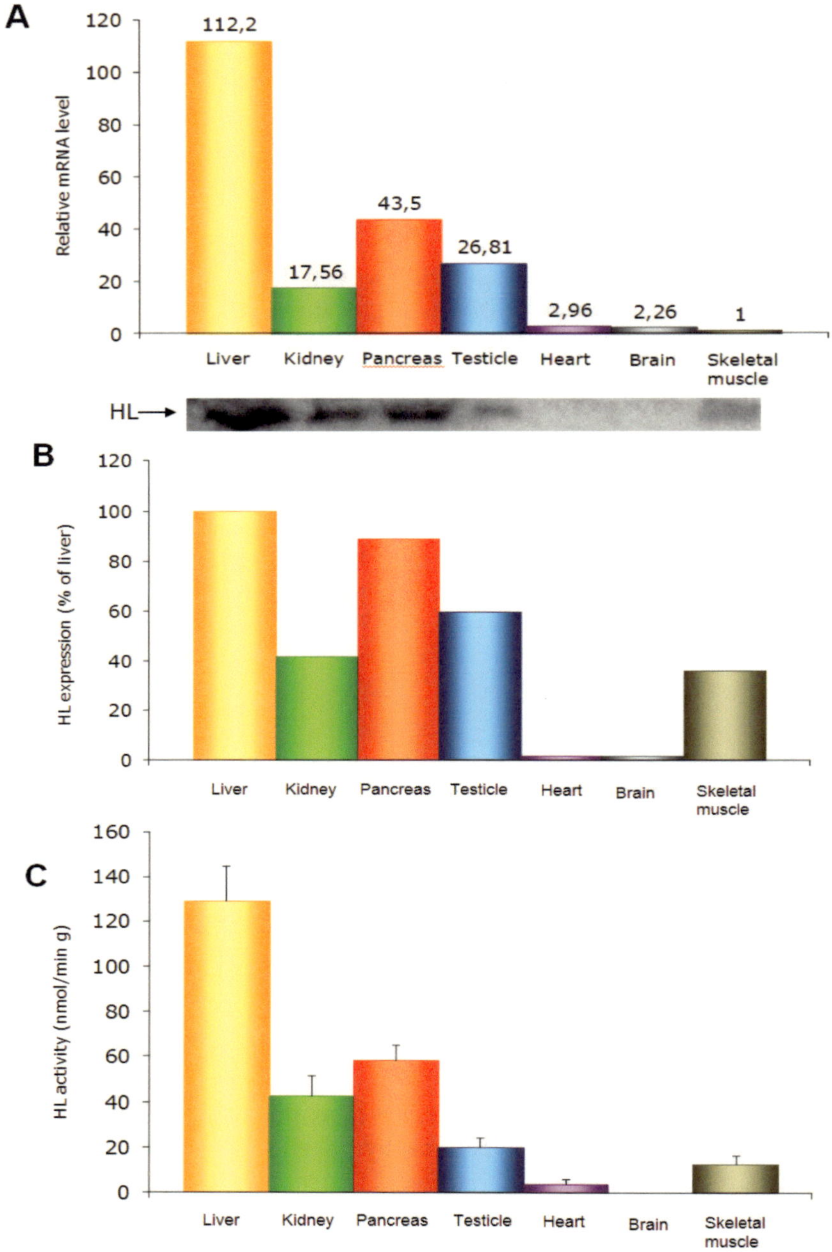

Fig. 4. Comparative analysis of mRNA levels, protein expression and enzymatic activity of HMG-CoA lyase in different human tissues. (A) Relative levels of mRNA HL expression in human tissues (B) HL protein expression measured in mitochondrial fraction from human tissues (C) HL activity was measured in the mitochondrial fraction of human tissues spectrophotometrically. Data are presented as mean ±SEM

Clinical manifestations in acute clinical episodes	
Vomiting Diarrhea Hipotonia Hypothermia Lethargy Apnea Coma	Frequent all of them if the clinical picture worsens
Laboratory test	
General biochemistry	
Metabolic acidosis	Always present
Hypoglycemia	Always present
Hypoketonemia	Always present
Ketonuria	Absent
Hyperammonemia	Elevated frequently
Hepatic transaminases	Elevated frequently
Bilirrubin	Elevated in some cases
Prothrombin time	Elevated in some cases
Organic acids	
3-hydroxy-3-methylglutaric	Elevated very frequently
3-methylglutaric	Elevated frequently
3-methylglutaconic	Elevated sometimes
3-hydroxyisovaleric	Elevated sometimes
HL enzyme activity	Less than 5%
Affected organs	
Brain	Macro o Microcephaly (infrequent) Alterations of the white matter (frequent) Epilepsy (infrequent) Cerebral infarction (infrequent)
Pancreas	Acute pancreatitis (infrequent)
Liver	Hepatomegaly (very frequent)
Heart	Dilated cardiomyopathy with arrythmia (infrequent)

Table 1. Clinical and laboratory findings of the HMG-CoA lyase deficiency

3.1.2 Chronic complications

Chronic complications are uncommon but include: hepatomegalia, macrocephalia (Gibson et al., 1988b; Stacey et al., 1985) microcephalia (Lisson et al., 1981) and delayed development (Gibson et al., 1994). It has been reported that organs such as the brain, the liver and occasionally the pancreas and the heart are affected (Gibson et al., 1994; Leung et al., 2009; Muroi et al., 2000a; Urganci et al., 2001; Wilson et al., 1984; Zafeiriou et al., 2007; Zoghbi et

al., 1986). Recently, a study of mRNA levels, protein expression and enzyme activity of human HMG-CoA lyase in kidney, pancreas, testis, heart, skeletal muscle and brain has contributed to better understanding of the enzyme function and of the involvement of these organs in 3-hydroxy-3-methylglutaric aciduria (Puisac et al., 2010).
The liver is the organ most frequently affected in this deficiency, although involvement is usually mild, with elevated transaminases and hepatomegaly (Urganci et al., 2001; Wysocki & Hahnel, 1986). Ketogenesis is more active in the liver and the blockage of this pathway could result in an accumulation of toxic intermediate metabolites.
Pancreatitis is a potential complication in patients with organic acidemias, (Kahler et al., 1994) and some cases have been reported in 3-hydroxy-3-methylglutaric aciduria (Muroi et al., 2000a; Wilson et al., 1984). The finding of higher enzymatic activity in pancreas (Puisac et al., 2010) indicates that it may be more susceptible to toxic accumulation of metabolites. Among the brain abnormalities in these patients, cerebral white matter involment is the most common reported finding (Lisson et al., 1981; Yalcinkaya et al., 1999; Zafeiriou et al., 2007) and also one case of prominent corticospinal tract and pontine involvement has also been reported (Yylmaz et al., 2006). HL is not found at different levels of mRNA, protein and enzymatic activity, in the mitochondria from human brain (Puisac et al., 2010). This suggests that the neurological alterations frequently associated with this deficiency, are related to hypoglycaemia and to the absence of the only alternative substrate to glucose for the brain, ketone bodies. Concomitantly, the organic acids would not be produced in situ, although they could cross the blood-brain barrier of an immature brain (Wajner et al., 2004) and cause damage.
Dilated cardiomyopathy has been described in two patients with 3-hydroxy-3-methylglutaric aciduria, one young male (Gibson et al., 1994) and one adult (Leung et al., 2009). In this last case, the authors suggest that the cardiomyopathy results from impaired ketogenesis, intracellular fatty acid accumulation and a secondary carnitine deficiency. However, very little HL was found in heart tissue (Puisac et al., 2010). This result does not support the hypothesis of local accumulation of organic acids or regulation the entry of fatty acids to the heart and thus prevent their accumulation as a cause of the cardiomyopathy. In HL deficiency heart disease could be caused by the lack of an alternative energy substrate. The heart is a continuously active muscle which uses various energy substrates depending on their availability (Kodde et al., 2007). Although ketone bodies are not an indispensable substrate, the added L-carnitine deficiency, which is caused by the HL deficiency, could alter the transport of fatty acids to the mitochondria for oxidation and the coupling between glycolysis and glucose oxidation (Allard et al., 2006).

3.2 Diagnosis

This deficiency should be suspected in children with hypoglycaemia, hipoketonemia and metabolic acidosis. A preliminary diagnosis is made from a characteristic pattern of organic acids in urine, with high levels of 3-hydroxy-3-methylglutaric acid, 3-hydroxy-isovaleric acid, 3-methylglutaric acid and 3-methylglutaconic acid (Table 1). The characteristic metabolite of this disease is the 3-hydroxy-3-methylglutaric acid, but can also occur in the deficiency of carbamyl phosphate synthetase or Leigh-like disease (Faull et al., 1976). The confirmation of HL deficiency requires direct assay of the enzyme activity in leukocytes (Wysocki et al., 1976a) fibroblasts (Wysocki et al., 1976b; Wanders et al., 1988a) or liver biopsy (Schutgens et al., 1979). In prenatal diagnosis the pattern of organic acids in amniotic liquid (Chalmers et al., 1979), in maternal urine (Duran et al., 1979) and measurements of HL activity in cultured amniocytes or chorionic villi (Mitchell et al., 1995; Chalmers et al., 1979) could be used as diagnostic tools. The molecular characterization of mutations in the gene *HMGCL*, including alterations in the mRNA, helps to complete the diagnosis.

3.3 Treatment

During acute episodes, treatment is based on symptoms and consists of intravenous administration of glucose to control hypoglycemia, and bicarbonate to correct acidosis. Maintenance therapy is based on restrictive protein and fat diet, whose aim is to reduce the formation of toxic metabolites. However, the most important concern is to avoid metabolic stress such as intercurrent illnesses and starvation. Carnitine treatment has been proposed to improve the patient´s general state by facilitating urinary excretion of toxic metabolites (Dasouki et al., 1979). Moreover, L-carnitine, can be essential to prevent the development of cardiomyopathy (Puisac et al., 2010).

3.4 Prognosis

Despite this disease belongs to a group of 29 genetic conditions for which effective treatment is currently available (Watson et al., 2006), HMG-CoA lyase deficiency is fatal in approximately 20% of the cases. Nevertheless, early and careful treatment may result in a good prognosis with normal growth and development. Besides, in absence of complications, illness tends to improve with time and adults are usually free of symptoms.

4. *HMGCL* gene

The *HMGCL* gene (Gen Bank NM_000191.2) located in the short arm of chromosome 1 (1p36.1-p35), between *FUCA1* and *TCEB3* encodes human HL. It has 9 exons and 8 introns (Figure 5) and a total of 24,336 base pairs. Its 5′-untranslated region bears the characteristic elements of a housekeeping gene, as well as a CpG island that contains binding sites for SP1. There is no evidence of the existence neither of a TATA box nor a CAAT box (Wang et al., 1996). Exons size varies between 64 and 527 base pairs (bp) and the introns range between 600 and 3400 bp. Exon 1 and part of exon 2 codify a 27 aminoacids array that forms the signal peptide for mitochondrial entering. Exon 9 codifies for 33 codons at the C-terminal ending and also has 406 bp from the 3′untranslated region (Mitchell et al., 1993). The polyadenylation signal in humans and mouse is ATTAAA. This gene is present in both eukaryotes and prokaryotes and it has been cloned and studied in a variety of organisms, including humans (Mitchell et al., 1993), chicken (Mitchell et al., 1993), mouse (Wang et al., 1993), the *Rhodospilirrum rubrum* (Baltscheffsky et al., 1997) and bacterial strains such as *Pseudomonas mevalonii* (Anderson et al., 1989), *Brucella mellitensis* and *Bacillus subtillus* (Forouhar et al., 2006).

The mRNA transcribed from *HMGCL* human gene has a size of 1.6 Kb and it has been found in all tissues studied albeit in widely differing amounts (Puisac et al., 2010) (Figure 4a) Tissues with the highest expression are liver 112.2 arbitrary units (100%) pancreas 43.5 (39%), kidney 17.56 (16%), testis 26.81 (24%), heart 2.96 (2,6%) brain 2.26 (2%) and skeletal muscle 1 (0.89%).

This gene presents a physiological splicing with three variants, one with all exons encoding the active protein and two with deletion of exons 5 and 6 and deletion of exons 5, 6 and 7 that encode inactive proteins (Muroi et al., 2000; Beatriz Puisac PhD thesis). These last two transcripts appear in tissues such as heart, brain and skeletal muscle which have little or no ketogenic potential.

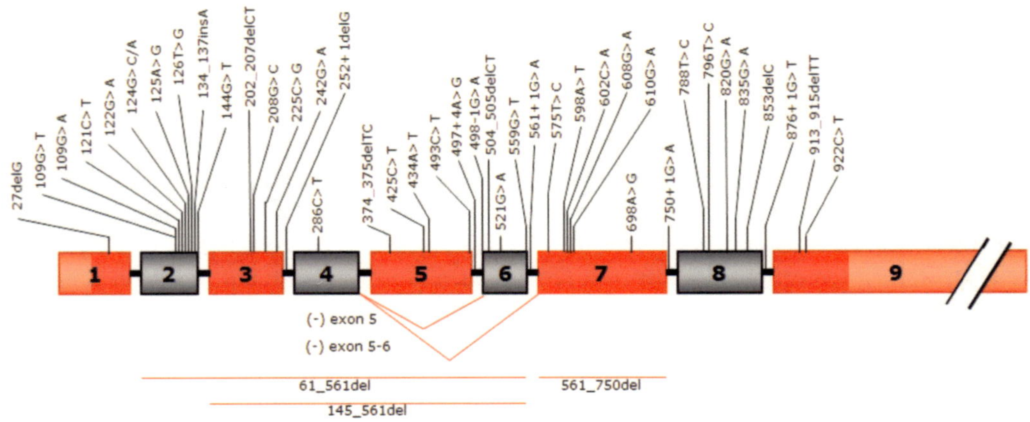

Fig. 5. Scheme of mutations located in the human *HMGCL* gene

4.1 Mutational update

To date 50 variant alleles in the *HMGCL* gene (48 mutations and 2 SNPs) in more than 100 patiens have been reported (Table 2). The missense mutations are the most frequent (25) followed by intronic mutations (7), frameshift deletions (6), nonsense mutations (6), large deletions (3) and insertions (1). The mutations are uniformly distributed along the gene sequences, although some clustering is observed in exon 2 and exon 7, suggesting that they could be hot spots for mutations (Figure 5).

Three mutations are more common than the rest: one is the c.122G>A (81 alleles, 43 patients: 38 homozygous, 5 heterozygous with an allele unknown), prevalent in Saudi Arabia, where 40 patients carry it (Mitchell et al., 1998; Al-Sayed et al., 2006) and that has also been found in a patient in Italy, another in Turkey (Mitchell et al., 1998) and one in the Tcheck Republic suggesting that this mutation may have arisen independently more than once (Pospisilova et al., 2003).

Allelic variant	Exon/ Intron	Aminoacid change/ Predicted effect	Patients	Mutant Aleles	Origin	References
Missense mutations						
c.109G>A	E2	E37K	2	4	2 Pakistani	Menao 2009
c.122G>A	E2	R41Q	43	81	1 Czech, 1 Italian (ht), 40 Saudi (4 ht), 1 Turkish	Al-Sayed 2006; Mitchell 1998; Pospisilova 2003
c.124G>A	E2	D42N	1	1	1 Brazilian (ht)	Vargas 2007
c.124G>C	E2	D42H	1	1	1 Cajun (ht)	Mitchell 1998
c.125A>G	E2	D42G	2	4	1 German, 1 Palestinian	Menao 2009; Mitchell 1998
c.126T>G	E2	D42E	1	2	1 Austrian	Mitchell 1998

Allelic variant	Exon/ Intron	Aminoacid change/ Predicted effect	Patients	Mutant Aleles	Origin	References
c.144G>T	E2	K48N	1	1	1 Spanish	Carrasco 2007
c.208G>C	E3	V70L	1	1	1 French-Canadian (ht)	Mitchell 1992
c.225C>G	E3	S75R	1	2	1 German	Casals 2003
c.425C>T	E5	S142F	1	1	1 Spanish (ht)	Menao 2009
c.434A>T	E5	E145V	1	1	1 Japanese (ht)	Muroi 2000
c.493C>T	E5	R165W	1	2	1 Turkish	Koling 2000
c.494G>A	E5	R165Q	1	1	1 French? (ht)	Pierron 2009
c.494G>T	E5	R165Q	1	1	1Tawianese (ht)	Lin 2009
c.521G>A	E6	C174Y	1	2	1 Palestinian	Menao 2009
c.575T>C	E7	F192S	1	2	1 Spanish	Menao 2009
c.598A>T	E7	I200F	1	2	1 French	Menao 2009
c.602C>A	E7	S201Y	1	2	1 English	Casals 2003
c.608G>A	E7	G203E	1	2	1 Italian	Mir 2006
c.610G>A	E7	D204N	2	3	1 Argentinean ,1 Portuguese (ht)	Casals 2003; Cardoso 2004
c.698A>G	E7	H233R	4	5	2 Czech (1ht), 1 French (ht), 1 English (ht)	Menao 2009; Pospisilova 2003; Roberts 1996; Zapater 1998
c.788T>C	E8	L263P	1	1	1 French (ht)	Zapater 1998
c.796T>C	E8	C266R	1	1	1 Greek (ht)	Zafeiriou 2007
c.820G>A	E8	G274R	1	1	1 French? (ht)	Pierron 2009
c.835G>A	E8	E279K	2	3	2 Japanese (1 ht)	Muroi 2000
Nonsense mutations						
c.109G>T	E2	E37X; Exon 2 skipping	31	55	1 Argentinian, 2 Moroccan, 13 Portuguese (4ht) , 11 Spanish (1ht), 1 Turkish, 3 portuguese-brazilian (2ht)	Cardoso 2004; Casale 1998; Menao 2009; Pié 1997; Puisac 2005
c.121C>T	E2	R41X	1	1	1 English/German (ht)	Mitchell 1998
c. 242G>A	E3	W81X	1	2	1 Ecuatorian	Menao 2009
c.286C>T	E4	Q96X	1	2	1 Italian	Funghini 2001
c.559G>T	E6	E187X	1	1	1 Spanish (ht)	Menao 2009
c.922C>T	E9	Q308X	1	2	1 Japanese	Muroi 2000

Allelic variant	Exon/ Intron	Aminoacid change/ Predicted effect	Patients	Mutant Aleles	Origin	References
Deletions/ insertions						
c.27delG	E1	P9P/ frameshift: stop codon 33	1	1	1 Czech (ht)	Pospisilova 2003
c.134-137insA	E2	N46K/frameshift: stop codon 47	2	4	2 Italian	Mitchell 1995
c.61-561del	E2,E3,E4,E5, E6	Deletes V21-E187 in frame	1	1	1 English	Wang 1996
c.202-207delCT	E3	S69C/ frameshift: stop codon 79	3	6	2 Acadian French-Canadian, 1 Spanish	Mitchell 1993
c.145-561del	E3,E4,E5, E6	Deletes E49-E187 in frame	1	1	1 Turkish	Wang 1996
c.374-375delTC	E5	V125D/frameshift: stop codon 150	1	1	1 Greek (ht)	Zafeiriou 2007
c.504-505delCT	E6	V168V/frameshift: stop codon 176; Exon 5 and 6, 6 skipping	10	11	3 Portuguese-brazilian (3ht), 2 Portuguese (2ht), 5 Spanish (4 ht)	Cardoso 2004; Casals 1997; Menao 2009; Vargas 2007
c.561-750del	E7	Deletes E187-Q250 in frame	1	2	1 Japanese	Muroi 2000
c.853delC	E8	Frameshift: stop codon 258	1	1	1 English (ht)	Menao 2009
c.913-915delTT	E9	F305Y/ frameshift: stop codon 314	3	6	3 Saudi	Al-Sayed 2006; Mitchell 1998
Intronic mutations						
IVS3+1Gdel	I3	Exon 3 deletion	1	2	1 Japanese	Muroi 2000
IVS3+1G>A	I3	Exon 3 deletion	1	1	1 Tawianese (ht)	Lin 2009
IVS5+4A>G	I5	Exon 5 deletion/ exon 5-6 deletion	1	1	1 English (ht)	Menao 2009
IVS6-1G>A	I5		1	1	1 Taiwanese (ht)	Lin 2009
IVS6+1G>A	I6		1	2	1 Saudi	Al-Sayed 2006
IVS7+1G>A	I7	r.slp	2	2	2 Spanish (2 ht)	Menao 2009
IVS8+1G>T	I8	Exon 8 deletion	1	2	1 Turkish	Buesa 1996

Allelic variant	Exon/ Intron	Aminoacid change/ Predicted effect	Patients	Mutant Aleles	Origin	References
Polimorfism						
c.252+34C>T	I3		1	1	1 Palestinian (ht)	Menao 2009
c.654A>G	E7	L218L	1	-	1 Spanish	Pié 1997
c.727A>G	E7	T243A	4	8	1 Moroccan, 1 Portuguese, 2 Spanish	Pié 1997

Table 2. Mutations and polymorphisms in the *HMGCL* gene. Position refers to the numbering of the HL cDNA sequence in Mitchell et al., 1993. ht, heterozygous

The second most frequent mutation is the c.109G>T (Mediterranean mutation) (55 alleles, 31 patients: 24 homozygous, 6 double heterozygous, 1 heterozygous with an allele unknown), found mostly in the Iberian Peninsula (13 patients in Portugal, 11 in Spain and 3 in brazilian-portugueses). It has also been described two cases in Morocco and another in Turkey (Pié et al., 1997; Casale et al., 1998; Cardoso et al., 2004; Puisac et al., 2005; Menao et al., 2009). It has been hypothesized that in Portugal and Spain the genetic hit was introduced during the Arabian invasions of the Iberian Peninsula in the eighth century. Further studies should be necessary to dillucidate if the mutation origin is the Iberian Peninsula itself or the Magreb (Pié et al., 2007).

The third most frequent mutation is c.504_505delCT (11 alleles, 10 patients: 1 homozygous, 9 double heterozygous), although its incidente is much lower than the first two. It seems to be exclusively located in the Iberian Peninsula, where 15% of Portuguese (2 cases) (Cardoso et al., 2004) and 27% of Spanish patients have it (Menao et al., 2009). This mutation is also present in 3 of the 4 molecularly diagnosed Brazilians patients, though they were of Portuguese origin (Vargas et al., 2007).

In most of the remaining countries, only a few patients are reported, with a high level of allelic heterogeneity. In Japan 4 mutations have been reported in 5 unrelated patients (Muroi et al., 2000b), in Taiwan 3 mutations in 2 patients (Lin et al., 2009) in Italy, 5 mutations in 5 patients (Mitchell et al., 1995; Mitchell et al., 1998; Funghini et al., 2001) in Turkey 4 mutations in 4 patients (Wang et al., 1996; Buesa et al., 1996; Pié et al., 1997; Mitchell et al., 1998) . In the United Kingdom 6 mutations in 5 patients, though one of them was of German origin (c.121C>T) (Wang et al., 1996; Mitchell et al., 1998; Casals et al., 2003; Menao et al., 2009), 3 mutations in 3 patients in the Tcheck Republic (Pospisilova et al., 2003) and in Germany 2 mutations in 2 patients (Mitchell et al., 1998; Casals et al., 2003). The French group, the Acadians (descendents of the 17th-century French colonists), the Cajuns (Acadians settled in Louisiana) and the French-Canadians, despite of their common origin, present a great allelic heterogenicity: 6 mutations in 6 patients (Mitchell et al., 1992; Mitchell et al., 1993; Zapater et al., 1998; Mitchell et al., 1998; Menao et al., 2009).

4.2 Genotype-phenotype correlations

The genotype-phenotype correlation is difficult to establish because the progress of the disease seems to be more related to the causes that produce hypoglycaemia (fasting or acute illness) than to a specific genotype. For example, patients carrying the same mutation, for

instance the so-called Mediterranean mutation (c.109G>T) may have from moderate to severe crises of lethal consequences. This is why in clinical practice it is fundamental to avoid situations that may cause hypoglycemia in these patients (Pié et al., 2007).
Several studies agree that studied missense mutations cause a loss of enzyme activity greater than 95% although these mutations often produce mild phenotypes (Mitchell et al., 1998; Carrasco et al., 2007; Menao et al., 2009). This suggests that the illness appears only in very severe genotypes, and that partial disruption of the enzyme is probably compatible with normal function. This adds more difficulties to establish genotype-phenotype correlations because we only see the effects of very severe genotypes.

5. Conclusion

Although 3-hydroxy-3-methylglutaric aciduria is a very rare disease, given the availability of an effective treatment, we recommend the screening of this disease in any child with hypoglycemia and metabolic acidosis. Moreover, in countries with a greater number of diagnosed cases (Saudi Arabia, Portugal and Spain), we also recommend to screen for the following mutations: c.122G>A, c.109G>T and c.504_505delCT. The high percentage of splicing mutations justifies including the measurement of the mRNA.

6. Acknowledgment

This study was supported by Spanish grants from: Diputación General de Aragón (Ref.# Grupo Consolidado B20) and University of Zaragoza (Ref.# PIF-UZ_2009-BIO-02). We also thank to "Biomol-Informatics SL -www.bioinfo.es-" for bioinformatic support.

7. References

Allard, ML., Jeejeebhoy, KN., & Sole, MJ. (2006). The management of conditioned nutritional requirements in heart failure. *Heart Failure Reviews,* Vol. 11, No. 1, (March 2006), pp. 75-82, ISSN 1382-4147

Al-Sayed, M., Imtiaz, F., Alsmadi, OA., Rashed, MS., & Meyer, BF. (2006). Mutations underlying 3-hydroxy-3-methylglutaryl CoA lyase deficiency in the Saudi population. *BMC Medical Genetics*, Vol. 16, No. 7, (December 2006), ISSN 1471-2350

Anderson, DH., & Rodwell, VW. (1989). Nucleotide sequence and expression in Escherichia coli of the 3-hydroxy-3-methylglutaryl coenzyme A lyase gene of Pseudomonas mevalonii. *Journal of Bacteriology*, Vol. 171, No. 12, (December 1989), pp. 6468-6472, ISSN 0021-9193

Ashmaina, LI., Rusnak, N., Miziorko, HM., & Mitchell, GA. (1994). 3-Hydroxy-3-methylglutaryl-CoA lyase is present in mouse and human liver peroxisomes. *The Journal of Biological Chemistry,* Vol. 269, No. 50 (December 1994), pp. 31929-31932, ISSN 0752-7399

Ashmarina, LI., Pshezhetsky, AV., Branda, SS., Isaya, G., & Mitchell, GA. (1999). 3-Hydroxy-3-methylglutaryl coenzyme A lyase: targeting and processing in peroxisomes and mitochondria. *Journal of Lipid Research,* Vol. 40, No. 1, (January 1999), pp. 70-75, ISSN 0022-2275

Bachhawat, BK., Robinson, WG., & Coon, MJ. (1955). The enzymatic cleavage of beta-hydroxy-beta-methylglutaryl coenzyme A to acetoacetate and acetyl coenzyme A. *Journal of Biological Chemistry,* Vol. 216, (August 1955), pp. 727-736, ISSN 0021-9258

Baltscheffsky, M., Brosché, M., Hultman, T., Lundvik, L., Nyrén, P., Sakai-Nore, Y., Severin, A., & Strid, A. (1997). A 3-hydroxy-3-methylglutaryl-CoA lyase gene in the photosynthetic bacterium Rhodospirillum rubrum. *Biochimica Biophysica Acta,* Vol. 1337, No. 1, (January 1997), pp. 113-122, ISNN 0005-2736

Biden, TJ., & Taylor, KW. (1983). Effects of ketone bodies on insulin release and islet-cell metabolism in the rat. *Biochemical Journal,* Vol. 212, No. 2, (May 1983), pp. 371-377, ISSN 0264-6021

Bischof, F., Nagele, T., Wanders, RJ., Trefz, FK., & Melms, A. (2004). 3-Hydroxy-3-methylglutaryl-coenzyme A lyase deficiency in an adult with leukoencephalopathy. *Annals of Neurology,* Vol. 56, No. 5, (November 2004), pp. 727-730. ISNN 0364-5134

Buesa, C., Pié, J., Barceló, A., Casals, N., Mascaró, C., Casale, CH., Haro, D., Duran, M., Smeitink, JA., Hegardt, FG. (1996). Aberrantly spliced mRNAs of the 3-hydroxy-3-methylglutaryl coenzyme A lyase (HL) gene with a donor splice-site point mutation produce hereditary HL deficiency. *Journal of Lipid Research,* Vol. 37, No.11, (November 1996), pp. 2420-2432, ISNN 0022-2275

Cardoso, ML., Rodrigues, MR., Leão, E., Martins, E., Diogo, L., Rodrigues, E., Garcia, P., Rolland, MO., & Vilarinho, L. (2004). The E37X is a common HMGCL mutation in Portuguese patients with 3-hydroxy-3-methylglutaric CoA lyase deficiency. *Molecular Genetics and Metabolism,* Vol. 82, No. 4, (August 2004), pp. 334-338, ISSN 1096-7192

Carrasco, P., Menao, S., López-Viñas, E., Santpere, G., Clotet, J., Sierra, AY., Gratacós, E., Puisac, B., Gómez-Puertas, P., Hegardt, FG., Pie, J., & Casals, N. (2007). C-terminal end and aminoacid Lys48 in HMG-CoA lyase are involved in substrate binding and enzyme activity. *Molecular Genetics and Metabolism,* Vol. 91, No. 2, (June 2007), pp. 120-127, ISSN 1096-7192

Casale, CH., Casals, N., Pié, J., Zapater, N., Pérez-Cerdá, C., Merinero, B., Martínez-Pardo, M., García-Peñas, JJ., García-Gonzalez, JM., Lama, R., Poll-The, BT., Smeitink, JA., Wanders, RJ., Ugarte, M., & Hegardt, FG. (1998). A nonsense mutation in the exon 2 of the 3-hydroxy-3-methylglutaryl coenzyme A lyase (HL) gene producing three mature mRNAs is the main cause of 3-hydroxy-3-methylglutaric aciduria in European Mediterranean patients. *Archives of Biochemistry and Biophysics,* Vol. 349, No.1, (January 2001), pp. 129-137, ISSN 0003-9861

Casals, N., Gomez-Puertas, P., Pie, J., Mir, C., Roca, R., Puisac, B., Aledo, R., Clotet, J., Menao, S., Serra, D., Asins, G., Till, J., Elias-Jones, AC., Cresto, JC., Chamoles, NA., Abdenur, JE., Mayatepek, E., Besley, G., Valencia, A., & Hegardt, FG. (2003). Structural (betaalpha)$_8$ TIM barrel model of 3-hydroxy-3-methylglutaryl-coenzyme A lyase. *Journal of Biological Chemistry,* Vol. 278, No. 31, (May 2003), pp. 29061-29023, ISSN 0021-9258

Chalmers, RA., Tracey, BM., Mistry, J., Stacey, TE., & McFadyen, IR. (1989). Prenatal diagnosis of 3-hydroxy-3-methylglutaric aciduria by GC-MS and enzymology on cultured amniocytes and chorionic villi. *Journal of Inherited Metabolic Disease,* Vol. 12, No. 3, pp. 286-292, ISSN 0141-8955

Clinkenbeard, KD., Reed, WD., Mooney, RA. (1975). Intracellular localization of the 3-hydroxy-3-methylglutaryl coenzyme A cycle enzymes in liver. Separate cytoplasmic and mitochondrial 3-hydroxy-3-methylglutaryl coenzyme A generating systems for cholesterogenesis and ketogenesis. *Journal of Biological Chemistry,* Vol. 250, No. 8, (April 1975), pp. 3108-3116, ISSN 0021-9258

Dasouki, M., Buchanan, D., Mercer, N., Gibson, KM., & Thoene, J. (1987). 3-Hydroxy-3-methylglutaric aciduria: response to carnitine therapy and fat and leucine restriction. *Journal of Inherited Metabolic Disease*, Vol. 10, No. 2, (1987), pp. 142-146, ISSN 0141-8955

Duran, M., Ketting, D., Wadman, SK., Jakobs, C., Schutgens, RB., & Veder, HA. (1978). Organic acid excretion in a patient with 3-hydroxy-3-methylglutaryl-CoA lyase deficiency: facts and artefacts. *Clinica Chimica Acta*, Vol. 90, No. 2, (December 1978), pp. 187-193, ISSN 0009-8981

Faull, KF., Bolton, PD., Halpern, B., Hammond, J., Danks, DM., Hähnel, R., Wilkinson, SP., Wysocki, SJ., & Masters, PL. (1976). Letter: Patient with defect in leucine metabolism. *New England Journal of Medicine*, Vol. 294, No. 18, (April 1976), pp. 1013, ISSN 0028-4793.

Forouhar, F., Hussain, M., Farid, R., Benach, J., Abashidze, M., Edstrom, WC., Vorobiev, SM., Xiao, R., Acton, TB., Fu, Z., Kim, JJ., Miziorko, HM., Montelione, GT., & Hunt, JF. (2006). Cristal structures of two bacterial 3-hydroxy-3-methylglutaryl-CoA lyases suggest a common catalytic mechanism among a family of TIM barrel metalloenzymes cleaving carbon-carbon bonds. *Journal of Biological Chemistry*, Vol. 281, No. 11, (March 2006), pp. 7533-7545, ISSN 0021-9258

Fu, Z., Runquist, JA., Forouhar, F., Hussain, M., Hunt, JF., Miziorko, HM., & Kim, JJ. (2006). Crystal structure of human 3-hydroxy-3-methylglutaryl-CoA Lyase: insights into catalysis and the molecular basis for hydroxymethylglutaric aciduria. *Journal of Biological Chemistry*, Vol. 281, No. 11, (March 2006), pp. 7526-7532, ISSN 0021-9258.

Fu, Z., Runquist, JA., Montgomery, C., Miziorko, HM., & Kim, JJ. (2010). Functional insights into human HMG-CoA lyase from structures of Acyl-CoA-containing ternary complexes. *Journal of Biological Chemistry*, Vol. 285, No. 34, (August 2010), pp. 26341-26349, ISSN 0021-9258

Funghini, S., Pasquini, E., Cappellini, M., Donati, MA., Morrone, A., Fonda, C., & Zammarchi, E. (2001). 3-Hydroxy-3-methylglutaric aciduria in an Italian patient is caused by a new nonsense mutation in the HMGCL gene. *Molecular Genetics and Metabolism*, Vol. 73, No. 3, (July 2004), pp. 268-275, ISSN 1096-7192

Gibson, KM., Breuer, J., & Nyhan, WL. (1988a). 3-Hydroxy-3-methylglutaryl-coenzyme A lyase deficiency: review of 18 reported patients. *European Journal of Pediatrics*, Vol. 148, No. 3, (December 1988), pp. 180-186, ISSN 0340-6199

Gibson, KM., Breuer, J., Kaiser, K., Nyhan, WL., McCoy, EE., Ferreira, P., Greene, CL., Blitzer, MG., Shapira, E., & Reverte, F. (1988b). 3-Hydroxy-3-methylglutaryl-coenzyme A lyase deficiency: report of five new patients. *Journal of Inherited Metabolic Disease*, Vol. 11, No. 1, pp. 76-87, ISNN 0141-8955

Gibson, KM., Cassidy, SB., Seaver, LH., Wanders, RJ., Kennaway, NG., Mitchell, GA., & Spark, RP. (1994). Fatal cardiomyopathy associated with 3-hydroxy-3-methylglutaryl-CoA lyase deficiency. *Journal of Inherited Metabolic Disease*, Vol. 17, No. 3, pp. 291-294, ISNN 0141-8955

Kahler, SG., Sherwood, WG., Woolf, D., Lawless, ST., Zaritsky, A., Bonham, J., Taylor, CJ., Clarke, JT., Durie, P., & Leonard, JV. (1994). Pancreatitis in patients with organic acidemias. *The Journal of Pediatrics*, Vol. 124, No. 2, (February 1994), pp. 239-243, ISSN 0022-3476

Kodde, IF., van der Stok, J., Smolenski, RT., & de Jong, JW. (2007). Metabolic and genetic regulation of cardiac energy substrate preference. *Comparative Biochemistry and Physiology*, Vol. 146, No. 1, (January 2007), pp. 26-39, ISSN 1095-6433

Kramer, PR., & Miziorko, HM. (1980). Purification and characterization of avian liver 3-hydroxy-3-methylglutaryl coenzyme A lyase. *Journal of Biological Chemistry,* Vol. 255, No. 22, (November 1980), pp. 11023-11028, ISSN 0021-9258

Krisans, SK. (1996). Cell compartmentalization of cholesterol biosynthesis. *Annals of the New York Academy of Sciences,* Vol. 804, (December 1999), pp. 142-164, ISSN 0077-8923

Leung, AA., Chan, AK., Ezekowitz, JA. & Leung, AK. (2009). A Case of Dilated Cardiomyopathy Associated with 3-Hydroxy-3-Methylglutaryl-Coenzyme A (HMG CoA) Lyase Deficiency. *Case Report in Medicine,* Vol. 2009, (2009), pp.1-3 ISSN 1687-9627

Lewin, TM., Granger, DA., & Kim, JH. (2001). Regulation of mitochondrial sn-glycerol-3-phosphate acyltransferase activity: response to feeding status is unique in various rat tissues and is discordant with protein expression. *Archives of Biochemistry and Biophysics,* Vol. 396, No. 1, (December 2001), pp. 119-127, ISSN 0003-9861

Lin, WD., Wang, CH., Lai, CC., Tsai, Y., Wu, JY., Chen, CP., & Tsai , FJ. (2009). Molecular analysis of Taiwanese patients with 3-hydroxy-3-methylglutaryl CoA lyase deficiency. *Clinica Chimica Acta,* Vol. 401, No. 1-2, (March 2009), pp. 33-36, ISNN 0009-8981

Lisson, G., Leupold, D., Bechinger, D., & Wallesch, C. (1981). CT findings in a case of deficiency of 3-hydroxy-3-methylglutaryl-CoA-lyase. *Neuroradiology,* Vol. 22, No.2, pp.99-101, ISSN 0028-3940

MacDonald, MJ., Smith, AD., & Hasan, NM. (2007). Feasibility of pathways for transfer of acyl groups from mitochondria to the cytosol to form short chain acyl-CoAs in the pancreatic beta cell. *Journal of Biological Chemistry,* Vol. 282, No. 42, (October 2007), pp. 30596-30606, ISSN 0021-9258

Malaisse, WJ., Lebrun, P., & Rasschaert, J. (1990). Ketone bodies and islet function: 86Rb handling and metabolic data. *American Journal of Physiology,* Vol. 259, (January 1990), pp. E123-E130, ISSN 0363-6135

Menao, S., López-Viñas, E., Mir, C., Puisac, B., Gratacós, E., Arnedo, M., Carrasco, P., Moreno, S., Ramos, M., Gil, MC., Pié, A., Ribes, A., Pérez-Cerda, C., Ugarte, M., Clayton, PT., Korman, SH., Serra, D., Asins, G., Ramos, FJ., Gómez-Puertas, P., Hegardt, FG., Casals, N., & Pié, J. (2009). Ten novel HMGCL mutations in 24 patients of different origin with 3-hydroxy-3-methyl-glutaric aciduria. *Human Mutation,* Vol. 30, No. 3, (March 2009), pp.E520-529, ISSN 1098-1004

Mitchell, GA., Robert, MF., Fontaine, G., Wang, S., Lambert, M., Cole, D., Lee, C., Gibson, M., & Miziorko, MH. (1992). HMG CoA lyase (HL) deficiency: detection of a causal mutation in an affected French-Canadian sibship. *American Journal of Human Genetics,* Vol.51, A173, ISSN 0002-9297

Mitchell, GA., Robert, MF., Hruz, PW., Wang, SP., Fontaine, G., Behnke, CE., Mende-Mueller, LM., Schappert, K., Lee, C., Gibson, KM., & Miziorko, HM. (1993). 3-Hydroxy-3-methylglutaryl coenzyme A lyase (HL). Cloning of human and chicken liver HL cDNAs and characterization of a mutation causing human HL deficiency. *Journal of Biological Chemistry,* Vol. 268, No. 6, (February 1993), pp. 4376-4381, ISSN 0021-9258

Mitchell, GA., Jakobs, C., Gibson, KM., Robert, MF., Burlina, A., Dionisi-Vici, C., & Dallaire, L. (1995). Molecular prenatal diagnosis of 3-hydroxy-3-methylglutaryl CoA lyase deficiency. *Prenatal Diagnosis,* Vol. 15, No. 8, (August 1995), pp. 725-729, ISSN 0197-3851

Mitchell, GA., Ozand, PT., Robert, MF., Ashmarina, L., Roberts, J., Gibson, KM., Wanders, RJ., Wang, S., Chevalier, I., Plöchl, E., & Miziorko, H. (1998). HMG CoA lyase deficiency: identification of five causal point mutations in codons 41 and 42, including a frequent Saudi Arabian mutation, R41Q. *American Journal of Human Genetics*, Vol. 62, No .2, (February 1998), pp. 295-300, ISSN 0002-9297

Montgomery, C., & Miziorko, HM. (2011). Influence of multiple cysteines on human 3-hydroxy-3-methylglutaryl-CoA lyase activity and formation of inter-subunit adducts. *Archives of Biochemistry and Biophysics,* Vol.511, No. 1-2, (April 2011), pp.48-55, ISSN 0003-9861.

Muroi, J., Yorifuji, T., Uematsu, A., & Nakahata, T. (2000a). Cerebral infarction and pancreatitis: possible complications of patients with 3-hydroxy-3-methylglutaryl-CoA lyase deficiency. *Journal of Inherited Metabolic Disease,* Vol. 23, No. 6, (September 2000), pp. 636-637, ISSN 0141-8955

Muroi, J., Yorifuji, T., Uematsu, A., Shigematsu, Y., Onigata, K., Maruyama, H., Nobutoki, T., Kitamura, A., & Nakahata, T. (2000b). Molecular and clinical analysis of Japanese patients with 3-hydroxy-3-methylglutaryl CoA lyase (HL) deficiency. *Human Genetics,* Vol. 107, No. 4, (October 2000), pp. 320-326, ISSN 0340-6717

Ozand, PT., Devol, EB., & Gascon, GG. (1992). Neurometabolic diseases at a national referral center: five years experience at the King Faisal Specialist Hospital and Research Centre. *Journal of Child Neurology,* Suppl. 7, (April 1992), pp.S4-S11, ISSN 0883-0738.

Pié, J., Casals, N., Casale, CH., Buesa, C., Mascaró, C., Barceló, A., Rolland, MO., Zabot, T., Haro, D., Eyskens, F., Divry, P., & Hegardt, FG. (1997). A nonsense mutation in the 3-hydroxy-3-methylglutaryl-CoA lyase gene produces exon skipping in two patients of different origin with 3-hydroxy-3-methylglutaryl-CoA lyase deficiency. *Biochemical Journal,* Vol. 323, No. 2, (April 1997), pp. 329-335, ISSN 0264-6021

Pié, J., López-Viñas, E., Puisac, B., Menao, S., Pié, A., Casale, C., Ramos, FJ., Hegardt, FG., Gómez-Puertas, P., & Casals, N. (2007). Molecular genetics of HMG-CoA lyase deficiency. *Molecular Genetics and Metabolism,* Vol. 92, No. 3, (November 2007), pp. 198-209, ISSN 1096-7192

Pospísilová, E., Mrázová, L., Hrdá, J., Martincová, O., & Zeman, J. (2003). Biochemical and molecular analyses in three patients with 3-hydroxy-3-methylglutaric aciduria. *Journal of Inherited Metabolic Disease,* Vol. 26, No. 5, (2003), pp. 433-441, ISSN 0141-8955

Puisac, B. (2004). Splicing variants and three-dimensional structure of human HMG-CoA lyase. Molecular and functional characterization of four new allelic variants. *PhD thesis. University of Zaragoza, Department of Pharmacology and Physiology* (September 2004).

Puisac, B., López-Viñas, E., Moreno, S., Mir, C., Pérez-Cerdá, C., Menao, S., Lluch, D., Pié, A., Gómez-Puertas, P., Casals, N., Ugarte, M., Hegardt, F., & Pié, J. (2005). Skipping of exon 2 and exons 2 plus 3 of HMG-CoA lyase (HL) gene produces the loss of beta sheets 1 and 2 in the recently proposed (beta-alpha) 8 TIM barrel model of HL. *Biophysical Chemistry,* Vol. 115, No. 2-3, (April 2005), pp. 241-245, ISSN 0301-4622

Puisac, B., Arnedo, M., Casale, CH., Ribate, MP., Castiella, T., Ramos, FJ., Ribes, A., Pérez-Cerdá, C., Casals, N., Hegardt, FG., & Pié, J. (2010). Differential HMG-CoA lyase expression in human tissues provides clues about 3-hydroxy-3-methylglutaric aciduria. *Journal of Inherited Metabolic Disease,* Vol. 33, No. 4, (August 2010), pp. 405-410, ISSN 1573-2665

Reimão, S., Morgado, C., Almeida, IT., Silva, M., Real, HC., & Campos, J. (2009). 3-Hydroxy-3-methylglutaryl-coenzyme A lyase deficiency: Initial presentation in a young adult. *Journal of Inherited Metabolic Disease,* (February 2009), ISSN 0141-8955

Rhodes, CJ., Campbell, IL., & Szopa, TM. (1985). Effects of glucose and D-3-hydroxybutyrate on human pancreatic islet cell function. *Clinical Science,* Vol. 68, No.5, (May 1985), pp. 567-572, ISSN 0143-5221

Roberts, JR., Narasimhan, C., Hruz, PW., Mitchell, GA., & Miziorko, HM. (1994). 3-Hydroxy-3-methylglutaryl coenzyme A lyase: Expression and isolation of the recombinant human enzyme and investigation of a mechanism for regulation of enzyme activity. *Journal of Biological Chemistry,* Vol. 269, No. 27, (July 1994), pp.17841-17846, ISSN 0021-9258

Roberts, JR., Narasimhan, C., & Miziorko, HM. (1995). Evaluation of cysteine 266 of human 3-hydroxy-3-methylglutaryl coenzyme A lyase as a catalytic residue. *Journal of Biological Chemistry,* Vol. 270, No. 31, (July 1995), pp. 17311-17316, ISSN 0021-9258

Roberts, JR., Mitchell, GA., & Miziorko, HM. (1996). Modeling of a mutation responsible for human 3-hydroxy-3-methylglutaryl-CoA lyase deficiency implicates histidine 233 as an active site residue. *Journal of Biological Chemistry,* Vol. 271, No. 40, (October 1996), pp. 24604-24609, ISSN 0021-9258

Robinson, AM., & Williamson, DH. (1980). Physiological roles of ketone bodies as substrates and signals in mammalian tissues. *Physiological Reviews,* Vol. 60, No. 1, (January 1980), pp. 143-187, ISSN 0031-9333

Scher, DS., & Rodwell, VW. (1989). 3-Hydroxy-3-methylglutaryl coenzyme A lyase from Pseudomonas mevalonii. *Biochimica and Biophysica Acta,* Vol. 1003, No. 3, (June 1989) pp. 321-326, ISSN 0304-4165

Schutgens, RB., Heymans, H., Ketel, A., Veder, HA., Duran, M., Ketting, D., & Wadman, SK. (1986). Lethal hypoglycemia in a child with a deficiency of 3-hydroxy-3-methylglutarylcoenzyme A lyase. *The Journal of Pediatrics,* Vol. 94, No. 1 (January 1979), pp. 89-91, ISSN 0022-3476

Stacey, TE., de Sousa, C., Tracey, BM., Whitelaw, A., Mistry, J., Timbrell, P., & Chalmers, RA. (1985). Dizygotic twins with 3-hydroxy-3-methylglutaric aciduria; unusual presentation, family studies and dietary management. *European Journal of Pediatrics,* Vol. 144, No. 2, (July 1985), pp. 177-181, ISSN 0340-6199

Sweetman, L., & William, JC. (1995). In: *The Metabolic and Molecular Basis of Inherited Disease,* C.R. Schreiver, A.L. Beaudet, W.S. Sly, D. Valle (Eds.), pp.1400-1402, McGraw-Hill, New York

Tuinstra, RL., Burgner, JW., & Miziorko, HM. (2002). Investigation of the oligomeric status of the peroxisomal isoform of human 3-hydroxy-3-methylglutaryl-CoA lyase. *Archives of Biochemistry and Biophysics,* Vol. 408, No. 2, (December 2001), pp. 286-294, ISSN 0003-9861

Urgançi, N., Arapoğlu, M., Evrüke, M., & Aydin, A. (2001). A rare cause of hepatomegaly: 3-hydroxy-3-methylglutaryl coenzyme-a lyase deficiency. *Journal of Pediatrics Gastroenterol & Nutrition,* Vol. 33, No. 3, (September 2001), pp. 339-41, ISSN 0277-2116

Vargas, CR., Sitta, A., Schmitt, G., Ferreira, GC., Cardoso, ML., Coelho, D., Gibson, KM., & Wajner, M. (2007). Incidence of 3-hydroxy-3-methylglutaryl-coenzyme A lyase (HL) deficiency in Brazil, South America. *Journal of Inherited Metabolic Disease,* (December 2007), ISSN 0141-8955

Wajner, M., Latini, A., Wyse, AT., & Dutra-Filho, CS. (2004). The role of oxidative damage in the neuropathology of organic acidurias: insights from animal studies. *Journal of Inherited Metabolic Disease,* Vol. 27, No. 4, (2004), pp. 427-448, ISSN 0141-8955

Wanders, RJ., Schutgens, RB., & Zoeters, PH. (1988a). 3-Hydroxy-3-methylglutaryl-CoA lyase in human skin fibroblasts: study of its properties and deficient activity in 3-hydroxy-3-methylglutaric aciduria patients using a simple spectrophotometric method. *Clinica Chimica Acta,* Vol. 171, No. 1, (January 1988), pp. 95-101, ISSN 0009-8981

Wanders, RJ., Schutgens, RB., & Zoeters, BH. (1988b). Prenatal diagnosis of 3-hydroxy-3-methylglutaric aciduria via enzyme activity measurements in chorionic villi, chorionic villous fibroblasts or amniocytes using a simple spectrophotometric method. *Journal of Inherited Metabolic Disease,* Vol. 11, No. 4, (1988), pp. 430, ISSN 0141-8955

Wang, SP., Robert, MF., Gibson, KM., Wanders, RJ., & Mitchell, GA. (1996). 3-Hydroxy-3-methylglutaryl CoA lyase (HL): mouse and human HL gene (*HMGCL*) cloning and detection of large gene deletions in two unrelated HL-deficient patients. *Genomics,* Vol. 33, No. 1, (April 1996), pp. 99-104, ISSN: 0888-7543

Wang, SP., Marth, JD., Oligny, LL., Vachon, M., Robert, MF., Ashmarina, L., & Mitchell, GA. (1998). 3-Hydroxy-3-methylglutaryl-CoA lyase (HL): gene targeting causes prenatal lethality in HL-deficient mice. *Human Molecular Genetics,* Vol. 7, No.13, (December 1998) pp. 2057-2062, ISSN 0964-6906

Watson, MS., Mann, MY., Lloyd-Puryear, MA., & Rinaldo, M. (2006). Newborn screening: toward a uniform screening panel and system. *Genetics in Medicine,* 8 Suppl 1: 1S-252S, ISSN 1098-3600

Wilson, WG., Cass, MB., Søvik, O., Gibson, KM., & Sweetman, L. (1984). A child with acute pancreatitis and recurrent hypoglycemia due to 3-hydroxy-3-methylglutaryl-CoA lyase deficiency. *European Journal of Pediatrics,* Vol. 142, No. 4, (September 1984), pp. 289-291, ISSN 0340-6199

Wysocki, SJ., & Hahnel, R. (1976a). 3-Hydroxy-3-methylglutaric aciduria: deficiency of 3-hydroxy-3-methylglutaryl coenzyme A lyase. *Clinica Chimica Acta,* Vol. 71, No. 2, (September 1976), pp.349-351, ISSN 0009-8981

Wysocki, SJ., & Hahnel. R. (1976b). 3-Hydroxy-3-methylglutaric aciduria: 3-hydroxy-3-methylglutaryl-coenzyme A lyase levels in leucocytes. *Clinica Chimica Acta,* Vol. 73, No. 2, (December 1976), pp. 373-375, ISSN 0009-8981

Wysocki, SJ., & Hähnel, R. (1986). 3-Hydroxy-3-methylglutaryl-coenzyme a lyase deficiency: a review. *Journal of Inherited Metabolic Disease,* Vol. 9, No. 3, (1986), pp. 225-233, ISSN 0141-8955

Yalçinkaya, C., Dinçer, A., Gündüz, E., Fiçicioğlu, C., Koçer, N., & Aydin, A. (2007). MRI and MRS in HMG-CoA lyase deficiency. *Pediatrics Neurology,* Vol. 20, No. 5, (May 2007), pp. 375-380, ISSN 0887-8994

Yýlmaz, Y., Ozdemir, N., Ekinci, G., Baykal, T., & Kocaman, C. (2006). Corticospinal tract involvement in a patient with 3-HMG coenzyme A lyase deficiency. *Pediatrics Neurology,* Vol. 35, No. 2, (August 2006), pp. 139-141, ISSN 0887-8994

Zafeiriou, DI., Vargiami, E., Mayapetek, E., Augoustidou-Savvopoulou, P., & Mitchell, GA. (2007). 3-Hydroxy-3-methylglutaryl coenzyme a lyase deficiency with reversible white matter changes after treatment. *Pediatrics Neurology,* Vol. 37, No.1, (July 2007), pp. 47-50, ISSN 0887-8994

Zapater, N., Pié, J., Lloberas, J., Rolland, MO., Leroux, B., Vidailhet, M., Divry, P., Hegardt, FG., & Casals, N. (2001). Two missense point mutations in different alleles in the 3-hydroxy-3-methylglutaryl coenzyme A lyase gene produce 3-hydroxy-3-methylglutaric aciduria in a French patient. *Archives of Biochemistry and Biophysics,* Vol. 358, No. 2, (October 1998), pp. 197-203, ISSN 0003-9861

Zoghbi, HY., Spence, JE., Beaudet, AL., O'Brien, WE., Goodman, CJ., & Gibson, KM. (1986). Atypical presentation and neuropathological studies in 3-hydroxy-3-methylglutaryl-CoA lyase deficiency. *Annals of Neurology,* Vol. 20, No. 3, (September 1986), pp. 367-369, ISSN 0364-5134.

9

Mitochondrial HMG–CoA Synthase Deficiency

María Arnedo, Mónica Ramos, Beatriz Puisac,
Mª Concepción Gil-Rodríguez, Esperanza Teresa, Ángeles Pié,
Gloria Bueno, Feliciano J. Ramos, Paulino Gómez-Puertas and Juan Pié
Unit of Clinical Genetics and Functional Genomics, School of Medicine,
University of Zaragoza
Spain

1. Introduction

The mitochondrial 3-hydroxy-3-methylglutaryl-CoA (HMG-CoA) synthase deficiency (MIM 600234) is an autosomic recessive inborn error of metabolism, hard to characterize and probably underdiagnosed (Thompson et al., 1997). The enzyme failure is caused by mutations in the gene *HMGCS2,* located in chromosome 1. The illness was first diagnosed in 1997 (Thompson et al., 1997), in a six-year old boy, who presented a semicomatose state after three days with gastroenteritis and diet (Bouchard et al., 2001). Up to date, only eight patients have been reported with an estimated incidence of <1/1,000,000, although it could be higher because some patients probably have been misdiagnosed as Reye syndrome.

The mitochondrial HMG-CoA synthase enzyme (mHS, EC 4.1.3.5) has a main role in the synthesis of the ketone bodies and in the HMG-CoA formation. Ketone bodies act as an alternative glucose fuel in a number of tissues as heart, muscle and brain, and have a critical role during metabolic stress and starving, situations where the symptoms of the disease appear.

2. Ketogenesis

The ketogenesis is a metabolic process that takes place inside the mitochondria. The acetyl-CoA, originated during the fatty acids β-oxidation, is converted to acetoacetate, β-hidroxybutyrate and acetone. These metabolites are known as ketone bodies and act as a glucose alternative fuel in many tissues as heart, skeletal muscle and brain. In brain, ketone bodies play an essential role in situations of hypoglycemia (Edmond, 1992; Zammit & Moir, 1994). Besides their alternative fuel role, ketone bodies are lipogenic precursors too. They play a role during the myelinating process in the neonates' brain (Nehlig & Pereira de Vasconcelos, 1993), and in a minor degree in the mammary gland during suckling (Zammit, 1981). Moreover, they seem to have some functions in metabolism regulation (Robinson & Williamson, 1980).

The main tissue where ketogenesis takes place is the liver (Zammit & Moir, 1994). However, it has been also found in kidney, adipose tissue (Thumelin et al., 1993), and intestine of suckling rats (Hahn & Taller, 1987) and, in a minor degree, in cortical astrocytes of newborn rats (Cullingford et al., 1998; Blázquez et al., 1998).

Ketone bodies can be elevated in physiological situations as: fasting, prolonged exercise, high-fat diet or pregnancy (Felig & Lynch, 1970), in the neonate (Hawkins et al., 1971); and in pathologic situations as: diabetes (Bates et al., 1968), obesity and disease of the glucose or glycogen metabolism (Mitchell et al., 1997).

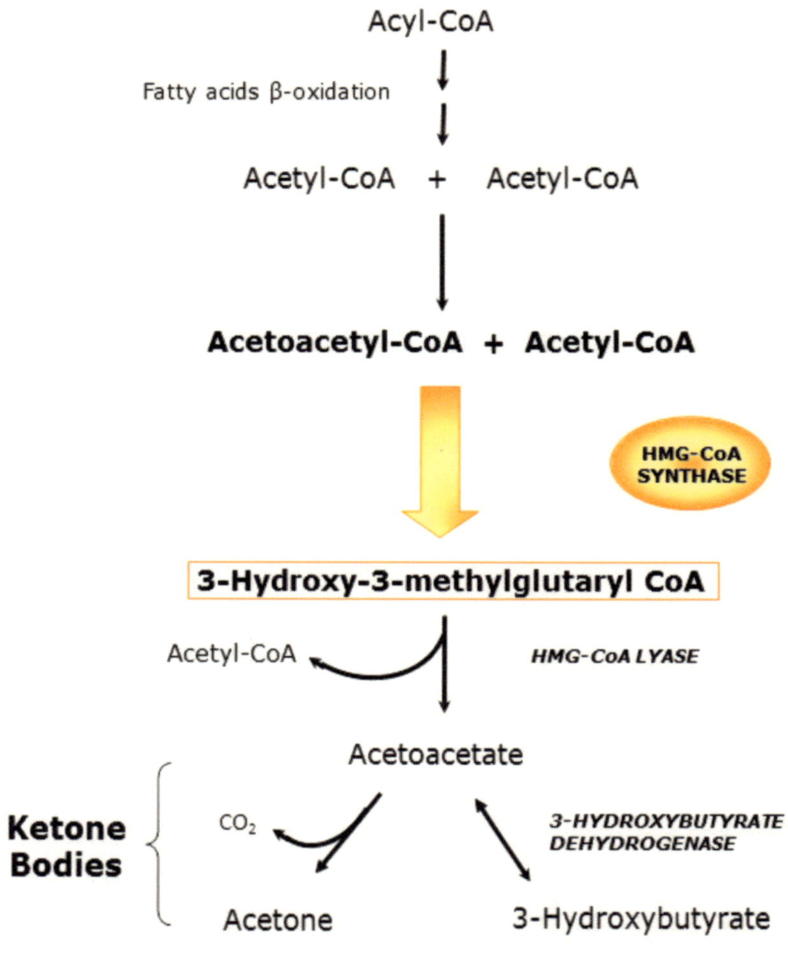

Fig. 1. Ketone bodies synthesis pathway

The main pathway of ketone bodies from acetyl-CoA includes the following reactions (Figure 1):

- In the first reaction, two acetyl-CoA molecules join to form acetoacetyl-CoA. This reaction is catalyzed by the acetoacetyl-CoA thiolase enzyme.
- Then, acetoacetyl-CoA reacts with another acetyl-CoA to produce the HMG-CoA. This is a condensation reaction where the mHS enzyme is involved, and whose failure is responsible of the disease.

- In the third reaction, the HMG-CoA is cleaved into acetoacetate, the first ketone body produced, and acetyl-CoA. This step is catalyzed by the HMG-CoA lyase (HL).
- Finally, in the last reaction, the acetoacetate is reduced to β-hydroxybutyrate, the second ketone body generated. The enzyme involved in this reaction is the β-hydroxybutyrate dehydrogenase. Acetone is formed by the spontaneous decarboxylation of acetoacetate.

There is an alternative ketogenic pathway different from the previously described, which takes place with substrates of aminoacids catabolism. Both pathways converge in the mitochondrial HL enzyme.

3. mHS enzyme

The mHS catalyzes the second reaction of the main pathway of the synthesis of ketone bodies and it is considered as the key enzyme of pathway regulation.

3.1 Enzymatic reaction

The mHS enzyme catalyzes the condensation of acetyl-CoA and acetoacetyl-CoA into HMG-CoA. The HMG-CoA, produced inside the mitochondria, drives towards the formation of ketone bodies. The mHS catalyzed reaction follows a Bi Bi Ping-Pong substitution mechanism (Cleland, 1963; Miziorko et al., 1975). This reaction has three steps (Miziorko et al., 1977) (Figure 2):

- Firstly, acetyl-CoA reacts with the thiol group of the catalytic Cys^{166} in order to produce a covalent intermediate form of the acetyl-enzyme. This is the limiting reaction step (Miziorko et al., 1977).
- Then, acetoacetyl-CoA (second substrate) condenses with the intermediate product to give HMG-CoA, which will be attached to the enzyme by a covalent bond.
- In the final step, HMG-CoA is released from the enzyme by hydrolysis.

High concentrations of acetoacetyl-CoA inhibit the first reaction step, because it competes with acetyl-CoA for the active site of the enzyme (Page & Tubbs, 1978). Magnesium can act as an inhibitor of the reaction too.

3.2 Protein structure

Human mHS has 508 amino acids and its structure is a homodimer formed by two identical monomers linked by a salt bridge (Figure 3). At the N-terminal end is the leader peptide, with 37 aa, which drives the protein to the mitochondria.

In 1985, the catalytic sequence of the enzyme was identified in a purified protein from chicken liver (Miziorko & Behnke, 1985). This sequence has 21 aa and a 100% homology with HMG-CoA synthases from other mammals. The catalytic aminoacid Cys^{129}, whose human homolog is the Cys^{166}, is located inside this region (Misra et al., 1995). The protein analysis shows three regions rich in proline, glutamine, serine and threonine, which could be PEST sequences (Pro-Glu-Ser-Thr) (Rogers et al., 1986). These regions are characterized by a quick turnover of proteins (Boukaftane et al., 1994; Ayté et al., 1990).

Recently, the human enzyme has been crystallized and its alpha/beta structure, with 17 beta sheets and 19 alpha helices, has been well characterized. The tunnel of substrate entry and product exit is located outside of the molecule, at the opposite side of the interaction between the two monomers (Shafqat et al., 2010).

A

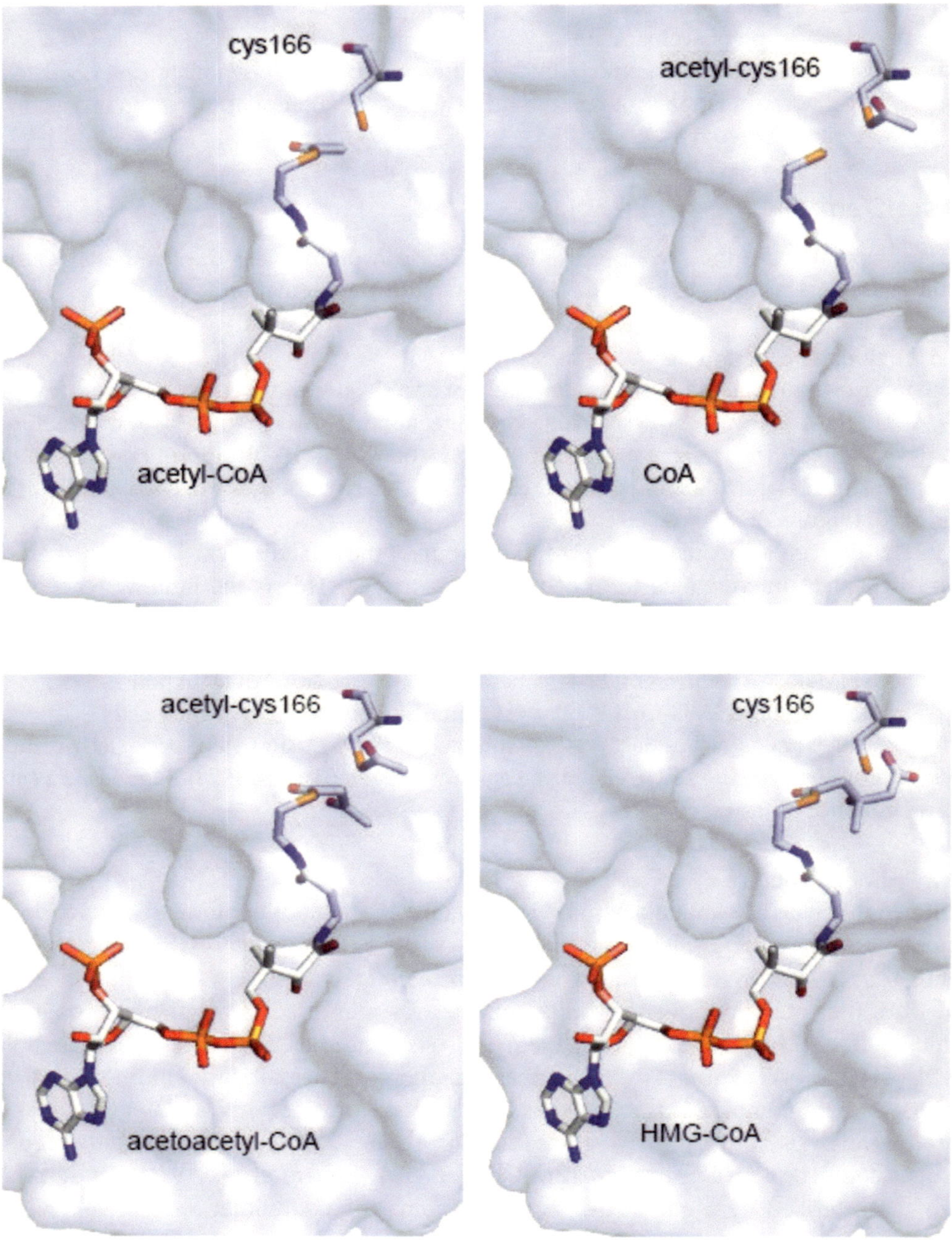

B

Fig. 2. A. Acetyl-enzyme intermediate formation. B. HMG-CoA formation

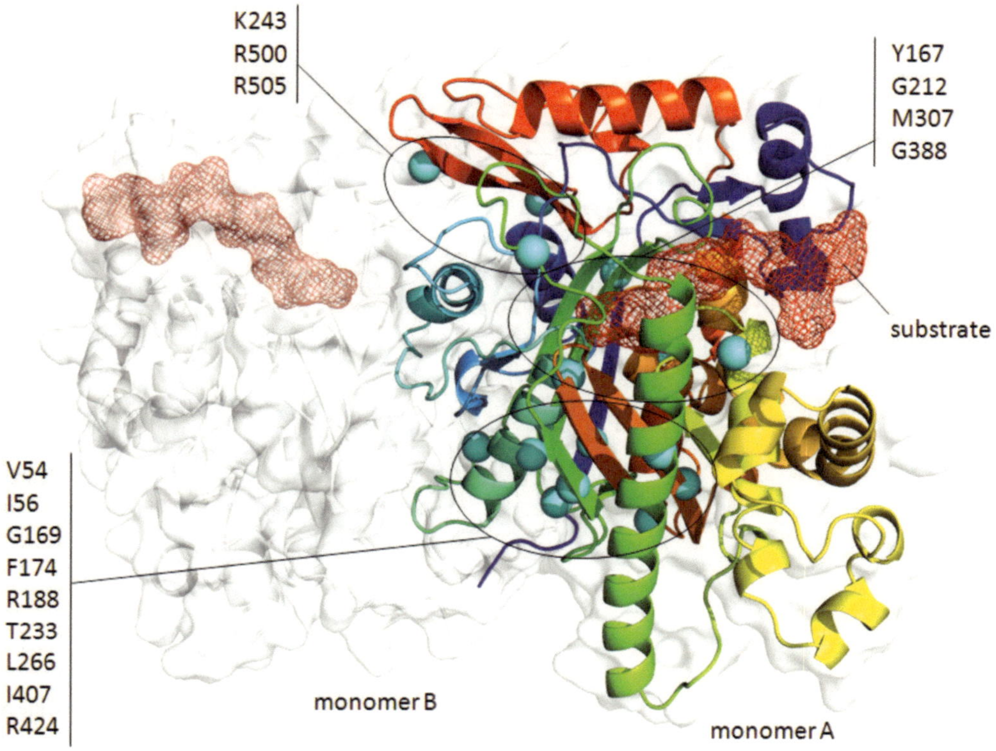

Fig. 3. Structural location of missense mutations in human mHS, represented as blue spheres

3.3 Enzyme expression

Studies of gene expression in human tissues in basal conditions showed a tissue-specific expression. High mRNA levels are detected in the liver, the organ with the highest ketogenic capacity. Expression is also high in colon, which is related to the fermentative processes that take place in it (Mascaró et al., 1995). A minor level of mRNA expression has been observed in heart, skeletal muscle, gonads, kidney and pancreas (Mascaró et al., 1995; Royo et al., 1993). Studies in rats have found mRNA expression in cortical astrocytes from newborns (Cullingford et al., 1998; Blazquez et al., 1998), and in the intestine of suckling animals (Bekesi & Williamson, 1990; Thumelin et al., 1993; Serra et al., 1993).

Changes in the level of gene expression have been reported during development. In suckling rats, the highest levels of expression were detected at the third day of life, decreasing progressively until weaning, when mRNA levels are similar to those of adult well fed rats (Serra et al., 1993).

3.4 Enzyme regulation

Production of ketone bodies in hepatic mitochondria is a complex and highly regulated process (Guzmán & Geelen, 1993; Zammit & Moir, 1994). Their synthesis increases in starving situations and in high fat intake, while it decreases after feeding or insulin administration and in the suckling-weaning transition (Williamson & Whitelaw, 1978; McGarry & Foster, 1980; Robinson et al., 1980).

Initially, the acyl-CoA input to the mitochondria was considered the principal check-point of ketogenesis (Guzman & Geelen, 1993; McGarry & Brown, 1997). However, later studies showed that the mHS enzyme can regulate ketogenesis (Williamson et al., 1968). Therefore, metabolic conditions that imply an increase of ketone bodies are linked to an increase of the levels of *HMGCS2* gene expression (Casals et al., 1992) and of the mHS enzyme (Serrá et al., 1993). Meanwhile, conditions that cause a decrease of the synthesis of ketone bodies are related to a decrease in the mRNA levels of the *HMGCS2* gene (Casals et al., 1992) and of the mHS enzyme (Serrá et al., 1993).

Currently, two check-points are recognized in the control of the synthesis of ketone bodies, one at the same step that of the Carnitine Palmitoyl Transferase 1 reaction, which provides the substrate acetyl-CoA, and another in the ketogenic pathway, at the step of the mHS enzyme (Williamson et al., 1968; Dashti & Ontko, 1979). Regulation of mHS is the most important step and depends on two mechanisms: a long term regulation of the transcription of the *HMGCS2* gene (Casals et al., 1992; Hegardt, 1999), and a short term regulation of the protein. This one depends on succinyl and desuccinyl enzymes reactions (Lowe & Tubbs, 1985; Quant et al., 1990). All of these mechanisms are influenced by nutritional and hormonal factors.

3.5 Isoenzymes

Two HMG-CoA synthase isoenzymes which catalyze the same reaction are known, however, they are located in different structures inside the cell. The mHS (Clinkenbeard et al., 1975) is involved in the synthesis of ketone bodies in the mitochondria, while the cytosolic HMG-CoA synthase (cHS) is critical for the synthesis of cholesterol (Clinkenbeard et al., 1975; Reed et al., 1975).

Expression pattern of cHS is different from the one described for mHS. The cytosolic enzyme is expressed in most of the tissues, and its gene is considered a house-keeping gene. High mRNA levels are observed in liver followed by heart, placenta and pancreas (Mascaró et al., 1995). Their transcriptional regulation is different from the mHS and it is negatively regulated by cholesterol and other isoprenoids (Hua et al., 1993).

The activity measures of the HMG-CoA synthase in a liver crude extract is divided between a 20-40% for the cHS and a 60-80% for the mHS (Clinkenbeard et al., 1975). Surprisingly, there is not reported any case with cHS deficiency.

4. mHS deficiency

Deficiency of mHS is an inborn error of metabolism that affects the synthesis of ketone bodies. It is a very rare autosomal recessive disorder reported in 1997 (Thompson et al., 1997), in a six year old boy. The patient had hypoglycemia, hypoketonemia and semicomatous state, after three days with gastroenteritis and dieting. Symptoms quickly reversed after intravenous administration of glucose. Liver biopsy showed a decrease in the activity of mHS. Molecular study of the gene confirmed the diagnosis (Bouchard et al., 2001). Generally, the disease shows unspecific clinical symptoms and metabolites excretion profile, sometimes attributed to a fatty acid β-oxidation enzyme defect and that makes it to be underdiagnosed. Some authors pointed out that it can be misdiagnosed as Reye syndrome and be associated with the sudden infant death syndrome (Thompson et al., 1997). Symptoms usually appear after situations of starving and/or high energy expenditure (fever, stress, exercise). In normal conditions, metabolic pathways that provide alternative glucose sources, as the synthesis of ketone bodies, are activated. A defect of ketogenesis can trigger a coma in the individual with low glucose availability.

4.1 Clinical features

In all the cases reported, clinical symptoms have appeared in childhood, specially during the first year of life; however, two of the 8 cases were diagnosed at the age of four and six years, respectively.

Clinical features of mHS deficiency are unspecific (Table 1), which makes it hard to diagnose. Initial symptoms include vomiting and lethargy that can progress to coma. In most cases these symptoms are accompanied with hepatomegaly (Thompson et al., 1997) and in some cases with respiratory disease and encephalopathy. These symptoms quickly improve after glucose administration. Up to date, all the reported cases have had a favorable outcome, despite severe acute episodes. All the reported patients with mHS deficiency are still alive.

4.2 Diagnosis

4.2.1 Biochemical data

Hypoglycemia is the main biochemical anomaly detected during an acute episode. Increase of the levels of plasmatic free fatty acids and urine dicarboxylic acids is also found. Plasma levels of acylcarnitines, lactate and ammonium are within normal limits (Morris et al., 1998). In some cases, metabolic acidosis has been reported (Table 1).

This disease, as opposite to the HL deficiency, does not show a characteristic organic acids pattern in urine. The mHS substrate does not accumulate because it can be metabolized to acetyl-CoA during the β-oxidation.

4.2.2 Enzyme activity

An enzymatic assay in liver biopsy is needed to confirm the mHS deficiency, because liver is the tissue with the highest enzyme expression. This method has several limitations, being the main one that in liver homogenate we cannot distinguish between mHS and cHS enzyme activity. This problem impairs the interpretation of the results and explains that the assay has only been carried out in two patients (Thompson et al., 1997; Morris et al., 1998). The possibility to use other tissues or alternative cells as lymphocytes or fibroblasts has been proposed, but the low expression levels in these tissues did not allow investigators to obtain valid measurable levels (Thompson et al., 1997).

4.2.3 Molecular diagnosis

Molecular analysis is the method of choice to confirm the clinical diagnosis. It is done from genomic DNA of the patient, by PCR amplification and sequencing of the *HMGCS2* gene.

4.2.4 Differential diagnosis with HMG-CoA lyase deficiency

The HL is the immediately posterior to mHS enzyme in the pathway of the ketone bodies synthesis. HL deficiency (3-hydroxy-3-methylglutaric aciduria) has very similar clinical manifestations to mHS deficiency, although there are significant differences that the clinicians should know in order to differentiate them.

	Signs and laboratory data	mHS deficiency	HL deficiency
SIGNS	Encephalopathy	+/-	+/-
	Hypotonia	-	+/-
	Lethargy	+/-	+/-
	Abnormal Breathing	+/-	+/-
	Coma	+/-	+/-
	Hepatomegaly	+	+/-
	Normal development	+	+/-
	Death	-	+/-
BIOCHEMICAL DATA	Hypoglycaemia	+	+
	Hypoketonemia	+	+
	Hyperammonemia	-	+/-
	Transaminase	+/-	+/-
	Metabolic acidosis	+/-	+
	High urine dicarboxylic acid	+	-
	High 3-hydroxy-3-methylglutaric, 3-hydroxyisovaleric, 3-methylglutaconic and 3-methylglutaric acids	-	+
	Normal level of carnitine	+	+/-

+Always; -Never; +/- Sometimes.

Table 1. Signs and Biochemical data of mHS and HL deficiency

Patients with HL deficiency may present acute crisis as well, during the neonatal or early infancy periods. Both diseases appear when exogenous supply of glucose fails (fasting periods), or when excessive glucose consumption exists (stress, fever or exercise). In the majority of patients with mHS deficiency, the acute crisis begins with hepatomegaly and superficial coma. However, in HL deficiency, or other β-oxidation enzymes, symptoms of the deficiency usually involve several tissues (Thompson et al., 1997). In the latter, most of the patients show muscular weakness and myopathy (Ribes et al., 2003). In the HL deficiency symptoms as dehydration, hypotonia, hypothermia, tachypnea, lethargy, coma and even death, have been reported (Wysocki & Hahnel, 1986; Menao et al., 2009). Up to date, no patient with mHS deficiency has died due to this disease.

Complications of 3-hydroxy-3-methylglutaric aciduria include, macrocephaly (Stacey et al., 1985), development delay and dilated cardiomyopathy with arrhythmia (Gibson et al., 1994). Microcephaly has been reported in one patient (Lisson et al., 1981). Up to date, no complications have been reported in patients with mHS deficiency.

The most important difference between both diseases is found in the urine profile of the organic acids, which is characteristic only in HL deficiency. Metabolites that accumulate in urine are the 3-hydroxy-isovaleric acid, the 3-methylcrotonyl glycine, the 3-methylglutaric acid, the 3-methylglutaconic acid and the 3-hydroxy-3-methylglutaric acid. Neither of these metabolites is increased in mHS deficiency. Clinical and biochemical data of both deficiencies are included in Table 1.

4.3 Treatment

Treatment is symptomatic during acute episodes and consists of intravenous administration of glucose to correct hypoglycemia. Long-term maintenance therapy includes low-fat diet and avoidance of fasting periods of more than 12 hours. It is also important to avoid situations of metabolic stress, mainly produced by recurrent illness that can be prevented by extra caloric intake (Morris et al., 1998).

5. *HMGCS2* gene

Although mHS is codified by a gene (Ayte et al., 1990) different from the cHS gene (Gil et al., 1986), their high homology suggests a common origin about 500 millions years ago, when vertebrates appeared (Boukaftane et al., 1994).
Human *HMGCS2* gene is located in chromosome 1 (1p12-p13), between the markers WI-7519 and D1S514. It has 10 exons and 9 introns, with a total size of 21,708 bp (Figure 4). Exons length oscillates between 107 and 846 bp, and the intron's size varies between 0.4 and 4.1 kDa. cDNA has a total size of 2,082 bp.
So far, no splice variants of the gene have been experimentally confirmed, although the current Expressed Sequence Tag database includes a variant with a deletion of exon 4.

5.1 Mutation update

Up to date, 8 patients have been diagnosed by molecular analysis. Among them nine allelic variants have been identified: seven missense variants, one nonsense and one intronic mutation (Figures 3 and 4). One of these variants, the Y167C, affects to a closed Cys^{166} amino acid, which is considered the catabolic site of the enzyme (Hegard, 1999). The nonsense variant R424X (Bouchard et al., 2001; Morris et al., 1998), produced a truncated protein of 424 amino acids that probably cannot be incorporated into the active protein dimer. The intronic mutation is located in the first nucleotide of the intron 5 (c.1016+1G>A). In general, this type of mutations produces the deletion of the affected exon (exon 5 in this case), although in this disease the mechanism has not been confirmed (Zschocke et al., 2002).
In order to prove the effect of the mutation in the enzyme activity, protein over-expression has been tried with recombinant DNA techniques although with no success (Bouchard et al., 2001).

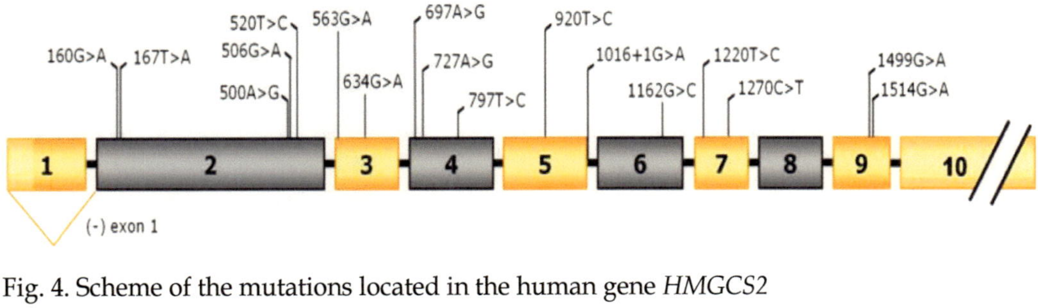

Fig. 4. Scheme of the mutations located in the human gene *HMGCS2*

Patient	Disease debut	Genotype	Symptoms and signs	Organic acids	Acylcarnitine	Reference
Patient 1	6 years	F174L/F174L	Gastroenteritis, hypoglycemia, hipoketonemia, superficial coma	Normal	Normal	Bouchard 2001; Thompson 1997
Patient 2	1 year and 4 months	R424X/unknown	Diarrhea, vomiting, hepatomegaly, hypoglycemia, hipoketonemia, coma	Dicarboxylic aciduria	Normal	Bouchard 2001; Morris 1998
Patient 3	11 months	G212R/R500H	Gastroenteritis, vomiting, hepatomegaly, hypoglycemia, hipoketonemia, coma	Dicarboxylic aciduria	Normal	Aledo 2001
Patient 4	9 months	G212R/IVS5+1G>A	Gastroenteritis, diarrhea, vomiting, hepatomegaly, hypoglycemia, hipoketonemia, coma	Dicarboxylic aciduria	Normal	Zschocke 2002
Patient 5	4 years and 6 months	V54M/Y167C	Gastroenteritis, diarrhea, vomiting, hypoglycemia, hipoketonemia, coma	Dicarboxylic aciduria	Normal	Wolf 2003
Patient 6	1 year and 7 months	V54M/Y167C	Hepatomegaly, normal hepatic function	Dicarboxylic aciduria	Normal	Wolf 2003
Patient 7	7 months	M307T/R188H	Vomiting, hepatomegaly, hipoglycemia hipoketonemia, encephalopathy.	Dicarboxylic aciduria	Normal	Aledo 2006
Patient 8	1 year	M307T/R188H	Vomiting, lethargy	Normal	Normal	Aledo 2006

Mutations G169D, T233A, K243E, L266S, I407T, R505Q, R84X and exon 1 deletion were reported by Pitt et al., at the 11th International Congress on Inborn Errors of Metabolism, San Diego CA and by Shafqat et al., 2010.
Mutations I56N, T233A, K243E and R84X were reported by Shafqat et al., 2010.
No clinical data were available from the patients who carried these mutations.

Table 2. Clinical findings and biochemical data from patients with mHS deficiency

Another approach consisted in studying, with an indirect method, the mutation effect in MEV-1 cell cultures (Aledo et al., 2001). These studies were based in the cell mevalonate auxotrophy correction when they are transfected with cDNA of the *HMGCS2* gene. The expression of the mHS gene gives to MEV-1 cells the capacity to synthesize HMG-CoA inside the mitochondria, which is transformed in mevalonate and cholesterol (Ortiz et al., 1994). As expected, the mutated mHS cDNA transfection does not correct the MEV-1 cells auxotrophy, which proves the deficiency of HMG-CoA synthesis.
Recently, new mutations in mHS deficiency patients have been reported, but no clinical information was given. There are 8 missense mutations and one nonsense (Shafqat et al., 2010).
In Table 2 an updated list of mutations reported in the *HMGCS2* gene is displayed, together with the patients´ clinical data.

6. Genotype-phenotype correlations

With the current knowledge available, it is difficult to establish strong genotype-phenotype correlations, among other reasons, for instance, because we ignore relevant information such as the levels of enzyme activity in affected patients. The seriousness of the disease may be more related to the agent that triggered hypoglycemia and to the time without treatment than with the mutation itself.

7. Conclusion

Although mHS deficiency is an extremely rare disease, it is likely underdiagnosed and its prevalence is higher than estimated. Pediatricians may suspect this disorder in infants with vomiting, mild hepatomegaly, hypoglycemia, metabolic acidosis, increased levels of plasmatic free fatty acids and dicarboxylic aciduria, specially if symptoms appeared after a situation of metabolic stress, usually due to dieting in a gastroenteritis or during an infection process. Currently, the only reliable diagnostic -confirmatory- test is the molecular analysis of the gene, since measurements of the levels of enzymatic activity are masked by the activity of isoenzyme cHS.

8. Acknowledgment

This study was supported by Spanish grants from: Diputación General de Aragón (Ref.# Grupo Consolidado B20) and University of Zaragoza (Ref.# PIF-UZ_2009-BIO-02). We also thank to "Biomol-Informatics SL -www.bioinfo.es-" for bioinformatic support.

9. References

Aledo, R., Zschocke, J., Pie, J., Mir, C., Fiesel, S., Mayatepek, E., Hoffmann, GF., Casals, N., & Hegardt, FG. (2001). Genetic basis of mitochondrial HMG-CoA synthase deficiency. *Human Genetics,* Vol. 1, No. 109, (July 2001), pp. 19-23, ISSN 11479731

Ayte, J., Gil-Gomez, G., Haro, D., Marrero, PF., & Hegardt, FG. (1990). Rat mitochondrial and cytosolic 3-hydroxy-3-methylglutaryl-CoA synthases are encoded by two different genes. *Proceedings of the National Academy of Sciences of the United States of America,* Vol. 10, No. 87, (May 1990), pp. 3874-3878, ISSN 1971108

Bates, MW., Krebs, HA., & Williamson, DH. (1968). Turnover rates of ketone bodies in normal, starved and alloxan-diabetic rats. *Biochemical Journal,* Vol. 110, No. 4, (December 1968), pp. 655-661, ISSN 5704813

Békési, A., & Williamson, DH. (1990). An explanation for ketogenesis by the intestine of the suckling rat: the presence of an active hydroxymethylglutaryl-coenzyme A pathway. *Biology of the Neonate,* Vol. 58, No. 3, (1990), pp. 160-165, ISSN 2279051

Blázquez, C., Sanchez, C., Velasco, G., & Guzman, M. (1998). Role of carnitine palmitoyltransferase I in the control of ketogenesis in primary cultures of rat astrocytes. *Journal of Neurochemistry,* Vol. 4, No. 71, (October 1998), pp. 1597-1606, ISSN 9751193

Bouchard, L., Robert, MF., Vinarov, D., Stanley, CA., Thompson, GN., Morris, A., Leonard, JV., Quant, P., Hsu, BY., Boneh, A., Boukaftane, Y., Ashmarina, L., Wang, S., Miziorko, H., & Mitchell, GA. (2001). Mitochondrial 3-hydroxy-3-methylglutaryl-CoA synthase deficiency: clinical course and description of causal mutations in two patients. *Pediatric Research,* Vol. 3, No. 49, (March 2001), pp. 326-331, ISSN 11228257

Boukaftane, Y., Duncan, A., Wang, S., Labuda, D., Robert, MF., Sarrazin, J., Schappert, K., & Mitchell, GA. (1994). Human mitochondrial HMG CoA synthase: liver cDNA and partial genomic cloning, chromosome mapping to 1p12-p13, and possible role in vertebrate evolution. *Genomics,* Vol. 3, No. 23, (October 1994), pp. 552-559, ISSN 7851882

Casals, N., Roca, N., Guerrero, M., Gil-Gómez, G., Ayté, J., Ciudad, CJ., & Hegardt, FG. (1992). Regulation of the expression of the mitochondrial 3-hydroxy-3-methylglutaryl-CoA synthase gene. Its role in the control of ketogenesis. *The Biochemical Journal,* Vol. 1, No. 283, (April 1992), pp. 261-264, ISSN 1348927

Cleland, WW. (1963). The kinetics of enzyme-catalyzed reactions with two or more substrates or products. I. Nomenclature and rate equations. *Biochimica et Biophysica Acta,* Vol. 67 (January 1968), pp. 104-137, ISSN 1402166

Clinkenbeard, KD., Reed, WD., Mooney, RA., & Lane, MD. (1975). Intracellular localization of the 3-hydroxy-3-methylglutaryl coenzyme A cycle enzymes in liver. Separate cytoplasmic and mitochondrial 3-hydroxy-3-methylglutaryl coenzyme A generating systems for cholesterogenesis and ketogenesis. *The Journal of Biological Chemistry,* Vol. 8, No. 250, (April 1975), pp. 3108-3116, ISSN 164460

Cullingford, TE., Bhakoo, KK., & Clark, JB. (1998). Hormonal regulation of the mRNA encoding the ketogenic enzyme mitochondrial 3-hydroxy-3-methylglutaryl-CoA synthase in neonatal primary cultures of cortical astrocytes and meningeal fibroblasts. *Journal of Neurochemistry,* Vol. 5, No. 71, (November 1998), pp. 1804-1812, ISSN 9798904

Dashti, N., & Ontko, JA. (1979). Rate-limiting function of 3-hydroxy-3-methylglutaryl-coenzyme A synthase in ketogenesis. *Biochemical Medicine,* Vol. 3, No. 22, (December 1979), pp. 365-374, ISSN 93966

Edmond J. (1992). Energy metabolism in developing brain cells. *Canadian Journal of Physiology and Pharmacoogyl,* Vol. 70, No. S1 (May 1992), pp. S118-S129, ISSN 1295662

Felig, P., & Lynch, V. (1970). Starvation in human pregnancy: hypoglycemia, hypoinsulinemia, and hyperketonemia. *Science,* Vol. 170, No. 961, (November 1970), pp.990-992, ISSN 5529067

Gibson, KM., Cassidy, SB., Seaver, LH., Wanders, RJ., Kennaway, NG., Mitchell, GA., & Spark, RP. (1994). Fatal cardiomyopathy associated with 3-hydroxy-3-methylglutaryl-CoA lyase deficiency. *Journal of Inherited Metabolic Disease,* Vol. 3, No. 17 (1994), pp. 291-294, ISSN 7807935

Gil, G., Goldstein, JL., Slaughter, CA., & Brown, MS. (1986). Cytoplasmic 3-hydroxy-3-methylglutaryl coenzyme A synthase from the hamster. I. Isolation and sequencing of a full-length cDNA. *The Journal of Biology Chemistry,* Vol. 261, No. 8, (March 1986), pp. 3710-3716, ISSN 286903

Guzmán, M., & Geelen, MJ. (1993). Regulation of fatty acid oxidation in mammalian liver. *Biochimical et Biophysucal Acta* Vol. 1167, No. 3 (April 1993), pp. 227-241, ISSN 8097

Hahn, P., & Taller, M. (1987). Ketone formation in the intestinal mucosa of infant rats. *Life Science,* Vol. 12, No. 41, (September 1987), pp. 1525-1528, ISSN 3626770

Hawkins, RA., Williamson, DH., & Krebs, HA. (1971). Ketone-body utilization by adult and suckling rat brain in vivo. *Biochemical Journal,* Vol. 122, No. 1, (March 1971), pp. 13-18, ISSN 5124783

Hegardt, FG. (1999). Mitochondrial 3-hydroxy-3-methylglutaryl-CoA synthase: a control enzyme in ketogenesis. *The Biochemical Journal,* Vol. 3, No. 338, (March 1999), pp. 569-582, ISSN 10051425

Hua, X., Yokoyama, C., Wu, J., Briggs, MR., Brown, MS., Goldstein, JL., & Wang, X. (1993). SREBP-2, a second basic-helix-loop-helix-leucine zipper protein that stimulates transcription by binding to a sterol regulatory element. *Proceedings of the National Academy of Sciences USA,* Vol. 90, No.24, (December 1993), pp. 11603-11607, ISSN 790345

Lisson, G., Leupold, D., Bechinger, D., & Wallesch, C. (1981). CT findings in a case of deficiency of 3-hydroxy-3-methylglutaryl-CoA-lyase. *Neuroradiology,* Vol. 22, No. 2, (1981), pp. 99-101, ISSN 6170906

Lowe, DM., & Tubbs, PK. (1985). Succinylation and inactivation of 3-hydroxy-3-methylglutaryl-CoA synthase by succinyl-CoA and its possible relevance to the control of ketogenesis. *The Biochemical Journal,* Vol. 1, No. 232, (November 1985), pp. 37-42, ISSN 2867762

Mascaró, C., Buesa, C., Ortiz, JA., Haro, D., & Hegardt, FG. (1995). Molecular cloning and tissue expression of human mitochondrial 3-hydroxy-3-methylglutaryl-CoA synthase. *Archives of Biochemistry and Biophysics,* Vol. 2, No. 317, (March 1995), pp. 385-390, ISSN 7893153

McGarry, JD., & Brown, NF. (1997). The mitochondrial carnitine palmitoyltransferase system. From concept to molecular analysis. *European Journal of Biochemistry,* Vol. 244, No. 1 (February 1997), pp. 1-14, ISSN 9063439

McGarry, JD., & Foster, DW. (1980). Regulation of hepatic fatty acid oxidation and ketone body production. *Annual Review of Biochemistry,* No. 49, (1980), pp. 395-420, ISSN 6157353

Menao, S., Lopez-Viñas, E., Mir, C., Puisac, B., Gratacós, E., Arnedo, M., Carrasco, P., Moreno, S., Ramos, M., Gil, MC., Pié, A., Ribes, A., Pérez-Cerda, C., Ugarte, M., Clayton, PT., Korman, SH., Serra, D., Asins, G., Ramos, FJ., Gómez-Puertas, P., Hegardt, FG., Casals, N., & Pié, J. (2009). Ten novel *HMGCL* mutations in 24 patients of different origin with 3-hydroxy-3-methyl-glutaric aciduria. *Human Mutation,* Vol. 3, No. 30, (March 2009), pp. E520-529, ISSN 19177531

Misra, I., Charlier, HA Jr., & Miziorko, HM. (1995). Avian cytosolic 3-hydroxy-3-methylglutaryl-CoA synthase: evaluation of the role of cysteines in reaction chemistry. *Biochemica et Biophysical Acta,* Vol. 1247, No. 2 (March 1995), pp. 253-259, ISSN 7696316

Mitchell, JB., DiLauro, PC., Pizza, FX., & Cavender, DL. (1997). The effect of preexercise carbohydrate status on resistance exercise performance. *International Journal of Sport Nutrition,* Vol. 7, No. 3, (1997), pp. 185-196, ISSN 9286742

Miziorko, HM., Clinkenbeard, KD., Reed, WD., & Lane, MD. (1975). 3-Hydroxy-3-methylglutaryl coenzyme A synthase. Evidence for an acetyl-S-enzyme intermediate and identification of a cysteinyl sulfhydryl as the site of acetylation. *The Journal of Biological Chemistry,* Vol. 250, No. 10 (August 1975), pp. 5768-5573, ISSN 238985

Miziorko, HM. & Behnke, CE. (1985). Active-site-directed inhibition of 3-hydroxy-3-methylglutaryl coenzyme A synthase by 3-chloropropionyl coenzyme A. *Biochemistry,* Vol. 13, No. 24, (June 1985), pp. 3174-3179, ISSN 2862911

Miziorko, HM., & Lane, MD. (1977). 3-Hydroxy-3-methylgutaryl-CoA synthase. Participation of acetyl-S-enzyme and enzyme-S-hydroxymethylgutaryl-SCoA intermediates in the reaction. *The Journal of Biological Chemistry,* Vol. 252, No. 4, (February 1977), pp. 1414-1420, ISSN 14151

Morris, AA., Lascelles, CV., Olpin, SE., Lake, BD., Leonard, JV., & Quant, PA. (1998). Hepatic mitochondrial 3-hydroxy-3-methylglutaryl-coenzyme a synthase deficiency. *Pediatric Research,* Vol. 3, No. 44, (September 1998), pp. 392-396, ISSN 9727719

Nehlig, A., & Pereira de Vasconcelos, A. (1993). Glucose and ketone body utilization by the brain of neonatal rats. *Progress in Neurobiology,* Vol. 40, No. 2 (February 1993), pp. 163-221, ISSN 8430212

Ortiz, JA., Gil-Gómez, G., Casaroli-Marano, RP., Vilaró, S., Hegardt, FG., & Haro, D. (1994). Transfection of the ketogenic mitochondrial 3-hydroxy-3-methylglutaryl-coenzyme A synthase cDNA into Mev-1 cells corrects their auxotrophy for mevalonate. *The Journal of Biological Chemistry,* Vol. 269, No. 46 (November 1994), pp.28523-28526 ISSN 7961793

Page, MA., & Tubbs, PK. (1978). Some properties of 3-hydroxy-3-methylglutaryl-coenzyme A synthase from ox liver. *Biochemical Journal,* Vol 173, No. 3, (September 1978), pp. 925-928, ISSN 39450

Quant, PA., Tubbs, PK., & Brand, MD. (1990). Glucagon activates mitochondrial 3-hydroxy-3-methylglutaryl-CoA synthase in vivo by decreasing the extent of succinylation of the enzyme. *European Journal of Biochemistry / FEBS,* Vol. 1, No. 187, (January 1990), pp. 169-174, ISSN 1967579

Reed, WD., Clinkenbeard, D., & Lane, MD. (1975). Molecular and catalytic properties of mitochondrial (ketogenic) 3-hydroxy-3-methylglutaryl coenzyme A synthase of liver. *The Journal of Biological Chemistry,* Vol. 8, No. 250, (April 1975), pp. 3117-3123, ISSN 804485

Ribes, A., Rodes, M., Gregersen, N., & Divry, P. (2003). Transtornos de la β-oxidación mitocondrial de los ácidos grasos. *Patología Molecular,* González-Sastre, F., Guinovart, JJ. pp. 333-359, Elseveir-Masson, ISBN 9788445812532

Robinson, AM., & Williamson, DH. (1980). Physiological roles of ketone bodies as substrates and signals in mammalian tissues. *Physiological Reviews,* Vol. 60, No. 1 (Janurary 1980), pp. 143-187, ISSN 6986618

Robinson, BH., Oei, J., Sherwood, WG., Slyper, AH., Heininger, J., & Mamer, OA. (1980). Hydroxymethylglutaryl CoA lyase deficiency: features resembling Reye syndrome. *Neurology,* Vol. 7 Pt 1, No. 30, (July 1980), pp. 714-718, ISSN 6156427

Rogers, S., Wells, R., & Rechsteiner, M. (1986). Amino acid sequences common to rapidly degraded proteins: the PEST hypothesis. *Science,* Vol 234, No. 4774 (October 1986), pp.364-368, ISSN 287651

Royo, T., Pedragosa, MJ., Ayte, J., Gil-Gómez, G., Vilaró, S., & Hegardt, FG. (1993). Testis and ovary express the gene for the ketogenic mitochondrial 3-hydroxy-3-methylglutaryl-CoA synthase. *Journal of Lipid Research,* Vol. 9, No. 34, (September 1993), pp. 867-874, ISSN 8102635

Serra, D., Casals, N., Asins, G., Royo, T., Ciudad, CJ., & Hegardt, FG. (1993). Regulation of mitochondrial 3-hydroxy-3-methylglutaryl-coenzyme A synthase protein by starvation, fat feeding, and diabetes. *Archives of Biochemistry and Biophysics,* Vol. 1, No. 307, (September 1993), pp. 40-45, ISSN 7902069

Shafqat, N., Turnbull, A., Zschocke, J., Oppermann, U., & Yue, WW. (2010). Crystal structures of human HMG-CoA synthase isoforms provide insights into inherited ketogenesis disorders and inhibitor design. *Journal of Molecular Biology,* Vol. 4, No. 398, (May 2010), pp.497-506, ISSN 20346956

Stacey, TE., de Sousa, C., Tracey, BM., Whitelaw, A., Mistry, J., Timbrell, P., & Chalmers, RA. (1985). Dizygotic twins with 3-hydroxy-3-methylglutaric aciduria; unusual presentation, family studies and dietary management. *European Journal of Pediatrics,* Vol. 2, No. 144, (July 1985), pp. 177-181, ISSN 2412823

Thompson, GN., Hsu, BY., Purr, JJ., Treacy, E., & Stanley, CA. (1997). Fasting hypoketotic coma in a child with deficiency of mitochondrial 3-hydroxy-3-methylglutaryc-CoA synthase. *The New England Journal of Medicine,* Vol.17, No.337, (October 1997), pp.1203-1207, ISSN 9337379

Thumelin, S., Forestier, M., Girard, J., & Pegorier, JP. (1993). Develpmental changes in mitochondrial 3-hydroxy-3-methylglutaryc-CoA synthase gene expression in rat liver, intestine and kidney. *The Biochemical Journal,* Vol.2 No. 192, (June 1993), pp.493-496, ISSN 8099282

Williamson, DH., & Whitelaw., E. (1978). Physiological aspects of the regulation of ketogenesis. *Biochemical Society symposium,* No. 43, (1978); pp.137-161, ISSN 571280

Williamson, DH., Bates, MW., & Krebs, HA. (1968). Activity and intracellular distribution of enzymes of ketone-body metabolism in rat liver. *The Biochemical Journal,* Vol. 3, No. 108, (July 1968), pp.353-361, ISSN 5667251

Wysocki, SJ., & Hahnel, R. (1986). 3-Hydroxy-3-methylglutaryc-coenzyme a lyase deficiency: a review. *Journal of Inherited Metabolic Disease,* Vol. 3, No. 9, (1986), pp. 225-233, ISSN 3099065

Zammit VA. (1981). Regulation of hepatic fatty acid metabolism. The activities of mitochondrial and microsomal acyl-CoA:sn-glycerol 3-phosphate O-acyltransferase and the concentrations of malonyl-CoA, non-esterified and esterified carnitine, glycerol 3-phosphate, ketone bodies and long-chain acyl-CoA esters in livers of fed or starved pregnant, lactating and weaned rats. *Biochemical Journal*, Vol. 198, No. 1 (July 1981), pp. 75-83 ISSN 7326003

Zammit, VA., & Moir, AM. (1994). Monitoring the partitioning of hepatic fatty acids in vivo: keeping track of control. *Trends of Biochemistry Science*, Vol. 19, No.8, (August 1994), pp.313-317, ISSN 7940674

Zschocke, J., Penzien, JM., Bielen, R., Casals, N., Aledo, R., Pié, J., Hoffmann, GF., Hegardt, FG., & Mayatepek, E. (2002). The diganosis of mitochondrial HMG-CoA synthase deficiency. *The Journal of Pediatrics*, Vol. 6, No. 140, (June 2002); pp.778-780, ISSN 12072887

10

Alström Syndrome

Cristina Maria Mihai[1], Jan D. Marshall[2] and Ramona Mihaela Stoicescu[3]
[1]*"Ovidius" University, Faculty of Medicine, Constanta,*
[2]*The Jackson Laboratory, Bar Harbor, ME,*
[3]*"Ovidius" University, Faculty of Pharmacy, Constanta*
[1,3]*Romania*
[2]*USA*

1. Introduction

Recent advancements in genetic research that have elucidated the function of some of the rare disease-causing genes have suggested that a large number of genetic disorders with widely divergent phenotypes, that were not previously identified as related, may be, in fact, highly related in cellular function or common pathways. A classic example of this is the recent category of disorders called ciliopathies. Cilia and flagella are ancient, evolutionarily conserved organelles that project from cell surfaces to perform diverse biological roles, including whole-cell locomotion; movement of fluid; chemo-, mechano-, and photosensation; and sexual reproduction. Over the past ten years, several studies demonstrated the connections between cilia, basal bodies and human diseases with a wide phenotypic spectrum, including randomization of body symmetry, obesity, cystic kidney diseases and retinal degeneration. Defects in ciliary structure or function can lead to a broader set of developmental and adult phenotypes, with mutations in ciliary proteins now associated with nephronophthisis, Joubert Syndrome, Meckel-Gruber Syndrome, Bardet-Biedl Syndrome, and Alström Syndrome (ALMS), [Badano et al., 2006]. Further study of these diverse ciliopathies could lead to an understanding of the phenotypic patterns that could potentially have predictive and therapeutic value. Alström Syndrome (ALMS; MIM #203800), first described by Carl-Henry Alström, in 1959 [Alström et al., 1959], is a rare condition that affects many body systems. ALMS is characterized by a constelation of serious or life-threatening medical problems including sensory deficits, obesity, type 2 diabetes mellitus, and multiple organ failure. The signs and symptoms of ALMS vary in severity, and not all affected individuals have all of the characteristic features of the disorder, making the diagnosis more difficult. Additionally, many of the signs and symptoms of this condition begin in infancy or early childhood, although some appear later in life. The major phenotypes usually observed in children with ALMS include cone–rod retinal dystrophy beginning in infancy and leading to juvenile blindness, sensorineural hearing impairment, insulin resistance, and obesity, and congestive heart failure (CHF) due to dilated cardiomyopathy (DCM). As patients reach adolescence, more of the major phenotypes develop, including type 2 diabetes mellitus, hypertriglyceridemia, hypothyroidism, and short adult stature. Males and females have hypogonadism and are infertile. Pulmonary, hepatic, and renal phenotypes are progressive [Marshall et al. 1997,

2005]. The primary cause of mortality among young affected patients is cardiac involvement from dilated cardiomyopathy whereas renal failure is the major cause of death among the older subgroup [Marshall et al., 1997]. Systemic fibrosis is commonly observed [Marshall et al., 2005]. About 700 affected individuals have been identified worldwide. The estimated prevalence is of <1: 5,000,000 [JD.Marshall, Personal communication]. Ethnically or geographically isolated populations have a higher-than-average frequency of Alström syndrome [Deeble et al., 2000 & Ozgül et al., 2007].

2. Diagnosis

2.1 Clinical diagnosis

The diagnosis of ALMS is usually established by clinical findings. Diagnosis may be delayed because some features begin at birth and others emerge as the child develops. Diagnosis can also be difficult due to variable expression of the severity of the clinical features both within and among families. It is important to note that, although some of the features are seen frequently, affected individuals may not have all of the symptoms discussed below.

2.1.1 Major features

Cone-rod dystrophy. The first symptoms are pendular or searching nystagmus and extreme photodysphoria or light sensitivity. The retinal dystrophy in ALMS often develops within a few weeks after birth and virtually all children exhibit low vision within the first year of life [Malm et al., 2008; Russell-Eggitt et al., 1998]. Fundus examination in the first decade may be normal or may show a pale optic disc and narrowing of the retinal vessels. Electroretinography (ERG), required to establish the diagnosis of cone-rod dystrophy, is abnormal from birth, eventually with impairment of both cone and rod function. Rod function is preserved initially but deteriorates as the individual ages. By 9 – 10 years of age, visual acuity is severely impaired. There is increasing constriction of visual fields, leading to total blindness with no light perception by age 16- 20 years [Marshall et al., 2007a, Michaud et al., 1996]. The severity and age of onset of the retinal degeneration vary among ALMS patients [Malm et al., 2008]. Retinal changes include attenuated vessels, pale optic discs, and partial atrophy of the retinal pigment epithelium. Pathological studies show a reduction of cell layers in the posterior retina and depletion of peripheral cells, the outer nuclear layer, and photoreceptors [Sebag et al., 1984, Vingolo et al., 2010]. Exudative retinopathy was described in Alström Syndrome [Gogi et al., 2007]. Vision may be aided in the first few years if the child is given prescription dark, red-tinted glasses. Cataract is a common finding and some patients might transiently benefit from its treatment/removal [Marshall et al., 2005, 2007, Satman et al., 2002].

Progressive bilateral sensorineural hearing impairment

Most patients develop mild-to-moderate bilateral sensorineural hearing loss in early childhood (<10 years) that is slowly progressive, particularly in the high-frequency range [Van den Abeele et al., 2001; Welsh 2007]. There is a high incidence of otitis media and fluid retention along with a high susceptibility to glue ear, which compounds the existing sensorineural impairment [Marshall et al. 2005, Michaud et al., 1997]. Hearing loss may be detected as early as age one year in some patients, although wide differences in acuity exist. Although bilateral hearing aids generally benefit most children, about 10% progress to profound deafness and must rely on tactile signing for communication [Marshall et al.,

2007a]. There is evidence that vestibular function is abnormal in some patients. [Möller, 2005]. Because hearing loss develops gradually and the onset is post-lingual, children typically do not experience the speech problems often associated with deafness. These early changes in neurosensory capabilities can have tremendous impact not only on the social development of the child but also on his/her adaptation to the external environment [Joyet al., 2007, Van den Abeele et al., 2001].

Obesity

Obesity in Alström Syndrome is an early and consistent feature observed in nearly all affected children [Marshall et al., 2005, 2007a]. Body Mass Index (kg/m^2) is typically greater than 25 or >95th centile, with the distribution of adipose tissue predominantly viscerally and subcutaneously [Paisey et al., 2008]. Birth weight is normal, but rapid weight gain usually begins at approximately 6 months to 1 year of age. In some individuals body weight tends to normalize, decreasing into the high-normal to normal range after adolescence. The moderation of weight does not seem to be correlated with the onset of other serious complications such as CHF, T2DM, or renal failure [Minton et al., 2006]. Wide shoulders, a barrel chest, a 'stocky' build, and truncal obesity are typical [Marshall et al., 2007a]. However, both waist circumference and body fat percentage (as measured using dual-energy X-ray absorptiometry) negatively correlated with age, and was independent of Body Mass Index, indicating the possible recruitment of more metabolically active fat stores [Minton et al., 2006]. The presence of hyperphagia has been controversial, although both hyperphagia and food obsession are common anecdotal complaints [Marshall et al., 1997, 2005].

Growth and development

Children grow rapidly and are initially tall for their age with a height >50th centile, with 2–3 years advanced bone age prior to puberty. However, early closure of the growth plates results in height below the 50th centile by age 14–16 years [Michaud et al., 1996]. Thoracic and lumbar scoliosis and kyphosis commonly develop in the early teenage years and can progress rapidly. Many patients have a 'buffalo hump' of increased fatty tissue above the shoulders [Marshall et al., 2005, 2007a]. Abnormalities of the insulin-like growth factor system (IGFs) of affected patients have been demonstrated [Maffei et al., 2007, Mihai et al., 2008, 2009]. Yet, the exact reasons for short stature remain to be determined.

Dilated cardiomyopathy

DCM can occur at any age, but is seen most typically during infancy. Onset, progression, and clinical outcome of the DCM vary, even within families [Hoffman et al., 2005, Makaryus et al., 2003]. Approximately 40% of affected infants have a transient but severe DCM with onset between age three weeks and four months [Marshall et al., 2005, Worthley & Zeitz, 2001]. Most of these children survive and make an apparently full recovery in infancy. The proportion of those with ALMS who develop infantile-onset DCM may be underestimated because some infants who succumb early may have undiagnosed Alström syndrome.

A subset of 10-15% of patients does not experience infantile DCM, but develop cardiomyopathy for the first time as adolescents or adults. These patients present with a progressive restrictive cardiomyopathy [Worthley & Zeitz, 2001], identified between the teens to late 30s. Although DCM is the most common underlying cause of death in the infantile period, survival for children with infantile-onset tends to be better than that for adult-onset. Marshall et al showed that while one-third of adult-onset DCM patients died, ~74% of infantile-onset DCM patients survived [Marshall et al., 2005]. As these children grow older, their cardiac function tends to be low-normal, and they remain at risk for a recurrence of CHF as adolescents or adults, with a poor prognosis. Postmortem myocardial fibrosis has been described [Minton et al., 2006]. Cardiac magnetic resonance imaging suggests myocardial fibrosis may be present both in clinically affected and asymptomatic individuals [Loudon et al., 2009].

Augmented aortic systolic pressure may also contribute to heart failure [Smith et al., 2007].

DCM in infants in the presence of nystagmus and photophobia should be a strong indicator of a diagnosis of ALMS.

Pulmonary disease

Chronic respiratory illness is one of the most frequent complaints and ranges in severity from frequent bronchial infections to chronic asthma, sinusitis/bronchitis, alveolar hypoventilation, and frequent episodes of pneumonia. The chronically inflamed airways are hyper-reactive and highly sensitive to triggering or irritating factors. In some patients, as inflammation continues, the lungs are infiltrated by fibrotic lesions and moderate to severe interstitial fibrosis has been reported [Marshall et al., 2005]. Pulmonary disease can be quite severe and include chronic obstructive pulmonary disease and pulmonary hypertension, secondary to pulmonary fibrosis. Respiratory infections with sudden reduced blood oxygen saturation have triggered sudden death. Acute hypoxia and acute respiratory distress syndrome in some older patients probably results from a combination of pulmonary fibrosis and severe scoliosis [Khoo et al., 2009; Florentzson et al., 2010].

Insulin resistance/type 2 diabetes mellitus

Two of the earliest metabolic changes in ALMS, insulin resistance and hyperinsulinemia, have been observed in patients as young as 1 year of age, sometimes before the onset of obesity [Marshall et al., 2005, 2007a]. Most children will eventually develop T2DM, some as early as age 4, but there is wide variability in the age of onset. The median age of onset is 16 years. T2DM in Alström syndrome is the result of tissue resistance to the actions of insulin, as demonstrated by an elevated plasma insulin concentration and glucose intolerance that usually present in childhood [Marshall et al., 2005, 2007a]. *Acanthosis nigricans,* a common feature in ALMS, consistent with severe insulin resistance, obesity, hyperinsulinemia, is described in about one-third of patients, whether or not they have diabetes [Marshall et al., 2005, 2007a]. However, in a small study of 12 unrelated individuals with ALMS, severe childhood obesity, BMI and waist circumference decreased with age, whereas insulin resistance increased [Minton et al., 2006]. Interestingly, ALMS patients with T2DM do not appear to develop typical peripheral sensory neuropathy symptoms and maintain good protective sensation despite comparable hyperglycemia and dyslipidemia seen in other types of diabetes. This suggests the *ALMS1* mutations might in some way protect against hyperglycemia-induced sensory neuropathy [Paisey et al., 2009]. However, studies of nerve conduction in these patients are needed to confirm these findings.

Hepatic disease

Nearly all patients with ALMS may have some degree of liver involvement that first presents with fatty liver. Initially, overt clinical manifestations are absent, but transaminases and gamma-glutamyl transpeptidase could be elevated. Ultrasound may show evidence of steatosis, steatohepatitis, and enlarged liver and spleen, which can progress in ALMS patients as they grow older. In some individuals, hepatic inflammation and fibrosis develops, with a highly variable age of onset, clinical course, and prognosis. As the disease progresses, liver function tests are further disturbed with altered prothrombin values or elevated International normalized ratio (INR) and ammonia. Progression to hepatic failure can occur in childhood [Quiros-Tejeira et al., 2001], but usually worsens in the second to third decades. Portal hypertension, hepatosplenomegaly, cirrhosis, esophageal varices, ascites, and liver failure are among the late clinical signs and the upper gastro-intestinal hemorrhage due to portal hypertension is a cause of death in some patients [Marshall et al., 2005, 2007a]. It is not yet known why the hepatic function becomes serious in some children, while others remain stable [Awazu et al., 1995, 1997, Connolly et al., 1991 & Marshall et al., 2005].

Liver biopsies and postmortem examination have revealed varying degrees of steatohepatitis, hepatic fibrosis, cirrhosis, chronic nonspecific active hepatitis with lymphocytic infiltration, patchy necrosis, [Marshall et al., 2005, Quiros-Tejeira et al., 2001]. Macrovesicular steatosis can be present or absent [Marshall et al., 2005]. Other gastrointestinal manifestations include upper gastrointestinal pain, chronic diarrhea, constipation, cecal volvulus, and gastroesophageal reflux [Marshall et al., 2005; Khoo et al., 2009].

Renal disease

The age of onset, progression rate, and severity of renal involvement are variable in ALMS, but most often becomes serious in adolescents or adults. Slowly progressive nephropathy, progressive glomerulofibrosis, and a gradual destruction of the kidneys are a major feature in adult patients with ALMS. Whether hypertension is a consequence of or contributes to renal dysfunction is uncertain, but it is present in ~30% of individuals [Marshall et al., 2005]. Patients may have symptoms ranging from chronic, mild kidney dysfunction to end-stage renal failure. Histopathologic changes include hyalinization of tubules and interstitial fibrosis [Goldstein and Fialkow, 1973, Marshall et al., 2005, 2007a]. There is evidence suggesting that the position of the alteration in *ALMS1* may play a role in the severity of the renal disease [Marshall et al., 2007b].

Hypogonadotropic hypogonadism

Male hypogonadotropic hypogonadism results in low plasma testosterone secondary to low plasma gonadotropin concentration. Males often have a small penis and testes, usually with gynecomastia in adolescence. Atrophic fibrotic seminiferous tubules are described [Marshall et al., 2007a]. Secondary sexual characteristics such as axillary and pubic hair are normal in both males and females. In female adolescents, sexual development usually progresses normally and menarche is not delayed (average age 12 years). In a few patients, precocious puberty has occurred (age 6–10) and breast development has been delayed. The external genitalia, uterus, and fallopian tubes are normal, but menstruation is often scant, sporadic, or irregular, sometimes accompanied by endometriosis. There can be reduced plasma gonadotropin concentrations. Baseline FSH and LH in female adolescents are usually in the normal range; however, some evidence of primary hypogonadism has been reported [Quiros-Tejeira et al., 2001]. Increased androgen production and hirsuitism are common [Kocova et al., 2010]. A relatively high frequency (>20% of female patients) of ovarian cysts is reported, which may be associated with obesity and hyperinsulinemia. No ALMS patients have been known to reproduce – the few cases where this is „reported" are in patients without a confirmed molecular diagnosis [Boor et al., 1993].

Hypertriglyceridemia

Hyperlipidemia, particularly hypertriglyceridemia, can be present from early childhood. In some patients, a sudden, rapid rise in triglycerides places them at risk for pancreatitis [Paisey et al., 2009, Wu et al., 2002]. Other features in Alström Syndrome, such as hyperinsulinemia, may also contribute to the elevated triglycerides [Maffei et al., 2002, 2007].

2.1.2 Minor features

Hypothyroidism

A hypothyroid condition, mostly primary (low free thyroxine (FT4), high thyroid-stimulating hormone (TSH)), is observed in approximately 20% of patients [Michaud et al., 1996]. Subclinical hypothyroidisms in about 30% of patients and isolated incidents of hyperthyroidism have been observed [Ozgül et al., 2007]. The mechanism of the hypothyroidism remains unknown, although it could be hypothesized that fibrotic infiltrations in the thyroid gland play a role.

Dental abnormalities

Dental anomalies include discolored teeth, gingivitis, a large space between the front teeth, and extra or missing teeth [Koray et al., 2001].

Hands and feet

Most children have characteristic wide, thick, flat feet, and short stubby fingers and toes with no polydactyly or syndactyly. Rare cases of digit anomalies have been reported [Marshall et al., 2007a].

Urological dysfunction

Males and females with ALMS can experience varying degrees of urinary problems. Minor symptoms include urinary urgency, difficulty initiating or poor flow, long intervals between voiding, incomplete voiding (urinary retention) or abdominal pain before or during urination [Marshall et al., 2005]. There can be an unusual changing presentation, switching from retention to increased frequency, and incontinence. Recurrent urinary tract infections or cystitis are common in both males and females. Urethral strictures have also been described and fibrotic infiltrations have been noted histopathologically. A subset of patients have developed more severe complications such as marked frequency and urgency, incontinence, and significant perineal or abdominal pain requiring surgical intervention [Charles et al., 1990, Marshall et al., 2005, 2007a]. Anatomical abnormalities can also occur in ALMS, including calyceal deformities, narrowed ureteropelvic angles, dilated ureters, and misalignment of the kidneys [Ozgül et al., 2007].

Developmental delay

Although delay of cognitive impairment is not a common feature of ALMS, delay in early developmental milestones is seen in ~45% of affected children. Motor milestones, in particular sitting, standing, and walking, are typically delayed by 1–2 years and there may be deficits in coordination, balance, and fine motor skills. Hearing and vision deficits probably contribute to the early developmental, expressive and receptive language, and learning delays seen in many young children with ALMS. Children with a receptive language deficit also tend to have an expressive language delay. Intellectual delays and behavioral issues in rare cases have resulted in a diagnosis of mental retardation. A range of autism-spectrum behavior has been observed in a subset of patients [Marshall et al., 2005, 2007a].

Other neurologic manifestations may include absence seizures and general sleep disturbances [Marshall et al., 2005, 2007a]. The frequency of mood and psychiatric disorders in ALMS-affected individuals has not been determined [Joy et al., 2007].

The combined effect of hearing loss and an accompanying multiple disabilities present a unique and complex problem to professionals and parents, different from the problems usually associated with any disability alone. A review of the literature yields surprisingly little specific information on educational programs for such children. The fact that there are many differences among children with multiple disabilities adds to the difficulties of providing appropriate programs.

2.2 Diagnostic criteria in Alström Syndrome

A major problem in arriving at a diagnosis of ALMS is the high phenotypic heterogeneity that can occur even within the same affected family [Ozgül et al., 2007, Hoffman et al., 2005 & Titomanilo et al., 2004]. Marshall and co-workers [Marshall et al., 2007a] provided a comprehensive guidance for diagnostic criteria in their 2007 publication, as summarized below:

Birth – 2 years: Diagnosis requires 2 major or 1 major and 2 minor criteria	
Major criteria:	1) *ALMS1* mutation in 1 allele and/or family history of Alström Syndrome 2) Vision pathology (nystagmus, photophobia).
Minor criteria:	1) Obesity 2) DCM with CHF.
Other variable supportive evidence	Recurrent pulmonary infections, normal digits, delayed developmental milestones.

3-14 years of age: diagnosis requires 2 major criteria or 1 major and 3 minor criteria	
Major criteria:	1) *ALMS1* mutation in 1 allele and/or family history of Alström Syndrome 2) Vision pathology (nystagmus, photophobia, diminished acuity). If old enough for testing: cone dystrophy by ERG.
Minor criteria:	1) Obesity and/or insulin resistance and/or T2DM 2) History of DCM with CHF 3) Hearing loss 4) Hepatic dysfunction 5) Renal failure 6) Advanced bone age

Other variable supportive evidence	Recurrent pulmonary infections, normal digits, delayed developmental milestones, hyperlipidemia, scoliosis, flat wide feet, hypothyroidism, hypertension, recurrent urinary tract infections, growth hormone deficiency

15 years – adulthood: 2 major and 2 minor criteria or 1 major and 4 minor criteria	
Major criteria:	1) ALMS1 mutation in 1 allele and/or family history of Alström Syndrome 2) Vision pathology (history of nystagmus in infancy/childhood, legal blindness, cone and rod dystrophy by ERG).
Minor criteria:	1) Obesity and/or insulin resistance and/or T2DM 2) History of DCM with CHF. 3) Hearing loss 4) Hepatic dysfunction 5) Renal failure 6) Short stature 7) Males: hypogonadism. Females: irregular menses and/or hyperandrogenism
Other variable supportive evidence	Recurrent pulmonary infections, normal digits, history of developmental delay, hyperlipidemia, scoliosis, flat wide feet, hypothyroidism, hypertension, recurrent urinary tract infections/urinary dysfunction, growth hormone deficiency, alopecia.

Table 1.

In conclusion, ALMS is a very complex disorder, being characterized by a constellation of progressive and highly variable disease symptoms. Diagnosis is made on the basis of clinical features observed, usually without genetic confirmation. Delay of onset of some of the characteristic features (type 2 diabetes mellitus, DCM/chronic heart failure, hepatic dysfunction, pulmonary, and renal disease) makes early differential diagnosis very difficult in young children, as many of the cardinal features do not become apparent until the teenage years. As the child grows, the characteristic pattern of ALMS evolves and the clinical picture becomes clearer.

2.3 Age of onset and incidence of common features of Alström Syndrome

Marshall and co-workers [Marshall et al., 2005] described the age of onset and the incidence of common features of Alstrom syndrome. Cone-rod dystrophy was diagnosed in 100% of ALMS patients between birth and 15 months. Obesity usually begins to develop during the first year, birth weight being normal. Hearing loss is progressive and presents in 88% of cases during the first 9 years. Dilated cardiomyopathy could be diagnosed in 42% of infants under 4 months of age. In adolescents and adults the pattern is often restrictive cardiomyopathy, with an overall incidence of 18%. Insulin resistance/type 2 diabetes can be diagnosed in children as young as 4 years of age. While urologic dysfunction can be seen at any age, chronic renal failure begins in adolescents and adults. About 25-30 % of ALMS patients are diagnosed with developmental delay, based on the assessment of early development milestones. Liver involvement develops variabily, between 8 and 30 years of age, in 23-98% of patients. Over 98% are diagnosed with short stature after puberty or in adulthood. Among the endocrine abnormalities, hypogonadotropic hypogonadism was diagnosed in 78% of males.

2.4 Genetic diagnosis

Alström Syndrome is the consequence of recessively inherited mutations in a single gene, *ALMS1,* located on the short arm of chromosome 2 [Collin et al., 2002, Hearn et al., 2002]. Parents are obligate carriers of a single copy of the altered gene and have no reported heterozygous phenotypic characteristics. Males and females are affected with equal probability (1:1 ratio). Although the incidence is greater in isolated or consanguineous communities, there is no one ethnic group more likely to carry *ALMS1* mutations [Marshall et al, 2007a].

ALMS1 is comprised of 23 exons. The longest *ALMS1* transcript potentially encodes a 461 kDa protein of 4169 amino acids. Exon 1 contains a tract of glutamic acid residues (aa 13–29), followed by a stretch of seven alanine residues (aa 30−36) [Collin et al., 2002, Hearn et al., 2002]. Exon 8, a large 6-kb exon, contains a large tandem repeat domain encoding 34 imperfect repeats of 45–50 amino acids. This domain constitutes 40% of the protein, a short polyglutamine segment, a leucine zipper domain and a conserved motif near the C-terminus.

The *ALMS1* protein is ubiquitously expressed and at least one isoform localizes to centrosomes and basal bodies of ciliated cells, perhaps playing an important role in cilia function and intraflagellar transport [Collin et al., 2005, Hearn et al., 2005; Knorz et al., 2010]. RNA interference knockdown experiments indicate that a total lack of *ALMS1* impairs cilia formation [Li G et al., 2007].

To date, the mutations reported in *ALMS1* have been nonsense and frameshift variations (insertions or deletions) and one reciprocal translocation that are predicted to cause premature protein truncation [Collin et al., 2002, Hearn et al., 2002]. Since 2002, more than 100 different mutations in *ALMS1* have been identified. The variants are primarily clustered in exons 16, 10, and 8, but less common mutations also occur in exons 12 and 18 [Marshall et al., 2007a; Joy et al., 2007; Pereiro, et al., 2010]. Founder effects are reported in families of English and Turkish descent. In addition, numerous single-nucleotide polymorphisms have been identified, the functional significance of which is unclear [Marshall et al., 2007a]. The mechanisms by which disease alleles of *ALMS1* cause the various pathologies observed in Alström Syndrome remain unknown and identification of pathogenic mutations in *ALMS1* has not led to any genotype-specific treatments [Hearn et al., 2005, Kinoshita et al., 2003, Li G et al., 2007, Minton et al., 2006 & Patel et al., 2006].

ALMS1 RNA is widely expressed by many tissues. Splice variants have been identified from human brain and testis which may suggest differing functions of theALMS1 protein between organs [Hearn et al., 2002].

The ubiquitous expression of *ALMS1* correlates with the wide range of organ dysfunction in ALMS and suggests that the C-terminal portion of the Alms1 protein that is missing in ALMS patients plays a critical role in disease causation [Girard & Petrovsky, 2010]. Because *ALMS1* is a very large gene, complete sequencing is time consuming and expensive. Therefore, we recommend a screening strategy that targets the regions of *ALMS1* where most of the mutations are seen (exons 16, 10, part of 8). If no mutation is identified in these areas, the remaining genomic regions can be sequenced on a research basis. The sensitivity of this approach is approximately 65%, that is, in about 42% of all patients both mutations will be detected, in about half of the patients, only one of the two mutations will be found, and in about 10% of the patients, none of the mutations will be found. The recent development of an-ALMS mutation array to detect known mutations in *ALMS1* (Asper Biotech (www.asperbio.com) can be used as an efficient and cost-effective first pass screening for known mutations *ALMS1* and 10 known Bardet-Biedl Syndrome (BBS) genes [Pereiro et al.,2010]. New technological developments including target capture and next generation sequencing will offer the possibility of efficient and cost-effective identification of novel *ALMS1* mutations and for carrier testing [Bell et al., 2011]

The possible results of genetic testing must be interpreted within the context of the clinical picture [Marshall et al., 2007a]:

- 2 mutations identified in ALMS1. Diagnosis: ALMS.
- 1 mutation in *ALMS1* together with clinical signs of Alström Syndrome. Diagnosis: very strong evidence for the confirmation of ALMS (although about 0.25% of all healthy individuals could also show this result).
- No ALMS1 mutation identified. This does not exclude the diagnosis, in the presence of clinical manifestations suggestive for ALMS.

3. Differential diagnosis of Alström Syndrome [Marshall et al., 2007a]

Cardiac	Vision	OMIM	
Yes	Cone dystrophy, photophobia	203800	*Alström Syndrome*
Congenital heart defects (5–10%)	Night blindness, rod–cone dystrophy (age 10-16)	209900	*Bardet–Biedl Syndrome (BBS #1-14)*
No	Cone dystrophy	216900 262300 139340	*Congenital achromatopsia*
No	Cone dystrophy (infancy)	204000	*Leber congenital amaurosis (LCA)*
No	Optic atrophy	222300	*Wolfram (DIDMOAD)*
No	Rod-cone dystrophy >5 years myopia, bulls-eye maculopathy, peripheral vision loss	216550	*Cohen Syndrome*
No	Coloboma, microphthalmia, aniridia, cataract	210350	*Biemond II Syndrome*

Mental development	Hypogonadism	Diabetes	Obesity	Renal	Neurosensory hearing loss	Respiratory	
Normal/delayed	Yes	T2DM (90%)	Yes	Glomerulo-sclerosis	Yes (90%)	Pulmonary failure, recurrent cough	*Alström Syndrome*
Mental retardation (50%)	Yes	T2DM (5–15%)	Yes	Structural renal abnormalities	Yes (5–20%)	No	*Bardet–Biedl Syndrome (BBS #1-14)*
Normal/ delayed	No	No	No	No	No	No	*Congenital achromatopsia*
Normal/ delayed	No	No	No	No	No	No	*Leber congenital amaurosis (LCA)*
Normal, behavior problems	No	Diabetes insipidus, insulin-dependent diabetes mellitus	No	Diabetic nephropathy	Yes	No	*Wolfram (DIDMOAD)*
Moderate-to-severe delay	No	No	Yes, abdominal obesity, thin arms and legs	No	No	No	*Cohen Syndrome*
Mental retardation	Yes	No	Yes	No	No	No	*Biemond II Syndrome*

Genetic	Head	Orthopedic	Urologic	Hepatic	
ALMS1 (2p13)	No	Short fingers, wide flat feet, scoliosis	Varying degrees of urinary problems (25%)	Steatosis cirrhosis	*Alström Syndrome*
BBS1, BBS2, ARL6/BBS3, BBS4, BBS5, MKKS/BBS6, BBS7, TTC8/BBS8, B1/BBS9, BBS10, TRIM32/BBS11, BBS12, MKS1/BBS13, CEP290/BBS14.	High-arched palate, hypodontia	Poly-, brachy-, and syndactyly		Steatosis	*Bardet–Biedl Syndrome (BBS #1-14)*
CNGA3 CNGB3GNAT2	No	Normal		No	*Congenital achromatopsia*
GUCY2D (LCA1), *RPE65* (LCA2), *SPATA7* (LCA3), *AIPL1* (LCA4), *LCA5* (LCA5), *RPGRIP1* (LCA6), *CRX* (LCA7), *CRB1* (LCA8), *CEP290* (LCA10), *IMPDH1* (LCA11), *RD3* (LCA12), and *RDH12* (LCA13).	No	Normal		No	*Leber congenital amaurosis (LCA)*
WFS1 (4p16)	No	Normal	Urinary atony	No	*Wolfram (DIDMOAD)*
COH1 (8q22)	Characteristic facial features	Narrow hands and feet, tapered fingers		No	*Cohen Syndrome*
	Absent incisors, microcephaly, characteristic facial features	Postaxial polydactyly, scoliosis		No	*Biemond II Syndrome*

Table 2.

4. Management

There is no treatment at this time that can cure ALMS or prevent or reverse the medical complications.

Early diagnosis is important to allow counseling of parents and institution of appropriate supportive medical treatment. In the absence of specific therapy to correct the underlying genetic defect, ALMS remains a progressive disease and regular intensive medical management is essential to track progression and to anticipate the emergence of new symptoms and disease manifestations.

Cardiac, renal and liver review should be routinely performed in all ALMS patients, even if asymptomatic.

The main causes of death in ALMS are from cardiomyopathy, pulmonary, kidney or liver failure [Marshall et al., 2005, Benso et al., 2002]. In the end stage, multiple organs are compromised, and sudden multiple organ failure is common.

4.1 Management of sensory deficits

Vision and hearing loss can impact the social and educational success of the child, so, management of the multiple sensory deficits in young children diagnosed with ALMS and social support at school are crucial [Marshall et al., 2007a].

4.1.1 Rod-cone dystrophy

Photophobia and nystagmus are serious problems, particularly in younger children. Regular ophthalmologic evaluations should be sought as soon as possible [Gogi et al., 2007]. Red-tinted prescription glasses are helpful in alleviating the distress children experience in bright lighting. No therapy for the progressive vision loss exists, but early evaluation of visual acuity facilitates the provision of visual aids and helps prepare the child for a future with little or no sight. Educational planning should anticipate future blindness, therefore, early mobility training and Braille or other non-visual language skills is critically important for the learning environment of the child. Computing skills (including voice recognition and transcription software), and the use of large print reading materials early on while vision is still present are crucial [Marshall et al 2010].

4.1.2 Progressive sensorineural hearing loss

Hearing evaluation should begin early in childhood, as otoacoustic emissions and audiometry may reveal subclinical hearing loss. Conductive loss is common in children as a result of chronic otitis media. Hearing can usually be effectively managed with bilateral digital hearing aids, but should be monitored regularly. Myringotomy has been helpful in individuals with recurrent "glue ear". Cochlear implantation has benefitted some patients, but surgeons should be aware of the risk of sudden hypoxia for these patients undergoing procedures requiring anesthesiology [Florentzson et al., 2010].

4.2 Obesity. Insulin resistance/Type 2 diabetes

The major clinical treatment focus is on control of obesity and T2DM.

Candidate therapeutic intervention to treat severe insulin resistance and possibly prevent the transition from insulin resistance to overt diabetes include insulin-sensitizing drugs (metformin and thiazolidinediones) [Sinha et al., 2007 as cited in Atabek, 2007, Nag S et al.,

2003] and beta cell-preserving drugs (incretins, thiazolidinediones) [Pagano et al., 2008, Paisey et al., 2009]. However, this requires close monitoring of liver, cardiac, and renal function. Glitazones are added to further reduce insulin resistance but must be avoided in the presence of active or treated heart failure and when the serum creatinine concentration exceeds 200 μmol/L. Exenatide, an incretin mimetic, an injectable analogue of glucagon-like peptide 1(GLP- 1) could be promising in adults with ALMS.

Weight loss exercises should play a pivotal role in weight reduction plan for ALMS patients, as in other patients diagnosed with dibetes and obesity, although could be challenging. Walking, hiking, biking, and swimming with partners and adaptations for the blind have been helpful. Peripheral sensor-motor neuropathy is a common complication of T2DM, but in a small clinical testing study in ALMS, a full preservation of protective foot sensation was demonstrated [Paisey et al., 2009]. The responsiveness to treatment of hyperglycemia is variable. Younger patients rarely require insulin, but some patients require insulin in very-high doses long term [Marshall et al., 2007a].

Caloric restriction helps control obesity, glucose tolerance and hyperinsulinemia [Holder et al., Lee et al., 2009 & Paisey et al. 2008], although as with children with other genetically acquired obesity syndromes, dietary compliance may be a major problem. Reducing dietary carbohydrates may prove more effective than fat restriction in control of hyperglycemia and hyperinsulinemia [Paisey et al., 2008]. No clinical experience has been reported in ALMS of use of specific appetite suppressant medication, such as duramine or sibutramine.

4.3 Hypertriglyceridemia

Insulin resistance, T2DM, dyslipidaemia and associated cardiac, renal and hepatic consequences coexist from a young age with considerable morbidity and reduction in life expectancy. ALMS patients can have potentially harmfully increased lipid levels. Hypertriglyceridemia can often be normalized by diet, exercise and Metformin. Some patients with severe hypertriglyceridemia responded to a combination of low-fat diet, statins and nicotinic acid [Paisey et al., 2004], very little data existing, however, about the safety and efficacy of such treatments before puberty.

Early introduction of preventative nutrition with low-carbohydrates, exercise and drug therapies (niacin extended-release and incretins) in ALMS could be beneficial [Paisey, 2009].

Pancreatitis should be treated as in the general population, but it is a challenge to treat a patient with multiple system involvement such as ALMS patients [Marshall et al., 2010, Paisey, 2009, Wu WC et al., 2003].

4.4 Impaired growth hormone (GH)-IGF1 axis function

There is an impaired growth hormone (GH)-IGF1 axis function in ALMS (Maffei et al., 2000, 2002), therefore, therapy with recombinant human Growth Hormone (rhGH) has been attempted in a small series of patients and isolated cases and has been reported to be beneficial for some metabolic parameters. Demonstrating growth hormone deficiency in a patient with ALMS, Tai and co-workers assessed the metabolic effects of growth hormone therapy concluding that rhGH therapy might have beneficial effects on body composition, liver fat content, lipid profiles, and insulin resistance in Alström Syndrome patients, with improvement of the glucose homeostasis [Tai et al., 2003]. Also, Maffei et al. found a reduction of ALS (acid labile subunit) and the increase of IGFBP-2 as expression of growth hormone deficiency condition in 15 young adults with ALMS [Maffei et al., 2000]. RhGH therapy should be considered still investigational [Marshall et al. 2007a]. Several studies are needed to prove that this therapy is cost-effective and without risk in patients with ALMS and severe insulin resistance.

4.5 Cardiomyopathy

Patients diagnosed with ALMS should be regularly monitored for cardiac function by echocardiography, even if asymptomatic [Makaryus et al., 2002, Zubrow et al., 2006]. Several authors [Loudon et al., 2009, Makaryus et al., 2007] stated the importance of serial cardiac magnetic resonance scanning in diagnosis of the underlying disease progression and responses to treatment. Long-term angiotensin-converting enzyme inhibition is indicated for the patient with cardiomyopathy. Many patients respond to other medications, which favorably affect heart function, such as diuretics, digitalis, beta-blockers, and spironolactone. Whether cardiac transplantation is a viable option is yet to be determined, due to the multisystemic involvement, particularly pulmonary, endocrine, and renal function. There has been one successful heart-lung transplantation reported in an adolescent patient with Alström Syndrome, but with no T2DM or significant renal failure [Görler et al., 2007]. A second successful heart transplant has been achieved in an infant prior to the onset of the endocrinological and renal disturbances [JD Marshall, Personal communication].

4.6 Thyroid

Replacement therapy with L-thyroxin, when needed, is very effective and well-tolerated in the majority of patients.
Thyroid function should be monitored closely in critical hospital settings [Marshall et al., 2007].

4.7 Urologic

Lack of coordination between bladder and urine outflow (detrusor-urethral dyssynergia) can be helped by intermittent self-catheterization of the bladder. Ileal diversion may be necessary in rare patients [Marshall et al., 2007; Charles, et al. 1990].

4.8 Hypogonadotropic hypogonadism

If abnormalities in pubertal development or menstrual abnormalities are present, the affected individual should be referred to an endocrinologist with expertise in sexual developmental abnormalities. Primary hypogonadism in ALMS males result in low levels of testosterone, treated with weekly or twice monthly injections of testosterone from puberty onwards. Treatment with cyclical oestrogen and progesterone is important and effective to regulate menstrual cycle and development.

4.9 Hepatic disease

Liver function parameters should be routinely monitored, beginning in childhood. Portal hypertension and varices may be aggressively treated with beta-blockers and sclerotherapy of the esophageal veins. Variceal banding could be useful to prevent upper gastro-intestinal hemorrhage. A transjugular intrahepatic portosystemic shunt (TIPS) is used to treat the complications of portal hypertension, when the patient has failed to respond to previous therapeutic measures. Patients with significant portal hypertension should be evaluated early for liver transplantation [Marshall et al., 2007].

4.10 Renal disease

Because renal insufficiency develops slowly as the patient ages, regular testing of renal function (plasma electrolytes, blood urea nitrogen, creatinine, and urea) is important, particularly in the older patient. Baseline values should be taken in children. Management of hypertension, a low-sodium and low-protein diet, avoidance of nephrotoxic drugs are very important in the preservation of renal function, as well as angiotensin-converting enzyme inhibitors prescribed according to general guidelines. Fibrosis and glomerulosclerosis in the kidneys may lead to eventual renal failure, requiring dialysis. Renal transplantation has been successful in several patients, although can be contraindicated in the presence of other complications including morbid obesity, uncontrolled diabetes, and cardiomyopathy [Marshall et al., 2007].

4.11 Pulmonary disease

Pulmonary fibrosis, dilated cardiomyopathy, and scoliosis can compromise cardio-respiratory function, particularly with concomitant respiratory infection or anesthesia in routine surgical procedures. Monitoring cardiac status and oxygenation during acute illness and postoperatively are mandatory, considering that ALMS patients can suddenly, without warning become critically hypoxic [Lynch et al., 2007, Tiwari et al., 2010]. Chronic obstructive airway disease and associated infection should be managed in line with appropriate national guidelines.

4.12 Other

4.12.1 Gastrointestinal

Reflux esophagitis should be diagnosed by barium swallow or upper gastrointestinal endoscopy, in the presence of suggestive symptoms and treated accordingly to the guidelines.

4.12.2 Orthopedic abnormalities

In the presence of flat feet, scoliosis, barrel chest, kyphoscoliosis the referral to an orthopedist is appropriate. Some patients have had surgical intervention for scoliosis, but care should be taken when undertaking surgical procedures, as previously mentioned.

4.12.3 Neurologic manifestations

ALMS patients should be examined for: absence seizures, autistic-spectrum behavioral abnormalities, excessive startle, unexplained joint or muscle pain, muscle dystonia, or hyporeflexia.

4.13 Prevention of secondary complications

There should be routine pediatric immunizations, especially against flu and hepatitis B virus infections.

Families should be encouraged to seek contact with good sources of support and information, such as Alström Syndrome International (www.alstrom.org) or other groups assisting families with this rare disorder.

5. Conclusion

Full understanding of the phenotypic characteristics, particularly with the help of existing mouse models [Collin et al., 2005, Arsov et al., 2006a, 2006b] will lead to better insight into the pathophysiology of *ALMS1*. By developing targeted therapies, certain debilitating aspects of ALMS could be prevented or treated earlier, improving the overall outcome in this complex disorder [Marshall et al., 2007]. Also, careful clinical and genetic studies can contribute to a better understanding of the disease evolution after different therapeutic attempts in Alström Syndrome.

6. References

Alström, C.H., Hallgren, B., Nilsson, L.B., & Åsander H. (1959). Retinal degeneration combined with obesity, diabetes mellitus and neurogenous deafness: a specific syndrome (not hitherto described) distinct from the Laurence-Moon-Bardet-Biedl syndrome: a clinical, endocrinological and genetic examination based on a large pedigree. *Acta psychiatrica et neurologica Scandinavica Supplementum*, Vol. 129, pp. 1-35, ISSN: 0365-5067.

Arsov, T., Larter, C.Z., Nolan, C.J., Petrovsky, N., Goodnow, C.C., Teoh, N..C, Yeh, M.M. & Farrell, G.C. (2006). Adaptive failure to high-fat diet characterizes steatohepatitis in Alms1 mutant mice. *Biochemichal and Biophysical Research Communications*. Vol. 342, No. 4 (April 2006), pp. 1152–1159. (a)

Arsov, T., Silva, D.G., O'Bryan, M.K., Sainsbury, A., Lee, N.J., Kennedy, C., Manji, S.S., Nelms, K., Liu, C., Vinuesa, C.G., de Kretser, D.M., Goodnow, C.C.& Petrovsky, N. (2006). Fat Aussie—a new Alström Syndrome mouse showing a critical role for Alms1 in obesity, diabetes and spermatogenesis. *Molecular Endocrinology*. Vol. 20, No. 7 (July 2006), pp. 1610–1622. (b)

Atabek, M.E. (2007). Re: "Effect of metformin and rosiglitazone in a prepubertal boy with Alström syndrome". *Pediatric Endocrinology & Metabolism*, Vol. 21, No. 1 (January 2008): 100; author reply 100-101.

Awazu, M., Tanaka, T., Yamazaki, K., Kato, S., Higuchi, M. & Matsuo, N. (1995). A 27-year-old woman with Alström syndrome who had liver cirrhosis. *The Keio Journal of Medicine*. Vol. 44, No. 2 (June 1995), pp. 67–73.

Awazu, M., Tanaka, T., Sato, S., Anzo, M., Higuchi, M., Yamazaki, K., & Matsuo, N. (1997). Hepatic dysfunction in two sibs with Alström syndrome: case report and review of the literature. *American journal of medical genetics*. Vol. 69, No. 1 (March 1997), pp. 13–16.

Badano, J.L., Mitsuma, N., Beales, P.L. & Katsanis, N. (2006). The ciliopathies: an emerging class of human genetic disorders. *Annual Review of Genomics and Human Genetics*, Vol.7, (September 2006), pp.125-148, ISSN: 1527-8204.

Bell,C.J., Dinwiddie, D.L., Miller, N.A., Hateley, S.L., Ganusova, E.E., Mudge, J., Langley, R.J., Zhang, L., Lee, C.C., Schilkey, F.D., Sheth, V., Woodward, J.E., Peckham, H.E., Schroth, G.P., Kim &R.W.,Kingsmore, S.F. (2011). Carrier testing for severe childhood recessive diseases by next-generation sequencing. *Science. Translational . Medicine.*, *3*, 65ra4.

Benso, C., Hadjadj, E., Conrath, J. & Denis, D. (2002). Three new cases of Alström syndrome. *Graefe's Archive for Clinical and Experimental Ophthalmology*. Vol. 240, No. 8 (August 2002), pp. 622-627.

Boor, R., Herwig, J., Schrezenmeir, J., Pontz, B.F. & Schönberger, W. (1993). Familial Insulin Resistant Diabetes Associated With Acanthosis Nigricans, Polycystic Ovaries, Hypogonadism, Pigmentary Retinopathy, Labyrinthine Deafness, and Mental

Retardation. *American Journal of Medical Genetics*. Vol. 45, No. 5 (March 1993), pp. 649-653.

Charles, S., Moore, A., Yates, J., Green, T. & Clark, P. (1990). Alström 's syndrome: further evidence of autosomal recessive inheritance and endocrinological dysfunction. *Journal of Medical Genetics*. Vol. 27, No. 9 (September 1990), pp. 590–592.

Collin, G.B., Marshall, J.D., Ikeda, A., W., So, V., Russell-Eggitt, I., Maffei, P., Beck, S., Boerkoel, C.F., Sicolo, N., Martin, M., Nishina, P.M. & Naggert, J.K. (2002). Mutations in ALMS1 cause obesity, type 2 diabetes and neurosensory degeneration in Alström syndrome. *Nature Genetics*. Vol. 31, (May 2002), pp. 74–78.

Collin, G.B., Cyr, E., Bronson, R., Marshall, J.D., Gifford, E.J., Hicks, W., Murray,. SA., Zheng, Q.Y., Smith, R.S., Nishina, P.M. & Naggert, J.K. (2005). Alms1-disrupted mice recapitulate human Alström syndrome. *Human Molecular Genetics*. Vol. 14, No. 16 (August 2005), pp. 2323–2333.

Connolly, M.B., Jan, J.E., Couch, R.M., Wong, L.T., Dimmick, J.E. & Rigg, J.M. (1991). Hepatic dysfunction in Alström disease. *American Journal of Medical Genetics*. Vol. 40, No. 4 (September 1991), pp. 421–424.

Deeble, V.J., Roberts, E., Jackson, A., Lench, N., Karbani, G. & Woods, C.G. (2000). The continuing failure to recognise Alström syndrome and further evidence of genetic homogeneity. *Journal of Medical Genetics*. Vol.37, No.3 (March 2000), pp. 219.

Florentzson, R., Hallén, K. & Möller, C. (2010). Alström syndrome and cochlear implantation. The first clinical experience. *10th International CI-conference June 27-July 1, 2010, Stockholm.*

Girard D. & Petrovsky, N. (2010). Alström syndrome: insights into the pathogenesis of metabolic disorders. *Nature Reviews. Endocrinology*. Vol. 7, No. 2 (February 2011), pp. 77-88.

Gogi, D., Bond, J., Long, V., Sheridan, E. & Woods, C.G. (2007). Exudative retinopathy in a girl with Alström syndrome due to a novel mutation. *The British Journal of Ophthalmology*. Vol. 91, No. 7 (July 2007), pp. 983–984.

Goldstein, J.L.& Fialkow, P.J. (1973). The Alström syndrome. Report of three cases with further delineation of the clinical, pathophysiological, and genetic aspects of the disorder. *Medicine*. Vol. 52, No. 1 (January 1973), pp. 53–71.

Goerler, H., Warnecke, G., Winterhalter, M., Müller, C., Ballmann, M., Wessel, A., Haverich, A., Strüber, M. & Simon, A. (2007). Heart-lung transplantation in a 14-year-old boy with Alström syndrome. *The Journal of Heart and Lung Transplantation*. Vol. 26, No. 11, pp: 1217-8

Hearn, T., Renforth, G.L., Spalluto, C., Hanley, N.A., Piper, K., Brickwood, S., White, C., Connolly, V., Taylor, J.F.N., Russell-Eggitt, I., Bonneau, D., Walker, M. & Wilson, D.I. (2002). Mutation of *ALMS1*, a large gene with a tandem repeat encoding 47 amino acids, causes Alström syndrome. *Nature Genetics*. Vol. 31, No. 1 (May 2002), pp. 79-83.

Hearn, T., Spalluto, C., Phillips, V.J., Renforth, G.L., Copin, N., Hanley, N.A. & Wilson, D.I.(2005). Subcellular localization of ALMS1 supports involvement of centrosome and basal body dysfunction in the pathogenesis of obesity, insulin resistance, and type 2 diabetes. *Diabetes*. Vol. 54, No. 5 (May 2005), pp. 1581-1587.

Hoffman, J.D., Jacobson, Z., Young, T.L., Marshall, J.D. & Kaplan, P. (2005). Familial variable expression of dilated cardiomyopathy in Alström syndrome: a report of four sibs. *American Journal of Medical Genetics*. Vol. 135A, No. 1 (May 2005), pp. 96–98.

Holder, M., Hecker, W. & Gilli, G. Impaired Glucose Tolerance Leads to Delayed Diagnosis of Alström Syndrome. *Diabetes Care*. Vol. 18, No. 5 (May 1995), pp. 698-700.

Joy, T., Cao, H., Black, G., Malik, R., Charlton-Menys, V., Hegele, R.A. & Durrington, P.N. (2007). Alström syndrome (OMIM 203800): a case report and literature review. *Orphanet Journal of Rare Diseases*. Vol. 2, No. 1 (December 2007): 49, Available from http://www.ojrd.com/content/2/1/49.

Khoo, E.Y., Risley, J., Zaitoun, A.M., El-Sheikh, M., Paisey, R.B., Acheson, A.G. & Mansell P.(2009): Alström syndrome and cecal volvulus in 2 siblings. *American Journal of Medical Sciences*. Vol. 337, No. 5 (May 2009), pp: 383-385.

Kinoshita, T., Hanaki, K., Kawashima, Y., Nagaishi, J., Hayashi, A., Okada, S., Murakami, J., Nanba, E., Tomonaga, R. & Kanzaki, S. (2003). A novel non-sense mutation in Alström syndrome: subcellular localization of its truncated protein. *Clinical Pediatric Endocrinology*. Vol. 12, No. 2, pp. 114.

Knorz, V.J., Spalluto, C., Lessard, M., Purvis, T.L., Adigun, F.F., Collin, G.B., Hanley, N.A., Wilson, D. &, Hearn, T.(2010). Centriolar association of ALMS1 and likelycentrosomal functions of the ALMS motif-containing proteins C10orf90 and KIAA1731. *Molecular biology of the cell*. Vol. 1, No. 21 (November 2010), pp:: 3617-3629.

Kocova, M., Sukarova-Angelovska, E., Kacarska, R., Maffei, P., Milan, G. & Marshall, J.D. (2010). The Unique Combination of Dermatological and Ocular Phenotypes in Alström Syndrome: Severe Presentation, Early Onset, and Two Novel *ALMS1* Mutations. *British Journal of Dermatology*. (December 2010) doi: 10.1111/j.1365-2133.2010.10157.x. [Epub ahead of print].

Koray, F., Dorter, C., Benderli, Y., Satman, I., Yilmaz, T., Dinccag, N. & Karsidag, K. (2001). Alström syndrome: a case report. *Journal of Oral Science*. Vol. 43, No. 3 (September 2001), pp. 221–224.

Lee, N., Marshall, J.D., Collin, G.B., Naggert, J.K., Chien, Y.H., Tsai, W.Y.& Hwu, W.L. (2009). Caloric restriction in Alström syndrome prevents hyperinsulinemia. *American Journal of Medical Genetics Part A*. Vol. 149A, No. 4 (February 2009), pp. 666-668.

Li, G., Vega, R., Nelms, K., Gekakis, N., Goodnow, C., McNamara, P., Wu, H., Hong, N. & Glynne, R. (2007). A Role for Alström Syndrome Protein, Alms1, in Kidney Ciliogenesis and Cellular Quiescence. *PLoS Genetics*. Vol. 3, No. 1 (January 2007): e8. doi:10.1371/journal.pgen.0030008.

Loudon, M.A., Bellenger, N.G., Carey, C.M. & Paisey, R.B. (2009). Cardiac magnetic resonance imaging in Alström syndrome. *Orphanet Journal of Rare Diseases*. Vol. 4 (June 2009):14. http://www.ojrd.com/content/4/1/14

Lynch, G., Clinton, S. & Siotia, A. (2007). Anaesthesia and Alström's Syndrome. *Anaesthesia and Intensive Care*. Vol. 35, No. 2 (April 2007), pp. 305-306.

Maffei, P., Munno, V., Marshall, J.D., Milanesi, A., Martini, C., De Carlo, E., Mioni, R., Pontoni, E., Menegazzo, C. & Sicolo, N. (2000). GH and IGF-I Axis in Alström Syndrome. *Journal of Endocrinological Investigation*. Vol. 23 (Suppl. to No. 6), pp. 29.

Maffei, P., Boschetti, M., Orsi, I., Marshall, J.D., Paisey, R.B., Beck, S., Munno, V., Minuto, F., Barreca, A.M. & Sicolo, N. (2002). The IGF system in Alström Syndrome. *Growth Hormone and IGF Research*. Vol. 12, No. 4, pp. 291.

Maffei, P., Munno, V., Marshall, J.D., Scandellari, C. & Sicolo, N. (2002). The Alström syndrome: is it a rare or unknown disease? *Annali Italiani di Medicina Interna*. Vol. 17, No. 4 (October-December 2002), pp. 221–228.

Maffei, P., Boschetti, M., Marshall, J.D., Paisey, R.B., Beck, S., Resmini, E., Collin, G.B., Naggert, J.K., Milan, G., Vettor, R., Minuto, F., Sicolo, N. & Barreca, A. (2007). Characterization of the IGF system in 15 patients with Alström syndrome. *Clinical endocrinology*. Vol. 66, No. 2 (February 2007), pp. 269–275.

Makaryus, A.N., Popowski, B., Kort, S., Paris, Y. & Mangion, J. (2003). A rare case of Alström syndrome presenting with rapidly progressive severe dilated cardiomyopathy diagnosed by echocardiography. *Journal of the American Society of Echocardiogr.aphy*. Vol. 16, No. 2 (February 2003), pp. 194–196.

Markaryus, A.N., Zubrow, M.E., Marshall, J.D., Gillam, L.D. &Mangion, J.R. (2007). Cardiac manifestations of Alström syndrome: echocardiographic findings. *Journal of American Society of Echocardiography*. Vol.20, No. 12, (December 2007), pp.1359-1363.

Malm, E., Ponjavic, V., Nishina, P.M., Naggert, J.K., Hinman, E.G., Andréasson, S., Marshall, J.D. & Möller, C. (2008). Full-field electroretinography and marked variability in clinical phenotype of Alström syndrome. *Archives of Ophthalmology*. Vol. 126, No. 1 (January 2008), pp. 51–57.

Marshall, J.D., Ludman, M.D., Shea, S.E., Salisbury, S.R., Willi, S.M., LaRoche, R.G. & Nishina, P.M. (1997). Genealogy, natural history, and phenotype of Alström syndrome in a large Acadian kindred and three additional families. American *Journal of Medical Genetics*.Vol.73, No.2 (December 1997), pp. 150–161.

Marshall, J.D., Bronson, R.T., Collin, G.B., Nordstrom, A.D., Maffei, P., Paisey, R.B., Carey, C., Macdermott, S., Russell-Eggitt, I., Shea, S.E., Davis, J., Beck, S., Shatirishvili, G., Mihai, C.M., Hoeltzenbein, M., Pozzan, G.B., Hopkinson, I., Sicolo, N., Naggert, J.K. & Nishina, P.M. (2005). *New Alström syndrome phenotypes based on the evaluation of 182 cases. Archives of internal medicine*. Vol. 165, No. 6 (March 2005), pp. 675–683.

Marshall, J.D., Beck, S., Maffei, P.& Naggert, J.K. 2007(a). Alström syndrome. *European Journal of Human Genetics*. Vol. 15, No.12 (December 2007), pp. 1193–1202.

Marshall, J.D., Hinman, E.G., Collin, G.B., Beck, S., Cerqueira, R., Maffei, P., Milan, G., Zhang, W., Wilson, D.I., Hearn, T., Tavares, P., Vettor, R., Veronese, C., Martin, M., So, W.V., Nishina, P.M. & Naggert, J.K. (2007). Spectrum of ALMS1 variants and evaluation of genotype–phenotype correlations in Alström syndrome. *Human Mutation*. Vol. 28, No. 11 (November 2007), pp. 1113-1123 (b).

Marshall, J.D., Paisey, R.B., Carey, C. & Macdermott, S. (Last update June 2010). *Alström Syndrome*. GeneReviews. NCBI Bookshelf. Available from http://www.ncbi.nlm.nih.gov/books/NBK1267/

Michaud, J.L., Héon, E., Guilbert, F., Weill, J., Puech, B., Benson, L., Smallhorn, J.F., Shuman, C.T., Buncic, J.R., Levin, A.V., Weksberg, R. & Brevière, G.M. (1996). Natural history of Alström syndrome in early childhood: Onset with dilated cardiomyopathy. *The Journal of Pediatrics*. Vol. 128, No. 2 (February 1996), pp. 225-229.

Mihai, C.M., Catrinoiu, D., Marshall, J.D., Stoicescu, R. & Tofolean, J.T. (2008). Cilia, Alström Syndrome - molecular concept, mechanisms and therapeutic perspectives. *Journal of Medicine and Life*. Vol. 1, No. 3 (July-September 2008), pp. 254-261.

Mihai, C.M., Catrinoiu, D., Toringhibel, M., Stoicescu, R.M., Negreanu-Pirjol, T. & Hancu, A. (2009). Impaired IGF1-GH axis and new therapeutic options in Alström Syndrome patients: a case series. *Cases Journal*. Vol. 2, No. 1 (January 2009): 19. http://www.casesjournal.com/content/2/1/19.

Minton, J.A., Owen, K.R., Ricketts, C.J., Crabtree, N., Shaikh, G., Ehtisham, S., Porter, J.R., Carey, C., Hodge, D., Paisey, R., Walker, M. & Barrett, T.G. (2006). Syndromic obesity and diabetes: changes in body composition with age and mutation analysis of ALMS1 in 12 United Kingdom kindreds with Alström syndrome. The Journal of Clinical Endocrinology and Metabolism. *Vol. 91, No. 8 (August* 2006), pp. 3110–3116.

Möller, C. (2005). Alström syndrome. *The National Swedish Board of Health and Welfare*. Nov 2005, *Available from http//www.sos.se*

Nag, S., Kelly, W.F., Walker, M. & Connolly, V. (2003). Type 2 diabetes in Alström syndrome: Targeting insulin resistance with a thiazolidinedione.*Endocrine Abstracts*. Vol. 5, pp. 104. British Endocrine Society, March 2003.

Paisey, R.B., Carey, C.M., Bower, L., Marshall, J., Taylor, P., Maffei, P. & Mansell, P. (2004). Hypertriglyceridaemia in Alström's syndrome: causes and associations in 37 cases. *Clinical Endocrinology*. Vol. 60, No. 2 (February 2004), pp. 228–231.

Paisey, R. B., Hodge, D. & Williams, K. (2008). Body fat distribution, serum glucose, lipid and insulin response to meals in Alström syndrome. *Journal of Human Nutrition and Dietetics*. Vol. 21, No. 3 (June 2008), pp. 268-274.

Paisey, R.B., Paisey, R.M., Thomson, M.P., Bower, L., Maffei, P., Shield, J.P., Barnett, S. & Marshall, J.D. (2009). Protection From Clinical Peripheral Sensory Neuropathy in Alström Syndrome in Contrast to Early-Onset Type 2 Diabetes. *Diabetes Care*. Vol. 32, No. 3 (March 2009b), pp. 462-464.

Paisey, R.B. (2009). New insights and therapies for the metabolic consequences of Alström syndrome. *Current Opinion in Lipidology*. Vol. 20, No. 4 (August 2009), pp. 315-230.

Quiros-Tejeira, R.E., Vargas, J. & Ament, M.E. (2001). Early-onset liver disease complicated with acute liver failure in Alström syndrome. *American Journal of Medical Genetics*. Vol. 101, No. 1 (June 2001), pp. 9–11.

Ozgül, R.K., Satman. I., Collin, G.B., Hinman, E.G., Marshall, J.D., Kocaman, O., Tütüncü, Y., Yilmaz, T. & Naggert, J.K. (2007). Molecular analysis and long-term clinical evaluation of three siblings with Alström syndrome. *Clinical Genetics*. Vol. 72, No.4 (October 2007), pp. 351–356.

Pagano, C., Romano, S., Maffei, P., Sicolo, N. & Vettor, R.(2008). Insulin resistance and diabetes in Alstrom syndrome. *5th International Scientific Congress. ALSTRÖM SYNDROME*. Padua - Venice , Italy, October 17-18, 2008.

Patel, S., Minton, J.A., Weedon, M.N., Frayling, T.M., Ricketts, C., Hitman, G.A., McCarthy, M.I., Hattersley, A.T., Walker, M. & Barrett, T.G. (2006). Common variations in the *ALMS1* gene do not contribute to susceptibility to type 2 diabetes in a large white UK population. *Diabetologia*, Vol. 49, No. 6 (June 2006), pp. 1209–1213.

Russell-Eggitt, I.M., Clayton, P.T., Coffey, R., Kriss, A., Taylor, D.S. & Taylor, J.F. (1998). Alström syndrome. Report of 22 cases and literature review. *Ophthalmology*. Vol. 105, No. 7, pp. 1274-1280.

Satman, I., Yilmaz, M.T., Gursoy, N., Karsidag, K., Dinccag, N., Ovali, T., Karadeniz, S., Uysal, V., Bugra, Z., Okten, A., & Devrim, S. (2002). Evaluation of insulin resistant diabetes mellitus in Alström syndrome: a long-term prospective follow-up of three siblings. Diabetes Research and Clinical Practice. *Vol. 56, No. 3 (June* 2002), pp. 189–196.

Sebag J, Albert DM & Craft JL (1984): The Alström syndrome: ophthalmic histopathology and renal ultrastructure. *British Journal of Ophthalmology* Vol. 68 No. 7, (July 1984) pp. 494-501.

Sinha, S.K., Bhangoo, A., Anhalt, H., Maclaren, N., Marshall, J.D., Collin, G.B., Naggert, J.K. & Ten, S. (2007). Effect of metformin and rosiglitazone in a prepubertal boy with Alström syndrome. *Journal of Pediatric Endocrinology & Metabolism*, Vol. 21, No. 1 (September 2007), pp. 1045-1052.

Smith, J.C., McDonnell, B., Retallick, C., McEniery, C., Carey, C., Davies, J.S., Barrett, T., Cockcroft, J.R. & Paisey, R (2007). Is arterial stiffening in Alström syndrome linked to the development of cardiomyopathy? *European Journal of Clinical Investigation.* Vol. 37, No. 2, (February 2007), pp. 99-105.

Tai, T.S., Lin, S.Y. & Sheu, W.H.H. (2003). Metabolic Effects of Growth Hormone Therapy in an Alström Syndrome Patient. *Hormone Research.* Vol. 60, No. 6, pp. 297-301.

Titomanlio, L., De Brasi, D., Buoninconti, A., Sperandeo, M.P., Pepe, A. & Andria, G. (2004). Alström syndrome: intrafamilial phenotypic variability in sibs with a novel nonsense mutation of the ALMS1 gene. *Clinical Genetics 2004.* Vol. 65, No. 2 (February 2004), pp. 156-157.

Tiwari, A., Awasthi, D., Tayal, S. & Ganguly, S, (2010). Alström syndrome: A rare genetic disorder and its anaesthetic significance. *Indian Journal of Anesthesiology.* Vol. 54, No. 2 (March 2010), pp. 154-156.

Van den Abeele, K., Craen, M., Schuil, J. & Meire, F.M. (2001). Ophthalmologic and systemic features of the Alström syndrome: report of 9 cases. *Bulletin de la Société Belge d'Ophtalmologie.* Vol. 281 (2001), pp. 67–72.

Vingolo, E.M., Salvatore, S., Grenga, P.L., Maffei, P., Milan, G. & Marshall J (2010). High-resolution spectral domain optical coherence tomography images of alström syndrome. *Journal pediatric ophthalmology strabismus* Vol. 47: e1-e3 (May 2010)Welsh, L. W. Alström Syndrome: Progressive Deafness and Blindness (2007). *The Annals of Otology, Rhinology & Laryngology.* Vol. 116, Vol. 4 (April 2007), pp. 281-285.

Worthley, M.I. & Zeitz, C.J. (2001). Case of Alström syndrome with late presentation dilated cardiomyopathy. *Internal Medicine Journal.* Vol. 31, No. 9 (December 2001), pp. 569-570.

Wu, W.C., Chen, S.C., Dia, C.Y., Yu, M.L., Hsieh, M.Y., Lin, Z.Y., Wang, L.Y., Tsai, J.F. & Chang, W.Y. (2002). Alström Syndrome with Acute Pancreatitis: A Case Report. *The Kaohsiung Journal of Medical Sciences.* Vol. 19, No. 7 (July 2003), pp. 358-360.

Zubrow, M.E., Makaryus, A., Marshall, J.D., Horowitz, S., Gillam, L.D. & Mangion, J.R. (2006). Echocardiographic Features of the Cardiomyopathy Associated With Alström Syndrome: A Retrospective Review. *American Society for Echocardiology Scientific Sessions*, Baltimore, MD, June, 2006.

11

Alpha One Antitrypsin Deficiency: A Pulmonary Genetic Disorder

Michael Sjoding and D. Kyle Hogarth
University of Chicago
U.S.A

1. Introduction

Alpha one antitrypsin protein (A1AT), is encoded on the SERPINA1 (serpin peptidase inhibitor, claude A, member 1 gene), (OMIM 107400), located on chromosome 14q32.1 and functions as inhibitor of the enzyme neutrophil elastase. People with a low serum level of this protein are described as having the alpha-1-antrypsin deficiency (A1ATD), (OMIM #613490), one of the most common heritable disorders. Having this disorder can predispose an individual to a variety of clinical diseases, with the lungs and the liver being the two organs most commonly affected. The A1AT protein is synthesized mainly in the liver by hepatocytes, secreted into the blood stream, and acts as an inhibitor of neutrophil elastase released primarily in the lung during inflammation. The most common allele for the SERPINA1 gene is named M (Middle), which encodes a normal A1AT protein identified in the middle on an isoelectric focusing gel. Over 120 allelic variants have been discovered and are named based on their position and movement on isoelectric gels, A-L if they exhibit faster migration than M, and N-Z if the proteins migrate more slowly. Rare mutations are often named after the discoverer or location of discover (Mmalton, Lowell, etc). A patient's genotype is notated as PI*Allele-Allele, and so patient homozygous for the wild-type A1AT protein is noted as being PI*M-M.

The most common allelic variation causing clinical disease is the Z protein, manifesting most often in the setting of the genotype PI*Z-Z. This mutated protein spontaneously misfolds and then polymerizes with other misfolded A1AT proteins, becoming trapped in large quantities in the endoplasmic reticulum of liver hepatocytes. This results in liver inflammation and fibrosis, and can lead to clinically significant cholestasis and cirrhosis. Not all allelic variants of A1ATD cause liver damage, however, as some encode truncated proteins which do not misfold or polymerize. Rare null mutations have also been discovered due to point mutations that introduce a premature stop codon within the DNA sequence. Patients with the genotype PI*Null-Null do not develop liver disease because they do not synthesize mutated protein, but are at extremely high risk for the development of lung disease because of their inability to inhibit neutrophil elastase.

In the case of the Z allele, the trapped protein is ineffectively secreted into the blood stream, resulting in a low serum concentration of A1AT. The mutated protein also has a reduced functional activity, making it a less effective inhibitor of neutrophil elastase. Without an appropriate level of functional A1AT in lung tissue, neutrophil elastase is free to break down elastin, a critical component of lung structure, which is thought to be the major

mechanism leading to lung damage and the development of emphysema. The lung injury is worsened in the setting of chronic tobacco use, making smoking cessation paramount in the management of people with the deficiency.
Clinical disease associated with the A1AT deficiency is highly variable, suggesting that many genetic modifiers and environmental exposures play a role in the disease expression. The typical symptoms of pulmonary disease include exertional shortness of breath, wheezing, and chronic cough. The cornerstone of disease management is ensuring total smoking abstinence in all patients, as smoking is associated with a much higher rate of decline in lung function in patients with A1AT deficiency. Replacement therapy with purified A1AT protein given intravenously has been approved in several countries as treatment of the deficiency state, and can prevent decline in lung function. Though many studies support its use and clinical benefit, true randomized placebo controlled studies have been limited in size and scope.

2. History of the disorder

In 1962 at the University of Lund, Sweden, Dr. Carl-Bertil Laurell (1919-2001) was examining the serum protein electrophoresis strips of patients with chronic obstructive pulmonary disease, when he noted an absence of the alpha-one band in a small group of patients. Dr. Sten Eriksson was a resident at the University hospital at the time and assisted Laurell in the study because of his previous experience with protein chemistry. Together, they discovered five cases that formed the basis of their first report of alpha one- antitrypsin deficiency. Three of the five patients in their report developed emphysema at an early age, leading to the conclusion that there must be an association between pulmonary disease and the alpha-one band deficiency (Laurell & Eriksson 1963).
It was later discovered that the major function of the alpha 1-antitrypsin protein was to inhibit the enzyme neutrophil elastase, a protease released by neutrophils in the lungs during inflammation. Neutrophil elastase was shown to induce experimental emphysema in animals. (Senior, et al. 1977). These findings lead to the first hypothesis describing the pathogenesis of lung disease, that an imbalance of proteases and anti-proteases could result in an unregulated destruction of critical components of lung structure, namely elastin, leading to the development of clinical lung disease. This hypothesis continues to be central to the understanding of lung disease pathogenesis to this day, and helps explain why patient deficient in A1AT, which could not regulate neutrophil elastase, would be predisposed to emphysema development.
Work by Dr. H. L. Sharp described the association between alpha one antitrypsin deficiency and liver disease in 10 children in 1969 (Sharp et al., 1969). Sharp discovered intracellular inclusions in the liver hepatocytes of A1ATD individuals, and further work found these inclusions to be polymers of the mutant Z allele of the A1AT protein. Evidence for A1ATD was also supported from the results of a large epidemiologic study published in 1976 by Sveger in Sweden (Sveger, 1976). After screening 200,000 infants for A1ATD he identified 127 infants and found that 14 developed cholestatic jaundice in infancy. These studies established the role of A1AT in liver disease pathogenesis.

3. Genetics

Alpha-1-antitrypsin deficiency has been described as an autosomal co-dominant disorder or as an autosomal recessive disorder. Patients who are heterozygote for the enzyme deficiency have roughly half the serum concentration of A1AT compared with normal individuals, and homozygote have a very low serum concentration of enzyme. This pattern of enzyme levels has lead many authors to describe the inheritance pattern as autosomal co-dominant, (see DeMeo's review on the genetics of A1ATD as one example (DeMeo & Silverman, 2004)). Heterozygotes have only a small increased risk for developing clinically significant disease, while homozygotes are at a much higher risk for developing disease, leading other authors to describe the deficiency as having autosomal recessive inheritance (see Alpha-1 antitrypsin deficiency page on the National Center for Biotechnology Information website as an example). We prefer to describe the inheritance pattern as autosomal co-dominant, as this highlights the fact that heterozygotes for the deficiency are at an increased risk for clinical disease when compared with the general population, especially in the setting of external risk factors for lung disease (e.g. smoking). Another important characteristic of the deficiency is its variable clinical expressivity. Some homozygotes for the deficiency do not develop impairment in the lung function and never develop symptoms related to the disease (Seersholm & Kok-Jensen 1998). Incomplete penetrance and variable clinical phenotype (expressivity) is one of the reasons why population studies estimating the number of individuals with the deficiency are much higher than the actual number of people who have been diagnosed. For unclear reasons, A1ATD is rarely tested for despite guidelines that recommend otherwise for clear patient types. Complicating A1ATD diagnosis is the continued low rate of diagnosis and management of Chronic Obstructive Pulmonary Disease (COPD).

More than 120 mutations in the SERPINA1 gene have been identified, although many do not cause a defect in the serum protein or function or relevant clinical disease (US National Library of Medicine August 2009). The allele most common to the general population is the M allele, and the most clinically relevant variants are the S and Z alleles. People with the PI*Z-Z genotype make up at least 95% of deficient individuals who present with clinical disease, and PI*M-Z heterozygotes on very rare occasion have any symptoms. The Z allele is caused by a glutamic acid to lysine substitution at position 342. A more common allelic variant is the S protein, caused by a glutamic acid to valine substitution at position 264. This protein is successfully degraded before accumulating in the liver and does not cause liver disease. PI*S-S individuals are not thought to be at risk for pulmonary disease, however the compound heterozygotes PI*S-Z or PI*S-null are at an increased risk for developing pulmonary symptoms. Null alleles are due to mutations that introduce an early stop codon, which prevents complete transcription of the gene. Patients who are homozygote for the null mutation (PI*null-null), or heterozygote with Z (PI*null-Z) are at the highest risk for developing severe pulmonary symptoms (Stoller & Aboussouan, 2005).

The Z allele occurs mainly within one haplotype, meaning that other genetic material surrounding the allele is similar, and suggests a single relatively recent origin in Caucasians (Cox et al., 1985). Its high frequency in southern Scandinavia and estimated origination date of approximately 2000 years ago suggests that the mutation originated in the Viking population and was spread across Europe by Viking raiders. Using the pooled epidemiological data on 75,390 individuals, researchers estimated the prevalence of both the Z and S mutation in 21 countries. With this information, they created a topographic map of the mutation prevalence, depicting how the mutation may have spread. The ZZ phenotype shows highest prevalence in the southern Scandinavian Peninsula, Latvia, and Denmark, and progressively decreases towards the South and the East of Europe. The S allele has its highest prevalence in the Iberian Peninsula, which includes modern day Portugal, and Spain, as well as Southern France and gradually decreases towards the North, South and

East of the continent. The S mutation appears to have originated within the Portuguese population, but its date of origin is unknown. It is assumed that both mutations were introduced to North America by mass migration.

Most Common Phenotypes and likely Pulmonary Consequences of A1AT alleles

Allele	Concentration of A1AT (micromoles/L)	COPD risk
Pi-MM	20-53	General population
Pi-MS	20-48	Very low/gen population
Pi-SS	15-33	Low
Pi-MZ	12-35	Low
Pi-SZ	9-19	Variable
Pi-ZZ	2.5-7	High
Pi-Z-null	<2.5	Very high
Pi-null-null	none	Very high

Fig. 1. Common alleles of the SERPINA1 gene (adapted from Hogarth & Rachelefsky, 2008)

4. Epidemiology

There is an estimated 1.1 million people with severe A1ATD and 116 million carriers in the world (Luisetti & Seersholm, 2004). Although previously consider a disease of Caucasians, recent data shows that A1ATD exists in all racial subgroups worldwide including African blacks, Arabs and Jews in the Middle East, as well as people from central, far east and south east Asia (de Serres, 2002). Determining the number of people in the United States with emphysema primarily due to A1ATD can made by taking the estimate of the number of Americans with COPD (3.1 million), and the estimate that about 1.9% of patients with emphysema are likely due to A1ATD (Lieberman et al., 1986). This results in an estimate that at least 59000 individuals in the United States have severe symptomatic COPD due to A1ATD. Large screening studies have also been undertaken, including the classic prevalence study done by Sveger, where 200,000 neonates were screened at birth in Sweden (Sveger 1974). The results demonstrated 1 in 1575 live births were homozygous for the Z mutation (PI*ZZ). A similar study undertaken in Oregon, USA screened 107,038 newborns and found the prevalence of the ZZ phenotype in that population to be 1 in 5097 (O'Brien et al., 1978). Among 20,000 healthy blood donors tested in St. Louis, Missouri in the United States, 1 in 2857 were homozygous for the Z mutation. With this information, the researchers estimated a total prevalence of 700 individuals in St. Louis with the deficiency, however they were only to locate 28 (4%) after contacting local doctors (Silverman, et al., 1989). Estimates from Central and Southern Africa based on limited data from screening studies estimated that 1 in 15 Africans are S carriers. Our own data on carrier rate in Americans of African Descent demonstrate 1 in 18 are S carriers. Epidemiologic data not only highlight that prevalence of the deficiency is high, but reinforce that the disease is significantly under diagnosed in most populations.

5. Pathophysiology

The SERPINA1 gene, previously known as the PI (proteasome inhibitor) gene, is located between 14q31.1-32.3 on the human genome, and encodes A1AT, which is a 52-kD glycoprotein composed of 394 amino acids. The active site is a single peptide bond, Met358-

Ser359. The protein is primarily synthesized and secreted by hepatocytes, but also in mononuclear cells, intestinal and lung epithelial cells. A1AT is an acute phase reactant with a normal concentration in serum of 20-53 micromole/L. Alpha one antitrypsin is a member of the serpin family of protease inhibitors, which regulate important proteolytic enzyme cascades including the coagulation cascade, complement cascade, and plasmin inhibition (Crowther et al., 2004). Serpins not only inhibit proteases but cause a conformational change in their structure readying them for destruction. A1AT's mechanism of inhibition has been likened to a mouse-trap. When neutrophil elastase attacks A1AT enzyme, it binds and then cleaves its reactive center loop, which causes a spring-like movement within the A1AT molecule to fling the elastase molecule across itself, inhibiting its function and altering its structure so it can be destroyed (Huntington et al., 2000).

5.1 Pulmonary pathophysiology

The prevailing theory describing the pathogenesis of emphysema in A1AT deficient individuals is of an imbalance in protease and anti-protease enzymes in lung tissue. Neutrophil elastase is released during inflammation and leads to an uncontrolled proteolytic attack on elastin, which is left unchecked by the low concentration of alpha one antitrypsin (Gadek et al., 1981). Furthermore, the circulating Z allele of A1AT has been shown to have a less functional active site, making the small amount of mutant protein a functionally ineffective inhibitor of neutrophil elastase (Ogushi et al., 1987). Elastin is the backbone of lung structure, and a critical component of the lungs ability to recoil. It is thought that elastin's destruction leads to lung hyperinflation and obstruction, leading to development of emphysema.

More recently, studies have shown that the mutated protein can form polymers within the lungs, similar to the polymerization occurring in the liver, and become chemoattractants for neutrophils resulting in excessive inflammation. Polymers of the mutated A1AT protein have been identified in the bronchial alveolar lavage fluid of individuals with the PiZZ phenotype (Mulgrew et al., 2004). These findings have lead to a possible evolutionary explanation for why alpha-one anti-trypsin deficiency became so prevalent in many populations. The argument for the selective advantage of being a carrier is that a less regulated pulmonary inflammatory response to an external noxious stimulus (e.g. infection) would lead to higher chances of recovery. Prior to the discovery of antibiotics for respiratory infections, the mortality rate from these illnesses was high. A more robust and unregulated inflammatory response in the lungs could have provided a survival advantage to the carriers (Lomas, 2006). In the modern antibiotic era, and the advent of mass-produced external noxious stimuli (smoking, pollution), this mutation does not appear to have a theoretical selective advantage anymore.

How cigarette smoke accelerates the decline of lung function in A1ATD has also been studied. When the methionine amino acid in the active site of A1AT protein is oxidized by cigarette smoke, the kinetics of neutrophil elastase inhibition is reduced (Ogushi et al., 1991). Newer experimental data shows A1AT may have other roles in the lung epithelium besides inhibiting neutrophil elastase. A1AT has recently been found to block the cigarette smoke mediated release of TNF-alpha and MMP-12 in alveolar macrophages (Churg at al., 2007). In cellular studies, A1AT has also been found to inhibit apoptosis through direct inhibition of activated Caspase-3 (Petrache et al., 2006). The link between A1AT and apoptosis has lead to new theories of emphysema development as both an inflammatory disorder and accelerated lung aging process.

5.2 Liver pathophysiology

People with the alpha one antitrypsin deficiency develop liver damage by a completely different mechanism. After being synthesized in hepatocytes, the mutated A1AT alleles bind together to form large polymers that result in inflammation and fibrosis. Liver disease caused by A1ATD has become the prototypical disease in a new category of diseases, termed the conformational diseases. Also included in this category of diseases are Alzheimer's and other forms of neurodegenerative dementias, which are caused by the aggregation of proteins in neurons (Carrell & Lomas, 2002). People with the PI*ZZ mutation of A1AT have a high concentration of the mutated alpha-one antitrypsin allele in the endoplasmic reticulum of liver cells. The Z mutation allows the protein to undergo a spontaneous structural change, which opens up the main sheets of the molecule and bind to the reactive center in the next molecule. These interactions can result in the formation of long polymers of mutated proteins (Lomas et al., 1992). The large protein structures aggregate in liver cells, which is thought to lead to inflammation, fibrosis and cirrhosis by a still unclear mechanism. The reason why some people with ZZ allele genotype do not develop clinically relevant liver disease is also not clear.

6. Clinical manifestations

A1ATD is often unrecognized despite the high prevalence of lung disease in the United States and the world. Alpha-1-related lung disease presents with common respiratory symptoms including dyspnea, decreased exercise tolerance, wheezing, cough, excess sputum production, frequent lower respiratory tract infections, and a history of suspected allergies and/or asthma (Needham & Stockley, 2004). These symptoms are often ascribed to other diseases for years prior to the correct diagnosis of alpha one antitrypsin deficiency. A 1994 mail survey found that on average it took 7.2 years after symptom onset before the diagnosis was made, and 44% of people saw three different physicians before a diagnosis was made (Stoller et al., 1994). A similar survey repeated in 2003 found the mean time to diagnosis was 5.6 years, however, the delay was more pronounced in older and female patients (Stoller et al., 2005). Since the diagnosis of A1ATD requires one simple blood test, clearly more effort needs to be made to educate both physicians and the public of the disease and the importance of a diagnosis.

There is significant variability in the age of symptom onset in people with A1ATD, and some smokers and non-smokers may never develop symptoms. This highlights the variability in disease penetrance among deficient individuals, and makes accurate descriptions of the common symptoms and other clinical characteristics of deficient individuals difficult to obtain. Most of the clinical characteristics and other features of the deficiency are obtained by studying large registries of patients with the disease. These data sets are often flawed by ascertainment bias. Most of the patients in the large A1ATD registries presented initially to a doctor with concerning pulmonary symptoms, eventually leading to a diagnosis of A1ATD. These patients are then referred to a specialist who will enroll them into the registry, and are termed index cases. Less often, asymptomatic individuals who are diagnosed after a family screening are enrolled (non-index cases). This was true of the large group of 1129 A1AT deficient individuals in the National Heart, Lung and Blood Institute Registry (McElvaney et al., 1997). 72% of the enrollees were index cases, receiving a diagnosis of the A1ATD after developing concerning pulmonary symptoms, and 20% were non-index cases, diagnosed by screening following an investigation of family members of individuals with A1ATD. In that registry, the remaining smaller percentage of people were diagnosed after they were discovered to have abnormal chest radiograph findings, abnormal pulmonary function tests, liver abnormalities, or other blood testing. therapy with the purified A1AT protein.

6.1 Pulmonary clinical manifestations

The NHLBI registry data provides the best clinical picture of the typical patients diagnosed with this deficiency. 97% of them had the PI*ZZ mutation, and most were diagnosed in the third or fourth decade of life. The most common symptom in this group was shortness of breath on exertion (83%). Other common symptoms included wheezing during an upper respiratory illness (75%), wheezing without upper respiratory illness (65%), recent lung infection (67%), and chronic productive cough (49%).

Pulmonary function testing of individuals in the NHLBI registry demonstrated a pattern consistent with emphysema: the median Forced Expiratory Volume in one second (FEV1) was 47% of predicted, the ratio of the FEV1/FVC (Forced Vital Capacity) was 43% of predicted, and the DLCO (which represents the amount of destruction in alveoli-capillary units) was 50% of predicted. These numbers highlight a common feature of people with A1ATD: the airflow obstruction (represented by low FEV1 and low FEV1/FVC) seen on pulmonary function testing seems to be out of proportion to the lifetime quantity of cigarettes they have smoked. Also in the NHLBI registry, 28% of people showed significant bronchodilator responsiveness (i.e., reversibility) of their airflow obstruction on pulmonary function tests during their initial visit, which is a characteristic of people with asthma (Eden et al., 2003). With these common symptoms and pulmonary function test characteristics, it is easy to see why patients with A1ATD are often misdiagnosed as having only uncomplicated asthma, emphysema or COPD.

In contrast to the above registry data, a study with high level of non-index cases (e.g. siblings of affected individuals) found that far fewer of this population had typical pulmonary symptoms of A1ATD (Seersholm & Kok-Jensen, 1998). After a mean follow-up of 8 years, only 46% of the non-index case patients reported symptoms of shortness of breath, 27% reported wheezing, and 14% reported a chronic cough. Also in this group, their average FEV1 was 100% of predicted, and their FEV1/FVC = 0.79, essentially normal pulmonary function tests.

Classically, severe A1ATD causes panlobar emphysema with lower lobe predominance on radiologic imagining studies (Guenter et al., 1968). However, with high-resolution chest CT scanning, bronchiectasis has also been found to be a common feature of patients with A1ATD. In a study of 74 people with the P*ZZ phenotype, 70 subjects had bronchiectasis changes on CT scan. 27% of the study participates were felt to have clinically significant bronchiectasis, which was described as 4 or more airway segments with bronchiectasis plus symptoms of regular sputum production (the most common symptom of people with bronchiectasis) (Parr et al., 2007).

Multiple studies have measured the rate of decline in lung function among patients with A1ATD using the forced expiratory volume in one second (FEV1) as a marker of lung disease progression. This measure is used regularly to quantify the severity and progression of patients with COPD and asthma. For non-smokers with normal levels of A1AT, the rate of FEV1 decline is around 20-30 mL/year. The decline in the FEV1 among a group of A1ATD patients who never smoked was 67 mL/year, was 54 mL/year in ex-smokers, and was 109 mL/year in current smokers (Alpha-1-antitrypsin deficiency study group, 1998). The first two numbers are not statistically significantly different, however the third is

significant, which highlights the extreme importance of smoking cessation in all people with A1ATD. The difference in the rate of decline of FEV1 between A1ATD and normal patients highlights the principle of augmentation therapy with replacement alpha-one protein.
Mortality in people with A1ATD is most frequently due to respiratory failure, followed by liver cirrhosis. The observed yearly mortality rate ranges between 1.7-3.5%. Factors associated with increased mortality include older age, lower education, lower FEV1, history of lung transplant, and people who were not receiving augmentation therapy with the purified A1AT protein (Stoller et al., 2005).

6.2 Liver clinical manifestations

A1ATD has a strong association with liver disease, leading to a recommendation that all individuals of any age with unexplained liver dysfunction should undergo testing for the deficiency. In the Swedish population screening study by Sveger, of 200,000 people, 18% of the 120 people found to be homozygote for the Z mutation had some evidence of liver dysfunction (Sveger, 1974). This included obstructive jaundice in 12%, and minor abnormalities in others. Among those with liver dysfunction, the risk of developing cirrhosis is high. It is possible that younger individuals more often have liver dysfunction because their hepatocytes are less well equipped to handle the polymerized A1AT proteins. In a small autopsy series of patients with A1AT disease, cirrhosis was observed in 34% of patients, and hepatocellular carcinoma was observed in 34% of those with cirrhosis (Eriksson, 1987).

6.3 Necrotizing panniculitis

Panniculitis is an uncommon skin disorder with a strong association with A1ATD. It is characterized by painful, cutaneous nodules at the sites of trauma, often on the trunk, back and thighs. On biopsy, areas of fat necrosis are interspersed with areas of normal tissue. The skin necrosis is felt to develop because of unopposed proteolysis, and augmentation therapy has been described as causing a rapid resolution of the disease (Dowd et al., 1995).

7. Testing for disease

Guidelines published by the American Thoracic Society and European Respiratory Society in 2003 have helped clarify who should undergo testing for A1ATD (American Thoracic Society, 2003). The guidelines divided people into categories for whom testing is recommended, those for whom testing could be discussed and considered, and those for whom testing was discouraged. For the following group of people testing should be recommended. These include: adults with emphysema, chronic obstructive pulmonary disease, or asthma with incompletely reversible airflow obstruction, people of all ages with otherwise unexplained liver disease, or adults with necrotizing panniculitis. In the following group of people testing could be considered and discussed: adults with bronchiectasis without an obvious etiology, adults with anti-proteinase 3-positive vasculitis (C-ANCA [anti-neutrophil cytoplasmic antibody]-positive vasculitis, formerly known as "Wegener's Granulomatosis"), adolescents with airflow obstruction on pulmonary function tests.
When family history is considered, the following recommendations were made. There is a strong recommendation for testing all siblings of an individual with A1ATD. There is also a recommendation to consider testing in the following situations: individuals with a family history of emphysema or liver disease, or anyone with a family history of A1ATD or A1ATD heterozygote. The 2003 guidelines recommended against routine population screening except

in the following circumstances - if the prevalence of A1ATD is greater than 1 in 1500 the population, smoking is prevalent, and adequate genetics counseling services are available.
Nephelometry or Rocket Immunodiffusion can measure serum levels of A1AT and is a reasonable screening test for the deficiency. However, this method is subject to errors because the protein is an acute phase reactant and rise with inflammation. The gold standard for diagnosis is "Phenotyping" of the protein is done via isoelectric focus gel analysis, which can only be performed at a few specialized laboratories within the United States. DNA Analysis of genotype is done to probe for the common S and Z genes. A1ATD testing can be done via serum and whole blood draw from the vein, but can also be done via a single finger-stick of blood placed onto a card that is mailed into a central lab for testing. A combination of measuring the serum A1AT concentration and performing a PCR based assay to identify S and Z alleles will accurately identify 96% of individuals as compared to the more difficult gold standard isoelectric focusing (Snyder, 2006).

8. Treatment

The corner stone of alpha one antitrypsin management is smoking cessation and smoke avoidance in all individuals with the deficiency. Guidelines for the management of the chronic airflow obstruction (COPD) have been published elsewhere (GOLD guidelines, ATS guidelines, etc.) Augmentation therapy is utilized to increase serum and lung epithelial lining fluid (ELF) levels of A1AT through the weekly intravenous infusion of purified human A1AT protein (Wewers et al., 1987).
It is FDA approved to treat for adult patients with A1ATD (protein concentration < 11 micromoles/dL) and evidence of air flow obstruction. The treatment can be very costly because it involves life-long regular infusions of a blood product, and it is not available worldwide. The treatment was approved based on two factors, that there is biochemical equivalence between exogenous replacement protein and protein found in normal human serum, and there is normalization of serum protein levels in deficient individuals who are receiving replacement. Many non-randomized prospective studies have demonstrated the effectiveness of augmentation via reduction in the annual rate of decline of lung function. Well-designed and adequately powered randomized trials have been limited to date. A recent meta-analysis of published human studies demonstrated augmentation therapy does reduce the annual rate of lung function decline (as measured by FEV_1) in A1ATD individuals (Chapman et al., 2009).

8.1 Future therapies

Ongoing work in areas of inhaled therapy, longer half-life protein, recombinant forms, small molecule chaperone inhibitors to increase liver secretion and gene transfer therapy continue. These studies and fields are all in various stages of development.

9. Conclusion

Alpha1- antitrypsin deficiency is a not uncommon disease, which is not limited to the European and Caucasian American population, but now affects all ethnic groups. Effective treatments for this disease, including smoking cessation, management of COPD/emphysema and other complications, and augmentation therapy with purified A1AT protein is well established. However, the disease remains under-diagnosed, and many times patients are diagnosed years after symptoms have developed. Future work to improve education among healthcare professionals to improve rates of diagnosis, as well as improved disease specific treatments are important steps in making this disease a more treatable illness.

10. References

Alpha-1-antitrypsin deficiency study group. (1998). Survival and FEV1 decline in individuals with severe deficiency of alpha1-antitrypsin. *Am J Respir Crit Care Med*, Vol. 158, No. 1, (July 1998). pp. 49-59.

American Thoracic Society/European Respiratory Society statement: standards for the diagnosis and management of individuals with alpha-1 antitrypsin deficiency. *Am J Respir Crit Care Med*, Vol. 168, No. 7, (October 2003). pp. 818-900.

Blanco, I., de Serres, FJ., Fernandex-Bustillo, E., Lara, B., & Miravitlles, M. (2006). Estimated numbers and prevalence of PI*S and PI*Z alleles of alpha 1-antitrypsin deficiency in European countries. *Eur Resp J*, Vol. 27, No. 1, (January 2006). pp. 77-84.

Carrell, RW. & Lomas, DA. (2002) Alpha 1-antitrypsin deficiency - a model for conformational disease. *NEJM* Vol. 346, No. 1 (January 2002), pp. 45-53.

Chapman, KR., Stockley, RA., Dawkins, C. Wilkes, MM., Navickis, RJ. (2009). Augmentation therapy for alpha1-antitrypsin deficiency: a meta analysis. *COPD*, Vol. 6, No. 3, (June 2009). pp. 177-18

Churg, A., Wang, X., Wang, RD., Meixner, SC. Pryzdial, EL., & Wright, JL. (2007) Alpha1-antitrypsin suppresses TNF-alpha and MMP-12 production by cigarette smoke-stimulated macrophages. *Am J Resp Cell Mol Bio*, Vol. 37, No. 2 (August 2007), pp. 144-151

Cox, DW., Woo, SL., & Mansfield, T. (1985). DNA restriction fragments associated with alpha 1-antitrypsin indicate a single origin for deficiency allele PI Z. *Nature*, Vol. 316, No. 6023, (July 1985). pp. 79-81

Crowther, DC., Belorgery, D., Miranda, E., Kinghorn, KJ., Sharp, LK., & Lomas, DA. (2004) Practical genetics: alpha1-antitrypsin deficiency and the serpinopathies. *Eur J of Human Gen*, Vol. 12, No. 3 (March 2004). pp. 167-172

de Serres, FJ. (2002). Worldwide racial and ethinic distribution of alpha1-antitrypsin deficiency. *Chest*, Vol. 122, No. 5 (November 2002). pp. 1818-1829.

DeMeo, DL, & Silverman, EK. (2004). Alpha1-Antitrypsin deficiency - 2: Genetic aspects of of alpha1-antitrypsin deficiency: phenotypes and genetic modifiers of emphysema risk. *Thorax*, Vol. 59, No. 3, (March 2004). pp. 259-264

Dowd, SK., Rodgers, GC., & Callen, JP. (1995). Effective treatment with alpha-protease inhibitor of chronic cutaneous vasculitis associated with alpha1-antitrypsin deficiency. *J Am Acad Dermatol*, Vol. 33, No. 5 pt 2, (November 1995). pp. 913-916.

Eden, E., Hammel, J., Rouhani, FN., Brantly, ML., Barker, AF., Buist, AS., Fallat, RJ., Stoller, JK., Crystal, RG., & Turino, GM. (2003). Asthma features in severe alpha1 antitrypsin deficiency: experience of the National heart , Lung, and Blood Institute Resistry. *Chest*, Vol. 123, No. 3, (March 2003). pp. 765-771.

Eriksson, S. (1987). Alpha 1-antitrypsin deficiecny and liver cirrhosis in adults: an analysis of 35 Swedish autopsied cases. *Act Med Scand*, Vol. 221, No. 5, pp. 461-67

Gadek, JE., Fells, GA., Zimmeran, RL. Rennard, SI., & Crystal, RG. (1981). Anti-elastase of the human alveolar structures: implications for the protease-antiprotease theory of emphysema. *J Clin Invest*, Vol. 68, No. 4 (October 1981), pp.889-898

Guenter, CA., Welch, MH., Russell TR, Hyde, RM., & Hammarsten, JF. (1968). The pattern of lung disease associated with alpha1-antitrypsin deficiency. *Arch Int Med*, Vol. 122, No. 3 (September 1968). pp. 254-257

Hogarth, KD., & Rachelefsky, G. (2008). Screening and Familial Testing of Patients for Alpha1 Antitrypsin Deficiency. *Chest*, Vol. 133, No. 4 (April 2008). pp. 981-988

Huntington, JA., Read, RJ., Carrell RW. (2000). Structure of a serpin-protease complex shows inhibition by deformation. *Nature*, Vol. 407, No. 6806 (October 2000). pp. 923-926

Laurell, CV., & Eriksson A. (1963) The electrophoretic alpha 1-globulin pattern of serum in alpha 1-antitrypsin deficiency. *Scandinavian Journal of Clinical Laboratory Investigation*, Vol. 15, pp. 132-40

Lieberman, J., Winter, B., & Sastre, A. (1986). Alpha1-antitrypsin Pi-types in 965 COPD patients. *Chest*, Vol. 89, No. 3 (March 1986). pp. 370-73.

Lomas, DA. (2006). The selective advantage of alpha 1-antitrypsin deficiency. *Am J Respir Crit Care Med*, Vol. 173, No. 10 (May 2006), pp. 1072-1077

Lomas, DA., Evans, DL., Finch, JT., & Carrell, RW. (1992). The mechanism of Z alpha1-antitrypsin accumulation in the liver. *Nature*, Vol. 357, No. 6379, (June 1992), pp. 605-607.

Luisetti, M., & Seersholm, N. (2004). Alpha1 antitrypsin deficiency: 1. Epidemiology of alpha1 antitrypsin deficiency. *Thorax*, Vol. 59, No. 2, (Febuary 2004). pp. 164-169.

McElvaney, NG., Stoller, JK., Buist, AS., Prakash, UB., Brantly, ML., Schluchter, MD., & Crystal, RD. (1997). Baseline Characteristics of Enrollees in the National Heart, Lung and Blood Institute Registry of Alpha-1 Antitripysin Deficiency. *Chest*, Vol. 111, No. 2, (Febuary 1997). pp. 394-403.

Mulgrew, AT., Taggart, CC., Lawless, MW., Greene, CM., Brantly, ML., O'Neill, SJ., McElvaney, NG. (2004). Z alpha1-antitrypsin polymerizes in the lung and acts as a neutrophil chemoattractant. *Chest*, Vol. 125, No. 5 (May 2004), pp. 1952-57

Needham, M. & Stockley, RA. (2004). Alpha1-antitrypsin deficiency - 3: clinical manifestations and natural history. *Thorax*, Vol. 59, No. 5, (May 2004), pp. 441-445

O'Brien, ML., Buist, NR., & Murphey (1978), WH. Neonatal screening for alpha 1-antitrypsin deficiency. *J Pediatr*, Vol. 92, No. 6 (June 1978). pp. 1006-1010.

Ogushi, F., Fells, GA., Hubbard, RC., Straus, SD., & Crystal, RG. (1987). Z-type alpha1-antitrypsin is less competent than M1-type alpha1-proteinase inhibitor as an inhibitor of neutrophil elastase. *J Clin Invest*, Vol. 80, No. 5 (November 1987), pp.1366-1374

Ogushi, F., Hubbard, RC., Vogelmeier, C., Fells, GA., & Crystal, RG. (1991) Risk factors for emphysema. Cigarette smoking is associated with a reduction in the association rate constant of alpha1 antitrypsin for neutrophil elastase. *J Clin Invest*, Vol. 87, No. 3 (March 1991), pp. 1060-1065.

Online Mendelian Inheritance in Man (July 2010). "MIM ID #613490: Alpha-1-Antitrypsin Deficiency. Available from http://www.ncbi.nlm.nih.gov/omim/613490, created 7/20/2010, accessed 3/14/2011

Online Mendelian Inheritance in Man (September 2010). MIM ID *107400: Serpin Peptidase Inhibitor, Clade A, Member 1; Serpina1. 3.14.2011. Available from http://www.ncbi.nlm.nih.gov/omim/613490. Accessed 3/14/2011

Parr, DG., Guest, PG., Reynolds, JH. Dowson, LJ. & Stockley, RA. (2007). Prevalence and Impact of Bronchiectasis in alpha 1-antitrypsin deficiency. *Am J Respir Crit Care Med*, Vol. 176, No. 12, (December 2007). pp. 1215-1221.

Petrache, I., Fijalkowska, I., Medler, TR., Skirball, J., Cruz, P., Zhen, L., Petrache, HI., Flotte, TR., & Tuder, RM. (2008). Alpha1-anti-trypsin Inhibits Caspase-3 Activity, Preventing Lung Endothelial Cell Apoptosis. *Am J of Path*, Vol. 169, No. 4 (October 2006), pp. 1155-1166.

Seersholm, N. & Kok-Jensen, A. (1998). Clinical features and prognosis of life time non-smokers with severe alpha1 antitrypsin deficiency. *Thorax*, Vol. 53, No. 4 (April 1998). pp. 265-268.

Seersholm, N., & Kok-Jensen A. (1998). Clinical features and prognosis of life time non-smokers with severe alpha1 antitrypsin deficiency. *Thorax*, Vol. 53, No. 4, (April 1998). pp. 265-268.

Senior, RM., Tegner, H., Kuhn, C., Ohlsson, K., Starcher, BC., & Pierce, JA. (1977). The induction of pulmonary emphysema with human leukocyte elastase. *Am Rev Respir Dis*, Vol. 166, No. 3, (September 1977). pp. (469-475)

Sharp, HL., Bridges, RA., Krivit, W., & Freier, ER. (1969). Cirrhosis associated with alpha1-antitrypsin deficiency: a previously unrecognized inherited disorder. *J Lab Clin Med*, Vol. 73, No. 6, (June 1969). pp. 934-939

Silverman, EK., Miletich, JP, Pierce, JA. Sherman, LA., Endicott, SK., Broze, GJ. & Campbell, EJ. (1989). Alpha1-antitrypsin deficiency: high prevalence in the St. Louis area determine by direct population screening. *Am Rev Respir Dis*, Vol. 140, No. 4 (October 1989). pp. 961-66

Snyder, MR., Katzmann, JA., Butz, ML., Wiley, C., Yang, P., Dawson, DB., Halling, KC., Highsmith, WE., & Thibodeau, SN. (2006). Diagnosis of alpha1-antitrypsin deficiency: an algorithm of quantitation, genotyping and phenotyping. *Clin Chem*, Vol. 52, No. 12, (December, 2006). pp. 2236-2242

Stoller, JK., & Aboussouan, LS. (2005). Alpha1-antitrypsin deficiency. *Lancet* , Vol. 365, No. 9478, (June 2005). pp. 2225-2236

Stoller, JK., Sandhaus, RA., Turino, G., Dickson, R., Rodgers, K. & Strange, C. (2005). Delay in diagnosis of alpha 1-antitrypsin deficiency: a continuing problem. *Chest*, Vol. 128, No. 4, (October 2005). pp. 1989-94.

Stoller, JK., Smith, P., Yang, P. & Spray, J. (1994). Physical and social impact of alpha 1-antitrypsin deficiency: results of a mail survey of the readership of a national newsletter. *Cleve Clin J Med*, Vol. 61, No. 6, (Nov-Dec 1994). pp. 461-467.

Stoller, JK., Tomashefski, J., Crystal, RG., Arroliga, A., Strange, C., Killian, DN., Schluchter, MD., & Wiedemann, HP., (2005). Mortality in individuals with severe deficiency of alpha1-antitrypsin. *Chest*, Vol. 127, No. 4, (April 2005). pp. 1196-1204.

Sveger, T. (1976). Liver disease in alpha 1-antitrypsin deficiency detected by screening of 200,000 infants. *N Enl J Med*, Vol. 294, No. 24, (June 1976). pp. 1316-1321

US National Library of Medicine, (August 2009) Genetics Home Reference, "SERPINA1" Available at http:/ghr.nlm.nih.gov/gene/SERPINA1, Accessed 3/14/2011

Wewers, MD., Casolaro, MA., Sellers, SE., Swayze, SC., McPhaul, KM., Wittes, JT., & Crystal, RG. (1987). Replacement therapy for alpha1-antitrypsin deficiency associated with emphysema. *NEJM*, Vol. 316, No. 17, (April 1987). pp. 1055-1062

12

Tangier Disease

Yoshinari Uehara[1], Bo Zhang[2] and Keijiro Saku[1]
[1]*Department of Cardiology, Fukuoka University Faculty of Medicine, Nanakuma, Jonan-ku, Fukuoka*
[2]*Department of Biochemistry, Fukuoka University Faculty of Medicine, Nanakuma, Jonan-ku, Fukuoka*
Japan

1. Introduction

Various clinical and epidemiological studies have demonstrated an inverse association between high-density lipoprotein (HDL) cholesterol and the risk of coronary events (von Eckardstein et al., 2001). However, it remains controversial whether this relationship is causal or only an epiphenomenon of a more general atherogenic disorder. HDL exerts various potential anti-atherogenic properties. For example, HDL particles transport cholesterol from cells of the arterial wall to the liver and steroidogenic organs, in which cholesterol is used for the synthesis of bile acids, lipoproteins, vitamin D, and steroid hormones (von Eckardstein et al., 2001). In contrast, low HDL cholesterol is frequently identified as a component of metabolic syndrome in many populations, i.e., together with overweight or obesity, glucose intolerance or overt diabetes mellitus, hypertriglyceridemia, and hypertension, which by themselves contribute to the pathogenesis of atherosclerosis (Despres and Marette, 1994). The most severe form of familial HDL deficiency is Tangier disease (TD), which is caused by a genetic disorder.

2. HDL metabolism and functions

HDL, isolated by ultracentrifugation, is a lipoprotein with a density in the range 1.063–1.21 g/ml (HDL_2, 1.063–1.125 g/ml; HDL_3, 1.125–1.21 g/ml) (Havel et al., 1955). However, HDL constitutes a heterogeneous group of particles differing in size, density, lipid composition, apolipoprotein content, and electrophoretic mobility. HDL can be separated into two main subfractions based on electrophoretic mobility, namely the major subfraction has the same mobility as alpha HDL, whereas the other subfractions migrate similar to pre-beta HDL. Most HDL particles in human plasma are alpha HDL, and pre-beta HDL represents only 2–14% of all apolipoprotein A-I (apoA-I) (Ishida et al., 1987; Kunitake et al., 1985).
HDL has a very complex metabolism associated with several HDL-related genes and is synthesized via a complex pathway. Although the underlying genetic defects in many cases of primary low HDL cholesterolemia are not clearly understood, mutations in three pivotal genes, namely apoA-I, lecithin:cholesterol acyltransferase, and ATP-binding cassette transporter A1 (ABCA1) are associated with low plasma HDL cholesterol levels (Miller et al., 2003). Some mutations of these genes are also associated with an increased risk of premature coronary artery disease (CAD).

3. Characters of TD

3.1 Clinical manifestations of TD

The most severe form of HDL deficiency is TD, first described by Fredrickson et al. (Fredrickson et al., 1961). The plasma lipid profiles in a typical TD patient (TD case 1) with peripheral neuropathy (Uehara et al., 2008a) and those of her younger brother are shown in Table 1. The biological hallmark of plasma in patients with TD is a deficiency of HDL cholesterol, low levels of low-density lipoprotein (LDL) cholesterol, and moderate hypertriglyceridemia. The concentration of apoA-I in plasma of patients with TD is 3% less than that in healthy subjects. TD is a rare autosomal recessive disorder characterized by the absence or extremely low levels of HDL cholesterol and apoA-I in plasma. Furthermore, cholesteryl esters accumulate in many macrophage-rich tissues including the tonsils, liver, spleen, peripheral nerves, lymph nodes, thymus, and arterial walls. Clinical symptoms in homozygotes include hyperplastic orange-yellow tonsils (Fig. 1), hepatosplenomegaly, corneal opacification, and premature CAD in 50% of cases, as well as relapsing peripheral neuropathy due to cholesteryl ester deposition in macrophages and Schwann cells (Assman et al., 1995; Fredrickson et al., 1961; Hobbs and Rader, 1999).

		Standard value	Tangier disease (Case)	Younger brother of case
Age, gender			50, Female	48, Male
Mutation with ABCA1 gene			homozygote, T940M	homozygote, T940M
Total Cholesterol	(mg/dl)	150-219	66	61
Triglyceride	(mg/dl)	50-149	204	191
HDL Choletserol	(mg/dl)	40-86	< 5	< 5
LDL Cholesterol	(mg/dl)	70-139	27	33
Apolipoprotein A-I	(mg/dl)	119-155	< 5	< 5
Apolipoprotein A-II	(mg/dl)	25.9-35.7	1.9	2
Apolipoprotein B	(mg/dl)	73-109	93	76
Apolipoprotein C-II	(mg/dl)	1.8-4.6	4.3	0.5
Apolipoprotein C-III	(mg/dl)	5.8-10.0	5.9	3.5
Apolipoprotein E	(mg/dl)	2.7-4.3	3.9	2.9
RLP cholesterol	(mg/dl)	< 7.5	3.4	5.5
Phospholipids	(mg/dl)	160-260	85	90
Total Bile Acids	(μmol/L)	< 10.0	38.8	22.0

Table 1. Serum lipid profiles in patient with Tangier disease

3.2 ABCA1 and TD

In 1999, TD was determined to be caused by a defect in the ABCA1 gene (formerly known as ABC1) (Brooks-Wilson et al., 1999; Rust et al., 1999; von Eckardstein et al., 2001) that is located on chromosome 9q31 and is composed of 50 exons spanning a region of approximately 149 kb (Remaley et al., 1999; Santamarina-Fojo et al., 2000). ABCA1 has been identified as a pivotal gene in the regulation of plasma levels of HDL cholesterol and cellular cholesterol homeostasis, which is defective in patients with TD. In these patients and their heterozygous relatives, ABCA1 gene mutations cause gene dose-dependent decreases in plasma levels of HDL cholesterol and in the capacity of skin fibroblasts and monocyte-derived macrophages to release cholesterol in the extracellular presence of apolipoproteins (Bodzioch et al., 1999; Brooks-Wilson et al., 1999; Lawn et al., 1999; Rust et al., 1999; von Eckardstein et al., 2001).

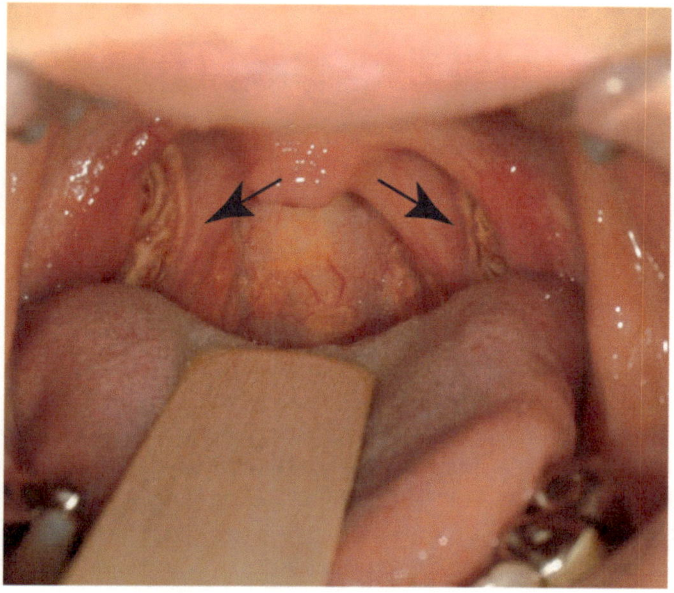

Fig. 1. Photograph of the oral cavity in a patient with Tangier disease reveals swollen orange colored tonsils with yellow lines (arrows). In a genetic sequence analysis, a homozygous missense point mutation was identified at nucleotide 2819 (mRNA position, AB055982) with a C to T mutation in exon 19. Thr940 was substituted by Met940 on the ATP-binding cassette transporter A1 (ABCA1) protein, which was found in the Walker-A motif, as the first nucleotide binding fold of the ABCA1 gene

ABC transporters are transmembrane proteins that facilitate the transport of specific substrates across the membrane in an ATP-dependent manner. ABCA1 is a member of the ABC transporter superfamily, which comprises 48 human transporters; the superfamily is divided into seven subfamilies, including full- or half-transporters, designated ABC A–G. ABC transporters are integral membrane proteins that transport various substrates such as lipids, peptides, amino acids, carbohydrates, vitamins, ions, glucuronides, glutathione conjugates, and xenobiotics to different cellular compartments (Dean and Annilo, 2005; Klein et al., 1999). ABC transporters are defined by the presence of nucleotide binding domains (NBD) that interact with ATP. These domains have two conserved peptide motifs, known as Walker-A and Walker-B, which are present in many proteins that utilize ATP (Walker et al., 1982). The ABC transporters also have a unique amino acid signature between the two Walker motifs that define ABC superfamilies (Klein et al., 1999).

Human ABCA1 belongs to the ABCA subfamily, which is composed of 12 full-transporters denoted ABCA1–13 (with the absence of a functional ABCA11) (Dean et al., 2001). All ABCA transporters are full-size transporters with 1543–5058 amino acids. Structurally, ABCA1 is a 2261 amino acid membrane transporter that is integrated into the membrane via transmembrane domains composed of six transmembrane helices. In addition, ABCA1 has two transmembrane domains and two nucleotide binding domains and is predicted to have an N-terminus oriented to the cytosol with two large extracellular loops (Fig. 2). ABCA1 is expressed in several human organs, with the highest expression levels occurring in the placenta, liver, lung, adrenal glands, and fetal tissues (Langmann et al., 1999).

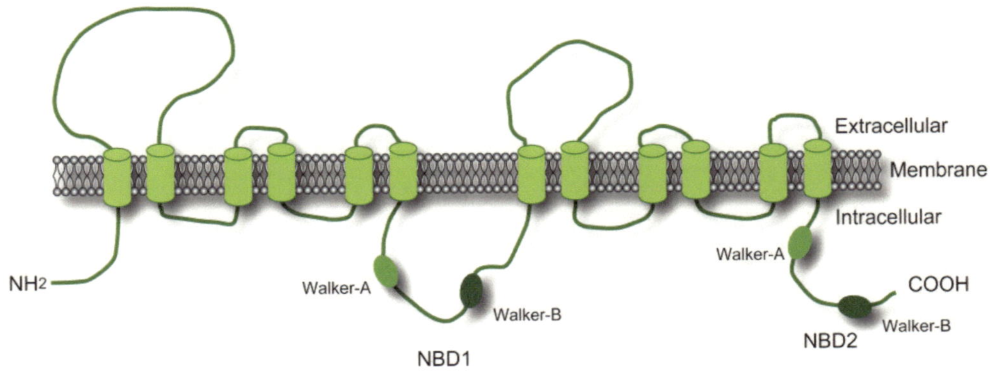

Fig. 2. Structure of the ATP-binding cassette transporter A1 (ABCA1) transporter. The ABCA1 protein consists of 2201 amino acids with two transmembrane domains composed of six transmembrane helices and two nucleotide binding domains (NBD-1 and NBD-2) containing two conserved peptide motifs known as Walker-A and Walker-B. It is predicted to have an N-terminus oriented into the cytosol and two large extracellular loops

4. Roles of ABC transporters in HDL metabolism

4.1 Functions of ABCA1 and its relationship to HDL metabolism

ABCA1 proteins transport cholesterol or phospholipids (PLs) from the membranous inner leaflet to the outer leaflet, and lipid-free or lipid-poor apoA-I subsequently takes up the transported cholesterol and PLs to form nascent HDL (Oram and Lawn, 2001). ABCA1 localizes to the plasma membrane and intracellular compartments, where it could potentially facilitate transport of lipids to either cell surface-bound (Neufeld et al., 2001) or internalized apolipoproteins (von Eckardstein and Rohrer, 2009). HDL metabolism has at least three steps. First, lipid-free or lipid-poor apoA-I removes free cholesterol from peripheral cells via ABCA1 to form nascent HDL. Second, nascent HDL is lipidated to mature HDL. Third, mature HDL interacts with other apoB containing triglyceride-rich lipoproteins (TRLs) such as very low density lipoprotein (VLDL) and intermediate-density lipoprotein (IDL). Therefore, ABCA1 is necessary to form nascent HDL and is an important key molecule in the initial step of the reverse cholesterol transport (RCT) pathway. Cultivated monocyte-derived macrophages from a normolipidemic healthy subject showed an approximately 125% increase in cholesterol efflux of lipid-free apoA-I, whereas macrophages derived from patients with TD did not respond to apoA-I during cholesterol efflux (Fig. 3A). Although cultivated monocyte-derived macrophages showed an increase in cholesterol efflux by lipid-free apoA-I in healthy subjects, the macrophages from patients with TD did not change apoA-I-mediated cholesterol efflux. These results demonstrate that apoA-I-mediated cholesterol efflux depends on ABCA1 in macrophages. Furthermore, ABCA1 plays a pivotal role in mediating PL and cholesterol efflux by lipid-free apoA-I, and thereby, in the formation of discoidal HDL precursors. However, ABCA1 interacts poorly with HDL_2 and HDL_3. Due to a genetic defect in ABCA1, patients with TD have an extremely low level of HDL and cannot form nascent HDL particles.

Disruption of the ABCA1 gene in mice results in an HDL deficiency and impaired cholesterol transport (McNeish et al., 2000; Orso et al., 2000), and overexpression of ABCA1 leads to increased apoA-I-mediated cholesterol efflux in transgenic mice (Singaraja et al., 2001; Vaisman et al., 2001). These results indicate that ABCA1 is a pivotal gene in the regulation of plasma HDL cholesterol and cellular cholesterol homeostasis.

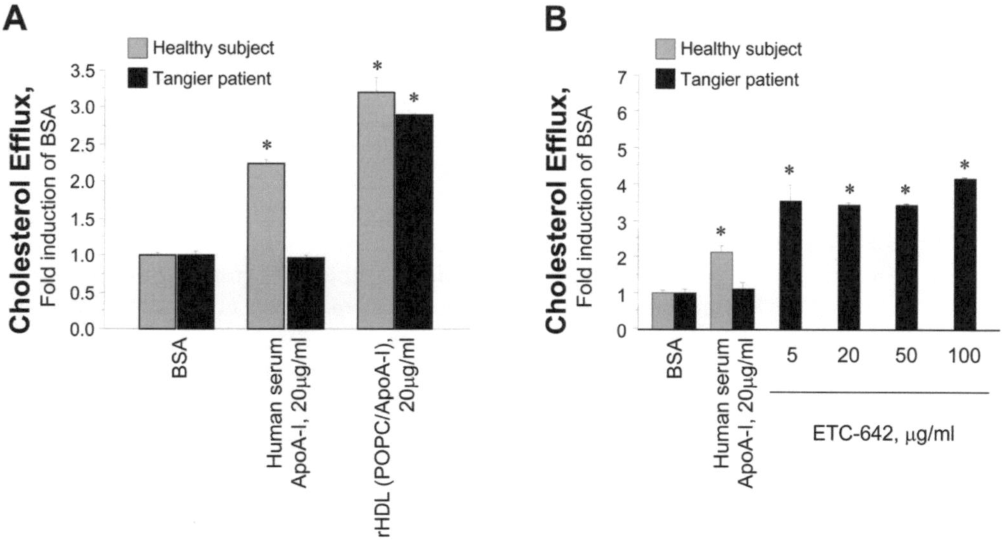

Fig. 3. Cellular cholesterol efflux from monocyte-derived macrophages in the peripheral blood of a patient with Tangier disease (TD). The human monocyte-derived macrophages from a healthy subject and a patient with TD were radiolabeled with ^{3}H-cholesterol. The cells were then equilibrated with 30 μg/ml cholesterol. Cholesterol efflux was induced by 4-h incubation with 20 μg/ml apolipoprotein A-I (apoA-I) and rHDL (POPC/apoA-I disc) (A) or ETC-642 (phospholipid (PL)/apoA-I mimetics) (B) using a previously modified method (Uehara et al.: *Diabetes* 2002;51:2922–8, Uehara et al.: *Atherosclerosis* 2008;197(1):283–9). rHDL, reconstituted HDL (POPC/apoA-I disc); ETC-642, synthetic peptide of 22 amino acids with 1,2-dipalmitoyl-sn-glycero-3-phosphocholine. n = 3–7; *P < 0.001 vs. BSA

4.2 Mechanisms of ABCA1 gene regulation

Cellular cholesterol efflux and ABCA1 expression are upregulated by cholesterol (Langmann et al., 1999; Lawn et al., 1999), oxysterols (Costet et al., 2000), rexinoids (Repa et al., 2000), and cAMP analogs (Bortnick et al., 2000; Lawn et al., 1999). The ABCA1 gene promoter has been analyzed (Costet et al., 2000; Santamarina-Fojo et al., 2000). Ligands of the nuclear transcription factor liver-X-receptors (LXRα and LXRβ) and retinoid-X-receptor alpha (RXRα), i.e., oxysterols and retinoids, respectively, have been identified as enhancers of ABCA1 gene expression (Costet et al., 2000; Oram et al., 2000; Repa et al., 2000; Venkateswaran et al., 2000). LXR and RXR form obligate heterodimers that preferentially bind to response elements within the ABCA1 gene promoter (Santamarina-Fojo et al., 2000; Wang et al., 2001). LXRα/β and RXRα bind to the response element direct repeat 4 (DR4)—two direct hexameric repeats separated by four nucleotides on the ABCA1 promoter that are activated by oxysterols and retinoic acid (Bungert et al., 2001; Willy et al., 1995). Binding of either one or both ligands activates ABCA1 transcription. Treating cells with either an oxysterol or 9-*cis*-retinoic acid induces ABCA1 expression, and their combined treatment has a marked synergistic effect (Schwartz et al., 2000). The activator of peroxisome proliferator activating receptor (PPAR)-α or -γ also enhances ABCA1 transcription in cultivated cells, but this stimulated ABCA1 transcription depends on an indirect effect by PPARs via upregulation of LXR expression. By contrast, the zinc finger protein ZNF202 transcription factor is a major repressor of ABCA1 transcription. Besides these regulatory factors, unsaturated fatty acids, but not saturated fatty acids, markedly inhibit ABCA1-mediated cholesterol efflux from macrophages because they act as antagonists during oxysterol binding to LXR (Uehara et al., 2002; Uehara et al., 2007). In addition to ZNF202 and unsaturated fatty acids, several potent transcription factors such as USF1, USF2, Fra2, and Sp3 are repressors of ABCA1 transcription (Yang et al., 2002).

4.3 Other ABC cholesterol transport proteins

ABCG1 (formerly known as ABC8), another member of the ABC transporter superfamily, has been mapped to chromosome 21q22.3 (Chen et al., 1996; Croop et al., 1997; Dean et al., 2001; Klucken et al., 2000; Savary et al., 1996; Walker et al., 1982). In contrast to ABCA1, ABCG1 is a half-transporter containing only one NBD and a transmembrane domain (Dean et al., 2001; Walker et al., 1982). Therefore, it is thought that ABCG1 requires a dimeric partner to become active. Wang et al. recently reported that ABCG1 and ABCG4 contribute to HDL_2- and HDL_3-dependent cellular cholesterol efflux (Wang et al., 2004) and appear to have an important function related to HDL lipidation (Smith, 2006; Uehara et al., 2008b; Wang et al., 2004).

Administering a high-fat high-cholesterol diet to ABCG1-deficient mice results in massive accumulation of lipids in tissue macrophages, whereas overexpression of human ABCG1 protects murine tissues from dietary fat-induced lipid accumulation (Kennedy et al., 2005). Furthermore, Mauldin et al. have shown that reduced ABCG1 function facilitates foam cell formation in type 2 diabetic mice (Mauldin et al., 2006). Transplantation of ABCG1-deficient ($ABCG1^{-/-}$) bone marrow into LDL receptor-deficient mice produces contrasting effects on atherosclerotic formation (Baldan et al., 2006; Out et al., 2006; Ranalletta et al., 2006). In contrast, a decrease in lesion formation and size has been observed in the absence of macrophage ABCG1 in mice (Baldan et al., 2006; Ranalletta et al., 2006). Total body expression of ABCG1 protects against the development of early atherosclerotic lesions (Out et al., 2007). However, the physiological roles of ABCG1 and its contribution to the progression of atherosclerosis in humans remain unclear. In addition to the nonspecific and passive pathway, mature-HDL particles, which are spherical and transport almost all HDL cholesterol, appear to induce cholesterol efflux via other ABC transporters, such as ABCG1 and ABCG4, rather than ABCA1 (Uehara et al., 2008b; Wang et al., 2004).

5. Lipoprotein profiles in TD measured by capillary isotachophoresis (cITP)

cITP is a newly established technique for characterizing plasma lipoprotein subfractions according to their electric charges. We have previously shown that plasma lipoproteins can be separated into eight fractions consisting of three HDL fractions with fast (fHDL), intermediate (iHDL), and slow (sHDL) electromobility, a fast VLDL fraction (fVLDL), a slow VLDL/IDL fraction (sVLDL),two LDL fractions with fast (fLDL) and slow (sLDL) electromobility, and a minor LDL fraction (mLDL) (Zhang et al., 2005) in normolipidemic (NL) subjects. Figure 4 shows the plasma lipoprotein profiles as characterized by cITP analysis in healthy NL subjects (Fig. 4A) and in two patients with TD (Fig. 4B and C). The plasma lipoprotein profiles have a characteristic lipoprotein pattern in patients with TD, namely their fasting plasma shows an extremely low signal in the three HDL fractions (peaks 1, 2, and 3) (Fig. 4B-a, B-d, C-a, and C-d). Moreover, while the sLDL fraction corresponding to native LDL (peak 7) was extremely reduced, the sVLDL and fLDL fractions corresponding to electronegative LDL (some oxidized LDL, βVLDL, small dense LDL, or modified LDL) were significantly enhanced. Interestingly, peaks 4 and 5, TRLs, were identified in the LDL subfraction of plasma from patients with TD, which is usually detected only in the VLDL/IDL subfraction but not in LDL in NL plasma. These findings indicate that patients with TD not only have a deficiency in HDL particles but also have a characteristic lipid composition for other lipoproteins such as triglyceride-rich LDL.

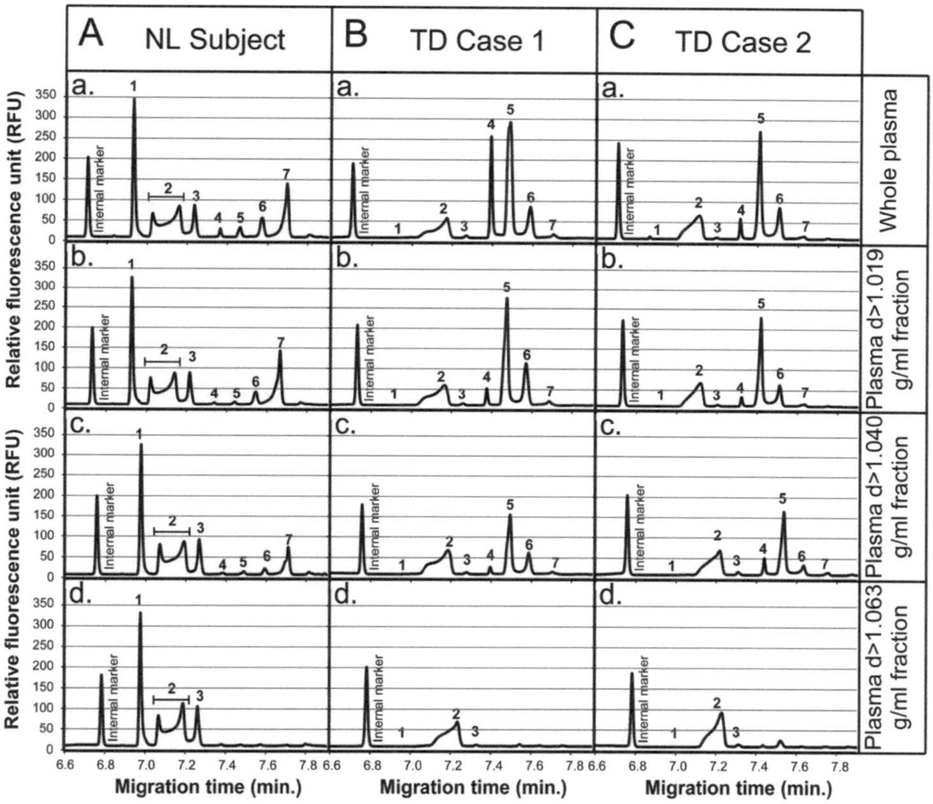

Fig. 4. Lipoprotein subfractions in whole plasma (a) and plasma density (d) > 1.019 g/ml (b), d > 1.040 g/ml (c), and d > 1.063 g/ml (d) fractions by ultracentrifugation in a normolipidemic (NL) subject (A) and two patients with Tangier disease (TD): Case 1, Thr940Met (B) and Case 2, Lys913X (C), as analyzed by capillary isotachophoresis. HDL peaks were not detected in whole plasma (a) or the HDL fraction (d) in patients with TD. Interestingly, peaks 4 and 5, triglyceride-rich lipoproteins (TRLs), were identified in the LDL subfraction of plasma from patients with TD, which was only detected in the VLDL/IDL subfraction but not in LDL in NL plasma. Peaks 1–3: fast-, intermediate-, and slow-migrating HDL; peaks 4 and 5 in a: fast- (fTRL) and slow-migrating (sTRL), respectively; peaks 4 and 5 in b, c: very-very-fast- and very-fast-migrating LDL (vvfLDL and vfLDL), respectively; peaks 6 and 7: fast- and slow-migrating LDL (fLDL and sLDL), respectively

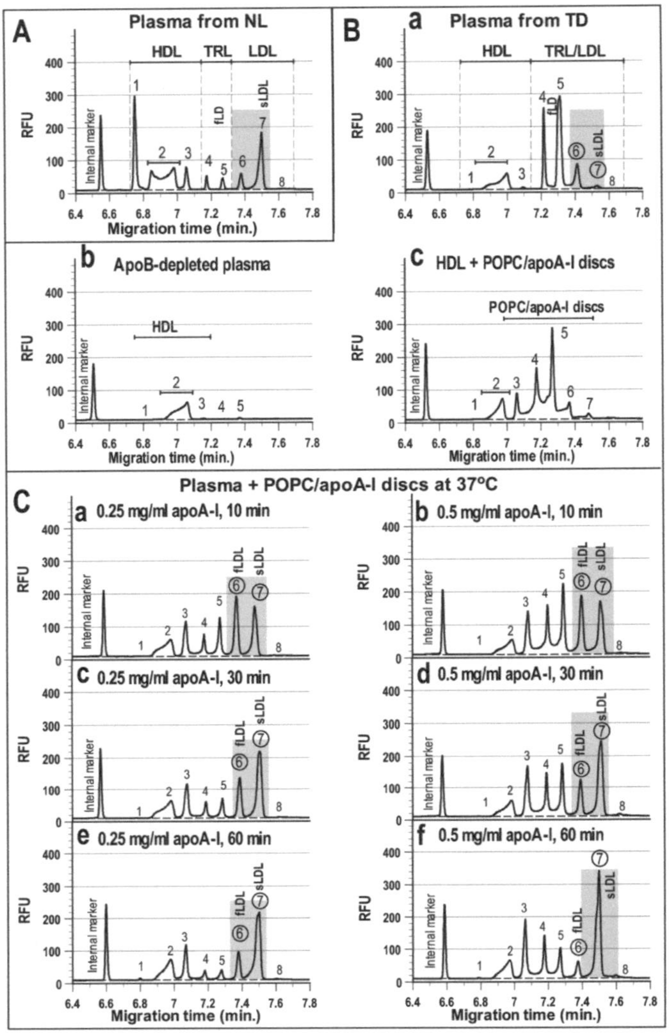

Fig. 5. Effects of 1-palmitoyl-2-oleoylphosphatidylcholine (POPC)/apolipoprotein A-I (apoA-I) discs on lipoprotein profiles in plasma from normolipidemic (NL) subjects (A) and a patient with Tangier disease (TD) (B) as characterized by capillary isotachophoresis (cITP). cITP lipoprotein profiles in apoB-depleted plasma from a patient with TD (B-b). Direct effects of discoidal reconstituted-HDL (rHDL) and the POPC/apoA-I disc (500 µg/ml) on the cITP lipoprotein profile in apoB-depleted plasma from a patient with TD (B-c). Time-dependent effects of rHDL and the POPC/apoA-I disc on the lipoprotein profiles by cITP (C). Lipoprotein profiles in plasma from a patient with TD in the presence (C-a–C-f) of POPC/apoA-I discs as characterized by cITP. Two doses (250 and 500 µg/ml) of POPC/apoA-I discs were incubated *in vitro* with whole plasma at 37°C from a patient with TD. The POPC/apoA-I discs were incubated with plasma for 10 min (C-a and C-b), 30 min (C-c and C-d), or 60 min (C-e and C-f), respectively.
Peaks 1–3, fast (fHDL), intermediate (iHDL), and slow (sHDL) fractions; peaks 4, 5, fast VLDL (fVLDL) and VLDL/IDL (sVLDL) fractions; peaks 6–8, fast (fLDL), slow (sLDL), and minor LDL (mLDL) fractions. TRL, triglyceride-rich lipoprotein

6. Therapeutic approach for HDL deficiency and TD

Although the inhibition of cholesteryl ester transfer protein, PL transfer protein, or scavenger receptor BI and activation of apoA-I or ABCA1 increase HDL cholesterol, the effects of such interventions on atherosclerosis are uncertain in light of studies on animal models and inborn errors of human HDL metabolism. However, no small molecule has been found that strongly stimulates apoA-I production. An LXR agonist is a candidate for increasing HDL cholesterol by increasing ABCA1 expression and HDL cholesterol levels, and RCT also induces hypertriglycemia as a result of the induction of hepatic VLDL production. Substituting or mimicking apoA-I and other potentially anti-atherogenic HDL components has been attempted. Intravenous infusion of an apoA-I variant called apoA-I Milano rapidly decreases atherosclerotic plaque volumes (Nissen et al., 2003). Because TD is a rare genetic disorder, the basic treatment for the disease is still unknown. The development of neuropathy or atherosclerosis in patients with TD is based on a disorder of cellular cholesterol excretion as the initial step of RCT. If the process is able to performed in vitro, it leads to the generation of HDL particle, which can take up the excessive cholesterol from peripheral cell, and it acts as a new therapeutic target without using gene therapy in patients with TD. Reconstituted HDL (rHDL), which is a complex of apoA-I or apoA-I mimetics with PL, must be disc shaped and may be a candidate medication for patients with TD. ApoA-I-mediated cholesterol efflux depends on ABCA1 in macrophages, and ABCA1 plays a pivotal role in mediating PL and cholesterol efflux to lipid-free apoA-I, and thereby, in the formation of discoidal HDL precursors. Mature HDL particles, which are spherical and transport almost all HDL cholesterol, appear to induce cholesterol efflux via other ABC transporters, such as ABCG1 and ABCG4, rather than ABCA1 (Wang et al., 2004). Therefore, we prepared a discoidal reconstituted HDL, which is a complex with apoA-I that contains 1-palmitoyl-2-oleoylphosphatidylcholine (POPC) (Rye et al., 1997). Interestingly, the apoA-I complex with POPC/apoA-I discs was able to take up cholesterol from macrophages in patients with TD and normal subjects (Fig. 3A). Moreover, ETC-642, a newly developed PL/apoA-I mimetic, is a synthetic peptide of 22 amino acids that contains 1, 2-dipalmitoyl-sn-glycero-3-phosphocholine and also works on cholesterol efflux in macrophages of patients with TD as well as the POPC/apoA-I disc (Fig. 3B).

rHDL and the POPC/apoA-I discs not only have a beneficial action on cholesterol efflux in macrophages but are also involved in lipoprotein–lipoprotein interactions in circulating plasma. To clarify the direct effects of the POPC/apoA-I discs in plasma from patients with TD, 250 and 500 μg/ml discs (final concentrations) were incubated with plasma at 37°C (Fig. 5C). After incubation, peaks 4 and 5 comprised TRLs, such as VLDL, and time dependently decreased in addition to an increase in peak 3 as sHDL. The POPC/apoA-I discs did not affect the native-LDL subfraction; however, surprisingly, the native-LDL subfraction was time dependently generated in plasma from patients with TD by incubating it with POPC/apoA-I discs at 37°C. von Eckardstein et al. have shown that lipid-poor HDL precursors are converted into mature, lipid-rich HDL by acquiring PLs and unesterified cholesterol from either cells or apoB-containing lipoproteins or through association with additional lipoprotein (von Eckardstein et al., 1998b). In contrast to normal subjects, the plasma of patients with TD does not convert preβ-HDL into α-HDL, which is believed to be related to the absence of a lipid transfer factor in the cells and plasma of patients with TD (Huang et al., 1995; von Eckardstein et al., 1998a). Thus, a deficiency in HDL composition leads to suppression of the interaction with lipoproteins, which may result in an increase in

TRLs and a decrease in native-LDL with cholesterol conversion among lipoproteins. Shahrokh et al. have shown that PL uptake by LDL contributes to form larger LDL particles (Shahrokh and Nichols, 1985), suggesting that the POPC/apoA-I discs might produce a large-sized LDL particle from a small-sized LDL particle using cholesterol-poor LDL in patients with TD. Although the plasma total concentrations of cholesterol and triglycerides do not change following incubation with POPC/apoA-I discs *in vitro*, the discs may transfer the cholesterol or triglycerides, resulting in changes in the lipoprotein components. These results suggest that the formation of mature-HDL particles by adding POPC/apoA-I discs led to physiological lipoprotein patterns such as higher native-LDL and lower TRLs in circulating plasma.

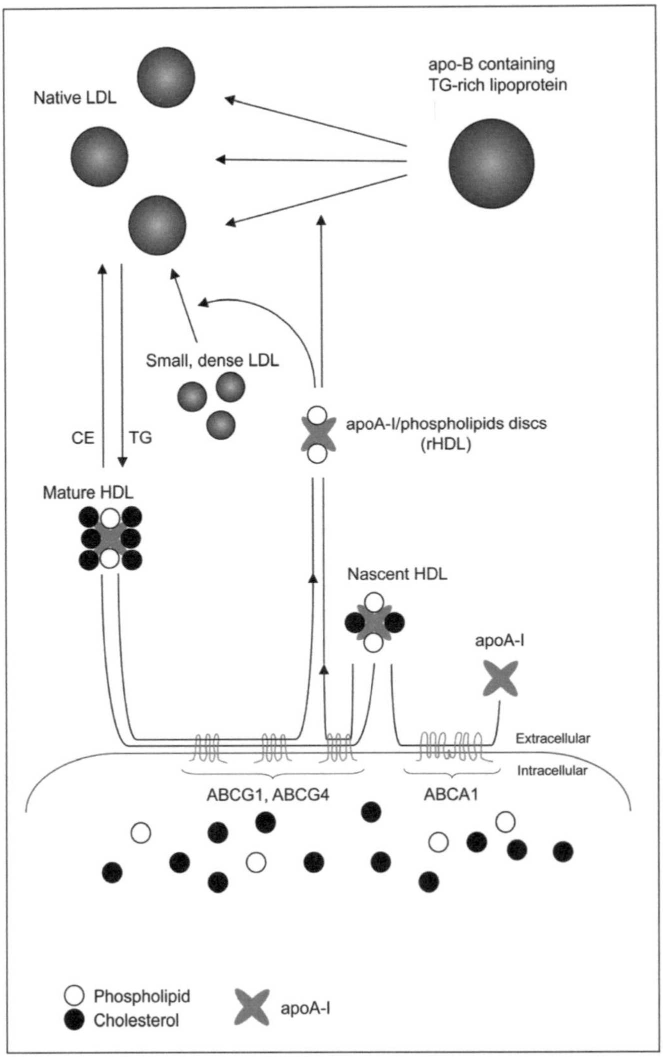

Fig. 6. Suggested function of phospholipid (PL)/apolipoprotein A-I (apoA-I) discs in HDL metabolism. apo, apolipoprotein; rHDL, reconstituted HDL; ABC, ATP-binding cassette transporter; CE, cholesteryl ester; TG, triglyceride

The suggested function of PL apoA-I discs in patients with TD is described in Fig. 6. rHDL and the apoA-I complex with PLs have beneficial effects for cholesterol efflux and lipoprotein components in patients with TD. Briefly, the PL/apoA-I discs acts to modulate lipoprotein metabolism via at least three different steps. 1) PL/apoA-I discs remove the cholesterol from peripheral cells through an ABCA1-independent pathway such as the ABCG1- and ABCG4-dependent pathway. 2) PL/ApoA-I discs form nascent HDL particles with cholesterol and PLs. 3) PL/ApoA-I discs interact with other lipoproteins such as apoB containing TRLs in circulating plasma. The discoidal apoA-I or apoA-I mimetics complex with PLs and potentially prevent or cure the symptoms of TD.

7. Conclusion

TD is a rare autosomal recessive disorder characterized by the absence or extremely low levels of HDL cholesterol and apoA-I in plasma. In addition, cholesteryl esters accumulate in many macrophage-rich tissues and organs. TD is caused by a defect in the ABCA1 gene, which is located on chromosome 9q31. ABCA1 has been identified as a pivotal gene in the regulation of plasma HDL cholesterol levels and cellular cholesterol homeostasis, which are defective in patients with TD. ABCA1 is a membrane protein that transports cholesterol and phospholipids from the membranous inner leaflet to the outer leaflet, and subsequently, lipid-free or lipid-poor apoA-I takes up the transported cholesterol and phospholipids to yield nascent HDL. Due to the ABCA1 genetic defect, patients with TD have an extremely low level of HDL cholesterol and cannot form nascent HDL particles. Namely, TD is based on a disorder of cellular cholesterol excretion as the initial step of RCT via ABCA1. If the process is able to performed in vitro, it leads to the generation of HDL particle, which can take up the excessive cholesterol from peripheral cell, and it acts as a new therapeutic target without using gene therapy in patients with TD.

8. References

Assman, G., von Eckardstein, A., Brewer, H.B.J. Eds., 1995. Familial high density lipoprotein deficiency: Tangier disease., New York: McGraw-Hill.

Baldan, A., Pei, L., Lee, R., Tarr, P., Tangirala, R.K., Weinstein, M.M., Frank, J., Li, A.C., Tontonoz, P., Edwards, P.A., 2006. Impaired development of atherosclerosis in hyperlipidemic Ldlr-/- and ApoE-/- mice transplanted with Abcg1-/- bone marrow. Arterioscler Thromb Vasc Biol. 26, 2301-7.

Bodzioch, M., Orso, E., Klucken, J., Langmann, T., Bottcher, A., Diederich, W., Drobnik, W., Barlage, S., Buchler, C., Porsch-Ozcurumez, M., Kaminski, W.E., Hahmann, H.W., Oette, K., Rothe, G., Aslanidis, C., Lackner, K.J., Schmitz, G., 1999. The gene encoding ATP-binding cassette transporter 1 is mutated in Tangier disease. Nat Genet. 22, 347-51.

Bortnick, A.E., Rothblat, G.H., Stoudt, G., Hoppe, K.L., Royer, L.J., McNeish, J., Francone, O.L., 2000. The correlation of ATP-binding cassette 1 mRNA levels with cholesterol efflux from various cell lines. J Biol Chem. 275, 28634-40.

Brooks-Wilson, A., Marcil, M., Clee, S.M., Zhang, L.H., Roomp, K., van Dam, M., Yu, L., Brewer, C., Collins, J.A., Molhuizen, H.O., Loubser, O., Ouelette, B.F., Fichter, K., Ashbourne-Excoffon, K.J., Sensen, C.W., Scherer, S., Mott, S., Denis, M., Martindale, D., Frohlich, J., Morgan, K., Koop, B., Pimstone, S., Kastelein, J.J., Hayden, M.R., et al., 1999. Mutations in ABC1 in Tangier disease and familial high-density lipoprotein deficiency. Nat Genet. 22, 336-45.

Bungert, S., Molday, L.L., Molday, R.S., 2001. Membrane topology of the ATP binding cassette transporter ABCR and its relationship to ABC1 and related ABCA transporters: identification of N- linked glycosylation sites. J Biol Chem. 276, 23539-46.

Chen, H., Rossier, C., Lalioti, M.D., Lynn, A., Chakravarti, A., Perrin, G., Antonarakis, S.E., 1996. Cloning of the cDNA for a human homologue of the Drosophila white gene and mapping to chromosome 21q22.3. Am J Hum Genet. 59, 66-75.

Costet, P., Luo, Y., Wang, N., Tall, A.R., 2000. Sterol-dependent transactivation of the ABC1 promoter by the liver X receptor/retinoid X receptor. J Biol Chem. 275, 28240-5.

Croop, J.M., Tiller, G.E., Fletcher, J.A., Lux, M.L., Raab, E., Goldenson, D., Son, D., Arciniegas, S., Wu, R.L., 1997. Isolation and characterization of a mammalian homolog of the Drosophila white gene. Gene. 185, 77-85.

Dean, M., Rzhetsky, A., Allikmets, R., 2001. The human ATP-binding cassette (ABC) transporter superfamily. Genome Res. 11, 1156-66.

Dean, M., Annilo, T., 2005. Evolution of the ATP-binding cassette (ABC) transporter superfamily in vertebrates. Annu Rev Genomics Hum Genet. 6, 123-42.

Despres, J.P., Marette, A., 1994. Relation of components of insulin resistance syndrome to coronary disease risk. Curr Opin Lipidol. 5, 274-89.

Fredrickson, D.S., Altrocchi, P.H., Avioli, L.V., Goodman, D.S., Goodman, H.C., 1961. Tangier disease combined clinical staff conference at the National Institutes of Health. Ann Intern Med. 55, 1016-1031.

Havel, R.J., Eder, H.A., Bragdon, J.H., 1955. The distribution and chemical composition of ultracentrifugally separated lipoproteins in human serum. J Clin Invest. 34, 1345-53.

Hobbs, H.H., Rader, D.J., 1999. ABC1: connecting yellow tonsils, neuropathy, and very low HDL. J Clin Invest. 104, 1015-7.

Huang, Y., von Eckardstein, A., Wu, S., Langer, C., Assmann, G., 1995. Generation of pre-beta 1-HDL and conversion into alpha-HDL. Evidence for disturbed HDL conversion in Tangier disease. Arterioscler-Thromb-Vasc-Biol. 15, 1746-54.

Ishida, B.Y., Frolich, J., Fielding, C.J., 1987. Prebeta-migrating high density lipoprotein: quantitation in normal and hyperlipidemic plasma by solid phase radioimmunoassay following electrophoretic transfer. J Lipid Res. 28, 778-86.

Kennedy, M.A., Barrera, G.C., Nakamura, K., Baldan, A., Tarr, P., Fishbein, M.C., Frank, J., Francone, O.L., Edwards, P.A., 2005. ABCG1 has a critical role in mediating cholesterol efflux to HDL and preventing cellular lipid accumulation. Cell Metab. 1, 121-31.

Klein, I., Sarkadi, B., Varadi, A., 1999. An inventory of the human ABC proteins. Biochim-Biophys-Acta. 1461, 237-62.

Klucken, J., Buchler, C., Orso, E., Kaminski, W.E., Porsch-Ozcurumez, M., Liebisch, G., Kapinsky, M., Diederich, W., Drobnik, W., Dean, M., Allikmets, R., Schmitz, G., 2000. ABCG1 (ABC8), the human homolog of the Drosophila white gene, is a regulator of macrophage cholesterol and phospholipid transport. Proc Natl Acad Sci U S A. 97, 817-22.

Kunitake, S.T., La Sala, K.J., Kane, J.P., 1985. Apolipoprotein A-I-containing lipoproteins with pre-beta electrophoretic mobility. J Lipid Res. 26, 549-55.

Langmann, T., Klucken, J., Reil, M., Liebisch, G., Luciani, M.F., Chimini, G., Kaminski, W.E., Schmitz, G., 1999. Molecular cloning of the human ATP-binding cassette transporter 1 (hABC1): evidence for sterol-dependent regulation in macrophages. Biochem Biophys-Res-Commun. 257, 29-33.

Lawn, R.M., Wade, D.P., Garvin, M.R., Wang, X., Schwartz, K., Porter, J.G., Seilhamer, J.J., Vaughan, A.M., Oram, J.F., 1999. The Tangier disease gene product ABC1 controls the cellular apolipoprotein-mediated lipid removal pathway. J Clin Invest. 104, R25-31.

Mauldin, J.P., Srinivasan, S., Mulya, A., Gebre, A., Parks, J.S., Daugherty, A., Hedrick, C.C., 2006. Reduction in ABCG1 in Type 2 diabetic mice increases macrophage foam cell formation. J Biol Chem. 281, 21216-24.

McNeish, J., Aiello, R.J., Guyot, D., Turi, T., Gabel, C., Aldinger, C., Hoppe, K.L., Roach, M.L., Royer, L.J., de Wet, J., Broccardo, C., Chimini, G., Francone, O.L., 2000. High density lipoprotein deficiency and foam cell accumulation in mice with targeted disruption of ATP-binding cassette transporter-1. Proc Natl Acad Sci U S A. 97, 4245-50.

Miller, M., Rhyne, J., Hamlette, S., Birnbaum, J., Rodriguez, A., 2003. Genetics of HDL regulation in humans. Curr Opin Lipidol. 14, 273-9.

Neufeld, E.B., Remaley, A.T., Demosky, S.J., Stonik, J.A., Cooney, A.M., Comly, M., Dwyer, N.K., Zhang, M., Blanchette-Mackie, J., Santamarina-Fojo, S., Brewer, H.B., Jr., 2001. Cellular localization and trafficking of the human ABCA1 transporter. J Biol Chem. 276, 27584-90.

Nissen, S.E., Tsunoda, T., Tuzcu, E.M., Schoenhagen, P., Cooper, C.J., Yasin, M., Eaton, G.M., Lauer, M.A., Sheldon, W.S., Grines, C.L., Halpern, S., Crowe, T., Blankenship, J.C., Kerensky, R., 2003. Effect of recombinant ApoA-I Milano on coronary atherosclerosis in patients with acute coronary syndromes: a randomized controlled trial. JAMA. 290, 2292-300.

Oram, J.F., Lawn, R.M., Garvin, M.R., Wade, D.P., 2000. ABCA1 is the cAMP-inducible apolipoprotein receptor that mediates cholesterol secretion from macrophages. J Biol Chem. 275, 34508-11.

Oram, J.F., Lawn, R.M., 2001. ABCA1. The gatekeeper for eliminating excess tissue cholesterol. J Lipid Res. 42, 1173-9.

Orso, E., Broccardo, C., Kaminski, W.E., Bottcher, A., Liebisch, G., Drobnik, W., Gotz, A., Chambenoit, O., Diederich, W., Langmann, T., Spruss, T., Luciani, M.F., Rothe, G., Lackner, K.J., Chimini, G., Schmitz, G., 2000. Transport of lipids from golgi to plasma membrane is defective in tangier disease patients and Abc1-deficient mice. Nat Genet. 24, 192-6.

Out, R., Hoekstra, M., Hildebrand, R.B., Kruit, J.K., Meurs, I., Li, Z., Kuipers, F., Van Berkel, T.J., Van Eck, M., 2006. Macrophage ABCG1 deletion disrupts lipid homeostasis in alveolar macrophages and moderately influences atherosclerotic lesion development in LDL receptor-deficient mice. Arterioscler Thromb Vasc Biol. 26, 2295-300.

Out, R., Hoekstra, M., Meurs, I., de Vos, P., Kuiper, J., Van Eck, M., Van Berkel, T.J., 2007. Total body ABCG1 expression protects against early atherosclerotic lesion development in mice. Arterioscler Thromb Vasc Biol. 27, 594-9.

Ranalletta, M., Wang, N., Han, S., Yvan-Charvet, L., Welch, C., Tall, A.R., 2006. Decreased atherosclerosis in low-density lipoprotein receptor knockout mice transplanted with Abcg1-/- bone marrow. Arterioscler Thromb Vasc Biol. 26, 2308-15.

Remaley, A.T., Rust, S., Rosier, M., Knapper, C., Naudin, L., Broccardo, C., Peterson, K.M., Koch, C., Arnould, I., Prades, C., Duverger, N., Funke, H., Assman, G., Dinger, M., Dean, M., Chimini, G., Santamarina Fojo, S., Fredrickson, D.S., Denefle, P., Brewer, H.B., Jr., 1999. Human ATP-binding cassette transporter 1 (ABC1): genomic organization and identification of the genetic defect in the original Tangier disease kindred. Proc Natl Acad Sci U S A. 96, 12685-90.

Repa, J.J., Turley, S.D., Lobaccaro, J.A., Medina, J., Li, L., Lustig, K., Shan, B., Heyman, R.A., Dietschy, J.M., Mangelsdorf, D.J., 2000. Regulation of absorption and ABC1-mediated efflux of cholesterol by RXR heterodimers. Science. 289, 1524-9.

Rust, S., Rosier, M., Funke, H., Real, J., Amoura, Z., Piette, J.C., Deleuze, J.F., Brewer, H.B., Duverger, N., Denefle, P., Assmann, G., 1999. Tangier disease is caused by mutations in the gene encoding ATP-binding cassette transporter 1. Nat Genet. 22, 352-5.

Rye, K.A., Hime, N.J., Barter, P.J., 1997. Evidence that cholesteryl ester transfer protein-mediated reductions in reconstituted high density lipoprotein size involve particle fusion. J Biol Chem. 272, 3953-60.

Santamarina-Fojo, S., Peterson, K., Knapper, C., Qiu, Y., Freeman, L., Cheng, J.F., Osorio, J., Remaley, A., Yang, X.P., Haudenschild, C., Prades, C., Chimini, G., Blackmon, E., Francois, T., Duverger, N., Rubin, E.M., Rosier, M., Denefle, P., Fredrickson, D.S., Brewer, H.B., Jr., 2000. Complete genomic sequence of the human ABCA1 gene: analysis of the human and mouse ATP-binding cassette A promoter. Proc Natl Acad Sci U S A. 97, 7987-92.

Savary, S., Denizot, F., Luciani, M., Mattei, M., Chimini, G., 1996. Molecular cloning of a mammalian ABC transporter homologous to Drosophila white gene. Mamm-Genome. 7, 673-6.

Schwartz, K., Lawn, R.M., Wade, D.P., 2000. ABC1 gene expression and ApoA-I-mediated cholesterol efflux are regulated by LXR. Biochem Biophys Res Commun. 274, 794-802.

Shahrokh, Z., Nichols, A.V., 1985. Interaction of human-plasma low-density lipoproteins with discoidal complexes of apolipoprotein A-I and phosphatidylcholine, and characterization of the interaction products. Biochim Biophys Acta. 837, 296-304.

Singaraja, R.R., Bocher, V., James, E.R., Clee, S.M., Zhang, L.H., Leavitt, B.R., Tan, B., Brooks-Wilson, A., Kwok, A., Bissada, N., Yang, Y.Z., Liu, G., Tafuri, S.R., Fievet, C., Wellington, C.L., Staels, B., Hayden, M.R., 2001. Human ABCA1 BAC transgenic mice show increased high density lipoprotein cholesterol and ApoAI-dependent efflux stimulated by an internal promoter containing liver X receptor response elements in intron 1. J Biol Chem. 276, 33969-79.

Smith, J.D., 2006. Insight into ABCG1-mediated cholesterol efflux. Arterioscler Thromb Vasc Biol. 26, 1198-200.

Uehara, Y., Engel, T., Li, Z., Goepfert, C., Rust, S., Zhou, X., Langer, C., Schachtrup, C., Wiekowski, J., Lorkowski, S., Assmann, G., von Eckardstein, A., 2002. Polyunsaturated Fatty Acids and Acetoacetate Downregulate the Expression of the ATP-Binding Cassette Transporter A1. Diabetes. 51, 2922-2928.

Uehara, Y., Miura, S., von Eckardstein, A., Abe, S., Fujii, A., Matsuo, Y., Rust, S., Lorkowski, S., Assmann, G., Yamada, T., Saku, K., 2007. Unsaturated fatty acids suppress the expression of the ATP-binding cassette transporter G1 (ABCG1) and ABCA1 genes via an LXR/RXR responsive element. Atherosclerosis. 191, 11-21.

Uehara, Y., Tsuboi, Y., Zhang, B., Miura, S., Baba, Y., Higuchi, M.A., Yamada, T., Rye, K.A., Saku, K., 2008a. POPC/apoA-I discs as a potent lipoprotein modulator in Tangier disease. Atherosclerosis. 197, 283-9.

Uehara, Y., Yamada, T., Baba, Y., Miura, S.I., Abe, S., Kitajima, K., Higuchi, M.A., Iwamoto, T., Saku, K., 2008b. ATP-binding cassette transporter G4 is highly expressed in microglia in Alzheimer's brain. Brain Res. 1217C, 239-246.

Vaisman, B.L., Lambert, G., Amar, M., Joyce, C., Ito, T., Shamburek, R.D., Cain, W.J., Fruchart-Najib, J., Neufeld, E.D., Remaley, A.T., Brewer, H.B., Jr., Santamarina-Fojo, S., 2001. ABCA1 overexpression leads to hyperalphalipoproteinemia and increased biliary cholesterol excretion in transgenic mice. J Clin Invest. 108, 303-9.

Venkateswaran, A., Laffitte, B.A., Joseph, S.B., Mak, P.A., Wilpitz, D.C., Edwards, P.A., Tontonoz, P., 2000. Control of cellular cholesterol efflux by the nuclear oxysterol receptor LXR alpha. Proc Natl Acad Sci U S A. 97, 12097-102.

von Eckardstein, A., Chirazi, A., Schuler-Luttmann, S., Walter, M., Kastelein, J.J., Geisel, J., Real, J.T., Miccoli, R., Noseda, G., Hobbel, G., Assmann, G., 1998a. Plasma and fibroblasts of Tangier disease patients are disturbed in transferring phospholipids onto apolipoprotein A-I. J Lipid Res. 39, 987-98.

von Eckardstein, A., Huang, Y., Kastelein, J.J., Geisel, J., Real, J.T., Kuivenhoven, J.A., Miccoli, R., Noseda, G., Assmann, G., 1998b. Lipid-free apolipoprotein (apo) A-I is converted into alpha-migrating high density lipoproteins by lipoprotein-depleted plasma of normolipidemic donors and apo A-I-deficient patients but not of Tangier disease patients. Atherosclerosis. 138, 25-34.

von Eckardstein, A., Nofer, J.R., Assmann, G., 2001. High density lipoproteins and arteriosclerosis. Role of cholesterol efflux and reverse cholesterol transport. Arterioscler Thromb Vasc Biol. 21, 13-27.

von Eckardstein, A., Rohrer, L., 2009. Transendothelial lipoprotein transport and regulation of endothelial permeability and integrity by lipoproteins. Curr Opin Lipidol. 20, 197-205.

Walker, J.E., Saraste, M., Runswick, M.J., Gay, N.J., 1982. Distantly related sequences in the alpha- and beta-subunits of ATP synthase, myosin, kinases and other ATP-requiring enzymes and a common nucleotide binding fold. Embo J. 1, 945-51.

Wang, N., Silver, D.L., Thiele, C., Tall, A.R., 2001. ATP-binding cassette transporter A1 (ABCA1) functions as a cholesterol efflux regulatory protein. J Biol Chem. 276, 23742-7.

Wang, N., Lan, D., Chen, W., Matsuura, F., Tall, A.R., 2004. ATP-binding cassette transporters G1 and G4 mediate cellular cholesterol efflux to high-density lipoproteins. Proc Natl Acad Sci U S A. 101, 9774-9.

Willy, P.J., Umesono, K., Ong, E.S., Evans, R.M., Heyman, R.A., Mangelsdorf, D.J., 1995. LXR, a nuclear receptor that defines a distinct retinoid response pathway. Genes Dev. 9, 1033-45.

Yang, X.P., Freeman, L.A., Knapper, C.L., Amar, M.J., Remaley, A., Brewer, H.B., Jr., Santamarina-Fojo, S., 2002. The E-box motif in the proximal ABCA1 promoter mediates transcriptional repression of the ABCA1 gene. J Lipid Res. 43, 297-306.

Zhang, B., Kaneshi, T., Ohta, T., Saku, K., 2005. Relation between insulin resistance and fast-migrating LDL subfraction as characterized by capillary isotachophoresis. J Lipid Res. 46, 2265-77.

13

Fabry Disease: A Metabolic Proteinuric Nephropathy

Jonay Poveda Nuñez[1], Alberto Ortiz[1], Ana Belen Sanz[2] and Maria Dolores Sanchez Niño[2]
[1]*IIS-Fundacion Jimenez Diaz and Universidad Autonoma de Madrid, Madrid,*
[2]*IdiPaz, Madrid*
Spain

1. Introduction

Fabry disease is a rare disease. However, Fabry disease is more common than other inherited lysosomal storage disorders, affecting 1 in 40,000 to 1 in 117,000 worldwide (Mehta et al., 2004, Germain, 2010). Fabry disease is the caused by an inherited deficiency of galactosylgalactosylglucosylceramidase" (EC 3.2.1.14), commonly referred to as α-galactosidase A (α-Gal A). As a result, there is progressive cellular accumulation of glycosphingolipids, leading to organ failure and premature death. For decades, only symptomatic therapy was available, that did not prevent the fatal evolution of the disease. In the last decade, two forms of Enzyme Replacement Therapy (ERT), that prevent disease progression as well as potentially reverse symptoms, have been developed. However, these drugs are expensive and do not cure the disease.

2. Fabry disease: concept

Fabry disease is an X-linked lysosomal storage disorder caused by mutations in the gene encoding the lysosomal enzyme α-galactosidase A (α-Gal A). α-galactosidase A catalyzes the hydrolytic cleavage of the terminal alpha-galactosyl moieties from globotriaosylceramide (Gb3) and glycoproteins. The deficiency of α-galactosidase leads to accumulation of Gb3 and other glycosphingolipids in plasma and different cell types throughout the body (Nance et al., 2006) (Figure 1). Glycosphingolipid storage may interfere with cellular membrane proteins, such as ion channels, become cytotoxic, or lead to accumulation of soluble cytotoxic metabolites (Schiffmann et al., 2002, Aerts et al., 2008, Sanchez-Niño et al., 2010), although the precise molecular link between lipid storage and disease manifestations is unclear. Progressive accumulation of Glycosphingolipid is associated with systemic disease, with a wide spectrum of clinical manifestations that reduce the life expectancy of patients.

3. Genetics

The α-galactosidase A gene (*GLA*) is located on the minus strand of the chromosome X on the locus Xq22.1. The *GLA* gene is 10,223 base pairs long and contains 7 exons. *GLA* gene may give rise to 7 different processed transcripts by alternative splicing. However, just one of these encodes the 429-aminoacid lysosomal α-Gal A with a molecular mass of 48.7 kD.

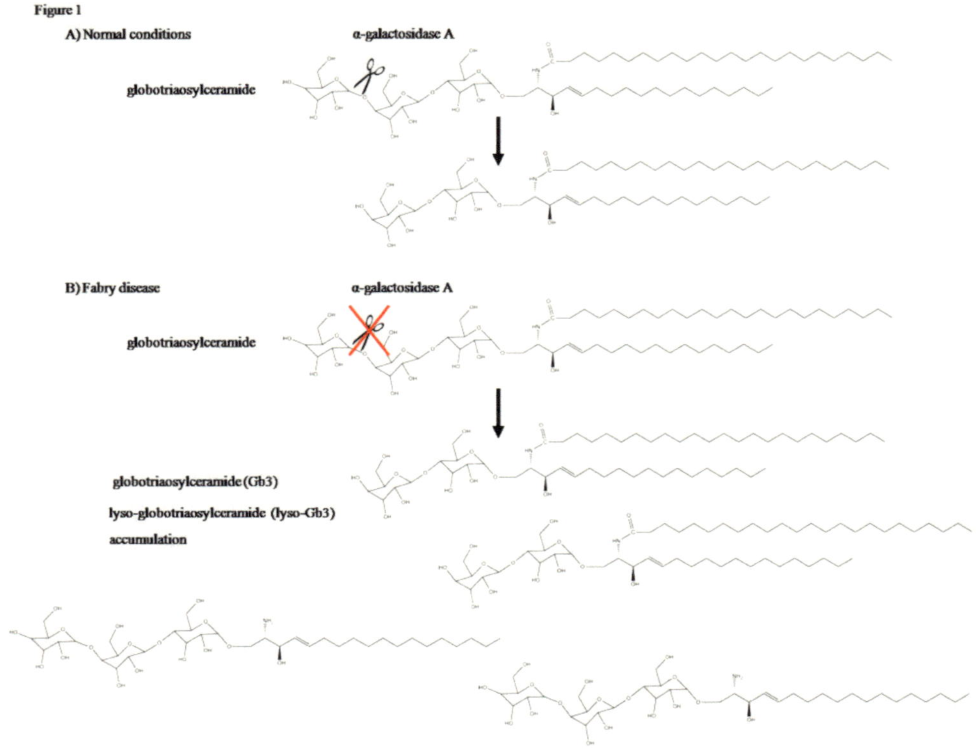

Fig. 1. A) α-galactosidase A catalyzes the hydrolytic cleavage of the terminal galactose from globotriaosylceramide (Gb3). B) The deficiency of α-galactosidase leads to accumulation of Gb3 and other glycosphingolipids, such as lyso-globotriaosylceramide (lyso-Gb3)

Within the coding region, 239 single nucleotide polymorphisms present in the general population and more than 400 *GLA* mutations that lead to Fabry disease have been found. Exons 5, 6 and 3 comprise the majority of point mutations respectively. Missense mutations may be classified in 3 groups in accordance with the effect they have on the protein function (Garman & Garboczi, 2004). First, mutations that alter the active site of the enzyme; second, mutation that interfere with the correct folding and stability of the protein; and finally, the remaining mutations that negatively affect the function of the enzyme. The nature of the mutation may influence therapeutic approaches. Most mutations are family-specific, which explains the marked variability in the residual enzyme activity and precludes the use of a single, fast genetic testing technique. Rather, the whole gene should be sequenced.

4. Clinical manifestations of Fabry disease

4.1 Early clinical features

Although glycolipid accumulation begins in the prenatal period, symptoms of the classic form of Fabry disease do not arise until childhood (Vedder et al., 2006). Symptoms include episodes of extremity pain or acroparesthesia, gastrointestinal symptoms, hypohidrosis and associated heat sensitivity (Cable et al., 1982; Ries et al., 2005; Rowe et al., 1974) (Table 1). Pain has been linked with small fiber neuropathy (Attal & Bouhassira, 1999) and is thought to be caused by either reduced perfusion of peripheral nerves or glycosphingolipid accumulation in neural or perineural cells (Gadoth & Sandbank, 1983; Gemignani et al., 1984). Pain has been described as burning and starts in the hands and feet but can radiate proximally. It may be present throughout the life of the patient, but frequently peaks in childhood or adolescence and then decreases. This has been attributed to end-stage nerve injury. Pain may be continuous or episodic, but is triggered by extreme temperature changes, fever, stress or physical exercise (MacDermot et al., 2001). Both, acute and chronic pains are difficult to deal with medically, requiring the use of narcotic or neuroleptic drugs respectively (Schiffmann & Scott, 2002).

Organ system	Sign/Symptom
Nervous system	Acroparesthesias Nerve deafness Heat intolerance, hypohidrosis Hearing loss, tinnitus
Gastrointestinal tract	Nausea, vomiting, diarrhea Postprandial bloating and pain, early satiety
Skin	Angiokeratomas
Eyes	Corneal and lenticular opacities Vasculopathy (retina conjunctiva)
Kidneys	Microalbuminuria, proteinuria Impaired concentration ability
Heart	Impaired heart rate variability ECG abnormalities (shortened PR interval) Mild valvular insufficiency Left ventricular hypertrophy

Table 1. Early signs and symptoms of Fabry disease

Gastrointestinal manifestations include nausea, vomiting, abdominal pain, early satiety, diarrhea and constipation (Hoffmann & Keshav, 2007). It has been proposed that delayed gastric emptying, in conjunction with lipid accumulation within ganglion cells of the autonomic nervous system, are responsible for the early satiety, whereas diarrhea has been linked to bacterial overgrowth (O'Brien et al., 1982).

Decreased sweating or hypohidrosis is another common feature of Fabry disease. It causes heat intolerance and inability to physical exercise. Hypohidrosis has also been attributed to autonomic neuropathy (Zarate & Hopkin, 2008). Less frequent than hypohidrosis is hyperhidrosis (excessive sweating), which is especially noticeable in the palms of the hands and soles of the feet (Zarate & Hopkin, 2008).

These symptoms highly reduce the quality of life of patients. However, the lack of physical findings frequently preclude the correct diagnosis in the absence of family history (Ries et al., 2005).

More characteristic disease manifestations arise in adolescence, such as angiokeratomas and corneal opacities. Angiokeratomas are reddish-purple vascular skin lesions, usually clustered around the swimming trunk region, which tend to increase in size and number with age (Zarate & Hopkin, 2008).

Corneal opacity (cornea verticillata) is the most characteristic ophthalmological abnormality observed in Fabry patients. They are the result of glycosphingolipids deposition between the basal membrane of the corneal epithelium and Bowman's membrane (Rodríguez-González-Herrero et al., 2008). Corneal opacities usually do not interfere with visual acuity. Other ophthalmological manifestations include conjunctival and retinal vascular tortuosity (Nguyen et al., 2005) and occlusion of retinal vessels (Utsumi et al., 1997).

Later in life many patients develop life-threatening complications including end-stage renal disease, heart and cerebrovascular diseases that may cause death (Table 2).

Organ system	**Sign/Symptom**
Central nervous system	Stroke
Kidneys	End-stage renal disease
Heart	Arrythmia, sudden death Ischemis Heart failure Heart fibrosis

Table 2. Life threatening signs and symptoms of Fabry disease

4.2 Life-threatening complications

Classical Fabry disease progresses to irreversible tissue damage and organ dysfunction, limiting life-expectancy in middle-age patients (Zarate & Hopkin, 2008). The main cause leading to death in men suffering from classic Fabry disease was renal failure before the widespread availability of renal replacement therapies, while now cardiac causes predominate (Mehta et al., 2006.).

Renal abnormalities include proteinuria, nephrotic range proteinuria, rarely nephrotic syndrome and chronic renal failure, requiring dialysis or kidney transplantation (Branton et al., 2002; Tsakiris et al., 1996, Ortiz et al., 2008, Ortiz et al., 2010)

Some patients develop end-stage renal disease at the same age as those with the classic form but lack other characteristic signs of the classical phenotype such as angiokeratomas, acroparesthesias or hypohidrosis, thus hindering the diagnosis of the condition (Nakao et al., 2003).

Cardiac disease may have several clinical manifestations. (Patel et al, 2011) The most frequent cardiac abnormality is progressive hypertrophic cardiomyopathy, although diastolic dysfunction, arrhythmia, myocardial fibrosis and short P-R are also seen (Linhart & Elliott, 2007). Fabry patients are frequently hypotensive. However, Fabry patients may have blood pressure that may be above recommended targets for chronic kidney disease patients (which are below 130 mmHg systolic and below 80 mmHg diastolic) (Ortiz et al., 2008). Cardiac symptoms may include palpitations, angina, shortness of breath and sudden death (Shah & Elliott, 2005).

The mechanisms leading to myocardial hypertrophy are not completely understood. The fact that only 1-2% of heart hypertrophy is attributable to actual storage of glycosphingolipids within the cardiac cells suggests that activation of signaling pathways leading to fibrosis play an important role (Linhart & Elliott, 2007). In this regard, much of the heart volume consists of fibrosis. Actual promoters of fibrosis are unknown. However, if we take a clue from the kidney, both death of myocardial cells and the presence of fibrogenic soluble mediators, such as lyso-gb3, that promote release of transforming growth factor beta 1 (TGFβ1), a fibrogenic cytokine, may be contributors (Sanchez-Niño et al, 2010).

A cardiac variant of Fabry disease has been described. In these patients, clinical manifestations and Gb3 storage are almost restricted to the heart (Ogawa et al., 1990). This is associated with residual α-galactosidase A activity or certain mutations. There is no clinical evidence of classical Fabry disease in other organs, although mild proteinuria has been observed (Ishii et al., 2002). Clinical manifestations appear later in life than in classical Fabry disease.

Cerebrovascular complications, mainly ischemic episodes, occur in Fabry disease (Sims et al. 2009). This is thought to be due to the accumulation of Gb3 in the cerebral blood vessels (Altarescu et al., 2001). However, the effect of sphingolipid storage is different depending on vessels' diameter. Thus, Gb3 deposition leads to progressive stenosis in small blood vessels, whereas in larger vessels weakened walls dilate, causing hyper-perfusion and tortuosity (Mitsias P, 1996). Clinical consequences of cerebrovascular injury include stroke, transient ischemic attacks, epilepsy, vertigo and headache (Mehta & Ginsberg, 2005).

Arterial remodeling and intima-media thickening have been described and may explain ischemic events. By contrast, classical atherosclerotic lesions are uncommon. It is unclear whether this is due to the relative young age of most patients or to a specific change in the vascular response to injury brought about the glycolipid accumulation or the metabolic consequences of the disease. In this regard, high HDL cholesterol levels have been described in Fabry patients (Cartwright et al., 2004). In at least in some Fabry patients HDL particles contribute disproportionately to carry glycosphingolipids (Clarke et al., 1976).

4.3 Other clinical manifestations

Additional clinical manifestations may include anemia, azoospermia, depression, facial dysmorphism, hypothyroidism, lymphoedema, parapelvic kidney cysts and priapism (Ries et al., 2004, Sunder-Plassmann, 2006), although there is discussion whether some of these, such as hypothyroidism, are real Fabry disease manifestations.

Tinnitus and substantial hearing loss have been described, especially in men (Hegemann et al., 2006). Hearing loss seems to be directly related to neuropathy (Ries et al., 2007).

Significant airflow reduction is common in Fabry patients. Respiratory involvement manifests as shortness of breath and dyspnea with exercise, chronic cough, and less frequently asthma (Rosenberg et al., 1980).

4.4 Fabry disease in women

Traditionally females were considered to be at low risk of clinical manifestations of Fabry disease. However, there is accumulating evidence that some females may suffer symptoms as severe as males (Wilcox et al., 2008). In this regard, Fabry disease may be considered as an X-linked disease with a high penetrance in females. Terms such as "recessive X-linked disease" are no longer used. It has been estimated that only 70% of women with *GLA* mutations develop clinical manifestations of the disease, which tend to be less severe and more variable than in men (Dobyns, 2006, Schiffmann R, 2009). As a result, it is likely that a large number of affected women remain undiagnosed. Women are affected because of the lack of cross-correction between cells with normal α-Gal A activity and cells with deficient α-Gal A (Romeo et al., 1975). Female cells have two X chromosomes, but one of them is randomly inactivated (lyonization). It is thought that the percentage of disease-carrying X chromosomes that are inactivated is a key factor contributing to disease expression variability in females (Dobrovolny et al., 2005).

5. Fabry nephropathy

5.1 Natural course

Fabry nephropathy is one of the most severe manifestations of Fabry disease and was the cause of death before the widespread availability of dialysis and kidney transplantation. Like most aspects of Fabry disease, kidney disease is thought to result from Gb3 accumulation in glomerular endothelial, mesangial and intersticial cells, podocytes and renal vasculature. Progressive intracellular accumulation of Gb3 is thought to cause glomerulosclerosis and interstitial fibrosis (Alroy J, 2002) as well as its urinary excretion together with other lipids (Branton MH, 2002). More recently a role of soluble glycolipid metabolites in the pathogenesis of podocyte injury has been suggested (Sanchez-Niño et al, 2010). As a result of lipid storage, kidneys may increase in size, although, as is the case with other renal disease characterized by enlarged kidney, such as diabetic nephropathy, in advanced renal failure the kidneys eventually shrink (Torra R, 2008).

Manifestations of kidney injury in Fabry disease include urinary concentrating defect, proteinuria, renal insufficiency and eventually renal failure requiring renal replacement therapy. The severity of kidney manifestations increases with age.

5.1.1 Renal function

Progressive loss of kidney function is characterized by elevated serum creatinine levels and decreasing glomerular filtration rates (GFR) (Ortiz et al, 2008). There is some debate as to the existence of an early hyperfiltration period, analogous to that observed in diabetic nephropathy, since assessment with of GFR by precise, research-grade technique is lacking. Early reports indicated that the loss of GFR was similar to that observed in diabetic nephropathy, around 10 ml/min/year (Branton et al., 2002). Lower rates have been described in recent times, that may be partially attributed to an overall better symptomatic control of chronic kidney disease aimed at proteinuria and blood pressure targets. Urinary protein excretion is the main predictor of GFR loss. Males with urinary protein/creatinine > 1.5 had a mean eGFR slope -5.6 ml/min per 1.73 m(2) per year, while this value was -1.3 ml/min per 1.73 m(2) per year for women with the highest urinary protein/creatinine (> 1.2) (Wanner et al., 2010).

Men with classical Fabry disease reach end-stage renal disease requiring dialysis or transplantation at a mean age of 40 years (Ortiz et al, 2010). Females reaching end-stage renal disease do so at the same mean age as males. However, there are ten-fold less females than males in both United States and European end-stage renal disease registries (Tsakiris et al., 1996, Thadhani et al, 2002). This suggests that in most females, Fabry nephropathy does not progress to reach end-stage renal disease, but in those in whom progression occurs, the time-course is similar to males.

5.1.2 Proteinuria

Early kidney injury is manifested as microalbuminuria which progresses to overt proteinuria (Schiffmann, 2009, Ortiz et al, 2008). Microalbuminuria is a misnomer that only indicates that pathological abnormalities may be detected by methods not available when the first tests to study albuminuria were commercialized. The term microalbuminuria indicates a urinary albumin excretion of > 30 mg/24h or >30 mg/g creatinine. In this regard, Fabry nephropathy usually recapitulates the sequence of events observed in diabetic nephropathy, another proteinuric nephropathy also consequence of a metabolic derangement. Overt proteinuria (>300 mg/24 h) was present in 43 and 26% of males and with early Fabry disease, respectively, and the proportions were higher with more severe kidney involvement (Ortiz et al, 2008). Established proteinuria (Albuminuria > 300 mg/day) is a sign of irreversible damage to the kidney (Zarate & Hopkin, 2008). Numerous experimental studies have shown a direct relationship between the degree of proteinuria and the rate of decline of renal functions (Tryggvason & Pettersson, 2003). Proteinuria is a consequence of glomerular damage but itself causes tubulointerstitial injury. Reabsorption of excess specific proteins filtered at the glomerulus by the proximal tubule activates these cells to release inflammatory factors and undergo apoptosis (Thomas ME, 1999). Thus, the magnitude of proteinuria could be used as a marker of glomerular damage. Interestingly, morphological studies, not specifically performed in Fabry disease, have confirmed a stronger correlation between tubulo-interstitial damage and renal function than between glomerular injury and renal function (Nath, 1992). Little is known about the factors that may speed up the process of Fabry nephropathy. Proteinuria is clearly a risk factor (Wanner et al., 2010). Thus, controlling proteinuria is thought to be important to for the progression of Fabry disease and evidence for this approach is discussed below.

5.1.3 Blood pressure

Hypertension is rarely found as an early symptom in Fabry disease but becomes more prevalent with the progression of the condition, indicating kidney declining function (Branton et al., 2002). Higher blood pressure values favor glomerular hyperperfusion as a compensatory response to nephron loss (Schieppati & Remuzzi, 2003). However, glomerular hypertension promotes kidney disease progression. Although not specifically tested in Fabry disease, lowering blood pressure to below 130 mmHg systolic AND 80 mmHg diastolic is recommended in patients with chronic kidney disease in order to slow the progression of nephropathy (K/DOQI clinical practice guidelines, 2004).

5.2 Heterogeneity

There is a great variability both in disease manifestations and the timing of kidney disease progression within and between families. Thus, the age at initiation of renal replacement therapy in the Fabry Registry data had a range of 15 to 79 years in males and 17 to 78 years in females (Ortiz A et al., 2010). The genetic or environmental factors that influence disease heterogeneity are unknown. However, unraveling them is a key priority since it will lead to a better understanding of the disease and potentially to novel therapeutic approaches.

5.3 Women

Most heterozygous women with Fabry disease used to be considered asymptomatic carriers. However, they may be as severely affected as men with the classic phenotype (Desnick et al., 2001, Wang et al., 2007, Wilcox et al., 2008). The clinical manifestation of Fabry disease in females tend to be less severe and to arise later than in males (Schiffmann. 2009). In this regard they may develop albuminuria and progressive renal dysfunction leading to the need of renal replacement therapy (Ortiz et al., 2008; Ortiz et al; 2010). If this occurs the mean age at initiation of renal replacemebt therapy is similar to men (Ortiz et al, 2010).

5.4 Diagnosis

In spite of the early onset of Fabry disease in some cases, the absence of family history, the variety of clinical manifestations and their similarity with those of other conditions may delay the diagnosis of Fabry disease, in some cases for years. Due to the availability of specific therapy, an early diagnosis would be desirable.

5.4.1 Diagnosis of Fabry disease

Diagnosis involves measuring residual enzyme activity in plasma, leukocytes or whole blood as well as sequencing of the gene to characterize the genetic defect (Ortiz et al., 2010b). Confirming the genetic defect may be important for the eligibility for treatment with novel approaches, such as chaperones. In the absence of family history, confirmation of the genetic defect by gene sequencing is mandatory in females when Fabry disease is suspected, since enzymatic assays may be normal even in the presence of Fabry disease due to random chromosome X inactivation. Genetic confirmation is also highly recommended in males.

A key, often forgotten aspect of Fabry disease, is the need to take a careful family history which allows the diagnosis of individuals in early stages of the disease.

5.4.2 Screening for Fabry disease

Screening by means of rapid and low-cost strategies to detect Fabry disease is indicated in high-risk populations (Oqvist et al., 2009). These include patients with unexplained left ventricular hypertrophy, younger patients with unexplained stroke and patients with chronic kidney disease of unknown etiology. However, neonatal screening has not yet been incorporated into routine clinical practice. Current screening methods are based on quantification of enzyme activity in dry blood spots. Performance for males is adequate. However, given the mosaicisms of females regarding X chromosome inactivation, Fabry women may have near normal whole blood enzyme activity and still have the disease. Thus, dried blood spot analysis is unable to detect about a 33% of heterozygous females leads to the need for more efficient strategies (Linthorst GE, 2005). Novel screening methods, such as proteomic analysis of urine, and quantification of urinary Gb3 or lyso-Gb3 are under study.

5.4.3 Renal biopsy for diagnosis of Fabry nephropathy

Kidney biopsy is recommended in Fabry patients exhibiting reduced GFR or proteinuria to confirm the diagnosis of Fabry kidney involvement (Ortiz et al., 2008b). In addition, renal biopsy for kidney disease of unknown origin may reveal unsuspected Fabry disease. Biopsies reveal typical Gb3 accumulation in tubular epithelial cells, glomerular and endothelial cells, and provide information on the extent of renal damage. In patients with Fabry disease, glomeruli present a striking white color under illumination in a stereomicroscope as a result of lipid-laden podocytes in contrast to the usual red color of normal glomeruli (Svarstad et al., 2004).

5.5 Pathogenesis and pathology

Fabry disease manifestations had traditionally been ascribed to intracellular accumulation of Gb3 and related glycosphingolipids (Figure 1). However, the precise pathways leading to tissue injury were unknown. Recent evidence suggests a role for more soluble molecules, such as lyso-Gb3, that may activate target tissue cells, such as podocytes, to release secondary mediators of injury that would be responsible for tissue injury and disease manifestations (Figure 2). This model (accumulation of a soluble metabolite with cytotoxic properties) would be analogous to the diabetes situation, where high glucose concentrations as a result of the metabolic derangement promote activation of target tissue cells to release mediators that cause tissue injury. If correct, this paradigm would greatly enhance research into novel therapeutic approaches to Fabry nephropathy by allowing the extrapolation of concepts from diabetic nephropathy, a better understood and more common disease (Sanchez- Niño et al., 2010b).

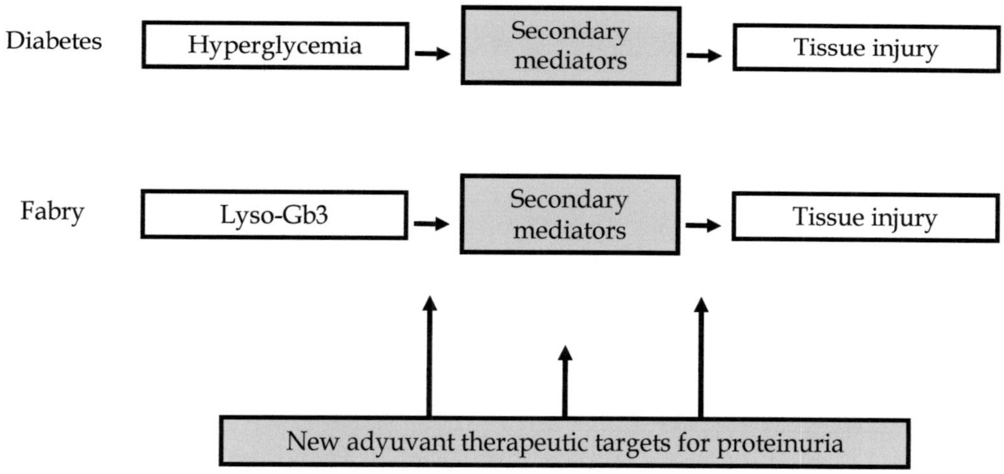

Fig. 2. Hypothetical similarities between the pathogenesis of diabetic nephropathy and Fabry disease nephropathy and potential therapeutic implications

Detailed descriptions of kidney pathology in children and adults with Fabry disease have recently been published (Tondel et al., 2008, Fogo et al., 2010, Najafian et al., 2010). There is widespread glycolipid accumulation in glomerular podocytes, mesangial and endothelial cells, as well as proximal and distal tubular cells, interstitial endothelial cells and other endothelial cells. While early pathogenic theories were centered in endothelial cell glycolipid accumulation, that was thought to lead to ischemic injury, the total early clearance of endothelial deposits by ERT, but persistence of proteinuria and chronic kidney disease progression despite this endothelial clearance have focused the attention to podocytes. In this regard, podocytes are the cells with a worse response to ERT in terms of glycolipid clearance (Germain et al, 2007). Only after 5 years of ERT a mild decrease in podocytes glycolipid deposition was noted. Furthermore, podocyte injury is a key feature of other proteinuric kidney diseases (Moreno et al., 2008). In addition, in children with early Fabry nephropathy the best pathological correlate of albuminuria was the presence and amount of podocytes glycolipid accumulation (Najafian et al., 2010). Thus, recent research into the pathogenesis of Fabry nephropathy has focused on the cell biology of the podocyte (Sanchez-Niño et al., 2010). The other key pathology feature of Fabry nephropathy is glomerular (glomerulosclerosis) and interstitial fibrosis, which is associated with loss of parenchymal renal cells (podocytes and tubular cells)(Fogo et al., 2010). Thus, there is renewed interest in the link between metabolites accumulated in Fabry disease and the synthesis and deposition of extracellular matrix components.

5.5.1 Metabolic initiators: Gb3 and lyso-Gb3

In Fabry disease, Gb3 is widely distributed in lysosomes and other cellular compartments such as the cell membrane, the ER or the nucleus (Askari et al., 2007). It was hypothesized that Gb3 may disrupt intracellular trafficking (Pagano RE, 2003) or alter the composition of membrane lipid rafts. Lipid rafts interact with other lipids and proteins that signal from cell surface receptors (Galbiati et al., 2001), such as endothelial nitric oxide synthase (eNOS) (Mogami et al., 2005). It was further hypothesized that cell stress due to Gb3 accumulation could promote the production of reactive oxygen species (ROS) that induce cell death (Shen et al., 2008).

Although Gb3 accumulation is widespread, serum Gb3 or Gb3 deposits do not necessarily correlate with clinical manifestations (Aerts et al., 2008). Instead, a new biologically active soluble glycolipid metabolite, globotriaosylsphingosine (lyso-Gb3), has been found in high serum, kidney and urinary concentrations in Fabry patients (Aerts et al., 2008, Auray-Blais et al., 2010, Togawa et al.2010b). Lyso-Gb3 is involved in vascular smooth muscle cell proliferation and induces in podocytes the production of mediators of glomerular injury such as TGF-β1, a critical mediator of extracellular matrix (ECM) production, fibrosis and podocyte injury (Alsaad & Herzenberg, 2007; Mason & Wahab, 2003; Pantsulaia. 2006; Park et al., 1997) (Sharma et al, 1997) and CD74, a MIF receptor that regulates the expression of lethal cytokines (Sanchez-Niño et al., 2009), suggesting a role in the pathogenesis of Fabry disease (Sanchez-Niño et al., 2010).

Lyso-Gb_3 seems to be involved in glomerular injury in Fabry disease by triggering the release of TGF-beta1 and CD74, both secondary mediators of glomerular injury common to diabetic nephropathy (Sanchez-Niño et al., 2010). TGF-beta1, in turn, leads to release of excess ECM components, including type IV collagen and fibronectin, by podocytes, contributing to the characteristic glomerulosclerosis of Fabry nephropathy. Further unpublished data suggest a more widespread release of inflammatory mediators by podocytes exposed to lyso-Gb3.

5.6 Therapy of Fabry nephropathy

The first therapies for Fabry disease were oriented to deal with the symptomatic effects of the disorder, such as pain, cardiac and cerebrovascular complications. However, most patients would die for ESRD unless kidney transplantation or renal dialysis was applied. Guidelines for the management of Fabry nephropathy have recently been published (Ortiz et al., 2008b).

5.6.1 Enzyme replacement therapy (ERT)

Until 2000, recognition of Fabry disease did not change the patient management or prognosis, since no specific treatment was available. However, in the last decade enzyme replacement therapy (ERT) is available and addresses the metabolic defect, although it does not cure the disease. ERT provides the chance to modify the natural history of Fabry disease. Two companies commercialize human recombinant α-galactosidase synthesized by genetically engineered cell lines.

Indications: ERT is indicated in every male with classical Fabry disease. In this population ERT should be initiated as early as possible. In addition, ERT should be prescribed to females with any evidence of injury to the heart, central nervous system or kidney and considered in females with symptoms in other organs and systems (Germain DP, 2010, Ortiz et al., 2010b). In case of a transitory limitation in ERT supplies, prioritization guidelines have been published (Linthorst et al., 2011). These guidelines should not be considered compelling indications in the absence of limited availability of treatment. Furthermore, these guidelines do not apply to a chronic limitation of resources since they take into account both the indication of ERT as well as the urgency of the need of ERT. Thus, they do not answer the question who should and should not be treated. They answer the question, if therapy is indicated but ERT availability is limited, who should be treated first, implying that not prioritized patients will also be treated but later, as soon as supplies are available.

There are currently two commercially available enzyme preparations for the treatment of Fabry disease: (1) Replagal® (agalsidase alfa; Shire Human Genetic Therapies, Inc., Cambridge, MA) and (2) Fabrazyme® (agalsidase beta; Genzyme Corporation, Inc., Cambridge, MA). Algasidase alfa is produced by cultured human fibroblasts, whereas agalsidase beta produced by the expression of human a-galactosidase cDNA in Chinese Hamster Ovary (CHO) cells. In the USA, only agalsidase β has been approved by the US Food and Drug Administration, while in Europe both enzymes are available for clinical use.

The approved doses of agalsidase-alfa and agalsidase-beta are 0.2 mg/kg and 1.0 mg/kg, given intravenously every 2 weeks, respectively. There is evidence that agalsidase-beta may be used at 0.3 mg/kg every two weeks for certain patients. This difference in dose remains unexplained by the molecular nature of the preparations and there is an ongoing debate whether they are similarly effective. The only published head-to-head clinical trial concluded that disease progression occurred when both enzymes where used at a dose of 0.2 mg/kg every two weeks (Vedder et al, 2007). We must emphasize that this dose is the approved one for agalsidase-alfa, but was 5-fold lower than the approved dose for agalsidase-beta. There is some indication, although the evidence is not strong, for a superiority of the higher dose in patients who develop anti-agalsidase antibodies. Furthermore a doubling of the approved agalsidase alfa dose provided further benefit in terms of nephroprotection for patients whose disease was progressing despite treatment with the approved dose. In addition, only agalsidase beta has shown a benefit on hard end-points in a phase IV randomized clinical trial (Banikazemi et al., 2007). Despite these considerations, a number of publications have documented that both enzymes at approved doses have proved effective in reducing glycolipid deposits and disease manifestations at least if used early (Eng et al, 2001, Schiffmann et al., 2001; Schiffmann et al., 2006; Germain et al., 2007; Mehta et al., 2009; Schaefer et al., 2009).

5.6.2 Benefits and unmet needs of ERT

ERT addresses the underlying metabolic cause of Fabry disease. ERT slows the loss of kidney function in patients with relatively preserved renal function and low proteinuria (Schiffmann et al., 2006) (Germain et al., 2007). However, progression occurs despite ERT in patients with more advanced renal disease, including those with proteinuria> 1g/d or glomeruloscerotic lesions in renal biopsyl, as ERT does not reduce proteinuria and may be unable to avoid its development in treated pediatric patients (Tøndel et al., 2008). Thus, since proteinuria is a major risk factor for progression of Fabry disease, it is advisable to combine antiproteinuric therapy with early institution of ERT.

5.6.3 Antiproteinuric approaches

ACEI/ARBs: the lesser efficacy of ERT once Fabry nephropathy has caused proteinuria or glomerulosclerosis (Germain et al., 2007) raises the need for adjuvant therapies that cooperate with ERT in improving outcomes. Co-treatment with angiotensin-converting enzyme (ACE) inhibitors and angiotensin-receptor blockers (ARB) decreases proteinuria (Tahir et al., 2007). These agents help to control hypertension when present, although in some case a low blood pressure may limit their use. To prevent unwanted blood pressure lowering effects initiation of therapy with low, fractionated doses is recommended.

Active vitamin D has pleiotropic effects that go well beyond the regulation of bone metabolism (Rojas-Rivera et al., 2010). Vitamin D receptor (VDR) activators such as calcitriol and paricalcitol prevent podocyte activation by lyso-Gb3 in podocytes (Sanchez-Niño et al., 2010). In this regard, there is some evidence that paricalcitol, a selective VDR activator, reduces proteinuria in diabetic nephropathy, even in patients treated with ACEIs or ARBs (Agarwal et al., 2005; Lambers Heerspink et al., 2009; de Zeeuw et al., 2010). Interestingly, patients suffering from chronic kidney disease frequently have deficiencies of both 25(OH) vitamin D and calcitriol. Vitamin D deficiencies should be corrected in these patients and VDR agonists are indicated for the prevention and treatment of secondary hyperparathyroidism in chronic kidney disease (Kidney Disease: Improving Global Outcomes (KDIGO) CKD-MBD Work Group. 2009) (National Kidney Foundation. 2003). Thus, VDR agonist therapy used to treat vitamin D deficiency or secondary hyperparathyroidism might be beneficial for proteinuria in Fabry disease.

5.6.4 Novel therapies in the horizon

The search for an ideal treatment of the underlying enzymatic defect is still ongoing. Current ERT is expensive, inconvenient and may not reach certain key cells such as the podocytes. Additional therapeutic approaches are being explored.

Substrate reduction therapy by small molecules may be associated with ERT to improve efficacy or reduce ERT dose. Gene therapy is also being explored. In addition certain mutations may benefit from novel therapeutic strategies. Thus, individuals carrying mutation that interfere with the correct folding and stability of the protein may benefit from small molecule chaperone therapy. In addition, an orally active small molecule, ataluren, might be useful in individuals carrying premature stop codons (Torra et al. 2010). Although never tested in Fabry disease, clinical trials in other genetic diseases are underway or have been completed (Kerem et al., 2008).

5.6.5 Monitoring therapy and disease progression

We lack reliable biomarkers that enable assessing disease progression, monitoring treatment response and individualizing ERT dose in Fabry disease. Biomarkers may represent lipid storage burden or target organ injury or response to therapy. Potential biomarkers of glycolipid storage include plasma or urine Gb3 and lyso-Gb3. Lyso-Gb_3 plasma and urinary levels are elevated in Fabry disease. Plasma lyso-Gb3 was found to be useful to diagnose Fabry disease (Rombach et al., 2010). Furthermore, while multiple regression analysis did not demonstrate correlation between plasma lyso-Gb3 concentration and total disease severity score in Fabry males, plasma lysoGb3 concentration did correlate with white matter lesions. In addition, in females, plasma lyso-Gb3 concentration correlated with overall disease severity (Rombach et al., 2010). In Fabry patients plasma lyso-Gb3 falls on ERT, and even more dramatically than Gb3 levels (Togawa et al., 2010, Van Breemen et al., 2011). Urinary lysoGb3 was also correlated with type of mutations, enzyme replacement therapy status and with a number of indicators of disease severity (Auray-Blais et al, 2010). Decreased urinary lyso-Gb3 may reflect decreased kidney lyso-Gb3 burden, since renal tissue lyso-Gb3 was decreased in Fabry mice upon ERT (Togawa et al., 2010b). Despite these promising observations, studies approaching the potential value of lyso-Gb3 concentrations to make clinical decisions regarding ERT dose have not been performed and, thus, it cannot be considered a biomarker for such purpose.

Albuminuria is a biomarker of kidney injury. Both in Fabry and non-Fabry kidney injury the magnitude of albuminuria predicts renal disease progression. In this regard there is solid evidence supporting targeting albuminuria as a therapeutic objective in non-Fabry disease. Anecdotal evidence suggests that this is the case too in Fabry disease, where lowering albuminuria is considered a target to be pursued through adjunctive antiproteinuric therapy (Tahir et al., 2007). A clinical trial (FAACET) is underway to test this hypothesis. Unfortunately, since albuminuria does not improve on ERT in adults, it cannot guide ERT dosing.

Finally promising preliminary data are available of the use of urinary protemics for the diagnosis and eventual monitoring of Fabry disease. The most promising technique is capillary electrophoresis coupled to mass spectrometry (CE-MS) (Mischak H et al., 2010).

6. Conclusions

Research in Fabry disease is very active in recent times and has led to a paradigm shift in our understanding of the disease and its management (Table 3). The advent of ERT has changed the prospects for Fabry disease patients. However, there are, still unsolved problems:

1. ERT does not modify proteinuria, a key risk factor for renal disease progression (Wanner et al., 2010), in adults and does not stop renal disease progression once a certain degree of renal injury, manifested as histological injury, decreased eGFR or proteinuria (>1g/d), has been reached (Germain DG et al., 2007).
2. Despite adequate endothelial cell clearance, ERT does not clear deposits in podocytes, key cells responsible for avoiding proteinuria (Germain DG et al., 2007). This and the correlation of early podocyte injury with proteinuria (Najafian et al., 2010) support a more central role of podocytes in the pathogenesis of renal disease than previously thought.

3. The lack of biomarkers of tissue injury activity and response to therapy hinders dose individualization, the follow-up of the therapeutic response and early identification of females most at risk for progressive disease.
4. The molecular link between the metabolic defect and tissue injury is still poorly characterized. This hinders the development of adjuvant therapies.

The full scope of these gaps in knowledge became evident during the global shortage on ERT availability, which took place in 2009-2010 (Linthorst et al, 2011). Hopefully this realization, as well as recent advances in the pathogenesis and treatment approaches for the disease will further improve the outcome of Fabry patients.

Classical concepts	New paradigms
Endothelium as key target cell	Podocyte as key target cell
Intracellular deposits cause injury	Soluble metabolites cause injury
Deposits injure cells containing them	Injury of distant or adjacent cells
Unknown tissue injury mechanisms	Recruitment of secondary mediators
ERT as only therapy	Need for adjuvant therapies
Same dose fits all	Individualize dose: biomarkers need
Therapeutic nihilism for advanced tissue injury	Target secondary mediators of injury in advanced tissue injury

Table 3. Classical concepts and new paradigms in Fabry nephropathy

7. Acknowledgements

Work by the authors was supported by FEDER funds FIS PS09/00447. JPN was supported by Fundacion Conchita Rabago and AO, MDSN and ABS by FIS.

8. References

Aerts, JM.; Groener, JE.; Kuiper, S.; Donker-Koopman, WE.; Strijland, A.; Ottenhoff, R.; van Roomen, C.; Mirzaian, M.; Wijburg, FA.; Linthorst, GE.; Vedder, AC.; Rombach, SM.; Cox-Brinkman, J.; Somerharju, P.; Boot, RG.; Hollak, CE.; Brady, RO. & Poorthuis, BJ. (2008). Elevated globotriaosylsphingosine is a hallmark of Fabry disease. *Proc Natl Acad Sci USA.,* Vol. 8, No. 105, (February 2008), pp. 2812-2817, ISSN 1091-6490

Agarwal, R.; Acharya, M.; Tian, J.; Hippensteel, RL.; Melnick, JZ.; Qiu, P.; Williams, L. & Batlle, D. (2005). Antiproteinuric effect of oral paricalcitol in chronic kidney disease. *Kidney Int.,* Vol. 6, No. 68, (December 2005), pp.2823-2828, ISSN 0085-2538

Alroy, J.; Sabnis, S. & Kopp, JB. (2002). Renal pathology in Fabry disease. *J Am Soc Nephro,.* Suppl. 2, No. 13, (June 2002), pp. 134-138, ISSN 1046-6673

Alsaad, KO. & Herzenberg, AM. (2007). Distinguishing diabetic nephropathy from other causes of glomerulosclerosis: an update. *J Clin Pathol.,* Vol. 1, No. 60, (January 2007), pp. 18-26, ISSN 1046-6673

Altarescu, G.; Moore, DF.; Pursley, R.; Campia, U.; Goldstein, S.; Bryant, M.; Panza, JA. & Schiffmann, R. (2001). Enhanced endothelium-dependent vasodilation in Fabry disease. *Stroke,* Vol. 7, No. 32, (July 2001), pp. 1559-1562, ISSN 1524-4628

Askari, H.; Kaneski, CR.; Semino-Mora, C.; Desai, P.; Ang, A.; Kleiner, DE.; Perlee, LT.; Quezado, M.; Spollen, LE.; Wustman, BA. & Schiffmann, R. (2007). Cellular and tissue localization of globotriaosylceramide in Fabry disease. *Virchows Arch.*, Vol. 4, No. 451, (October 2007), pp. 823-834, ISSN 0945-6317

Attal, N. & Bouhassira, D. (1999). Mechanisms of pain in peripheral neuropathy. *Acta Neurol Scand.*, No. 173, (1999), pp. 12-24, ISSN 0945-6317

Banikazemi, M.; Bultas, J.; Waldek, S.; Wilcox, WR.; Whitley, CB.; McDonald, M.; Finkel, R.; Packman, S.; Bichet, DG.; Warnock, DG. & Desnick, RJ.; Fabry Disease Clinical Trial Study Group. (2007). Agalsidase-beta therapy for advanced Fabry disease: a randomized trial. *Ann Intern Med.*, Vol. 2, No. 146, (January 2007), pp. 77-86, ISSN 1539-3704

Branton, MH.; Schiffmann, R.; Sabnis, SG.; Murray, GJ.; Quirk, JM.; Altarescu, G.; Goldfarb, L.; Brady, RO.; Balow, JE.; Austin Iii, HA. & Kopp, JB. (2002). Natural history of Fabry renal disease: influence of alpha-galactosidase A activity and genetic mutations on clinical course. *Medicine (Baltimore)*, Vol. 2, No. 81, (March 2002), pp. 122-138, ISSN 0025-7974

Branton, M.; Schiffmann, R. & Kopp, JB. (2002). Natural history and treatment of renal involvement in Fabry disease. *J Am Soc Nephrol.*, Suppl. 2, No. 13, (June 2002), pp. 139-143, ISSN 1046-6673

Cable, WJ.; Kolodny, EH. & Adams, RD. (1982) Fabry disease: impaired autonomic function. *Neurology*, Vol. 5, No. 32, (May 1982), pp. 498-502, ISSN 0028-3878

Cartwright, DJ.; Cole, AL.; Cousins, AJ. & Lee, PJ. (2004). Raised HDL cholesterol in Fabry disease: response to enzyme replacement therapy. *J Inherit Metab Dis.*, Vol. 6, No. 27, (2004), pp. 791-793, ISSN 0141-8955

Clarke JT; Stoltz JM & Mulcahey MR. (1976).Neutral glycosphingolipids of serum lipoproteins in Fabry's disease. *Biochim Biophys Acta.*, Vol. 2, No. 431, (May 1976), pp. 317-325, ISSN 0006-3002

de Zeeuw, D.; Agarwal, R.; Amdahl, M.; Audhya, P.; Coyne, D.; Garimella, T.; Parving, HH.; Pritchett, Y.; Remuzzi, G.; Ritz, E. & Andress, D. (2010). Selective vitamin D receptor activation with paricalcitol for reduction of albuminuria in patients with type 2 diabetes (VITAL study): a randomised controlled trial. *Lancet*, Vol. 9752, No. 376, (Novemer 2010), pp. 1543-1551, ISSN 1474-547X

Desnick, RJ.; Ioannou, YA. & Eng, CM. (2001) Alpha-Galactosidase A deficiency: Fabry disease. In: *The Metabolic Bases of Inherited Disease*, Scriver CR., pp. 3733-3774 McGraw-Hill, ISBN 0071163360, New York

Dobrovolny, R.; Dvorakova, L.; Ledvinova, J.; Magage, S.; Bultas, J.; Lubanda, JC.; Elleder, M.; Karetova, D.; Pavlikova, M. & Hrebicek, M. (2005) Relationship between X-inactivation and clinical involvement in Fabry heterozygotes. Eleven novel mutations in the alpha-galactosidase A gene in the Czech and Slovak population. *J Mol Med.*, Vol. 8, No. 83, (August 2005), pp. 647-654, ISSN 0946-2716

Dobyns, WB. (2006) The pattern of inheritance of X-linked traits is not dominant or recessive, just X-linked. *Acta Paediatr* , Vol 451, No. 95, (April 2006), pp. 11-15, ISSN 0803-5326

Eng, CM.; Guffon, N.; Wilcox, WR.; Germain, DP.; Lee, P.; Waldek, S.; Caplan, L.; Linthorst, GE. & Desnick, RJ.; International Collaborative Fabry Disease Study Group. (2001). Safety and efficacy of recombinant human alpha-galactosidase A--replacement therapy in Fabry's disease. *N Engl J Med.*, Vol. 1, No. 345, (July 2001), pp. 9-16, ISSN 0028-4793

Fogo, AB.; Bostad, L.; Svarstad, E.; Cook, WJ.; Moll, S.; Barbey, F.; Geldenhuys, L.; West, M.; Ferluga, D.; Vujkovac, B.; Howie, AJ.; Burns, A.; Reeve, R.; Waldek, S.; Noël, LH.; Grünfeld, JP.; Valbuena, C.; Oliveira, JP.; Müller, J.; Breunig, F.; Zhang, X. & Warnock, DG; all members of the International Study Group of Fabry Nephropathy (ISGFN). (2010). Scoring system for renal pathology in Fabry disease: report of the International Study Group of Fabry Nephropathy (ISGFN). *Nephrol Dial Transplant.*, Vol. 7, No. 25, (July 2010), pp. 2168-2177, ISSN 1460-2385

Gadoth, N. & Sandbank, U. (1983) Involvement of dorsal root ganglia in Fabry's disease. *J Med Genet.*, Vol. 4, No. 20, (August 1983), pp. 309-312, ISSN 0022-2593

Galbiati, F. ; Razani, B. & Lisanti, MP. (2001) Emerging themes in lipid rafts and caveolae. *Cell*, Vol. 4, No. 16 (August 2001), pp. 403-411, ISSN 0092-8674

Garman, SC. & Garboczi, DN. (2004) The molecular defect leading to Fabry disease: structure of human α-galactosidase. *J Mol Biol.*,Vol. 2, No. 337, (March 2004), pp. 319-335, ISSN 0022-2836

Gemignani, F.; Marbini, A.; Bragaglia, MM. & Govoni, E. (1984) Pathological study of the sural nerve in Fabry's disease. *Eur Neurol.*, Vol. 3, No. 23, (1984), pp. 173-181, ISSN 0014-3022

Germain, DP.; Waldek, S.; Banikazemi, M.; Bushinsky, DA.; Charrow, J.; Desnick, RJ.; Lee, P.; Loew, T.; Vedder, AC.; Abichandani, R.; Wilcox, WR. & Guffon, N. (2007) Sustained, long-term renal stabilization after 54 months of agalsidase beta therapy in patients with Fabry disease. *J Am Soc Nephrol.*, Vol. 5, No. 18, (May 2007), pp. 1547-1557, ISSN 1046-6673

Germain, DP. (2010). Fabry disease. *Orphanet J Rare Dis.*, No. 5, (Novemer 2010), pp. 30, ISSN 1750-1172

Hegemann, S.; Hajioff, D.; Conti, G.; Beck, M.; Sunder-Plassmann, G.; Widmer, U.; Mehta, A. & Keilmann, A. (2006) Hearing loss in Fabry disease: data from the Fabry Outcome Survey. Eur *J Clin. Invest.*,Vol. 9, No, 36, (September 2006), pp. 654-662, ISSN 0014-2972

Hoffmann, B. & Keshav S. (2007) Gastrointestinal symptoms in Fabry disease: everything is possible, including treatment. *Acta Paediatr.*, Vol. 455, No. 96, (April 2007), pp. 84-86, ISSN 0803-5326

Ishii, S.; Nakao, S.; Minamikawa-Tachino, R.; Desnick, RJ. & Fan, JQ. (2002) Alternative splicing in the α-galactosidase A gene: increased exon inclusion results in the Fabry cardiac phenotype. *Am J Hum Genet.*,Vol.4, No. 70, (April 2002), pp. 994-1002, ISSN 0002-9297

Kerem, E.; Hirawat, S.; Armoni, S.; Yaakov, Y.; Shoseyov, D.; Cohen, M.; Nissim-Rafinia, M.; Blau, H.; Rivlin, J.; Aviram, M.; Elfring, GL.; Northcutt, VJ.; Miller, LL.; Kerem, B. & Wilschanski, M. (2008). Effectiveness of PTC124 treatment of cystic fibrosis caused by nonsense mutations: a prospective phase II trial. *Lancet*, Vol. 9640, No. 372, (August 2008), pp. 719-727, ISSN 1474-547X

Kidney Disease: Improving Global Outcomes (KDIGO) CKD-MBD Work Group. (2009) KDIGO clinical practice guideline for the diagnosis, evaluation, prevention, and treatment of Chronic Kidney Disease-Mineral and Bone Disorder (CKD-MBD). *Kidney Int Suppl.*, No. 113, (August 2009), pp. 1-130, ISSN 0098-6577

Kidney Disease Outcomes Quality Initiative (K/DOQI). (2004). K/DOQI clinical practice guidelines on hypertension and antihypertensive agents in chronic kidney disease. *Am J Kidney Dis.*, Vol. 5, No. 53, (May 2004), pp. 1-290, ISSN 1523-6838

Lambers Heerspink, HJ.; Agarwal, R.; Coyne, DW.; Parving, HH.; Ritz, E.; Remuzzi, G.; Audhya, P.; Amdahl, MJ.; Andress, DL. & de Zeeuw, D. (2009) The selective vitamin D receptor activator for albuminuria lowering (VITAL) study: study design and baseline characteristics. *Am J Nephrol.*, Vol. 3, No. 30, (June 2009), pp. 280-286, ISSN 1421-9670

Linhart, A. & Elliott, PM. (2007) The heart in Anderson-Fabry disease and other lysosomal storage disorders. *Heart*, Vol. 4, No. 93, (April 2007), pp. 528-535, ISSN 1468-201X

Linthorst, GE.; Vedder, AC.; Aerts, JM. & Hollak, CE. (2005) Screening for Fabry disease using whole blood spots fails to identify one-third of female carriers. *Clin Chim Acta.*, Vol 1-2, No. 353, (March 2005), pp. 201-203, ISSN 0009-8981

Linthorst, GE.; Germain, DP.; Hollak, CE.; Hughes, D.; Rolfs, A.; Wanner, C. & Mehta, A. (2011). Expert opinion on temporary treatment recommendations for Fabry disease during the shortage of enzyme replacement therapy (ERT). *Mol Genet Metab.*, Vol. 1, No. 102, (January 2011), pp. 99-102, ISSN 1096-7206

MacDermot, KD.; Holmes, A. & Miners, AH. (2001) Anderson–Fabry disease: clinical manifestations and impact of disease in a cohort of 98 hemizygous males. *J Med Genet.*, Vol. 11, No. 38, (November 2001), pp. 750-760, ISSN 1468-6244

Mason, RM. & Wahab, NA. (2003) Extracellular matrix metabolism in diabetic nephropathy. *J Am Soc Nephrol.* Vol. 5, No. 14, (May 2003), pp. 1358-1373, ISSN 1046-6673

Mehta, A.; Ricci, R.; Widmer, U.; Dehout, F.; Garcia de Lorenzo, A.; Kampmann, C.; Linhart, A.; Sunder-Plassmann, G.; Ries, M. & Beck, M. (2004) Fabry disease defined: baseline clinical manifestations of 366 patients in the Fabry Outcome Survey. *Eur J Clin Invest.*, Vol. 3, No. 34, (March 2004), pp. 236-242, ISSN 0014-2972

Mehta, A.; Ginsberg, L.; FOS Investigators. (2005) Natural history of the cerebrovascular complications of Fabry disease. *Acta Paediatr.*, Vol. 447, No. 94, (March 2005), pp 24-27, ISSN 0803-5326

Mehta, A.; Beck, M. & Sunder-Plassmann, G. (2006). *Fabry Disease: Perspectives from 5 Years of FOS.* Oxford: Oxford PharmaGenesis, ISBN-10: 1-903539-03-X

Mehta, A.; Beck, M.; Elliott, P.; Giugliani, R.; Linhart, A.; Sunder-Plassmann, G.; Schiffmann, R.; Barbey, F.; Ries M & Clarke, JT.; Fabry Outcome Survey investigators. (2009). Enzyme replacement therapy with agalsidase alfa in patients with Fabry's disease: an analysis of registry data. *Lancet*, Vol. 9706, No. 374, (December 2009), pp. 1986-1996, ISSN 1474-547X

Mischak, H.; Delles, C.; Klein, J. & Schanstra, JP. (2010). Urinary proteomics based on capillary electrophoresis-coupled mass spectrometry in kidney disease: discovery and validation of biomarkers, and clinical application. *Adv Chronic Kidney Dis.*, Vol. 6, No. 17, (November 2010), pp. 493-506, ISSN 1548-5609

Mitsias, P. & Levine SR. (1996) Cerebrovascular complications of Fabry's disease. *Ann Neurol.*, Vol. 1, No. 40, (July 1996), pp. 8-17, ISSN 0364-5134

Mogami, K.; Kishi, H. & Kobayashi, S. (2005) Sphingomyelinase causes endothelium-dependent vasorelaxation through endothelial nitric oxide production without cytosolic Ca(2+) elevation. *FEBS Lett.*, Vol. 2, No. 579, (January 2005), pp. 393-397, ISSN 0014-5793

Moreno, JA.; Sanchez-Niño, MD.; Sanz, AB.; Lassila, M.; Holthofer, H.; Blanco-Colio, LM.; Egido, J.; Ruiz-Ortega, M. & Ortiz, A. (2008). A slit in podocyte death. *Curr Med Chem.*, Vol. 16, No. 15, (2008), pp. 1645-1654, ISSN 0929-8673

Najafian. B.; Svarstad, E.; Bostad, L.; Gubler, MC.; Tøndel, C.; Whitley, C.& Mauer, M. (2011). Progressive podocyte injury and globotriaosylceramide (GL-3) accumulation in young patients with Fabry disease. *Kidney Int.*, Vol. 6, No. 79, (March 2011), pp. 663-670, ISSN 1523-1755

Nakao, S.; Kodama, C.; Takenaka, T.; Tanaka, A.; Yasumoto, Y.; Yoshida, A.; Kanzaki, T.; Enriquez, AL.; Eng, CM.; Tanaka, H.; Tei, C. & Desnick RJ. (2003). Fabry disease: detection of undiagnosed hemodialysis patients and identification of a "renal variant" phenotype. *Kidney Int.*, Vol. 3, No. 64, (September 2003), pp. 801-807, ISSN 0085-2538

Nance, CS.; Klein, CJ.; Banikazemi, M.; Dikman, SH.; Phelps, RG.; McArthur, JC.; Rodriguez, M. & Desnick, RJ. (2006) Later-onset Fabry disease: an adult variant presenting with the cramp-fasciculation syndrome. *Arch Neurol.*, Vol. 3, No. 63, (March 2006), pp. 453-457, ISSN 0003-9942

Nath, KA. (1992) Tubulointerstitial changes as a major determinant in the progression of renal damage. *Am J Kidney Dis.*, Vol. 1, No. 20, (July1992), pp. 1-17, ISSN 0272-6386

National Kidney Foundation. (2003) K/DOQI clinical practice guidelines for bone metabolism and disease in chronic kidney disease. *Am J Kidney Dis.*,Vol. 4, No. 42, (October 2003), pp. 1-201, ISSN 1523-6838

Nguyen, TT.; Gin, T.; Nicholls, K.; Low, M.; Galanos, J. & Crawford, A. (2005) Ophthalmological manifestations of Fabry disease: a survey of patients at the Royal Melbourne Fabry Disease Treatment Centre. *Clin Experiment Ophthalmol.*, Vol. 2, No. 33, (April 2005), pp. 164-168, ISSN 1442-6404

O'Brien, BD.; Shnitka, TK.; McDougall, R.; Walker, K.; Costopoulos, L.; Lentle, B.; Anholt, L.; Freeman, H. & Thomsom, AB. (1982) Pathophysiologic and ultrastructural basis for intestinal symptoms in Fabry's disease. *Gastroenterology*. Vol. 5, No. 82, (May 1982), pp. 957-962, ISSN 0016-5085

Ogawa, K.; Sugamata, K.; Funamoto, N.; Abe, T.; Sato, T.; Nagashima, K. & Ohkawa, S. (1990). Restricted accumulation of globotriaosylceramide in the hearts of atypical cases of Fabry's disease. *Hum Pathol.*, Vol. 10, No. 21, (October 1990), pp. 1067-1073, ISSN 0046-8177

Oqvist, B.; Brenner, BM.; Oliveira, JP.; Ortiz, A.; Schaefer, R.; Svarstad, E.; Wanner, C.; Zhang, K. & Warnock, DG. (2009). Nephropathy in Fabry disease: the importance of early diagnosis and testing in high-risk populations. *Nephrol Dial Transplant.*, Vol. 6, No. 24, (June 2009), pp. 1736-1743, ISSN 1460-2385

Ortiz, A.; Oliveira, JP.; Waldek, S.; Warnock, DG.; Cianciaruso, B. & Wanner, C.; Fabry Registry. (2008). Nephropathy in males and females with Fabry disease: cross-sectional description of patients before treatment with enzyme replacement therapy. *Nephrol Dial Transplant.*, Vol. 5, No. 23, (May 2008), pp. 1600-1167, ISSN 1460-2385

Ortiz, A.; Oliveira, JP.; Wanner, C.; Brenner, BM.; Waldek, S. & Warnock, DG. (2008). Recommendations and guidelines for the diagnosis and treatment of Fabry nephropathy in adults. *Nat Clin Pract Nephrol.*, Vol. 6, No. 4, (June 2008), pp. 327-336, ISSN 1745-8331

Ortiz, A.; Cianciaruso, B.; Cizmarik, M.; Germain, DP.; Mignani, R.; Oliveira, JP.; Villalobos, J.; Vujkovac, B.; Waldek, S.; Wanner, C. & Warnock, DG. (2010). End-stage renal disease in patients with Fabry disease: natural history data from the Fabry Registry. *Nephrol Dial Transplant.*, Vol. 3, No. 25, (March 2010), pp. 769-775, ISSN 1460-2385

Pagano, RE. (2003) Endocytic trafficking of glycosphingolipids in sphingolipid storage diseases. *Philos Trans R Soc Lond B Biol Sci.*, Vol. 1433, No. 358, (May 2003), pp. 885-891, ISSN 0962-8436

Pantsulaia, T. (2006) Role of TGF-beta in pathogenesis of diabetic nephropathy. *Georgian Med News.*, No.131, (February 2006), pp. 13-18, ISSN 1512-0112

Park, IS.; Kiyomoto, H.; Abboud, SL. & Abboud, HE. (1997) Expression of transforming growth factor-beta and type IV collagen in early streptozotocin-induced diabetes. *Diabetes*, Vol. 3, No. 46, (March 1997), pp. 473-480, ISSN 0012-1797

Patel, MR.; Cecchi, F.; Cizmarik, M.; Kantola, I.; Linhart, A.; Nicholls, K.; Strotmann, J.; Tallaj, J.; Tran, TC.; West, ML.; Beitner-Johnson, D. & Abiose, A. (2011).Cardiovascular events in patients with fabry disease natural history data from the fabry registry. *J Am Coll Cardiol.*, Vol. 9, No. 57, (March 2011), pp. 1093-1099, ISSN 1558-3597

Ries, M.; Bettis, KE.; Choyke, P.; Kopp, JB.; Austin, HA 3rd.; Brady, RO. & Schiffmann, R. (2004). Parapelvic kidney cysts: a distinguishing feature with high prevalence in Fabry disease. *Kidney Int.*, Vol. 3, No. 66, (September 2004), pp. 978-982, ISSN 0085-2538

Ries, M.; Gupta, S.; Moore, DF.; Sachdev, V.; Quirk, JM.; Murray, GJ.; Rosing, DR.; Robinson, C.; Schaefer, E.; Gal, A.; Dambrosia, JM.; Garman, SC.; Brady, RO. & Schiffmann, R. (2005). Pediatric Fabry disease. *Pediatrics*, Vol. 3, No. 115, (March 2005), pp. 344-355, ISSN 1098-4275

Ries, M.; Kim, HJ.; Zalewski, CK.; Mastroianni, MA.; Moore, DF.; Brady, RO.; Dambrosia, JM.; Schiffmann, R. & Brewer. CC. (2007). Neuropathic and cerebrovascular correlates of hearing loss in Fabry disease. *Brain*, Vol. 1, No. 130, (January 2007), pp. 143-150, ISSN 1460-2156

Rodríguez-González-Herrero, ME.; Marín-Sánchez, JM.; Gimeno, JR.; Molero-Izquierdo, C.; De-Casas-Fernández, A.; Rodríguez-González-Herrero, B.; San-Román, I.; Lozano, J.; De-la-Morena, G. & Llovet-Osuna, F. (2008). Ophthalmological manifestations in Fabry's disease. Four clinical cases showing deficient alpha-galactosidase-A activity. *Arch Soc Esp Oftalmol.*, Vol. 12, No. 83, (December 2008), pp. 713-717, ISSN 1989-7286

Rojas-Rivera, J.; De La Piedra, C.; Ramos, A.; Ortiz, A. & Egido, J. (2010). The expanding spectrum of biological actions of vitamin D. *Nephrol Dial Transplant.*, Vol. 9, No. 25, (September 2010), pp. 2850-2865, ISSN 1460-2385

Rombach, SM.; Dekker, N.; Bouwman, MG.; Linthorst, GE.; Zwinderman, AH.; Wijburg, FA.; Kuiper, S.; Vd Bergh Weerman, MA.; Groener, JE.; Poorthuis, BJ.; Hollak, CE. & Aerts, JM. (2010). Plasma globotriaosylsphingosine: diagnostic value and relation to clinical manifestations of Fabry disease. *Biochim Biophys Acta.*, Vol. 9, No. 1802, (Septemer 2010), pp. 741-748, ISSN 0006-3002

Romeo, G.; D'Urso, M.; Pisacane, A.; Blum, E.; De Falco, A. & Ruffilli, A. (1975). Residual activity of alpha-galactosidase A in Fabry's disease. *Biochem Genet.*, Vol. 9-10, No. 13, (October 1975), pp.615-628, ISSN 0002-9343

Rosenberg, DM.; Ferrans, VJ.; Fulmer, JD.; Line, BR.; Barranger, JA.; Brady, RO. & Crystal, RG. (1980). Chronic airflow obstruction in Fabry's disease. *Am J Med.*, Vol. 6, No. 68, (June 1980), pp. 898-905, ISSN 0002-9343

Rowe, JW.; Gilliam, JI. & Warthin, TA. (1974). Intestinal manifestations of Fabry's disease. *Ann Intern Med.*, Vol. 5, No. 81, (November 1974), pp. 628-631, ISSN 0003-4819

Sanchez-Niño, MD.; Sanz, AB.; Ihalmo, P.; Lassila, M.; Holthofer, H.; Mezzano, S.; Aros, C.; Groop, PH.; Saleem, MA.; Mathieson, PW.; Langham, R.; Kretzler, M.; Nair, V.; Lemley, KV.; Nelson, RG.; Mervaala, E.; Mattinzoli, D.; Rastaldi, MP.; Ruiz-Ortega, M.; Martin-Ventura, JL.; Egido, J. & Ortiz, A. (2009). The MIF receptor CD74 in diabetic podocyte injury. *J Am Soc Nephrol.*, Vol. 2, No. 20, (February 2009), pp. 353-362, ISSN 1533-3450

Sanchez-Niño, MD.; Sanz, AB.; Carrasco, S.; Saleem, MA.; Mathieson, PW.; Valdivielso, JM.; Ruiz-Ortega, M.; Egido, J. & Ortiz, A. (2010). Globotriaosylsphingosine actions on human glomerular podocytes: implications for Fabry nephropathy. *Nephrol Dial Transplant.*, (May 2010) [Epub ahead of print], ISSN 1460-2385

Sanchez-Niño, MD.; Benito-Martin, A. & Ortiz, A. (2010). New paradigms in cell death in human diabetic nephropathy. *Kidney Int.*, Vol. 8, No. 78, (October 2010), pp. 737-744, ISSN 1523-1755

Schaefer, RM.; Tylki-Szymańska, A. & Hilz, MJ. (2009). Enzyme replacement therapy for Fabry disease: a systematic review of available evidence. *Drugs*, Vol. 16, No. 69, (November 2009), pp. 2179-2205, ISSN 0012-6667

Schieppati, A. & Remuzzi, G. (2003). Proteinuria and its consequences in renal disease. *Acta Paediatr Suppl.*, Vol. 443, No. 92, (December 2003), pp. 9-13, ISSN 0803-5326

Schiffmann, R.; Kopp, JB.; Austin, HA 3rd.; Sabnis, S.; Moore, DF.; Weibel, T.; Balow, JE. & Brady, RO. (2001). Enzyme replacement therapy in Fabry disease: a randomized controlled trial. *JAMA.*, Vol. 21, No. 285, (June 2001), pp. 2743-2749, ISSN 0098-7484

Schiffmann, R. & Scott, LJ. (2002) Pathophysiology and assessment of neuropathic pain in Fabry disease. *Acta Paediatr Suppl.*, Vol. 439, No. 91, (2002), pp. 48-52, ISSN 0803-5326

Schiffmann, R.; Ries, M.; Timmons, M.; Flaherty, JT. & Brady, RO. (2006). Long-term therapy with agalsidase alfa for Fabry disease: safety and effects on renal function in a home infusion setting. *Nephrol Dial Transplant.*, Vol. 2, No. 21, (February 2006), pp. 345-354, ISSN 0931-0509

Schiffmann, R.; Rapkiewicz, A.; Abu-Asab, M.; Ries, M.; Askari, H.; Tsokos, M. & Quezado, M. (2006). Pathological findings in a patient with Fabry disease who died after 2.5 years of enzyme replacement. *Virchows Arch.*, Vol. 3, No. 448, (March 2006), pp. 337-343, ISSN 0945-6317

Schiffmann, R. (2009). Fabry disease. *Pharmacol Ther.*, Vol. 1, No. 122, (April 2009), pp. 65-77, ISSN 1879-016X

Schiffmann, R.; Warnock, DG.; Banikazemi, M.; Bultas, J.; Linthorst, GE.; Packman, S.; Sorensen, SA.; Wilcox, WR. & Desnick, RJ. (2009). Fabry disease: progression of nephropathy, and prevalence of cardiac and cerebrovascular events before enzyme replacement therapy. *Nephrol Dial Transplant.*, Vol. 7, No. 24, (July 2009), pp. 2102-2111, ISSN 1460-2385

Shah, JS. & Elliott, PM. (2005). Fabry disease and the heart: an overview of the natural history and the effect of enzyme replacement therapy. *Acta Paediatr Suppl.*, Vol. 447, No. 94, (March 2005), pp. 11-14, ISSN 0803-5326

Sharma, K.; Ziyadeh, FN.; Alzahabi, B.; McGowan, TA.; Kapoor, S.; Kurnik, BR.; Kurnik, PB. & Weisberg, LS. (1997). Increased renal production of transforming growth factor-beta1 in patients with type II diabetes. *Diabetes.* Vol. 5, No. 46, (May 1997), pp. 854-859, ISSN 0012-1797

Shen, JS., Meng, XL., Moore, DF., Quirk, JM., Shayman, JA., Schiffmann, R. & Kaneski, CR. (2008) Globotriaosylceramide induces oxidative stress and up-regulates cell adhesion molecule expression in Fabry disease endothelial cells. *Mol Genet Metab.*, Vol. 3, No. 95, (November 2008), pp. 163-168, ISSN 1096-7206

Sims, K.; Politei, J.; Banikazemi, M. & Lee, P. (2009). Stroke in Fabry disease frequently occurs before diagnosis and in the absence of other clinical events: natural history data from the Fabry Registry. *Stroke*, Vol. 3, No. 40, (March 2009), pp. 788-794, ISSN 1524-4628

Sunder-Plassmann, G. (2006). Renal manifestations of Fabry disease, In: *Fabry Disease: Perspectives from 5 Years of FOS,* Mehta, A.; Beck M. & Sunder-Plassmann G., Oxford: Oxford PharmaGenesis, ISN 190353903X, Oxford

Svarstad, E., Iversen, BM. & Bostad, L. (2004). Bedside stereomicroscopy of renal biopsies may lead to a rapid diagnosis of Fabry's disease. *Nephrol Dial Transplant.*, Vol. 12, No. 19, (December 2004), pp. 3202-3203.

Tahir, H.; Jackson, LL. & Warnock, DG. (2007). Antiproteinuric therapy and fabry nephropathy: sustained reduction of proteinuria in patients receiving enzyme replacement therapy with agalsidase-beta. *J Am Soc Nephrol.*, Vol. 9, No. 18, (September 2007), pp. 2609-2617, ISSN 1046-6673

Thadhani, R.; Wolf, M.; West, ML.; Tonelli, M.; Ruthazer, R.; Pastores, GM. & Obrador, GT. (2002). Patients with Fabry disease on dialysis in the United States. *Kidney Int.*, Vol. 1, No. 61, (January 2002), pp. 249-255, ISSN 0085-2538

Thomas, ME.; Brunskill, NJ.; Harris, KP.; Bailey, E.; Pringle, JH.; Furness, PN. & Walls, J. (1999). Proteinuria induces tubular cell turnover: A potential mechanism for tubular atrophy. *Kidney Int.*, Vol. 3, No. 55, (March 1999), pp. 890-898, ISSN 0085-2538

Togawa, T.; Kodama, T.; Suzuki, T.; Sugawara, K.; Tsukimura, T.; Ohashi, T.; Ishige, N.; Suzuki, K.; Kitagawa, T. & Sakuraba, H. (2010). Plasma globotriaosylsphingosine as a biomarker of Fabry disease. *Mol Genet Metab.*, Vol. 3, No. 100, (July 2010), pp. 257-261, ISSN 1096-7206

Togawa, T.; Kawashima, I.; Kodama, T.; Tsukimura, T.; Suzuki, T.; Fukushige, T.; Kanekura, T. & Sakuraba, H. (2010). Tissue and plasma globotriaosylsphingosine could be a biomarker for assessing enzyme replacement therapy for Fabry disease. *Biochem Biophys Res Commun.*, Vol. 4, No. 399, (September 2010), pp. 716-720, ISSN 1090-2104

Tøndel, C.; Bostad, L.; Hirth, A. & Svarstad, E. (2008). Renal biopsy findings in children and adolescents with Fabry disease and minimal albuminuria. *Am J Kidney Dis.*, Vol. 5, No. 51, (May 2008), pp. 767-776, ISSN 1523-6838

Torra, R. (2008). Renal manifestations in Fabry disease and therapeutic options. *Kidney Int.*, No. 111, (December 2008), pp. 23-32, ISSN 0098-6577

Torra, R.; Oliveira, JP. & Ortiz, A. (2010). UGA hopping: a sport for nephrologists too? *Nephrol Dial Transplant.*, Vol. 8, No. 25, (August 2010), pp. 2391-2395, ISSN 1460-2385

Tryggvason, K. & Pettersson, E. (2003) Causes and consequences of proteinuria: the kidney filtration barrier and progressive renal failure. *J Intern Med.*, Vol. 3, No. 254, (September 2003), pp. 216-224, ISSN 0954-6820

Tsakiris, D.; Simpson, HK.; Jones, EH.; Briggs, JD.; Elinder, CG.; Mendel, S.; Piccoli, G.; dos Santos, JP.; Tognoni, G.; Vanrenterghem, Y. & Valderrabano, F. (1996). Report on management of renal failure in Europe, XXVI, 1995. Rare diseases in renal replacement therapy in the ERA-EDTA Registry. *Nephrol Dial Transplant.*, Suppl. 7, No. 11, (1996), pp. 4-20, ISSN 0931-0509

Utsumi, K.; Yamamoto, N.; Kase, R.; Takata, T.; Okumiya, T.; Saito, H.; Suzuki, T.; Uyama, E. & Sakuraba, H. (1997). High incidence of thrombosis in Fabry's disease. *Intern Med.*, Vol. 5, No. 36, (May 1997), pp. 327-329, ISSN 0918-2918

van Breemen, MJ.; Rombach, SM.; Dekker, N.; Poorthuis, BJ.; Linthorst, GE.; Zwinderman, AH.; Breunig, F.; Wanner, C.; Aerts, JM. & Hollak, CE. (2011). Reduction of elevated plasma globotriaosylsphingosine in patients with classic Fabry disease following enzyme replacement therapy. *Biochim Biophys Acta.*, Vol. 1, No. 1812, (January 2011), pp. 70-76, ISSN 0006-3002

Vedder, AC.; Strijland, A.; vd Bergh Weerman, MA.; Florquin, S.; Aerts, JM. & Hollak, CE. (2006). Manifestations of Fabry disease in placental tissue. *J Inherit Metab Dis.*, Vol. 1, No. 29, (February 2006), pp. 106-111, ISSN 0141-8955

Vedder, AC.; Linthorst, GE.; Houge, G.; Groener, JE.; Ormel, EE.; Bouma, BJ.; Aerts, JM.; Hirth, A. & Hollak, CE. (2007). Treatment of Fabry disease: outcome of a comparative trial with agalsidase alfa or beta at a dose of 0.2 mg/kg. *PLoS One*, Vol. 7, No. 2, (July 2007), pp. 598, ISSN 1932-6203

Wang, RY.; Lelis, A.; Mirocha, J. & Wilcox, WR. (2007). Heterozygous Fabry women are not just carriers, but have a significant burden of disease and impaired quality of life. *Genet Med.*, Vol. 1, No. 9, (January 2007), pp. 34-45, ISSN 1098-3600

Wanner, C., Oliveira, JP., Ortiz, A., Mauer, M., Germain, DP., Linthorst, GE., Serra, AL., Maródi, L., Mignani, R., Cianciaruso, B., Vujkovac, B., Lemay, R., Beitner-Johnson, D., Waldek, S. & Warnock, DG. (2010). Prognostic indicators of renal disease progression in adults with Fabry disease: natural history data from the Fabry Registry. *Clin J Am Soc Nephrol.*, Vol. 12, No. 5, (December 2010), pp. 2220-2228, ISSN 1555-905X

Wilcox, WR.; Oliveira, JP.; Hopkin, RJ.; Ortiz, A.; Banikazemi, M.; Feldt-Rasmussen, U.; Sims, K.; Waldek, S.; Pastores, GM.; Lee, P.; Eng, CM.; Marodi, L.; Stanford, KE.; Breunig, F.; Wanner, C.; Warnock, DG.; Lemay, RM. & Germain, DP; Fabry Registry. (2008). Females with Fabry disease frequently have major organ involvement: lessons from the Fabry Registry. *Mol Genet Metab.*, Vol. 2, No. 93, (February 2008), pp. 112-128, ISSN 1096-7206

Zarate, YA. & Hopkin, R J. (2008). Fabry's disease. *Lancet.* Vol. 9647, No. 372, (October 2008), pp. 1427-1435, ISSN 1474-547X

14

Fabry Cardiomyopathy: A Global View

Rocio Toro Cebada, Alipio Magnas and Jose Luis Zamorano
Departamento de Medicina de la Universidad de Cadiz, c/DR Marañon S/N, Cadiz
Spain

1. Introduction

Fabry disease (FD) is a lysosomal storage disease (LSD). It has been stated that the second most common LSD after Gaucher disease is Fabry disease; its worldwide incidence is from approximately 1 in 40 000 to 1 in 117 000 live newborns for the classic form of the disease, but the precise prevalence is unknown. Wide variations in the prevalence of FD have been reported in different countries and, with increasing awareness and screening, it is likely that the actual prevalence may be higher than previously recorded, particularly when late-onset phenotypes are taken into account. An accurate estimation of its epidemiology is difficult to make because FD is clinically very heterogeneous and its early classic manifestations tend to be non-specific and often unrecognized. Patients are therefore frequently mis-diagnosed, or not diagnosed until late in life. Recently a newborn screening showed an incidence of one in 3100 live-newborns, and according to this study, the later-onset forms of FD present a surprisingly high incidence [1].

Lysosomal biogenesis involves ongoing synthesis of lysosomal hydrolases, membrane constitutive proteins, and new membranes. Lysosomes originate in the fusion of trans-Golgi network vesicles (TGN) with late endosomes. Progressive vesicular acidification accompanies the maturation of the TGN vesicles and this gradient facilitates the pH-dependent dissociation of receptors and ligands, as well as activation of lysosomal hydrolases.

Abnormalities at any stage of the biosynthesis can impair enzyme activation and lead to lysosomal storage disorder. Lysosomal integral or associated membrane proteins are sorted to the membrane or interior of the lysosome by several different signals. Phosphorylation, sulfation, additional proteolytic processing, and macromolecular assembly of heteromers occur concurrently. These are critical to enzyme function, and defects can result in multiple enzyme / protein deficiencies.

The common pathway for LSD is the accumulation of specific macromolecules within tissues and cells that normally have a high flux of these substrates. The majority of lysosomal enzyme deficiencies result from point mutations or genetic arrangements at a locus that encodes a single lysosomal hydrolase[3-5].

Most LSDs are inherited as autosomal recessive disorders, except Hunter and FD. The latter is an X-linked inherited lysosomal storage disorder that results from mutations in the α-galactosidase gene. The gene encoding human α-galactosidase A enzyme (α-Gal A), located at Xq22.1, spans genomic sequences of approximately 13 kb, containing seven exons, which have been isolated and characterized [6,7].

Alpha-galactosidase A is a lysosomal exoglycohydrolase. The mature α-Gal A enzyme polypeptide is 398 amino acids and contains three functional N-glycosylation sites. The active enzyme is a homodimer of approximately 101 kd. This mutation has significant consequences in glycosphingolipid catabolism resulting from deficient or absent activity of the lysosomal enzyme α-gal A. This enzyme helps to break down and remove glycolipids. The enzymatic defect leads to progressive accumulation of the glycolipid globotriaosyl ceramide (Gb3 or Gl3), or ceramide trihexoside, in the lysosomes in the cells of most organs. Substrate accumulation leads to lysosomal distortion, which has significant pathologic consequences [8-9].

Up to now, more than 300 mutations that cause FD have been identified, including missense, nonsense, small deletions and insertions, large gene rearrangements, and splice mutations. Most mutations are private and unique, occurring in one or a few affected families. In the cardiac variant of FD all individuals to date have missense or splicing mutations that express residual α-Gal A activity. All renal variants identified to date have been associated with missense mutations. Three mutations (p.Arg112His, p.Arg301Gln, and p.Gly328Arg) have been identified in individuals with the classic phenotype and the cardiac variant phenotype, suggesting that other modifying factors are involved in disease expression. Therefore it is necessary to sequence the entire α-gal A gene and adjacent regions to identify the FD mutation in a family [10-14].

FD is considered highly penetrating in males, although variable in its expression. In affected males, the clinical diagnosis is confirmed by α-gal A deficiency. The majority of males with FD have absent or very low enzyme activity (1–2% of normal level) and classical phenotype with multiple disease manifestations. Males who show higher residual enzyme activity, approximately 3–10% of normal level, appear to have milder expression of FD. These individuals are diagnosed with FD later in life, after cardiomyopathy of unknown etiology (in most cases, hypertrophic cardiomyopathy - HMC) is discovered [4].

About 60–70% of females heterozygous for a Fabry disease mutation have some disease manifestations, and approximately 10% of these heterozygous females have severe manifestations, similar to the phenotype in males. Enzyme activity is not reliable for determining female carrier status because women who are obligate carriers have variable levels of α-gal A that can overlap with enzyme levels found in healthy controls. Therefore it is necessary to sequence the entire α-gal A gene and adjacent regions to identify the Fabry disease mutation in a family. The absence of family history suggestive of FD, or de novo mutations documented, does not rule out the diagnosis of FD. The rate of new mutations is unknown [8].

2. Cellular physiopathology

Many theories have been proposed with respect to the pathology of FD. It has been hypothesized that the overloading of lysosomes with Gb3 simply leads to the apoptosis of the cell [15]. Another theory argues that the inflammation process is related to the accumulation of Gb3. This theory has been defended based on the parallel structure between Gb3 and CD77, which is supposed to play an important role in apoptosis and necrosis [16]. Finally, Gb3-accumulation has been reported to induce oxidative stress and/or the formation reactive oxygen species (ROS). Another gateway into alteration of endothelial function may be given by the Nitric-Oxide-Synthase-3-genotypes. Endothelium-derived nitric oxide (eNO), produced by eNO synthase (eNOS), is a key regulator of vessel wall function and cardiovascular homeostasis[17]. Furthermore, the possible relationship between the relative thickness of the left posterior wall and endothelium-derived nitric oxide synthase has been demonstrated. These are the first data showing a significant association of non-GLA-derived sequence variants with the cardiac phenotype in Fabry disease that may, in part, explain the great phenotypic variability of the disease[18].

3. Clinical presentation

Clinically, FD may present as cardiomyopathy, renal disease or neurological small-vessels disease. The age range at which FD presents is quite broad and extends from childhood to the forties, depending on the enzyme residual activity.

Nephropathy is one of the major complications of FD: the nephropathy is progressive and is marked by a persistent insidious development. An analysis of the causes of death reported for 181 affected relatives and 42 patients (699 males and 754 females), enrolled in the Fabry outcome survey (FOS) indicates that the incidence of renal disease as a cause of death appears to be decreasing, while the incidence of cardiac disease is increasing; these trends probably reflect improvements in the management of renal disease in these patients. By adulthood, renal failure frequently becomes a major complication of FD, with more than 50% of male and more than 20% of female patients eventually developing advanced renal disease or end-stage renal disease (ESRD) [19-20].

Effects on the renal system in FD can and need to be detected in the earlier years of life. Renal involvement has previously been categorized as the second phase of the disease and, as stated by West et al.,[21] older patients are more likely to be diagnosed with severe Fabry nephropathy on their first consultation.

Microalbuminuria is one of the first signs of impairment of renal function, and overt proteinuria may start as early as 10 years of age. Biopsy studies have shown that glomerular and vascular changes are present before progression to overt proteinuria, although chronic kidney lesions may already be present. In young patients, glomerular hyperfiltration can mask the detection of early decline in the glomerular filtration rate (GFR) to the extent that a critical number of nephrons become damaged and cannot maintain adequate glomerular filtration.

The decline in GFR typically commences once proteinuria is established but may precede it. Overt proteinuria is more prominent in men than in women. Proteinuria is a risk factor for progression of nephropathy.

Progression to ESRD is common in hemizygous males (in the third to fifth decades of life), and this population group presents more rapid rates of FD progression than those who do not suffer ESRD. The survival of patients with FD in dialysis is better than that of diabetic patients, but it is clearly decreased compared with uremic patients with other nephropathies, despite a lower mean age of uremia. The outcome of kidney transplantation is similar to that found in other patients with ESRD, despite controversial issues published in the past. The use of a kidney donor with normal α-Gal-A activity in the control of the metabolic systemic disease is unproven. The recurrence of Gb3 deposits in the kidney graft has been documented only rarely [20].

Cardiac involvement is very common and is the most frequent cause of death not only in hemizygote males but also in female heterozygote carriers with α-Gal A deficiency, with a reduction of life expectancy of approximately 20 and 15 years respectively. The heart may be the only organ affected in the classic phenotype of FD, and this is designated the "cardiac variant". Within the heart, the myocites, vascular endothelium, conducting system and valves can all be affected. Abnormal storage of the lipid in the blood vessels, with eventual occlusion of the small arterioles, leads to most of the clinical manifestations. Although cardiac involvement of FD begins early, the average age for presenting clinically overt cardiac symptoms (including dyspnea, reduced exercise tolerance, angina, chest pain, palpitations, ventricular arrhythmias, syncope, transient ischemic attacks, stroke and heart failure) has been reported to be 32 years in men and 40 years in women. Cardiovascular manifestations include renovascular and systemic hypertension, aortic root dilatation, mitral prolapse and congestive heart failure [22].

Although angina is often reported, the incidence of epicardial coronary stenosis is not a dominant feature, and is probably related to coronary microvascular dysfunction. In respect of arrhythmias, a broad spectrum can be seen including shortened or prolonged PR-intervals, AV blocks of different degrees and, sometimes, malignant ventricular arrhythmias. The most frequent cardiac manifestations of the disease are permanent and paroxysmal atrial fibrillation and intermittent ventricular tachycardia. Moreover, an impairment of autonomic control of the heart in boys with FD increases heart variability and may be responsible for the increased cardiac morbidity [23].

LV hypertrophy is detected in more than 50% of patients. It is more frequent and has an earlier age of onset in males than in females. LVH is a hallmark of FD that can initially present with preserved ventricular function, as has been reported in 3% of men with LVH, and in up to 6% of men and 12% of women with late-onset hypertrophic cardiomyopathy (HCM). LVH is generally symmetrical, although asymmetric septal hypertrophy has been described, and the condition can mimic the phenotypical and clinical features of HCM.

FD is a relatively prevalent cause of HCM and is associated with significant morbidity and early death due to heart failure or ventricular arrhythmias. HCM, mainly characterized by LVH and conduction abnormalities, may in fact be the major presenting feature of the disease.

The electrocardiogram may show LV hypertrophy, P-wave abnormalities, conduction defects, and ventricular dysrhythmias. Typically the echocardiogram shows marked increases in wall thickness and ventricular dilatation later in the disease process. Leaflet and cuspid thickening can be seen, and this produces valve impairment that usually does not require surgical treatment [24] .

Tissue Doppler Imaging (TDI) and strain rate echocardiography represent new echocardiographic tools. In particular, with TDI allow measuring myocardial contraction and relaxation velocities can be measured, thus providing an objective assessment of both diastolic and systolic ventricular function. In addition, it has been demonstrated that specific TDI parameters (E\Ea ratio) provide a good estimate of left ventricular and atrial filling pressure. The study of left ventricular hypertrophy and cardiomyopathies represents one of the most important fields of application for this imaging technique. TDI can detect the first sign of myocardial damage in a patient with FC and normal cardiac wall thickness. Furthermore, Tissue Doppler (TD) studies have been shown to be useful in detecting cardiac involvement in female carriers with no systemic manifestations of Fabry disease. TDI analysis in mutation-positive patients can enable professionals to recognize preclinical cardiac damage in Fabry disease: a reduction of TDI velocities may represent the first sign of initial intrinsic myocardial impairment.

The clinical usefulness of TD echocardiography includes a predictive role, in a proper clinical setting. TDI has demonstrated cardiac impairment in patients without LVH, and the correlation between hypertrophy and severity of baseline dysfunction as measured by TDI supports the specificity of this technique. In addition, an inverse relationship between LVH and myocardial systolic velocity (Sa) has been found. Data suggest that Sa correlates very closely with LV wall thickness. In studies, the IVCT was significantly shorter in the group without LVH, compared with the control group, but showed a tendency to be longer in the group with LVH. This may be attributable to the onset of compensating mechanisms as a result of myocardial impairment, due to the stored vacuolated material being mostly confined to the perinuclear zone, with no or only mild instances of fibrosis in this population [26,27].

Cardiac magnetic resonance imaging (c-MRI) with delayed enhancement may be useful in the non-invasive recognition of myocardial fibrosis, in the context of cardiac involvement of FD. With delayed gadolinium enhancement, c-MRI can identify areas of myocardial damage in HCM and in FD. The evaluation of the myocardial location and distribution patterns of delayed enhancement helps in the identification of the two causes of LV hypertrophy, HCM and LVH associated with Fabry cardiomyopathy.

Furthermore, the myocardial T2 relaxation time is prolonged in patients with Fabry's disease compared with that in hypertrophic patients, and its measurement could be complementary to the delayed enhancement technique [28,29].

Dermatological lesions usually appear in hemizygotous patients, but less frequently in children and women. The earliest clinical signs of Fabry disease often manifest as dermatological disturbances such as angiokeratomas, hypohidrosis, acroparesthesias, and impaired thermal and vibration detection. These disturbances are caused by accumulation of cellular globotriaosylceramide in the skin due to deficient lysosomal α-galactosidase A activity.

The simplest recognizable, but not pathognomonic, characteristics are angiokeratomas, described mostly (66%) in males but also (33%) in females. Angiokeratomas, which are another hallmark of FD, are red papulomatous lesions occurring in groups on the buttocks and in umbilical areas, the thighs and genital areas. Telangiectasias have been described, again mostly in men. Some authors have described the typical "FD rash" that includes angiokeratomas and telangiectasias. It has been established that there is an association between these dermatological lesions and other early signs such as proteinuria, paresthesias and cornea verticillata. Facial dysmorphism with a characteristic coarsening of the facial features is increasingly recognized[30, 31].

Xeroderma has also been described; reduced production of tears and saliva affect 50 % of this population. Although hypohidrosis/anhidrosis is a classic feature of FD, it has been detected in only 11.9% of females and 6.4% of males, and is also reported in childhood.

With respect to ocular and auditory symptoms, the most characteristic manifestation is increased vascular tortuosity. Located in the superficial layer of the cornea, using a slit lamp, a haze has been described as the most frequent cornea abnormality. Some authors have suggested that the haze is the natural evolution of cornea verticillata. This latter condition has been described in the majority of patients affected with FD (70%); it is termed cornea verticillata because the deposits are distributed in a vortex pattern. Two types of lens opacity have been described in FD: one type is anterior capsular and subcapsular cataracts, which are always bilateral, and the other type is posterior subcapsular cataracts, which have been described more rarely but specifically, hence these latter have been designated "Fabry cataracts". Vascular lesions are demonstrated using ocular fundus examination [32-34]

High frequency sensorineural hearing loss is common in FD, and affects males earlier in life. Hearing is worse in patients with FD than in the general population, but clinically relevant hearing impairment only affects16% of patients. Sensorineural hearing loss is less common in children than previously reported, although tinnitus appeared to correlate significantly with severity of clinical presentation in children

The earliest neurological manifestation is painful neuropathy observed in the majority of the patients, mean age of onset 9-14 years in males and 16-20 years in females. Most invalidating neuropathic pain is described as acroparesthesias, which can affect the whole body, but are reported mostly in the hands and feet. Fabry neuropathy has a typical neurophysiological pattern that enables it to be differentiated from other neuropathies. The incidence of carpal tunnel syndrome appears higher than in the general population. Gastrointestinal manifestations of autonomous nervous system involvement may range from abdominal pain to diarrhoea and, more rarely, constipation; in women, abdominal pain may be considered, erroneously, to be of gynecological origin. Altered sweating function is a frequent and classic feature. High temperature increases poor tolerance: fever, and high environmental temperature, as well as physical exercise, can trigger acute pain at the extremities with weakness, which is often intense, and generalized malaise. The central nervous system can be affected, and this contributes to earlier mortality, with a median age of 50 years. As happens with the heart, men will typically be affected in their forties, and women ten years later.

Cerebrovascular events (TIAs, stroke), are present in over 25% of FD cases; in FD they occur at a rather early age and increase progressively. The areas most affected are those supplied by posterior circulation. Renal and cardiac disease can co-exist with cerebrovascular disease, and may predispose patients with FD disease to neurological disability and stroke; however, recent data show that most patients (70.9% of males and 76.9% of females) had not experienced renal or cardiac disease before their first stroke. In addition, 50% of males and 38.3% of females had their first stroke before being diagnosed with FD. In female FD patients, who were for a long time considered to be merely "carriers", and so less affected, the prevalence of cerebrovascular events reported now seems to be as high as in male patients. Differences in cerebral blood velocity have been shown in these patients. These observations have been confirmed after the patients had been treated for a long period of time. Typically, MRI may show lesions attributable to small infarctions, and diffuse alteration of the white matter, especially in deeper sections, with images suggestive of arteriolar involvement of the perforating arteries (lacunar infarctions and leukoaraiosis). The 'pulvinar sign' is a characteristic MRI manifestation of FD; it is a symmetric hyperintensity image in both pulvinar nuclei [1, 35-36].

Fabry patients, even those with marked structural alterations of the brain, show only mild cognitive deficits.

Neuro-psychiatric symptoms have been demonstrated in patients affected with FD. Depression is a frequent and under- diagnosed problem. Depression can have a serious effect on quality of life in patients with FD. The high frequency of depression in FD is likely

to be related to the general burden of this chronic multi-organic hereditary disease, but not to the structural brain alterations typical of FD.
Other symptoms associated with FD are gastrointestinal (GI) symptoms. Abdominal pain (often after eating) and diarrhoea are the most frequent manifestations, but other GI symptoms include constipation, nausea and vomiting. The median age of onset of many GI symptoms is before the age of 15 years. FD may be complicated by osteopenia of the lumbar spine and femoral neck.

4. Diagnosis of FD

Diagnosis of FD is often delayed by at least 3 years, and often by 20 years, after the onset of clinical instauration. Male patients with a family member affected need a biochemical analysis in order to measure the plasma or urinary Gb3(lys-Gb3), or α-galactosidase A activity. In addition, genetic analysis of the GLA gene can confirm the diagnosis.
For suspected heterozygotous females, demonstration of markedly decreased α-Gal A enzyme activity in plasma and/or isolated leukocytes confirms the carrier state in a female. In those women with normal α-Gal A enzyme activity, molecular genetic testing is necessary to clarify genetic status. Some studies have confirmed the need for direct sequencing in females, instead of other screening strategies.
Those patients with symptoms suggestive of FD require a screening based on the measurement of the accumulated substrate, Gb3, in the urine, especially male patients. Measurement of enzyme levels and assessment of mutational status using blood spots are increasingly utilized. Similarly, quantifying the enzyme in urine samples by enzyme-linked immunoabsorbent assay (ELISA) shows promise, although such diagnostic methods are only reliable in males[3].
Molecular prenatal diagnosis has become feasible in families with known mutations, or by analysis of intragenetic and closely-linked markers. The prenatal diagnosis of FD is performed using cultured amniocytes, direct and cultured chorionic villi, or blastomeres for preimplantation diagnosis. As soon as the fetal sex is known, the α-Gal A activity or mutation analyses are performed. Chorionic villus sampling is the optimal procedure, providing fresh fetal tissues after the first trimester[37] .

5. Treatment of FD

Specific pharmacologic therapy for FD with enzyme replacement therapy (ERT) is endorsed by health regulatory agencies. Two authorized drugs are available in Europe for ERT.
ERT supplies recombinant GLA to cells and reverses several of the metabolic and pathologic abnormalities. ERT has been available for the treatment of FD since 2001 with the introduction of two products, agalsidase-α (Repaglal@, ShireHGT Inc) and agalsidase β (Fabrazyme, Genzyme Corp).
Agalsidase-α is purified from a stably transfected human cell line 120 and is infused at a dose of 0.2 mg/kg over a period of 40 min, every two weeks. The extra efficacy of agalsidase alpha administered at 0.2 mg/kg in weekly infusions may be beneficial in some patients.
Agalsidase-β is produced in Chinese hamster ovary cells and is infused at a dose of 1.0 mg/kg over a period of up to 4 h, every 2 weeks. The use of a lower maintenance dose of agalsidase beta, 0.3 mg/kg, has been shown to maintain Gb3 clearance in the short term in some patients but not all.

Emerging treatment strategies for FD involve molecular chaperone therapy, and these are very promising for specific mutations. Pharmaceutical chaperones, currently in phase 3 clinical trials, are small molecular ligands that can be administered orally and which bind selectively to the mutant enzyme, promoting correct folding and delivery of the enzyme to the lysosome. In the case of FD, use of the chaperone 1-deoxygalactojirimycin hydrochloride has been shown to increase the activity of several a-galactosidase A-responsive mutants and to reduce urinary levels of Gb3 in those patients who have missense mutations. Recent studies have shown that chemical chaperones can improve the efficacy of ERT.

Substrate reduction therapy (SRT) circumvents enzyme replacement /modification by inhibiting synthesis of globotriaosyl ceramide. This approach involves the use of a glucosyl ceramide synthase inhibitor, which would slow the rate of Gb3 synthesis, and thus decrease lysosomal storage. Combinatorial therapy using ERT and SRT is being considered as a treatment strategy. Enzyme activators may increase the residual activity of mutant GLA in the lysosomes of patients with FD, thereby lessening lysosomal storage of the substrate and alleviating symptoms. However, these activators may not be beneficial if their efficacy is not high enough or if the residual activity of mutant GLA is inadequate.

Specific small molecule promoter activators may increase the amount of GLA in lysosomes by stimulating expression of the target protein. This would result in an increased amount of GLA in the lysosomes, as the enhancement of mutant enzyme expression may proportionally increase protein trafficking to the lysosome. Therefore, in Fabry patients with significant residual GLA enzyme activity, a small molecule promoter activator may correct lysosomal storage by amplifying the amount of enzyme in lysosomes.

Another future treatment strategy involves altering the proteostasis network in cells; this network consists of many highly-regulated biological pathways that influence protein synthesis, folding, trafficking, disaggregation and degradation In addition, the combination of proteostasis regulators with small molecule chaperones may further increase the amount of folded protein trafficked to lysosomes and thus enhance the therapy, although this hypothesis needs to be tested.

In addition to ERT, the standard treatment strategy, many symptoms of FD can be managed through supportive and palliative approaches. Daily prophylactic doses of neuropathic pain agents, such as phenytoin, carbamazepine, and gabapentin are effective in decreasing the frequency and severity of pain episodes in many patients.

Some patients need more potent analgesics, such as opioids, for pain management while avoiding potential dependency problems. For gastrointestinal disturbances, metoclopramide, H2 blockers, loperamide and hydrochloride can be beneficial. Therapeutic management primarily focuses on the control of blood pressure, lipids, and proteinuria. ACE inhibitors and ARA II /or blockers should be used in patients with proteinuria. Hypertension and hypercholesterolemia should be managed appropriately as usual. Prophylaxis with anti-aggregants is important in patients who have had ischemic attacks or stroke, and permanent cardiac pacing should be considered in high-risk patients. Furthermore, patients need to be encouraged to maintain a healthy lifestyle. While renal failure is the most frequent cause of death in classic FD, in patients with advanced renal disease, dialysis or transplantation can prolong life. However, in FD, even with the engrafted kidneys, other organ system damage continues, particularly vascular disease affecting the heart and brain. It is clear that, even with ERT, other treatments and preventative measures are necessary to manage Fabry disease [38-40].

6. Efficacy of ERT

Generally, ERT normalizes Gb3 levels in a wide variety of organs in most patients, and may be associated with symptomatic benefits. Overall measures of FD severity have shown a general reduction in disease severity after at least 1 year of ERT.

The efficacy of ERT in Fabry cardiomyopathy can be evaluated as the stabilization or decrease of the LV mass and regional myocardial function after 1 year of this treatment, and better exercise capacity at 3 years of therapy in those patients without fibrosis. In addition, clearance of Gb3 from cardiac interstitial capillary endothelial cells has been seen after ERT with agalsidase beta, although not in other cardiac cells such as cardiomyocites. The long-term effects of ERT on Fabry cardiomyopathy are related to the extent of myocardial fibrosis at baseline, when therapy is started. Fabry patients at an early stage of the disease have virtually no myocardial fibrosis. These patients with no detectable fibrosis and mild hypertrophy at baseline have shown a normalization of LV wall thickness and mass during ERT. Subsequently, the patients with no fibrosis have also improved in exercise capacity, which might be related, at least partly, to the positive effects of ERT on the Fabry cardiomyopathy

Concerning the optimal time for starting enzyme replacement therapy, prospective clinical trials in affected males and female carriers still in a preclinical phase using TDI and strain rate to assess non-invasively the efficacy of therapy are required to establish the benefits of starting treatment as soon as the diagnosis is reached. Strain-rate imaging based on tissue Doppler is superior to global parameters, like ejection fraction, in monitoring and quantifying LV function in patients with Fabry disease. The increase in peak systolic strain rate appears to be more specific for regional contractility and rather independent of wall thickness

In relation to renal function, the initiation of ERT before the development of significant proteinuria may be critical for preventing future kidney disease in these patients. Thus, creatinine clearance and eGFR have remained stable after ERT. Treatment with agalsidase alpha for 3 years has been shown to be effective in slowing the deterioration of renal function in patients with Fabry nephropathy. Even in patients with advanced renal disease or in kidney transplant recipients, ERT, by addressing the underlying metabolic deficiency, may slow the progression or development of extra-renal signs and symptoms of the disease.

Neither of the synthetic enzymes cross the blood brain barrier (BBB). Treatments can, therefore, only act on the endothelial cells of the cerebral arterial circulation, at least when the BBB is intact (in aggressive and aseptic meningitis-like forms of Fabry disease with lacunar infarcts, BBB may be seriously altered). More studies are necessary to provide evidence of the efficacy of ERT in preventing new cerebrovascular events.

7. References

[1] Germain DP. Fabry disease. *Orphanet J Rare Dis.* 2010; 22;5:30-36.

[2[Fuller M, Tucker JN, Lang DL, Dean CJ, Fietz MJ, Meikle PJ, Hopwood JJ. Screening patients referred to a metabolic clinic for lysosomal storage disorders. *J Med Genet.*

[3] Mehta A, Beck M, Eyskens F, Feliciani C, Kantola I, Ramaswami U, Rolfs A, Rivera A, Waldek S, Germain DP. Fabry disease: a review of current management strategies. QJM. 2010 ;103(9):641-59.

[4] Spada M, Pagliardini S, Yasuda M, Tukel T, Thiagarajan G, Sakuraba H, Ponzone A, Desnick RJ. High incidence of later-onset fabry disease revealed by newborn screening. *Am J Hum Genet.* 2006 ;79(1):31-40.
[5] Schiffmann R , Brady RO. New prospects for the treatment of lysosomal storage diseases. *Drugs* 2002; 62: 733-735.
[6] Froissart R, Guffon N, Vanier MT, Desnick RJ, Maire I. Fabry disease: D313Y is an alpha-galactosidase A sequence variant that causes pseudodeficient activity in plasma. *Mol Genet Metab.* 2003 ;80(3):307-14
[7] Desnick DP. Enzyme replacement and beyond. J Inherit Metab Dis. 2001;24(2):251-65.
[8] Desnick RJ, Wasserstein MP . Fabry disease: clinical features and recent advances in enzyme replacement therapy. *Adv Nephrol Necker Hosp.* 2001;31:317-39
[9] Germain DP. Fabry disease: recent advances in enzyme replacement therapy. *Expert Opin Investig Drugs.* 2002;11(10):1467-76.
[10] Rodríguez-Marí A, Coll MJ, Chabás A. Molecular analysis in Fabry disease in Spain: fifteen novel GLA mutations and identification of a homozygous female. *Hum Mutat.* 2003;22(3):258.
[11] Shabbeer J, Yasuda M, Benson SD, Desnick RJ. Fabry disease: identification of 50 novel alpha-galactosidase A mutations causing the classic phenotype and three-dimensional structural analysis of 29 missense mutations. *Hum Genomics.* 2006 ;2(5):297-30
[12] Nakao S, Kodama C, Takenaka T, Tanaka A, Yasumoto Y, Yoshida A, Kanzaki T, Enriquez AL, Eng CM, Tanaka H, Tei C, Desnick RJ. Fabry disease: detection of undiagnosed hemodialysis patients and identification of a "renal variant" phenotype. *Kidney Int.* 2003 ;64(3):801-7.
[13] Ashton-Prolla P, Tong B, Shabbeer J, Astrin KH, Eng CM, Desnick RJ. Fabry disease: twenty-two novel mutations in the alpha-galactosidase A gene and genotype/phenotype correlations in severely and mildly affected hemizygotes and heterozygotes. *J Investig Med.* 2000;48(4):227-35.
[14] MacDermot KD, Holmes A, Miners AH. Natural history of Fabry disease in affected males and obligate carrier females. *J Inherit Metab Dis.* 2001;24 Suppl 2:13-4; discussion 11-2.
[15] Valbuena C, Carvalho E, Bustorff M, Ganhão M, Relvas S, Nogueira R, Carneiro F,Oliveira JP. Kidney biopsy findings in heterozygous Fabry disease females with early nephropathy. *Virchows Arch.* 2008 ;453(4):329-38
[16] Safyan R, Whybra C, Beck M, Elstein D, Altarescu G. An association study of inflammatory cytokine gene polymorphisms in Fabry disease. *Eur Cytokine Netw.* 2006;17(4):271-5.
[17] Pastores GM, Hughes DA. To see a world in a grain of sand: elucidating the pathophysiology of Anderson-Fabry disease through investigations of a cellular model. *Kidney Int.* 2009;75(4):351-3
[18] Rombach SM, Twickler TB, Aerts JM, Linthorst GE, Wijburg FA, Hollak CE. Vasculopathy in patients with Fabry disease: current controversies and research directions. *Mol Genet Metab.* 2010;99(2):99-108.)
[19] Joosten H, Strunk AL, Meijer S, Boers JE, Ariës MJ, Abbes AP, Engel H, Beukhof JR. An aid to the diagnosis of genetic disorders underlying adult-onset renal failure: a literature review. *Clin Nephrol.* 2010;73(6):454-72.

[20] Feriozzi S, Schwarting A, Sunder-Plassmann G, West M, Cybulla M; International Fabry Outcome Survey Investigators. Agalsidase alpha slows the decline in renal function in patients with Fabry disease. *Am J Nephrol.* 2009;29(5):353-61.

[21] West M, Nicholls K, Mehta A, Clarke JT, Steiner R, Beck M, Barshop BA, Rhead W, Mensah R, Ries M, Schiffmann R. Agalsidase alpha and kidney dysfunction in Fabry disease. *J Am Soc Nephrol.* 2009;20(5):1132-9.

[22.] Gambarin FI, Disabella E, Narula J, Diegoli M, Grasso M, Serio A, Favalli BM, Agozzino M, Tavazzi L, Fraser AG, Arbustini E. When should cardiologists suspect Anderson-Fabry disease? *Am J Cardiol.* 2010 ;106(10):1492-9

[23] Perrot A, Osterziel KJ, Beck M, Dietz R, Kampmann C. Herz. Fabry disease: focus on cardiac manifestations and molecular mechanisms. 2002;27(7):699-702

[24] Hoigné P, Attenhofer Jost CH, Duru F, Oechslin EN, Seifert B, Widmer U, Frischknecht B, Jenni R. Simple criteria for differentiation of Fabry disease from amyloid heart disease and other causes of left ventricular hypertrophy. *Int J Cardiol.* 2006 ;111(3):413-22.

[25] Weidemann F, Linhart A, Monserrat L, Strotmann J. Cardiac challenges in patients with Fabry disease. *Int J Cardiol.* 2010 ;14:141(1):3-10.

[26] Pieroni M, Chimenti C, Russo A, Russo MA, Maseri A, Frustaci A. Tissue Doppler imaging in Fabry disease. *Curr Opin Cardiol.* 2004;19(5):452-7.

[27] Toro R, Perez-Isla L, Doxastaquis G, Barba MA, Gallego AR, Pintos G, Barbados FJ,Mangas A, Zamorano JL. Clinical usefulness of tissue Doppler imaging in predicting preclinical Fabry cardiomyopathy. *Int J Cardiol.* 2009;132(1):38-44.

[28] De Cobelli F, Esposito A, Belloni E, Pieroni M, Perseghin G, Chimenti C, Frustaci A, Del Maschio A. Delayed-enhanced cardiac MRI for differentiation of Fabry's disease from symmetric hypertrophic cardiomyopathy. *AJR Am J Roentgenol.* 2009 ;192(3):W97-102.

[29] Imbriaco M, Spinelli L, Cuocolo A, Maurea S, Sica G, Quarantelli M, Pisani A,Liuzzi R, Cianciaruso B, Sabbatini M, Salvatore M. MRI characterization of myocardial tissue in patients with Fabry's disease. *AJR Am J Roentgenol.* 2007;188(3):850-3.

[30] Germain DP. Fabry disease in 2004. *Rev Prat.* 2003;53(20):2215-20.

[31] Lidove O, Jaussaud R, Aractingi S. Dermatological and soft-tissue manifestations of Fabry disease: characteristics and response to enzyme replacement therapy. In: Mehta A, Beck M, Sunder-Plassmann G, editors. Fabry Disease: *Perspectives from 5 Years of FOS*. Oxford: Oxford PharmaGenesis; 2006. Chapter 24.

[32] Oussaud C, Dufier JL, Germain DP. Ocular manifestations in Fabry disease: a survey of 32 hemizygous male patients. *Ophtalmic genetics* 2003, Vol. 24, 3 , 129-139

[33] Hirano K, Murata K, Miyagawa A, Terasaki H, Saigusa J, Nagasaka T. et al. Histopathologic findings of cornea verticillata in a woman heterozygous for Fabry's disease. *Cornea.* 2001;20:233–6

[34] Sodi A, Sloannindis A, Metha A, Davey C, Beck Michael, Pitz Suzanne. Ocular manifestations of Fabry´s disease: data from the Fabry Outcome Survey. *Br J Ophtalmol* 2007; 91: 210-214

[35] Schiffmann R, Moore DF. Nervous system manifestations of Fabry disease: data from FOS – the Fabry Outcome Survey. In: Mehta A, Beck M, Sunder-Plassmann G, editors. Fabry Disease: Perspectives from 5 Years of FOS. Oxford: *Oxford PharmaGenesis*; 2006. Chapter 22.

[36] Dütsch M, Hilz MJ. Neurological complications in Fabry disease. *Rev Med Interne.* 2010;31 Suppl 2:S243-50.
[37] Desnick RJ. Prenatal diagnosis of Fabry disease. *Prenat Diagn*;2007; (8):693-4.
[38] Motabar O, Sidransky E, Goldin E, Zheng W. Fabry disease - current treatment and new drug development. *Curr Chem Genomics.* 2010 : 23;4:50-6.
[39] Rozenfeld PA. Fabry disease: treatment and diagnosis. *IUBMB Life.* 2009;61(11):1043-50.
[40] Weidemann F, Niemann M, Breunig F, Herrmann S, Beer M, Störk S, Voelker W, Ertl G, Wanner C, Strotmann J. Long-term effects of enzyme replacement therapy on Fabry cardiomyopathy: evidence for a better outcome with early treatment. *Circulation.* 2009;119(4):524-9.

15

The Multifaceted Complexity of Genetic Diseases: A Lesson from Pseudoxanthoma Elasticum

Daniela Quaglino, Federica Boraldi, Giulia Annovi and Ivonne Ronchetti
University of Modena and Reggio Emilia
Italy

1. Introduction

Pseudoxanthoma elasticum (PXE), also known as Grönblad-Strandberg syndrome, is an autosomal recessive disorder mainly affecting skin, eyes and the cardiovascular system due to progressive mineralization of elastic fibres (Gheduzzi et al., 2003) in the presence of normal levels of calcium and phosphorus in blood and urine.

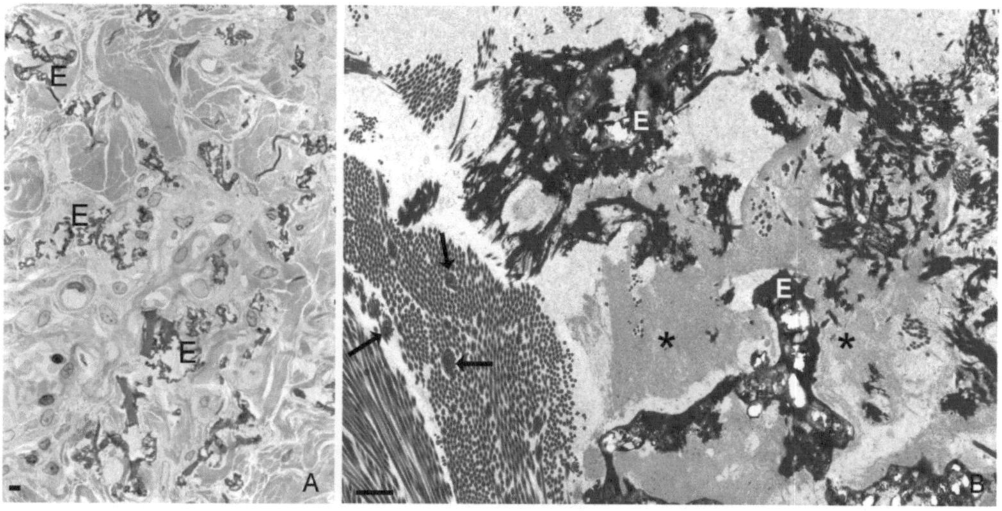

Fig. 1. Dermal biopsy from a patient affected by pseudoxanthoma elasticum (PXE).
A) Semi-thin section stained with toluidine blue and observed by light microscopy.
B) Ultrathin section stained with uranyl acetate and lead citrate visualized by transmission electron microscopy. Deformed, fragmented and mineralized elastic fibres (E) are clearly visible in the reticular dermis of the patient both at low and high magnifications. Collagen flowers (arrows) and electron-dense amorphous aggregates (*) can be recognized at the ultrastructural level. Bar= 1 μm

Although the elastic component is dramatically modified in terms of structural characteristics and functional properties, many other components of the extracellular matrix,

although not calcified, appear altered. Collagen fibrils, for instance, can be laterally fused giving rise to collagen flowers, whereas glycoproteins, abnormally secreted within connective tissues, are deposited in form of large amorphous aggregates (Gheduzzi et al., 2003; Pasquali-Ronchetti et al. 1981) (Figure 1).
The disease is due to mutations in the *ABCC6* gene, encoding for a transmembrane protein (MRP6) highly expressed in liver, kidney and at a lesser extent in several other tissues, although clinically affected. The physiological substrate of MRP6 is still elusive, even though functional studies reported that the protein may be involved in the transport of complex molecules as glutathione S-conjugate leukotriene C4 and of the synthetic cyclopentapeptide BQ123 (an endothelin 1 receptor antagonist) (Belinski et al., 2002; Ilias et al., 2002). Therefore, despite the exponentially increased number of studies performed in the last decade, the pathogenesis of ectopic calcifications in PXE is a still unresolved puzzle (Uitto et al. 2010).
PXE is present in all world's populations, with an estimated prevalence of 1 in 25.000–50.000 and a 2:1 female to male ratio (Neldner & Struk, 2002). Carriers of only one mutated allele do not develop evident clinical manifestations, however they cannot be considered completely healthy carriers, since they may be, for instance, at higher risk for cardiovascular complications (Vanakker et al., 2008).

2. Clinical manifestations

The clinical expression of PXE is heterogeneous, with considerable variation in age of onset, progression and severity of the disease, even within the same family and in the presence of identical mutations (Gheduzzi et al., 2004; Hu et al., 2003a).

2.1 Skin

Patients usually develop skin lesions, mainly at puberty, starting at the posterior side of the neck and in flexural areas such as armpits, antecubital and popliteal fossae, which may later expand to the inguinal region and the periumbilical area. Alterations are usually in form of round yellowish papules, 1–3 mm in diameter, that may coalesce with time into larger protruding plaques. In a relevant number of cases, the skin becomes wrinkled and redundant hanging in folds (Neldner & Struk, 2002) (Figure 2).
In the most severely affected patients, lesions on the mucosal membranes, especially on the inner side of the lower lip, can be observed. Occasionally, calcium deposits may extrude from the skin in advanced state of the disease, a condition described as "perforating PXE" (Lund & Gilbert, 1976). Other unusual clinical presentations of PXE include acneiform lesions (Heid et al., 1980), chronic granulomatous nodules (Heyl, 1967) and brown macules in a reticulate pattern (T.H. Li et al., 1996).

2.2 Cardiovascular system

Cardiovascular manifestations, although not frequent, can be observed already before the third or fourth decade of life and are mainly related to calcium deposition and degeneration of the elastic laminae of medium sized arteries (Mendelsohn et al., 1978). The most common cardiovascular complications, in approximately 20-25% of PXE patients, are: diminished or absent peripheral vascular pulsations, early onset of reno-vascular hypertension, echographic opacities due to calcification of arteries (especially in kidneys, spleen and pancreas), arterial hypertension, angina pectoris, intermittent claudication (often regarded as the first sign of accelerated atherosclerosis), gastrointestinal haemorrhages, arteriosclerosis and increased risk of myocardial and cerebral infarction (Neldner & Struk, 2002). Marked calcification of valves and of atrial and ventricular myocardium, as well as calcified thrombi, which can result in mitral valve prolapse or stenosis and restrictive cardiomyopathy, can be clearly revealed by echocardiography (Rosenzweig et al., 1993).

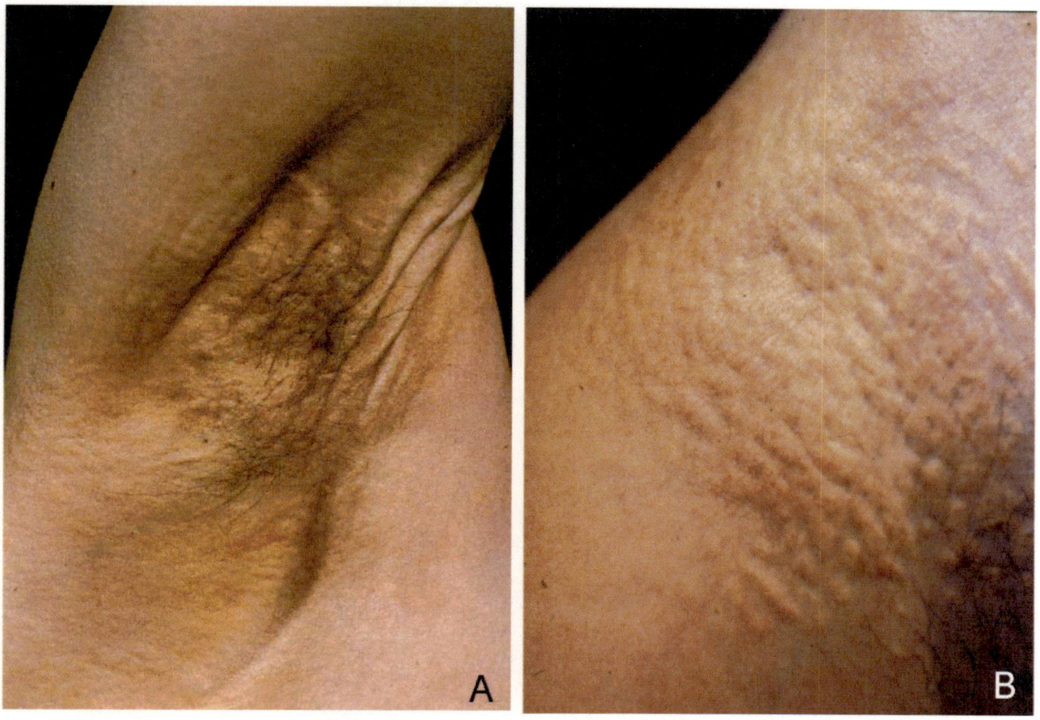

Fig. 2. Typical dermal alterations in PXE.
Papules (B) as well as wrinkled and redundant skin (A) are classical dermal lesions observed in PXE patients

About 10% of PXE patients experience bleeding complications, especially gastrointestinal haemorrhages, due to fragility of calcified submucosal vessels (Golliet-Mercier et al., 2005). Bleeding may infrequently affect other organs such as urinary tract, uterus, joints and the cerebrovascular system (Bock & Schwegler, 2008; Heaton & Wilson, 1986).

2.3 Eyes

PXE is also characterized by severe ocular alterations due to calcification of the Bruch's membrane, that is a thin layer of connective tissue bridging the pigmented retinal epithelium to the choriocapillaries and that consists of a network of interwoven elastic and collagen fibres (Booij et al., 2010). Eye abnormalities are firstly represented by peau d'orange (diffuse mottling of the fundus) that, on an average to 1 to 8 years, precedes angioid streaks (greyish irregular lines radiating outward from the optic papilla corresponding to breaks of the calcified Bruch's membrane) (Figure 3). Within 20 years from diagnosis, almost all PXE patients develop angioid streaks, that, in the course of the disease, may become pale and give way to a generalized atrophy of the adjacent tissue. In later stages, fibrovascular tissue as well as secondary choroidal neovascularization may develop. These new vessels have brittle walls, and this may cause recurrent, spontaneous, or trauma-induced retinal haemorrhages resulting in disciform scarring of the macula, which is responsible for decreased central visual acuity up to legal blindness (Georgalas et al., 2011).

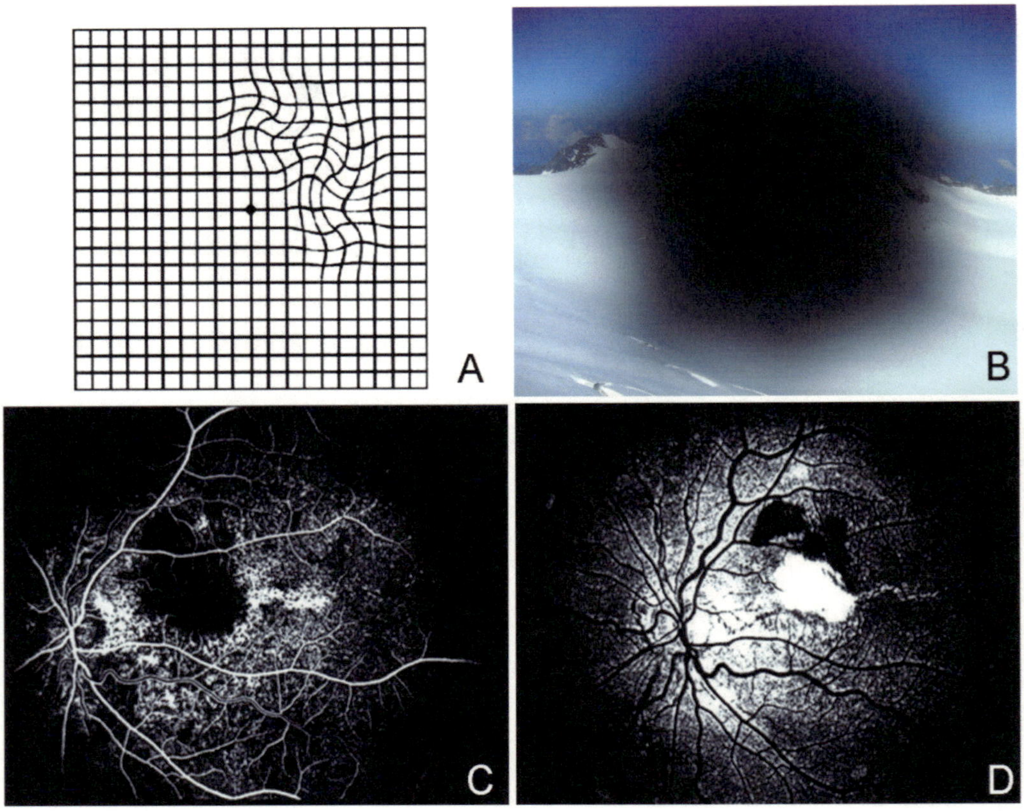

Fig. 3. Typical ocular alterations in PXE.
Elastic fibre mineralization within the Bruch's membrane, haemorrhage, neovascularization and fibrosis (C-D) are the major causes of visual abnormalities. Distortion of the Amsler grid (A) is generally the first clinical sign of ocular involvement. Progression of the disease will end up with central vision loss (B) up to legal blindness

2.4 Other organs

Interestingly, microcalcifications can be detected in several organs, as testis and breast (Bercovitch et al. 2003; Vanakker et al., 2006), as well as in liver, kidneys and spleen (59% of patients and 23.5% of healthy carriers). On renal and abdominal ultrasonography, for instance, a characteristic hyperechogenicity with dotted pattern, possibly reflecting the calcified elastic layers of arteries, has been frequently reported (Suarez et al., 1991), as well as bilateral nephrocalcinosis (Chraïbi et al., 2007). To be noted, however, that parameters of kidney and liver functions are always normal in PXE patients, suggesting that calcification does not affect the activity of these organs (Vanakker et al., 2006).

During pregnancy, the placenta is abnormal, being hypoplastic and atrophic with focal calcifications; moreover, striking anomalies of the elastic lamellae are found in the maternal vessels (Gheduzzi et al., 2001). These alterations do not negatively affect pregnancy, however early delivery can be recommended if foetus stops growing.

3. Genetics

Pseudoxanthoma elasticum is inherited in an autosomal recessive manner. As a general rule, each parent of an individual with an autosomal recessive condition carries one copy of the mutated gene, without showing or showing very mild signs and symptoms of the disorder. In a few cases, however, an affected individual may have one parent without signs and the other parent with some sign of the disease. Also these cases have to be considered autosomal recessive because the normal-appearing parent, in fact, carries an *ABCC6* gene mutation, and the affected offspring inherits two altered genes, one from each parent (Ringpfeil et al., 2006). This situation is called pseudodominance, because it resembles autosomal dominant inheritance, in which one copy of an altered gene is sufficient to cause a disorder.

Because PXE is characterized by calcification of elastic fibres, genes involved in the synthesis and assembly of the elastic fibre network were initially considered as primary candidates for mutations. These included elastin (ELN) on chromosome 7, elastin-associated microfibrillar proteins, such as fibrillin 1 and fibrillin 2 (FBN1 and FBN2) on chromosomes 15 and 5, and lysyl oxidase (LOX) also on chromosome 15. However, genetic linkage analyses excluded all these chromosomal regions (Christiano et al., 1992; Raybould et al., 1994). Subsequent studies, employing positional cloning approaches, provided strong evidence for linkage to the short arm of chromosome 16, limiting a region of approximately 500 kb (Le Saux et al., 1999).

Examination of the existing genome database revealed that this candidate region contained four genes, none of which had actually an obvious connection to elastic fibres or more generally to the extracellular matrix, but after a long systematic sequencing approach, it appeared that the *ABCC6* gene (16p.13.1) is the main site of mutations in PXE (Bergen et al., 2000; Le Saux et al., 2000; Ringpfeil et al., 2000) (Figure 4).

This gene, spanning ~73 kb genomic DNA, is composed of 31 exons, belongs to the subfamily C of the ABC genes (ATP-binding cassette) and encodes for MRP6 (a transmembrane protein of 1503 aminoacids) composed of three hydrophobic membrane segments comprising five, six, and six transmembrane spanning domains, respectively, and two evolutionary conserved intracellular nucleotide binding folds (NBFs). The NBFs contain conserved Walker A and B domains, and a C motif critical for ATP binding and transmembrane transporter functions (Chassaing et al., 2005; Hu et al., 2003b) (Figure 5).

So far, approximately 300 different mutations have been reported in *ABCC6* (Costrop et al., 2010; Gheduzzi et al., 2004; Miksch et al,. 2005; Plomp et al., 2008) and more than 80 have been detected in Italian PXE patients. The most frequent sequence changes are missense (55%) and nonsense (15%) mutations, as well as small deletions (15%), whereas less frequent alterations are represented by splicing errors, large deletions and insertions. Although the consequences of splicing mutations have not been investigated, at least 30% of all mutations cause a frameshift and the introduction of a stop-codon, which leads to premature chain termination. At protein level, the vast majority of mutations involve the cytoplasmatic domains and the carboxy-terminal end of MRP6. Mutations especially target the NBF1 and

NBF2 domains, and the 8th intracellular loop, consistent with the critical role of NBFs in ATP-driven transport. Functional studies have already shown that MRP6 transport is abolished by missense mutations located in NBF2 (Ilias et al., 2002).

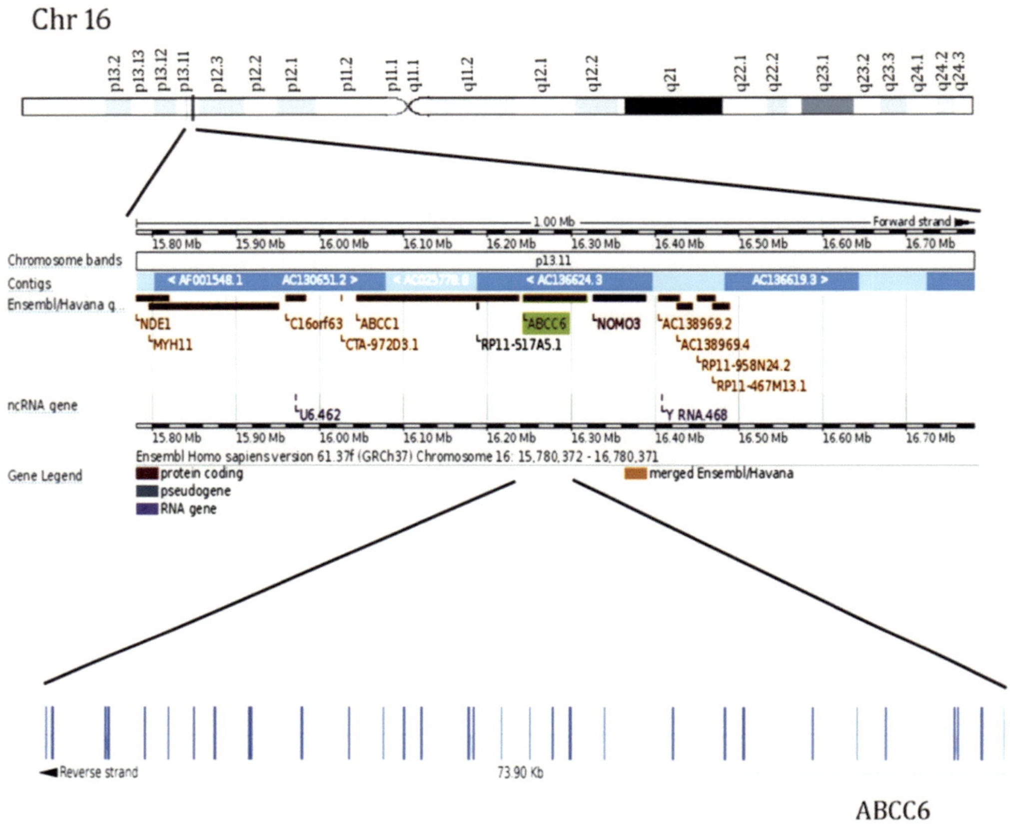

Fig. 4. Localization and structure of the *ABCC6* gene on chromosome 16

Two *ABCC6* mutations, R1141X and del (ex23_29), occur very frequently, probably due to founder effects and genetic drift. R1141X may produce an instable mRNA which is rapidly degraded by nonsense mediated RNA decay (Hu et al., 2003a; Le Saux et al., 2000). The frequency of these two recurrent mutations differs according to the population studied: of the detected mutations, ex23_29del is observed with a frequency of 28% in USA and 4% in Europe, whereas R1141X has a frequency of 4% in USA and 28% in Europe (Le Saux et al., 2001), with additional differences among European Countries, being 30% in Dutch patients (Bergen et al., 2004; Hu et al., 2003b) and about 26% and 13% in Italian and French patients, where a common founder effect was identified (Chassaing et al., 2004; Gheduzzi et al., 2004).

By contrast, in Japanese patients, neither R1141X nor ex23_29del mutations were identified, whereas mutations 2542delG and Q378X account for 53% and 25%, respectively (Noji et al., 2004). In South African families of Afrikaaners, mutation R1339C represents more than half of the detected mutations, with a common haplotype indicating, also in this case, a founder effect (Le Saux et al., 2002).

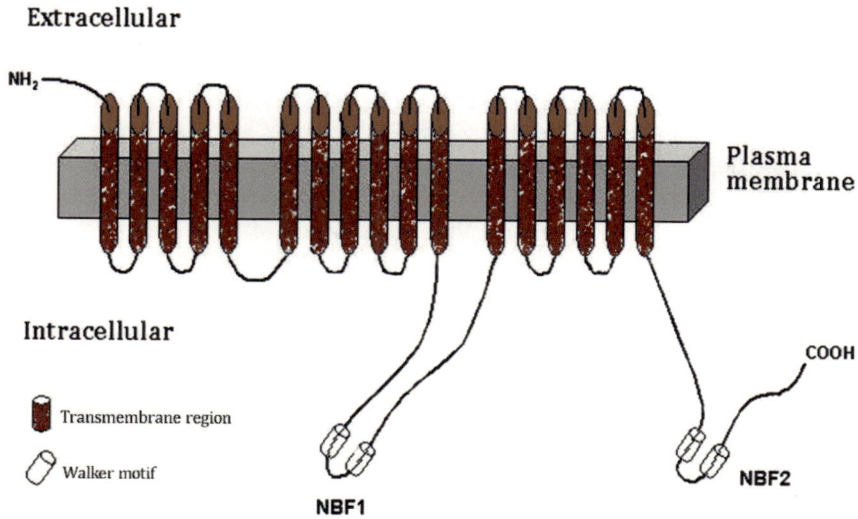

Fig. 5. Schematic drawing showing the typical transmembrane organization of the MRP6 protein

The *ABCC6* mutation detection rate is around 80-90%, since there are cases in which mutations cannot be identified in the coding region on one of the alleles, although the other allele harbours a recessive mutation (Chassaing et al., 2004; Gheduzzi et al., 2004); moreover, lack of mutation detection in some patients could reflect the occurrence of deletions (for example, deletion of exon 15 or deletion of the whole gene).

To date, no correlations have been established between the clinical phenotype and the nature or the position of the mutations (Pfender et al., 2007).

4. Pathogenesis

The physiological function and the natural substrate(s) of MRP6 are currently unknown, however, because of its homology to MRP1, it has been classified as a multidrug resistance associated protein, thus belonging to the large family of membrane proteins that transport organic anions and/or other molecules against a concentration gradient at the cost of ATP hydrolysis (Borst & Elferink, 2002; Haimeur et al., 2004). The role of MRP6 in drug resistance is actually limited to low-level resistance of a small number of chemicals, like etoposide, teniposide, doxorubicin and daunorubicin (Belinsky et al., 2002; Kool et al., 1999). Consistently with its assumed functional role, MRP6 is highly expressed in liver and kidneys being localized to the basolateral side of hepatocytes and of proximal kidney tubules, suggesting that it may transport biomolecules from cells into the blood (Bergen et al., 2000; Kool et al., 1999; Scheffer et al., 2002).

However, in spite of the high level of *ABCC6* expression, liver and kidney do not suffer from mutations in this gene. By contrast, tissues as skin, retina and vessels, which are deeply altered in PXE, express very low levels of MRP6 (Bergen et al., 2000; Kool et al., 1999). These findings raised a still unsolved dilemma concerning the pathogenesis of PXE: how do mutations in a gene expressed primarily in the liver result in the mineralization of peripheral connective tissues?

To explain the putative mechanisms leading to ectopic calcifications from *ABCC6* mutations under normal calcium and phosphorus homeostatic conditions, two theories have been reported in the literature (Uitto et al., 2010): "the liver metabolic hypothesis" and "the peripheral cell hypothesis". The metabolic hypothesis considers liver dismetabolism the only responsible for ectopic calcifications, whereas the peripheral cell hypothesis points to the role of mesenchymal cell metabolism on the homeostatic control of connective tissue calcifications in PXE.

The liver metabolic hypothesis postulates that the absence of functional MRP6 activity in hepatocytes results in deficiency of circulating factor(s) physiologically required to prevent aberrant mineralization (Jiang & Uitto, 2006; Uitto et al., 2010). In support of this hypothesis are clinical and experimental observations in PXE patients, as well as in the *Abcc6*$^{-/-}$ mouse (Klement et al., 2005), that serves as a model for human PXE. Firstly, clinical findings in PXE patients are rarely present at early childhood and the onset of clinical manifestations as well as the slow progression of the disease, due to continued accumulation of minerals in soft connective tissues of affected organs, can be regarded as the typical consequence of metabolic impairments that worsen with time. Secondly, serum from PXE patients, as well as from *Abcc6*$^{-/-}$ mice, lacks the capacity to prevent calcium/phosphate precipitation in an *in vitro* assay with smooth muscle cell cultures (Jiang et al., 2007). Furthermore, serum from PXE patients, when added to the culture medium, has been shown to modify the organization of elastic fibres without altering gene expression, thus suggesting the involvement of specific circulating factors directly acting on the assembly of elastic fibres (Le Saux et al., 2006), even if these changes occur in the absence of any *in vitro* calcification. Finally, recent skin grafting studies in wild-type and *Abcc6*$^{-/-}$ mice have further focused on the importance of circulating factor(s), hypothesizing that the mineralization process can be countered or even reversed by modifications of the homeostatic milieu (Jiang et al., 2009). In particular, it has been shown that the *Abcc6*$^{-/-}$ mouse skin graft does not develop mineralization, when placed onto the *Abcc6*$^{+/+}$ mouse, but calcification occurs in the skin of wild-type mouse after grafting onto the *Abcc6*$^{-/-}$ mouse, indicating that circulating factors in the recipient's blood could play a critical role in determining the degree of mineralization, irrespective of the graft genotype. However, in these skin graft experiments the possible modulation of fibroblast metabolism upon effect of circulating factors cannot be ruled out.

Actually, several studies have reported alterations in circulating factors in PXE patients, such as proteoglycans (Götting et al., 2005; Passi et al., 1996), plasma lipoproteins (Wang et al., 2001) and mineralization inhibitors, such as fetuin-A and Matrix Gla Protein (MGP) (Hendig et al., 2006, 2008). Moreover, a number of circulating molecules have been shown to be modified in the plasma of PXE patients by effect of a systemic altered redox balance (Garcia-Fernandez et al., 2008).

However, a number of questions remain to be elucidated. First of all, in PXE patients, despite of the absence and/or of the presence of one or more circulating factor(s), mineralization affects only a certain number of elastic fibres and only in peculiar areas of the body. Calcification seems, in fact, a rather specific phenomenon, since in PXE patients extracellular matrix components other than elastin (i.e. collagens or matrix glycoproteins) never undergo mineralization, furthermore, not all elastic fibres are calcified and not all areas of affected tissues are clinically involved (Gheduzzi et al.,2003; Pasquali-Ronchetti et al., 1981). In addition, the observation that patient's serum interferes with elastin assembly is in agreement with the above mentioned plasma modifications in PXE patients and especially with the abnormalities in glycosaminoglycan's content and species (Maccari et al., 2003, 2008;

Passi et al., 1996; Tiozzo Costa et al 1998), since it is well known that these matrix constituents are capable to greatly influence tropoelastin assembly (Gheduzzi et al., 2005; Tu & Weiss, 2008). Finally, if changes in the circulating environment can effectively modify the extent of ectopic calcifications, it is not clear why PXE mesenchymal cells, as dermal fibroblasts, maintain their abnormal phenotype even when they are cultured *in vitro* in optimal nutritional supplements and conditions far from their original environment (Boraldi et al., 2009).

Actually, in support to the "peripheral cell hypothesis", it has been demonstrated that *in vitro* skin fibroblasts isolated from PXE patients exhibit a modified biosynthetic expression profile, altered cell-cell and cell-matrix interactions associated with changes in proliferative capacity (Boraldi et al., 2009; Quaglino et al., 2000), abnormal synthesis of elastin and of glycosaminoglycan/proteoglycan complexes (Passi et al., 1996) and enhanced degradation potential due to elevated matrix metalloproteinase-2 activity (Quaglino et al., 2005). Consistently, histopathological and ultrastructural observations showed that, in PXE, mineralization occurs only on elastic fibres (Gheduzzi et al., 2003; Pasquali-Ronchetti et al., 1981), suggesting a peculiar composition and/or organization of elastic fibre components (Lebwohl et al.,1993; Sakuraoka et al., 1994). By immuno-electron microscopy, it has been demonstrated that aberrant matrix proteins known for their high affinity for calcium and normally involved in mineralization processes (such as alkaline phosphatase, vitronectin, fibronectin, bone sialoprotein, osteonectin and proteoglycans) are accumulated within PXE elastic fibres (Contri et al., 1996; Kornet et al., 2004; Passi et al., 1996).

All these data undoubtedly highlight the importance of mesenchymal cells in the pathogenesis of ectopic calcifications, never the less it is still unclear whether these changes depend or not upon the expression of the *ABCC6* gene in mesenchymal cells (Matsuzaki et al., 2005). It has to be noted, in fact, that even normal fibroblasts, possibly due to aberrant splicings, do not seem to express the full MRP6 protein (Matsuzaki et al., 2005) and that immunologically positive epitopes have been recognized only on membranes of the endoplasmic reticulum of isolated dermal fibroblasts (Boraldi et al., 2009). What could be the significance and importance of the presence of at least part of MRP6 in the endoplasmic reticulum of mesenchymal cells have not been investigated.

However, in the light of these observations, changes in membrane transport properties described in PXE cultured fibroblasts (Boraldi et al., 2003) would seem likely the result of the high level of reactive oxygen species (ROS) on the structural organization of cell membranes (Boraldi et al., 2009) and consequently on cell permeability. It has been in fact demonstrated *in vitro* (Pasquali-Ronchetti et al., 2006) and *in vivo* (Garcia-Fernandez et al., 2008) that PXE is characterized by an altered redox balance. At cellular level, the chronic oxidative stress condition is due, at least in part, to the loss of mitochondrial membrane potential ($\Delta\Psi$ (m)) with overproduction of ROS. Consistently, cultured fibroblasts produce more malondialdehyde, a product of lipid peroxidation, and accumulate higher amounts of carbonylated proteins compared to controls (Boraldi et al., 2009; Pasquali-Ronchetti et al., 2006). Likewise, in the circulation of patients, the redox unbalance leads to significantly high amount of oxidised proteins and lipids, which might have relevant effects on peripheral mesenchymal cells (Garcia-Fenandez et al., 2008).

Interestingly, among the molecular pathways which are sensitive to the redox potential is the vitamin K-cycle that, within connective tissues, is essential for the γ-glutamyl carboxylation of MGP (Matrix Gla Protein), a potent inhibitor of calcification in soft connective tissues (Schurgers et al., 2008). Consistently, in PXE fibroblasts (Gheduzzi et al., 2007) and in the *Abcc6* $^{-/-}$ mice (Li et al., 2007) there is a reduced carboxylation of MGP.

A recent characterization of the PXE fibroblast's protein profile revealed that numerous endoplasmic reticulum-associated proteins are differentially expressed in pathological cells. Among these proteins, calumenin and disulfide isomerase are involved in the recycling of vitamin K, leaving open the question if insufficient carboxylation of MGP in PXE cells could be due to reduced availability or to diminished recycling of vitamin K (Boraldi et al., 2009) (Figure 6).

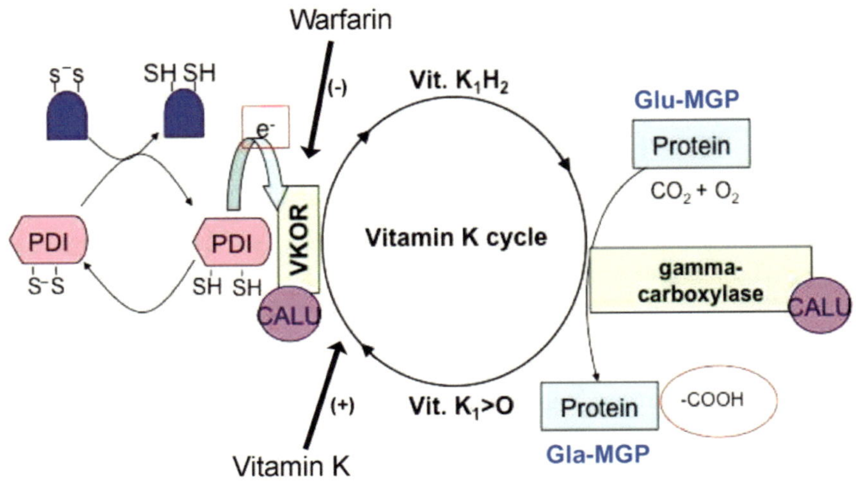

Fig. 6. Drawing illustrating the numerous factors involved in vitamin K cycle.
Vitamin K represents an important cofactor of protein carboxylation. Within the endoplasmic reticulum of mesenchymal cells, MGP (Matrix Gla protein) is activated by gamma-carboxylase from the inactive form (Glu-MGP) to the active form (Gla-MGP). Protein disulfide isomerase (PDI) and calumenin (CALU) are important modulators of these reactions. Warfarin, by inhibiting the action of vitamin K epoxide reductase, reduces the efficiency of the carboxylation process and favours the development of vascular calcifications. Modified from Wajih (Wajih et al., 2007)

To further confirm the importance of efficient MGP carboxylation in controlling the mineralization process, there are experimental evidences showing that antibodies specific for carboxylated (Gla-MGP) and non-carboxylated MGP (Glu-MGP) are differently localized within human dermal elastic fibres. In particular, both forms of MGP are rather heterogeneously distributed within elastin of control subjects, whereas in PXE patients Glu-MGP is markedly present in calcified areas and Gla-MGP is exclusively localized at the mineralization front (Gheduzzi et al., 2007). Although it has been suggested that MRP6 could function as a vitamin K transporter from the liver to the periphery, and that, in PXE, the mutated protein may prevent connective tissue from an adequate supply of the vitamin necessary for efficient carboxylation processes (Borst et al., 2008; Vanakker et al., 2010), *in vivo* and *in vitro* treatments with different forms of vitamin K do not appear to interfere and/or to inhibit the mineralization process (Jiang et al., 2011; Annovi et al., 2011).
Therefore, it could be suggested that mutated MRP6 in liver and kidney is responsible for the altered release in the circulation of factors that modify plasma components, among which proteins, lipids and, eventually, other constituents, thus contributing to produce an abnormal environment at the periphery, and to influence mesenchymal cell behaviour and

metabolism. Among peripheral alterations it would appear that there is an imbalance between production and degradation of oxidant species, abnormal protein and glycosaminoglycan synthesis, changes in post-translational protein modifications and abnormal DNA-methylation (Boraldi et al., 2009). Moreover, the alterations in the *in vitro* behaviour of PXE fibroblasts may suggest that permanent epigenetic changes have occurred, thus causing the inability of these cells to produce mature inhibitors and/or modulators of calcification (Figure 7).

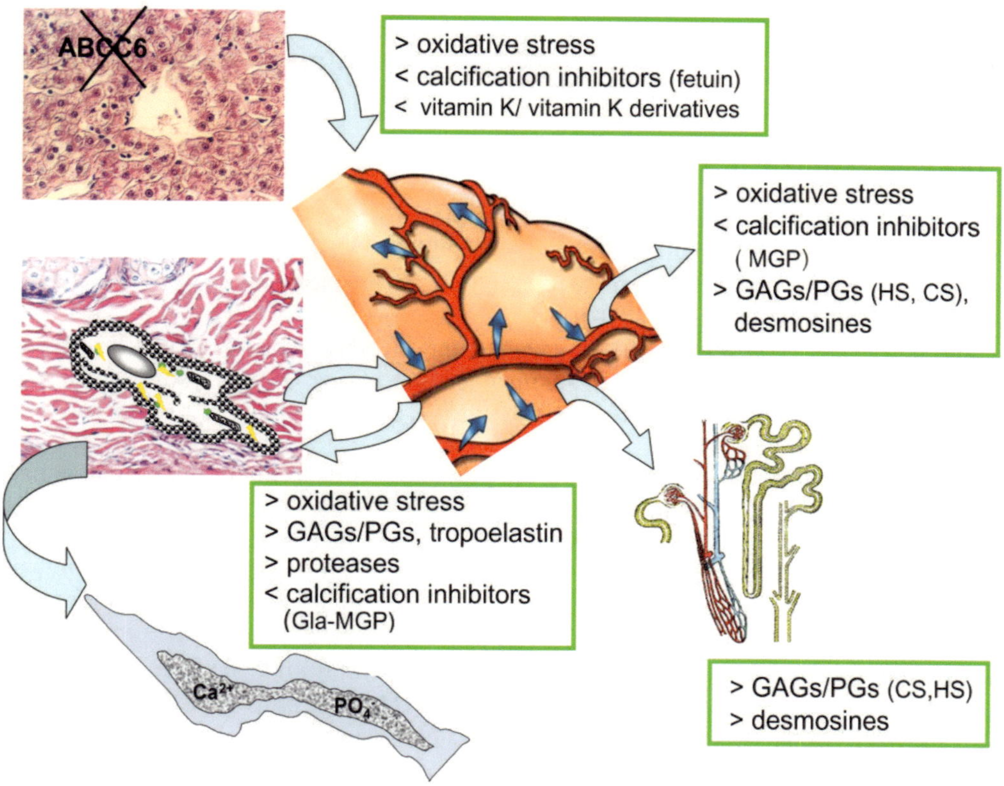

Fig. 7. Drawing that summarizes the major metabolic abnormalities observed in PXE and the relationships between organs and tissues possibly involved in the pathogenesis of elastic fibre calcification.
Absent or altered expression of the *ABCC6* gene in hepatocytes may be responsible for abnormal extrusion in the circulation of still unknown factor/s which is/are responsible for or contributing to oxidative stress, to ineffective inhibition of ectopic calcification, to reduced levels of vitamin K and/or vitamin K derivatives. Therefore, through the circulation, abnormal signals could reach mesenchymal cells epigenetically modifying their phenotype, i.e. chronic oxidative stress, altered synthesis of tropoelastin, production of glycosaminoglycans (GAGs) or proteoglycans (PGs) with peculiar physical-chemical properties, augmented proteolytic potential, lower expression of carboxylated Matrix Gla Protein (Gla-MGP), thus causing accumulation of calcium (Ca^{2+}) and phosphate (PO_4^-) mineral precipitates on elastic fibres. Abnormal products from mesenchymal cells can be found in the circulation or in the urine, i.e. parameters of redox balance, desmosines as indicators of elastin degradation, heparan sulfate (HS) and chondroitin-sulfate (CS) GAGs and inhibitors of calcification as MGP

The various levels of mineralization, even within the same tissue, could be explained by the heterogeneity of different mesenchymal cell subtypes and their peculiar functional imprinting related to structural and functional requirements of organs and tissues (Jelaska et al., 1999; Sorrell & Caplan, 2004).

On the basis of all these considerations, both "the liver metabolic" and "the peripheral cell" hypotheses, together, can actually help to understand the pathogenesis of clinical manifestations in PXE. On one side, there is the involvement of the liver that, expressing MRP6, has an important role in controlling metabolic processes and plasma composition, on the other side it cannot be underestimated the crucial role of peripheral mesenchymal cells, as fibroblasts, in regulating connective tissue homeostasis.

5. The role of modifier genes

Understanding PXE pathogenesis is further complicated by the fact that the age of disease onset and the expression of clinical symptoms are highly variable (Gonzales et al., 2009) and marked phenotypic variations have been observed in affected siblings bearing the same *ABCC6* mutation (Gheduzzi et al. 2004).

Although, there is no evidence for the involvement of other genes in the pathogenesis of PXE (Li et al., 2009), however, a number of modifying factors, both genetic and environmental, have been suggested to play a role in the phenotypic expression of the disease (Hovnanian, 2010).

One recently identified genetic factor involves polymorphisms in the promoter region of the *SPP1* gene (secreted phosphoprotein 1, also known as osteopontin) (Hendig et al., 2007). Osteopontin is a secreted, highly acidic phosphoprotein that is involved in immune cell activation, wound healing, bone morphogenenesis (Denhardt et al., 2001), thus playing a major role in regulating the mineralization process in various tissues, including skin and aorta, where osteopontin is localized to elastic fibres (Baccarani-Contri et al., 1994). Higher expression of this protein has been observed in skin biopsies from PXE patients compared to samples from unaffected regions or from healthy individuals (Contri et al., 1996) and also in mice suffering from dystrophic cardiac calcification, suggesting that its expression is influenced by the *Dyscalc1* locus on chromosome 7 (Aherrahrou et al., 2004). Although several polymorphisms in the *SPP1* gene have been described and associated with various disorders such as systemic lupus erythematosus and arteriosclerosis (Giacopelli et al., 2004), the role of osteopontin in regulating the calcification process, strongly suggested that sequence variations in the *SPP1* promoter region might account for the higher expression observed in PXE patients, thus affecting the disease outcome. Consistently, mutational screening revealed nine different sequence variations, and three *SPP1* promoter polymorphisms (c.-1748A>G, c.-155_156insG and c.244_255insTG), in particular, were significantly associated with PXE. Until now, no functional studies have been carried out with the *SPP1* promoter polymorphisms c.-1748>G, whereas the polymorphism variant c.244_245ins TG does not have a major regulatory effect. By contrast, the discovery that polymorphism c.155_156insG generates a Runx2-binding site opened a new field of investigations, since Runx2-binding sites are in fact very important for regulating *SSP1* expression in bone tissue (Giacopelli et al., 2004). A constitutive expression of Runx2, combined with a glucocorticoids' supplementation, results in a strong upregulation of *SPP1* expression and finally in a biological matrix mineralization by primary dermal fibroblasts (Phillips et al., 2006). Therefore, polymorphisms in the *SPP1* promoter may represent a genetic risk factor contributing to PXE susceptibility.

Other studies have correlated the incidence of cardiovascular complications in PXE with polymorphisms of genes encoding for xylosyltransferase 1 (*XT-1*) and xylosyltransferase 2 (*XT-2*), a set of key enzymes involved in proteoglycan biosynthesis and considered biochemical markers of fibrosis (Schön et al., 2006). The altered proteoglycan metabolism, already observed *in vitro* (Passi et al., 1996) and *in vivo* (Maccari et al., 2003), suggests that enzymes from these pathways may function as genetic co-factors in the severity of PXE. Furthermore, PXE patients have elevated serum XT-I activity. On the basis of these observations Authors suggested a connection between the severity of the disease and genetic variations in the *XYLT* genes (Schön et al., 2006).

More recent studies have shown that polymorphisms in genes associated with redox balance as catalase (*CAT*), superoxide dismutase 2 (*SOD2*) and glutathione peroxidase 1 (*GPX1*) are associated with early onset of clinical manifestations (Zarbock et al., 2007), whereas polymorphisms of the *VEGF* gene (vascular endothelial growth factor) are involved in the pathogenesis of ocular manifestations (Zarbock et al., 2009). The distribution of 10 single nucleotide polymorphisms (SNPs) in the promoter and coding region of the *VEGFA* gene has been evaluated in DNA samples from 163 German patients affected by PXE and in 163 healthy subjects. Five SNPs showed significant association with severe retinopathy. The most significant association was with polymorphism c.-460C>T. In the light of these results *VEGF* gene polymorphisms might be considered useful prognostic markers for the development of PXE-associated retinopathy, thus allowing earlier therapeutic intervention in order to prevent loss of central vision, one of the most devastating consequences of PXE (Zarbock et al., 2009).

By contrast, very few data are available on the role of *ABCC6* polymorphisms on the occurrence and/or severity of clinical manifestations in PXE patients. The *ABCC6* pR1268Q polymorphism has been associated with lower plasma triglycerides and higher plasma HDL-cholesterol, suggesting that *ABCC6* may contribute to modulate plasma lipoproteins and possibly cardiovascular complications (Wang et al., 2001). In a larger study conducted on a German cohort of PXE patients, in addition to the complete screening of the *ABCC6* gene, the *ABCC6* promoter region was also analyzed and the following polymorphisms were found: c.-127C>T, c.-132C>T and C.-219A>C. Interestingly, the difference in the c.-219A>C frequencies between PXE patients and controls was statistically significant and this polymorphism appeared located in a transcriptional activator sequence of the *ABCC6* promoter, functioning as a binding site for a transcriptional repressor predominantly found in genes involved in lipid metabolism (Schulz et al., 2006), further sustaining a possible correlation between *ABCC6* and lipid metabolism.

Surprisingly, the observation that the c.3421C>T loss-of-function mutation on one allele of *ABCC6* (R1141X) is significantly associated to coronary artery disease (CAD), in the apparently normal population (Köblös et al., 2010), was not confirmed in a cohort of Italian PXE patients (Quaglino, unpublished data), further sustaining the difficulty to perform a genotype-phenotype correlation, although not excluding the possibility that carriers of *ABCC6* loss-of-function mutations may benefit from cardiovascular prevention programs (Vanakker etal., 2008).

6. Diagnosis and treatments

In spite of the impressive progress in understanding the genetic/molecular basis of inherited diseases, also in PXE, similarly to other genetic disorders, there have been limited improvements in terms of treatment and cure. Major advances concern diagnosis, due to ability to recognize a continuously increased number of mutations (mutation detection rate varies from 80-90%). Attempts to establish genotype/phenotype correlations have yielded little clinically useful information other than the fact that, as PXE patients age, symptoms get worse, probably because of progressive accumulation of mineralized elastic fibres, associated to other age-related degenerative features (Garcia-Fernandez et al., 2008).

PXE is an important cause of blindness and of early death from cardiovascular manifestations (Neldner, 1988), therefore an early diagnosis is important in order to minimise the risk of systemic complications. One of the major problems encountered by patients affected by rare diseases, as PXE, is the difficulty to find physicians who are aware of the disorder and of the possible related complications. Therefore, strenuous efforts are necessary to spread the knowledge on these disorders not only in the scientific community, but also among practitioners, who represent the first medical reference point for patients. An additional help may derive from the definition of commonly accepted criteria for clinical diagnosis, which, in the case of PXE, include the presence of retinal angioid streaks (a fluorescein angiogram may be necessary) in combination with characteristic skin lesions (calcification of fragmented elastic fibres confirmed by von Kossa stain in a biopsy of lesional skin) (Figure 8) with or without a positive family history of PXE (two or more family members clinically diagnosed). It is however important to note that mild forms of the disorder can be easily overlooked and a negative family history does not exclude the diagnosis.

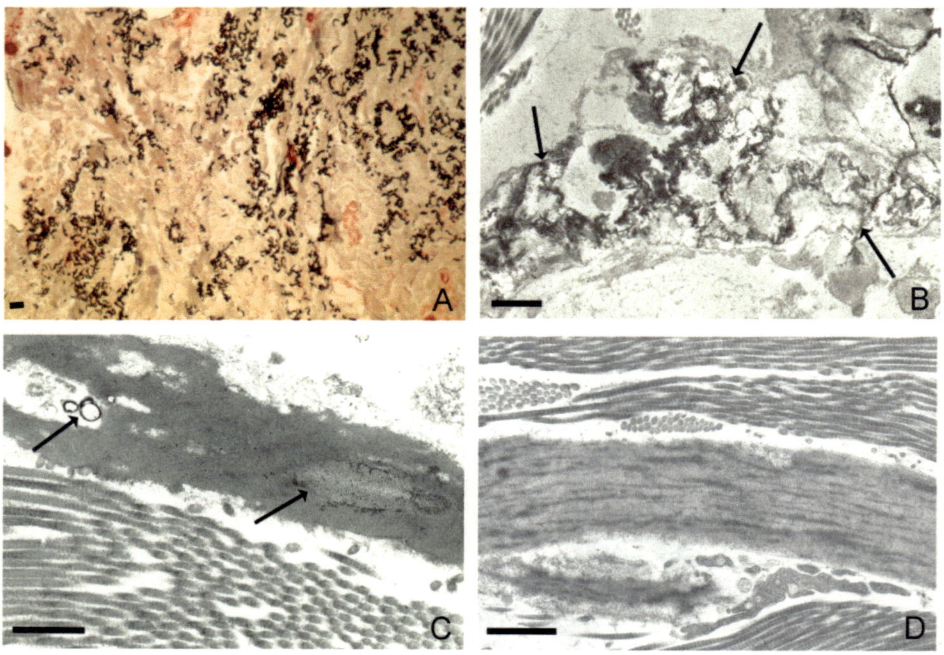

Fig. 8. Demonstration of mineralized elastic fibres is the gold standard diagnostic criteria in PXE.

A) Light microscopy of a dermal biopsy from a PXE patient stained with Von Kossa for the visualization of brownish calcified elastin. B-D) Transmission electron microscopy showing dramatically deformed and mineralized elastic fibres (arrows) in the dermis of a PXE patient (B) and small clinically irrelevant alterations (arrows) in the skin of PXE carriers (C), compared to the typical amorphous structure of normal elastic fibres (D). Bars: 1μm

Since the discovery of *ABCC6* as the PXE associated gene in 2000 (Bergen et al., 2000; Le Saux et al., 2000; Ringpfeil et al., 2000), molecular genetic testing have been rapidly developed and, although frequently limited to research laboratories or to highly specialized centres, they may represent an important diagnostic assessment. The techniques most frequently used are sequence analysis and mutation scanning, which are capable to detect missense, nonsense and frameshift mutations as well as small deletions and insertions. Testing strategies usually involve a first screening of exons in which a large number of mutations are located (i.e. exons 24 and 28), and, in case of negative results, the sequencing of the other coding regions. Moreover, since a 16.4 kb deletion involving exons 23-29 is another recurrent mutation, a specific deletion analysis can be required.

Analyses performed so far revealed that there is a considerable spectrum of genetic mutations (>300), with wide inter- and intra-familial phenotypic variations, and an extreme variability in terms of progression of the disease as well as of severity and extent of clinical manifestations. It must be reminded that PXE is a systemic disorder and therefore management of PXE requires coordinated input from a multidisciplinary team of specialists including dermatologist, primary care physician, ophthalmologist, cardiologist, vascular surgeon, plastic surgeon, genetics professional, and a nutritionist.

Moreover, once a diagnosis of PXE has been established, in order to delay and eventually manage ocular and cardiovascular complications, patients are encouraged to have clinical/instrumental examinations whose frequency may depend on the age of patient, age at diagnosis and severity of clinical manifestations. In particular, it is advisable to perform a complete dilated eye examination by a retinal specialist, particularly looking for *peau d'orange* and angioid streaks and baseline cardiovascular examination with periodic follow-up including: echocardiography, cardiac stress testing, and Doppler evaluation of peripheral vasculature.

At present, no specific treatment for PXE exists, in the sense that mineralization of elastic fibres cannot be delayed or reverted. Never the less, skin surgery has been successfully applied for cosmetic improvement (Ng et al., 1999), as well as peripheral and coronary arteries interventions in order to limit vascular complications (Donas et al., 2007; Shepherd & Rooke, 2003).

The only stage of the disease where therapy for ocular complications is possible and indicated is whenever a choroidal neovascularization (CNV) has developed (Georgalas et al., 2011). Traditional therapeutic options consist of laser photocoagulation (used to halt the progression of CNVs, although characterized by high rate of recurrence, visual loss, and central scotomas) (Pece et al., 1997) or of photodynamic therapy (PDT) (used to arrest the progression of CNVs, even though results appeared less encouraging then expected) (Heimann et al., 2005). Experimental surgical procedures, such as macular translocation or subfoveal CNV excision (Roth et al., 2005), appeared unsuccessful. More recently, taking advantage from the experience on macular degeneration, the intraocular injection of anti-angiogenic drugs, as avastin and lucentis, actually appeared to be the most effective therapeutic options for ocular complications (Verbraak, 2010).

In the absence of effective treatments specifically targeting pathways leading to ectopic calcifications, anectodical reports can be found in the literature concerning the use of drugs or of nutritional supplements. For instance, it has been suggested that pentoxifylline and cilostazol may ameliorate intermittent claudication (Muir, 2009), however, controlled studies of these drugs in PXE patients have not been performed. Interestingly, the ARED (Age Related Eye Disease) study suggested that a regimen of antioxidant vitamins could be beneficial in patients with macular degeneration. Given the similarities with PXE (i.e. ocular manifestations and altered redox balance) it is possible that the same recommendation can be valuable also for PXE (Lecerf & Desmettre, 2010), even though further investigations are required to support this hypothesis. By contrast, more promising perspectives, at least in the mouse model, seem to be represented by a diet supplemented with an excess of magnesium, although the mechanisms of reduced calcifications are still unknown (Gorgels et al., 2010; LaRusso et al, 2009) and the effects of long-term treatments with high doses of magnesium in humans have not been yet investigated.

7. PXE-like diseases

Even though no other phenotypes are known to be associated with mutations in the *ABCC6* gene, PXE-like clinical features, including aberrant mineralization of elastic fibres, have been reported in a number of apparently unrelated acquired and genetic clinical conditions (Neldner, 1988).

7.1 Acquired conditions

Among the acquired conditions, PXE-like cutaneous changes may be associated with multiple pregnancy, longstanding end-stage renal disease (Lewis et al., 2006), L-tryptophan induced eosinophilia myalgia syndrome (Mainetti et al., 1991), and amyloid elastosis (Sepp et al., 1990) as well as after D-penicillamine treatment, cutaneous exposure to calcium salts (Neldner & Martinez-Hernandez, 1979), and salpeter (Nielsen et al., 1978). In these cases, mineralization of skin may result from metabolic abnormalities affecting calcium and/or phosphate homeostasis or from direct deposition of mineral salts on collagen or elastic fibres. However, the pathomechanistic details and the role of predisposing genetic factors are unknown.

In papillary dermal elastolysis, white-yellow papules resembling PXE can be observed in aged women (60–80 years), although, in contrast to PXE, these lesions are histologically characterized by loss of elastin in the papillary dermis (Ohnishi et al., 1998).

Moreover, elastic fibres similar to those of PXE have been observed in the lesional skin of patients with a variety of inflammatory skin diseases in the absence of clinical evidence of PXE (Bowen et al., 2007), in calcific elastosis, lipedema, lipodermatosclerosis, granuloma annulare, lichen sclerosus, morphea profunda, erythema nodosum, septal panniculitis, basal cell carcinoma and fibrosing dermatitis (Bowen et al., 2007; Taylor et al., 2004).

Even though sporadically, ocular lesions similar to those typical of PXE, have also been reported in Paget's disease, Marfan's and Ehlers–Danlos syndromes (Gurwood & Mastrangelo, 1997) and calcifications of retina, retina vessels and the presence of osseous metaplasia have also been noted in patients with renal failure, Coats' disease, tuberous sclerosis and retinocytomas (Miller et al., 2004; Patel et al., 2002).

Finally it has to be mentioned that ectopic calcifications may occur in the vascular system during physiological aging, in atherosclerosis and hypercholesterolemia, hypertension, smoking, calcific aortic stenosis, Marfan syndrome, diabetes, renal failure and in smokers (Proudfoot & Shanahan, 2001). There are two types of calcifications that occur in arteries: the intimal calcification, characteristic of the atherosclerotic plaque and associated with cells and collagen, and the medial calcification (also known as Mönckeberg sclerosis) mainly associated with elastin. Patients with chronic kidney disease (CKD) frequently display both forms of calcification. Another form of vascular calcification also occurs nearly exclusively in CKD patients: calciphylaxis or calcific uremic arteriolopathy. This is a disorder of medial calcification of the small arterioles of the skin, resulting in skin necrosis (Moe & Chen, 2003).

7.2 Genetic conditions

Unexpectedly, PXE-like cutaneous changes have also been found in approximately 20% of patients with beta-thalassemia (beta-thal) and sickle cell anaemia (SCD), that are well known severe congenital forms of anemia resulting from the deficient or altered synthesis of haemoglobin beta chains (Baccarani-Contri 2001; Fabbri et al., 2009). The first report suggesting a link between beta-thal and PXE was based on the observation that angioid streaks were actually present in both diseases (Aesopos et al., 1989). Subsequent studies confirmed that PXE-like syndrome in beta-thalassemias and SCD, although less severe, is histopathologically and clinically identical to inherited PXE consisting of indistinguishable cutaneous, ocular and vascular abnormalities due to elastic fibre calcification (Baccarani-Contri et al., 2001; Bercovitch & Terry, 2004; Hamlin et al., 2003) (Figure 9). In particular, it has been observed that beta-thal patients have calcifications of the posterior tibial artery (55%), typical skin lesions (20%), angioid streaks (52%) and that one or more of the three manifestations are actually present in 85% of the patients (Aessopos et al., 1998). Cardiovascular complications have been only sporadically observed, although they include intracranial haemorrhages, ischemic strokes, coronary arterial calcification complicated by unstable angina, myocardial infarction, mitral valve prolapse, valve calcification and leaflet thickening, pericardial thickening, renal artery calcification with arterial hypertension and peripheral arterial abnormalities complicated by gastric haemorrhage and intestinal infarcts (Aessopos et al., 1997,1998, 2001; Cianciulli et al., 2002; Farmakis et al., 2003).

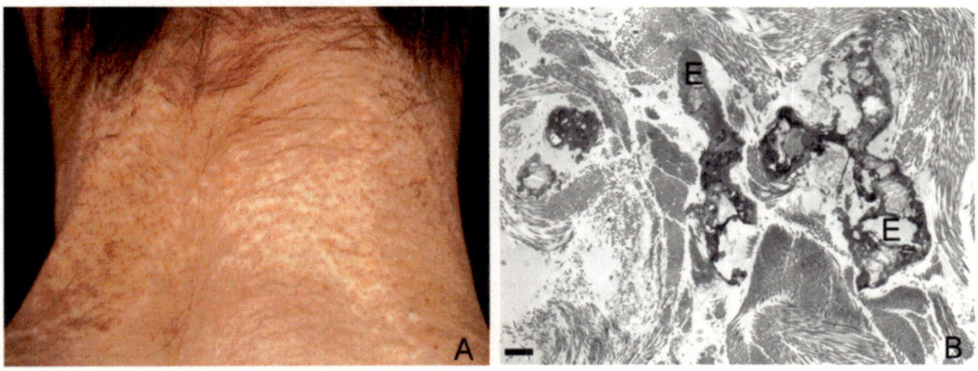

Fig. 9. PXE-like alterations in a patient affected by beta-thalassemia.
In these patients, papules and skin folds in typical areas of the neck (A) are associated to mineralized elastic fibres (E) in the dermis, as visualized by transmission electron microscopy (B). Bar: 1 μm

A genetic link between beta-thalassemia or SCDs and PXE is unlikely. In first instance, no mutations in the *ABCC6* gene were found in a cohort of beta-thal patients (Hamlin et al., 2003), moreover, *ABCC6* as well as other genes encoding for elastin or elastin associated molecules (i.e. fibrillins 1 and 2, elastin-related glycoproteins and lysyl-oxidase) are located on chromosomes different from that of the β-globin gene (Ringpfeil et al., 2000) and family members who do not have a haemoglobinopathies fail to show any PXE stigmata (Aessopos et al., 1994).

Never the less, in a study by Martin and coworkers (2006), fifty PXE patients have been investigated with the aim to determine the incidence of haemoglobin abnormalities typical of thalassemia. No cases of beta thalassemia were diagnosed in this cohort of patients, however in 20% of cases a significant but isolated (i.e. without microcytic anemia) increase of haemoglobin A2 (HbA2) was observed. The severity of clinical manifestations, other than the extent of cutaneous involvement, appeared independent from levels of haemoglobin. Therefore, *ABCC6* plus beta-globin digenism was ruled out of the pathogenesis of PXE, but it could be hypothesized a functional epigenetic reaction between *ABCC6* and the beta-globin locus, even though reciprocal interactions are clearly unequal since the change in *ABCC6* transcription occurring during the course of beta thalassaemia is responsible for a PXE phenotype, while increased HbA2 during the course of PXE has no haematological clinical consequences.

Interestingly, it has been recently demonstrated that a mouse model of beta-thal (*Hbb(th3/+)*) exhibits a NF-E2-induced transcriptional down-regulation of liver *ABCC6* (Martin et al., 2011), even though there are no evidence for spontaneous calcifications. It has been therefore suggested that decreased expression of mrp6 occurring later in life is probably insufficient to promote mineralization in the *Hbb(th3/+)* mouse C57BL/6J genetic background. However, these data may indicate that i) other factors, beside *ABCC6* expression are involved in the pathogenesis of calcifications, ii) responsive fibroblasts or other mesenchymal cells are required in order to modify connective tissue homeostasis, and iii) independently from the primary gene defect, common pathways may be involved in these disorders.

Within this context, it has been suggested that the elastic tissue injury in these patients may be the result of an oxidative process, induced by the combined and interactive effects of different factors (Aessopos et al., 1998; Garcia-Fernandez et al., 2008; Pasquali-Ronchetti et al., 2006). Plasma membrane microparticles, derived from the oxidative damage of red cell membranes by the effect of denatured hemoglobin products and free iron (Olivieri, 1999), as well as unbound fractions of hemoglobin and haem, which exceed the binding capacity of haptoglobin and hemopexin in the context of chronic hemolysis, have been considered to elicit inflammatory and oxidative reactions (Belcher et al., 2000; Gutteridge & Smith, 1988). The accumulated and prolonged effects of ROS/free radicals may result in disturbance of mesenchymal cell metabolism with structural deterioration of elastic fibres (Bunda et al., 2005). Accordingly, oxidative stress constitutes a potential acquired mechanism affecting the same molecular pathways, which are implicated in the pathogenesis of hereditary PXE.

The recent observation that a PXE-like phenotype can be observed in patients with pronounced deficiency of the vitamin K-dependent clotting factors raises the intriguing and exiting possibility that there might an additional pathway, independent of *ABCC6*, leading to the PXE phenotype (Vanakker et al. 2007).

Congenital deficiency of the vitamin K-dependent factors (VKCFD) is a rare bleeding disorder that can be caused either by mutation in the gamma-glutamyl carboxylase gene (*GGCX*) or in the vitamin K epoxide reductase complex(*VKORC*) (Oldenburg et al, 2000; Pauli et al, 1987). Moreover, acquired forms of the disorder can occur more frequently due to intestinal malabsorption of vitamin K (Djuric et al., 2007) or after prolonged treatments with vitamin K antagonists as warfarin (Palaniswamy et al., 2011). Vitamin K undergoes oxidation-reduction cycling within the endoplasmic reticulum, donating electrons to activate specific proteins via enzymatic gamma-carboxylation of glutamate groups before being enzymatically re-reduced (Figure 6).

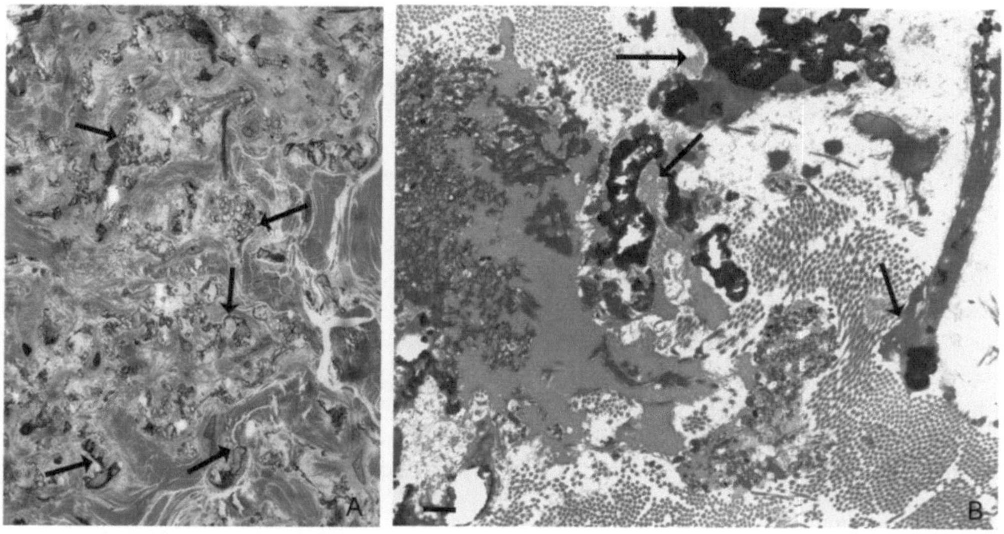

Fig. 10. Mineralized elastic fibres in a patient affected by VKFCD.
A) Light and B) transmission electron microscopy of a skin biopsy. Heavy mineralized elastic fibres (arrows) can be seen. Bar: 1μm

In addition to coagulation factors (II, VII, IX, X, and prothrombin) vitamin K activates protein C and protein S, osteocalcin (OC), matrix Gla protein (MGP), periostin, Gas6, and other vitamin K-dependent (VKD) proteins that, within bones, support calcium homeostasis and the mineralization process, whereas in vessel walls, and possibly in other peripheral soft connective tissues, they inhibit calcification, favouring endothelial integrity, cell growth and tissue renewal (Kidd, 2010).
Clinical overlap of PXE and VKCFD was obvious from the skin manifestations of yellowish papules or leathery plaques, with dot-like depressions, angioid streaks and/or ocular *peau d'orange*, as well as fragmentation and calcification of elastic fibres in the dermis. Important phenotypic differences from PXE included much more severe skin laxity with involvement of the trunk and limbs with thick, leathery skin folds rather than confinement to flexural areas, and no decrease in visual acuity. By light microscopy, changes in the reticular dermis were identical to those typical of PXE, consisting in polymorphous, fragmented, and mineralized elastic fibres, as shown by von Kossa stain. At the ultrastructural level, however, elastin had a more fragmented and mottled appearance than that typically observed in PXE (Vanakker et al., 2007) (Figure 10). In the light of these observations, it has been demonstrated *in vitro* (Gheduzzi et al., 2007) and *in vivo* (Li et al., 2007) that PXE is characterized by low levels of carboxylated-Matrix Gla Protein (Gla-MGP), thus suggesting that these changes may play a role in the pathogenesis of PXE, as described in more details in paragraph 4.

8. Conclusions

Pseudoxanthoma elasticum (PXE) is a rare genetic disorder characterized by mineralization of elastic fibres within all connective tissues, although the most important clinical manifestations affect skin, eyes and the cardiovascular system. Despite the dramatic involvement of the extracellular matrix, the first attempts made by researchers to find out the gene defect among those coding for matrix molecules failed and in 2000 three groups, independently, demonstrated that PXE is due to mutations in the *ABCC6* gene, that belongs to the ABC membrane transporters. To date the physiological substrate of this transporter is not known and still elusive are the pathogenetic mechanisms linking a defective cellular transporter, mainly expressed in liver and kidney, to ectopic calcification of connective tissues. This disease may therefore represent a very interesting example for investigating the complexity that regulates molecular pathways and the influence of metabolism on several organs/systems. Moreover, there is also evidence that similar endpoints (i.e. clinical and histological alterations) can be observed in some patients starting from gene defects different from *ABCC6* (i.e. beta-thalassemia, vitamin-K dependent coagulation deficiency). These data support the importance of using wide-spread technologies as transcriptomic or proteomic analyses to have a broader view of the molecular pathways that may be involved in the pathogenesis of elastic fibre calcification. Moreover recent findings in the literature highlights the role of polymorphisms in other genes that could be responsible for phenotypic changes and for a different severity of clinical manifestations in this monogenic disorder.

9. Acknowledgments

Authors gratefully acknowledge FCRM (EctoCal), PXE International and PXE Italia Onlus for their support.

10. References

Aesopos, A., Stamatelos, G., Savvides, P., Rombos, I., Tassiopoulos, T., & Kaklamanis, P. (1989). Pseudoxanthoma elasticum and angioid streaks in two cases of beta-thalassaemia. *Clin Rheumatol*, Vol. 8, No 4, pp. 522-527, ISSN 0770-3198

Aessopos, A., Voskaridou, E., Kavouklis, E., Vassilopoulos, G., Rombos, Y., Gavriel, L., & Loukopoulos, D. (1994). Angioid streaks in sickle-thalassemia. *Am J Ophthalmol*, Vol. 117, No 5, pp. 589-592, ISSN 0002-9394

Aessopos, A., Farmakis, D., Karagiorga, M., Rombos, I., & Loucopoulos, D. (1997). Pseudoxanthoma elasticum lesions and cardiac complications as contributing factors for strokes in beta-thalassemia patients. *Stroke*, Vol. 28, No 12, pp. 2421-2424, ISSN 0039-2499

Aessopos, A., Samarkos, M., Voskaridou, E., Papaioannou, D., Tsironi, M., Kavouklis, E., Vaiopoulos, G., Stamatelos, G., & Loukopoulos, D. (1998). Arterial calcifications in beta-thalassemia. *Angiology*, Vol. 49, No 2, pp. 137-143, ISSN 0003-3197

Aessopos, A., Farmakis, D., Karagiorga, M., Voskaridou, E., Loutradi, A., Hatziliami, A., Joussef, J., Rombos, J., & Loukopoulos, D. (2001). Cardiac involvement in thalassemia intermedia: a multicenter study. *Blood*, Vol. 97, No 11, pp. 3411-3416, ISSN 0006-4971

Aherrahrou, Z., Axtner, S.B., Kaczmarek, P.M., Jurat, A., Korff, S., Doehring, L.C., Weichenhan, D., Katus, H.A., & Ivandic, B.T. (2004). A locus on chromosome 7 determines dramatic up-regulation of osteopontin in dystrophic cardiac calcification in mice. *Am J Pathol*, Vol. 164, No 4, pp. 1379-1387, ISSN 0002-9440

Annovi, G., Boraldi, F., Guerra, D., Schurgers, L.J., Tiozzo, R., Pasquali-Ronchetti, I., & Quaglino, D. (2011). Does Vitamin K Supplementation Affects Vitamin K Cycle in

Control and PXE Fibroblasts? In: XXX Italian Society for the Study of Connective Tissues (SISC) Meeting, October 27-29, 2010, Palermo, Italy. *Connect. Tissue Res*, vol.52, No 4, pp.255-289, ISSN 0300-8207

Baccarani-Contri, M., Vincenti, D., Cicchetti, F., Mori, G., & Pasquali-Ronchetti, I. (1994). Immunochemical identification of abnormal constituents in the dermis of pseudoxanthoma elasticum patients. *Eur J Histochem*, Vol. 38, No 2, pp. 111-123, ISSN 1121-760X

Baccarani-Contri, M., Bacchelli, B., Boraldi, F., Quaglino, D., Taparelli, F., Carnevali, E., Francomano, M.A., Seidenari, S., Bettoli, V., De Sanctis, V., & Pasquali-Ronchetti, I. (2001). Characterization of pseudoxanthoma elasticum-like lesions in the skin of patients with beta-thalassemia. *J Am Acad Dermatol*, Vol. 44, No 1, pp. 33-39, ISSN 0190-9622

Belcher, J.D., Marker, P.H., Weber, J.P., Hebbel, R.P., & Vercellotti, G.M. (2000). Activated monocytes in sickle cell disease: potential role in the activation of vascular endothelium and vaso-occlusion. *Blood*, Vol. 96, No 7, pp. 2451-2459, ISSN 0006-4971

Belinsky, M.G., Chen, Z.S., Shchaveleva, I., Zeng, H., & Kruh, G.D. (2002). Characterization of the drug resistance and transport properties of multidrug resistance protein 6 (MRP6, ABCC6). *Cancer Res*, Vol. 62, No 21, pp. 6172-6177, ISSN 0008-5472

Bercovitch, L., Schepps, B., Koelliker, S., Magro, C., Terry, S., & Lebwohl, M. (2003). Mammographic findings in pseudoxanthoma elasticum. *J Am Acad Dermatol*, Vol. 48, No 3, pp. 359-366, ISSN 0190-9622

Bercovitch, L., & Terry, P. (2004). Pseudoxanthoma elasticum 2004. *J Am Acad Dermatol*, Vol. 51, No 1 Suppl, pp. S13-14, ISSN 0190-9622

Bergen, A.A., Plomp, A.S., Schuurman, E.J., Terry, S., Breuning, M., Dauwerse, H., Swart, J., Kool, M., van Soest, S., Baas, F., ten Brink, J.B., & de Jong, P.T. (2000). Mutations in ABCC6 cause pseudoxanthoma elasticum. *Nat Genet*, Vol. 25, No 2, pp. 228-231, ISSN 1061-4036

Bergen, A.A., Plomp, A.S., Gorgels, T.G., & de Jong, P.T. (2004). From gene to disease; pseudoxanthoma elasticum and the ABCC6 gene. *Ned Tijdschr Geneeskd*, Vol. 148, No 32. pp. 1586-1589, ISSN 0028-2162

Bock, A., & Schwegler, G. (2008). Intracerebral haemorrhage as first manifestation of pseudoxanthoma elasticum. *Clin Neurol Neurosurg*. Vol. 110, No 3, pp. 262-264, ISSN 0303-8467

Booij, J.C., Baas, D.C., Beisekeeva, J., Gorgels, T.G., & Bergen, A.A. (2010). The dynamic nature of Bruch's membrane. *Prog Retin Eye Res*, Vol. 29, No 1, pp. 1-18, ISSN 1350-9462

Boraldi, F., Quaglino, D., Croce, M.A., Garcia Fernandez, M.I., Tiozzo, R., Gheduzzi, D., Bacchelli, B., & Pasquali Ronchetti, I. (2003). Multidrug resistance protein-6 (MRP6) in human dermal fibroblasts. Comparison between cells from normal subjects and from Pseudoxanthoma elasticum patients. *Matrix Biol*, Vol. 22, No 6, pp. 491-500, ISSN 0945-053X

Boraldi, F., Annovi, G., Guerra, D., Paolinelli Devincenzi, C., Garcia-Fernandez, M.I., Panico, F., De Santis, G., Tiozzo, R., Ronchetti, I., & Quaglino, D. (2009). Fibroblast protein profile analysis highlights the role of oxidative stress and vitamin K recycling in the pathogenesis of pseudoxanthoma elasticum. *Proteomics Clin Appl*, Vol. 3, No 9, pp. 1084-1098, ISSN 1862-8346

Borst, P., & Elferink, R.O. (2002). Mammalian ABC transporters in health and disease. *Annu Rev Biochem*, Vol. 71, pp. 537-592, ISSN 0066-4154

Borst, P., van de Wetering, K., & Schlingemann, R. (2008). Does the absence of ABCC6 (multidrug resistance protein 6) in patients with Pseudoxanthoma elasticum prevent the liver from providing sufficient vitamin K to the periphery? *Cell Cycle*, Vol. 7, No 11, pp. 1575-1579, ISSN 1538-4101

Bowen, A.R., Götting, C., LeBoit, P.E., & McCalmont, T.H. (2007). Pseudoxanthoma elasticum-like fibers in the inflamed skin of patients without pseudoxanthoma elasticum. *J Cutan Pathol*, Vol. 34, No 10, pp. 777-781, ISSN 0303-6987

Bunda, S., Kaviani, N., & Hinek, A. (2005). Fluctuations of intracellular iron modulate elastin production. *J Biol Chem*, Vol. 280, No 3, pp. 2341-2351, ISSN 0021-9258

Chassaing, N., Martin, L., Mazereeuw, J., Barrié, L., Nizard, S., Bonafé, J.L., Calvas, P., & Hovnanian, A. (2004). Novel ABCC6 mutations in pseudoxanthoma elasticum. *J Invest Dermatol*, Vol. 122, No 3, pp. 608-613, ISSN 0022-202X

Chassaing, N., Martin, L., Calvas, P., Le Bert, M., & Hovnanian, A. (2005). Pseudoxanthoma elasticum: a clinical, pathophysiological and genetic update including 11 novel ABCC6 mutations. *J Med Genet*, Vol. 42, No 12, pp. 881-892, ISSN 0022-2593

Chraïbi, R., Ismaili, N., Belgnaoui, F., Akallal, N., Bouhllab, J., Senouci, K., & Hassam, B. (2007). Pseudoxanthoma elasticum and nephrocalcinosis. *Ann Dermatol Venereol*, Vol. 134, No 10 Pt 1, pp. 764-766, ISSN 0151-9638

Christiano, A.M., Lebwohl, M.G., Boyd, C.D., & Uitto, J. (1992). Workshop on pseudoxanthoma elasticum: molecular biology and pathology of the elastic fibers. Jefferson Medical College, Philadelphia, Pennsylvania, June 10, 1992. J *Invest Dermatol*, Vol. 99, No 5, pp. 660-663, ISSN 0022-202X

Cianciulli, P., Sorrentino, F., Maffei, L., Amadori, S., Cappabianca, M.P., Foglietta, E., Carnevali, E., & Pasquali-Ronchetti, I. (2002). Cardiovascular involvement in thalassaemic patients with pseudoxanthoma elasticum-like skin lesions: a long-term follow-up study. *Eur J Clin Invest*, Vol. 32, No. 9, pp. 700-706, ISSN 0014-2972

Contri, M.B., Boraldi, F., Taparelli, F., De Paepe, A., & Pasquali Ronchetti, I. (1996). Matrix proteins with high affinity for calcium ions are associated with mineralization within the elastic fibers of pseudoxanthoma elasticum dermis. *Am J Pathol*, Vol. 148, No 2, pp. 569-567, ISSN 0002-9440

Costrop, L.M., Vanakker, O.O., Van Laer, L., Le Saux, O., Martin, L., Chassaing, N., Guerra, D., Pasquali-Ronchetti, I., Coucke. P.J., & De Paepe, A. (2010). Novel deletions causing pseudoxanthoma elasticum underscore the genomic instability of the ABCC6 region. *J Hum Genet*, Vol. 55, No 2, pp. 112-117, ISSN 1434-5161

Denhardt, D.T., Giachelli, C.M., & Rittling, S.R. (2001). Role of osteopontin in cellular signaling and toxicant injury. *Annu Rev Pharmacol Toxicol*, Vol. 41, pp. 723-749, ISSN 0362-1642

Djuric, Z., Zivic, S., & Katic, V. (2007). Celiac disease with diffuse cutaneous vitamin K-deficiency bleeding. *Adv Ther*, Vol. 24, No 6, pp. 1286-1289, ISSN 0741-238X

Donas, K.P., Schulte, S., & Horsch, S. (2007). Balloon angioplasty in the treatment of vascular lesions in pseudoxanthoma elasticum. *J Vasc Interv Radiol*, Vol. 18, No 3, pp. 457-459, ISSN 1051-0443

Fabbri, E., Forni, G.L., Guerrini, G., & Borgna-Pignatti, C. (2009). Pseudoxanthoma-elasticum-like syndrome and thalassemia: an update. *Dermatol Online J*, Vol. 15, No 7, pp. 7, ISSN 1087-2108

Farmakis, D., Moyssakis, I., Perakis, A., Rombos, Y., Deftereos, S., Giakoumis, A., Polymeropoulos, E., & Aessopos, A. (2003). Unstable angina associated with coronary arterial calcification in a thalassemia intermedia patient with a pseudoxanthoma elasticum-like syndrome. *Eur J Haematol*, Vol. 70, No 1, pp. 64-66, ISSN 0902-4441

Garcia-Fernandez, M.I., Gheduzzi, D., Boraldi, F., Paolinelli DeVincenzi, C., Sanchez, P., Valdivielso, P., Morilla, M.J., Quaglino, D., Guerra, D., Casolari, S., Bercovitch, L., & Pasquali-Ronchetti, I. (2008). Parameters of oxidative stress are present in the circulation of PXE patients. *Biochim Biophys Acta*, Vol. 1782, No 7-8, pp. 474-481, ISSN 0925-4439

Georgalas, I., Tservakis, I., Papaconstaninou, D., Kardara, M., Koutsandrea, C., & Ladas, I. (2011). Pseudoxanthoma elasticum, ocular manifestations, complications and treatment. *Clin Exp Optom*, Vol. 94, No 2, pp. 169-180, ISSN 0816-4622

Gheduzzi, D., Taparelli, F., Quaglino, D. Jr, Di Rico, C., Bercovitch, L., Terry, S., Singer, D.B., & Pasquali-Ronchetti, I. (2001). The placenta in pseudoxanthoma elasticum: clinical, structural and immunochemical study. *Placenta*, Vol. 22, No 6, pp. 580-590, ISSN 0143-4004

Gheduzzi, D., Sammarco, R., Quaglino, D., Bercovitch, L., Terry , S., Taylor, W., & Pasquali Ronchetti, I. (2003). Extracutaneous ultrastructural alterations in pseudoxanthoma elasticum. *Ultrastruct Pathol*, Vol. 27, No 6, pp. 375-384, ISSN 0191-3123

Gheduzzi, D., Guidetti, R., Anzivino, C., Tarugi, P., Di Leo, E., Quaglino, D., & Ronchetti, I.P. (2004). ABCC6 mutations in Italian families affected by pseudoxanthoma elasticum (PXE). *Hum Mutat*, Vol. 24, No 5, pp. 438-439, ISSN 1059-7794

Gheduzzi, D., Guerra, D., Bochicchio, B., Pepe, A., Tamburo, A.M., Quaglino, D., Mithieux, S., Weiss, A.S., & Pasquali Ronchetti, I. (2005). Heparan sulphate interacts with tropoelastin, with some tropoelastin peptides and is present in human dermis elastic fibers. *Matrix Biol*, Vol. 24, No 1, pp.15-25, ISSN 0945-053X

Gheduzzi, D., Boraldi, F., Annovi, G., Paolinelli DeVincenzi, C., Schurgers, L.J., Vermeer, C., Quaglino, D., & Pasquali Ronchetti, I. (2007). Matrix Gla protein is involved in elastic fiber calcification in the dermis of pseudoxanthoma elasticum patients. *Lab Invest*, Vol. 87, No 10, pp. 998-1008, ISSN 0023-6837

Giacopelli, F., Marciano, R., Pistorio, A., Catarsi, P., Canini, S., Karsenty, G., & Ravazzolo, R. (2004). Polymorphisms in the osteopontin promoter affect its transcriptional activity. *Physiol Genomics*, Vol. 20, No 1, pp. 87-96, ISSN 0888-7543

Golliet-Mercier, N., Allaouchiche, B., & Monneuse, O. (2005). Pseudoxanthoma elasticum with severe gastrointestinal bleeding. *Ann Fr Anesth Reanim*, Vol. 24, No 7, pp. 833-834, ISSN 0750-7658

Gonzalez, M.E., Votava, H.J., Lipkin, G., & Sanchez, M. (2009). Pseudoxanthoma elasticum. *Dermatol Online J*, Vol. 15, No 8, pp. 17, ISSN 1087-2108

Gorgels, T.G., Waarsing, J.H., de Wolf, A., ten Brink, J.B., Loves, W.J., & Bergen, A.A. (2010). Dietary magnesium, not calcium, prevents vascular calcification in a mouse model for pseudoxanthoma elasticum. *J Mol Med*, Vol. 88, No 5. pp. 467-475, ISSN 0946-2716

Götting. C,, Hendig, D., Adam, A., Schön, S., Schulz, V., Szliska, C., Kuhn, J., & Kleesiek, K. (2005). Elevated xylosyltransferase I activities in pseudoxanthoma elasticum (PXE)

patients as a marker of stimulated proteoglycan biosynthesis. *J Mol Med*, Vol. 83, No 12, pp. 984-992, ISSN 0946-2716

Gurwood, A.S., & Mastrangelo, D.L. (1997). Understanding angioid streaks. *J Am Optom Assoc*, Vol. 68, No 5, pp. 309-324, ISSN 0003-0244

Gutteridge, J.M., & Smith, A. (1988). Antioxidant protection by haemopexin of haem-stimulated lipid peroxidation. *Biochem J*, Vol. 256, No 3, pp. 861-865, ISSN 0264-6021

Haimeur, A., Conseil, G., Deeley, R.G., & Cole, S.P. (2004). Mutations of charged amino acids in or near the transmembrane helices of the second membrane spanning domain differentially affect the substrate specificity and transport activity of the multidrug resistance protein MRP1 (ABCC1). *Mol Pharmacol*, Vol. 65, No 6, pp. 1375-1385, ISSN 0026-895X

Hamlin, N., Beck, K., Baccelli, B., Cianciulli, P., Pasquali-Ronchetti, I., & Le Saux, O. (2003). Acquired Pseudoxanthoma elasticum-like syndrome in beta-thalassaemia patients. *Br J Haematol*, Vol. 122, No 5, pp. 852-854, ISSN 0007-1048

Heaton, J.P., & Wilson, J.W. (1986). Pseudoxanthoma elasticum and its urological implications. *J Urol, Vol* 135, No 4, pp. 776-777, ISSN 0022-5347

Heid, E., Eberst, E., Lazrak, B., & Basset, A. (1980). Pseudoxanthoma elasticum and acneiform lesions. *Ann Dermatol Venereol*, Vol. 107, No. 6, pp. 569-567, ISSN 0151-9638

Heimann, H., Gelisken, F., Wachtlin, J., Wehner, A., Völker, M., Foerster, M.H., & Bartz-Schmidt, K.U. (2005) Photodynamic therapy with verteporfin for choroidal neovascularization associated with angioid streaks. *Graefes Arch Clin Exp Ophthalmol*, Vol. 243, No 11, pp. 1115-1123, ISSN 0721-832X

Hendig, D., Schulz, V., Arndt, M., Szliska, C., Kleesiek, K., & Götting, C. (2006). Role of serum fetuin-A, a major inhibitor of systemic calcification, in pseudoxanthoma elasticum. *Clin Chem*, Vol. 52, No 2, pp. 227-234, ISSN 0009-9147

Hendig, D., Arndt, M., Szliska, C., Kleesiek, K., & Götting, C. (2007). SPP1 promoter polymorphisms: identification of the first modifier gene for pseudoxanthoma elasticum. *Clin Chem*, Vol. 53, No 5, pp. 829-836, ISSN 0009-9147

Hendig, D., Zarbock, R., Szliska, C., Kleesiek, K., & Götting, C. (2008). The local calcification inhibitor matrix Gla protein in pseudoxanthoma elasticum. *Clin Biochem*, Vol. 41, No 6, pp. 407-412, ISSN 0009-9120

Heyl T. (1967). Psedoxanthoma elasticum with granulomatous skin lesions. *Arch Dermatol*, Vol 96, No 5, pp.528-531, ISSN 0003-987X

Hovnanian, A. (2010). Modifier genes in pseudoxanthoma elasticum: novel insights from the Ggcx mouse model. *J Mol Med*, Vol. 88, No 2, pp. 149-153, ISSN 0946-2716

Hu, X., Peek, R., Plomp, A., ten Brink, J., Scheffer, G., van Soest, S., Leys, A., de Jong, P.T., & Bergen, A.A. (2003a). Analysis of the frequent R1141X mutation in the ABCC6 gene in pseudoxanthoma elasticum. *Invest Ophthalmol Vis Sci*, Vol. 44, No 5, pp. 1824-1829, ISSN 0146-0404

Hu, X., Plomp, A., Wijnholds, J., Ten Brink, J., van Soest, S., van den Born, L.I., Leys, A., Peek, R., de Jong, P.T., & Bergen, A.A. (2003b). ABCC6/MRP6 mutations: further insight into the molecular pathology of pseudoxanthoma elasticum. *Eur J Hum Genet*, Vol. 11, No 3, pp. 215-224, ISSN 1018-4813

Iliás, A., Urbán, Z., Seidl, T.L., Le Saux, O., Sinkó, E., Boyd, C.D., Sarkadi, B., & Váradi, A. (2002). Loss of ATP-dependent transport activity in pseudoxanthoma elasticum-associated mutants of human ABCC6 (MRP6). *J Biol Chem*, Vol. 277, No 19, pp. 16860-16867, ISSN 0021-9258

Jelaska, A., Strehlow, D., & Korn, J.H. (1999). Fibroblast heterogeneity in physiological conditions and fibrotic disease. *Springer Semin Immunopathol*, Vol. 21, No 4, pp. 385-395, ISSN 0344-4325

Jiang, Q., & Uitto, J. (2006). Pseudoxanthoma elasticum: a metabolic disease? *J Invest Dermatol*, Vol. 126, No 7, pp. 1440-1441, ISSN 0022-202X

Jiang, Q., Li, Q., & Uitto, J. (2007). Aberrant mineralization of connective tissues in a mouse model of pseudoxanthoma elasticum: systemic and local regulatory factors. *J Invest Dermatol*, Vol. 127, No 6, pp. 1392-1402, ISSN 0022-202X

Jiang, Q., Endo, M., Dibra, F., Wang, K., & Uitto, J. (2009). Pseudoxanthoma elasticum is a metabolic disease. *J Invest Dermatol*, Vol. 129, No 2, pp. 348-354, ISSN 0022-202X

Jiang, Q., Li, Q., Grand-Pierre, A.E., Schurgers, L.J., & Uitto, J. (2011). Administration of vitamin K does not counteract the ectopic mineralization of connective tissues in Abcc6 (-/-) mice, a model for pseudoxanthoma elasticum. *Cell Cycle*, Vol. 10, No 4, pp. 701-707, ISSN 1538-4101

Kidd, P.M. (2010). Vitamins D and K as pleiotropic nutrients: clinical importance to the skeletal and cardiovascular systems and preliminary evidence for synergy. *Altern Med Rev*, Vol. 15, No 3, pp.199-222, ISSN 1089-5159

Klement, J.F., Matsuzaki, Y., Jiang, Q.J., Terlizzi, J., Choi, H.Y., Fujimoto, N., Li, K., Pulkkinen, L., Birk, D.E., Sundberg, J.P., & Uitto, J. (2005). Targeted ablation of the abcc6 gene results in ectopic mineralization of connective tissues. *Mol Cell Biol*, Vol. 25, No 18, pp. 8299-8310, ISSN 0270-7306

Köblös, G., Andrikovics, H., Prohászka, Z., Tordai, A., Váradi, A., & Arányi, T. (2010). The R1141X loss-of-function mutation of the ABCC6 gene is a strong genetic risk factor for coronary artery disease. *Genet Test Mol Biomarkers*, Vol. 14, No 1, pp. 75-78, ISSN 1945-0265

Kool, M., van der Linden, M., de Haas, M., Baas, F., & Borst, P. (1999). Expression of human MRP6, a homologue of the multidrug resistance protein gene MRP1, in tissues and cancer cells. *Cancer Res*, Vol. 59, No 1, pp. 175-182, ISSN 0008-5472

Kornet, L., Bergen, A.A., Hoeks, A.P., Cleutjens, J.P., Oostra, R.J., Daemen, M.J., van Soest, S., & Reneman, R.S. (2004). In patients with pseudoxanthoma elasticum a thicker and more elastic carotid artery is associated with elastin fragmentation and proteoglycans accumulation.*Ultrasound Med Biol*, Vol. 30, No 8, pp. 1041-1048, ISSN 0301-5629

LaRusso, J., Li, Q., Jiang, Q., & Uitto, J. (2009). Elevated dietary magnesium prevents connective tissue mineralization in a mouse model of pseudoxanthoma elasticum (Abcc6(-/-)). *J Invest Dermatol*, Vol. 129, No 6, pp. 1388-1394, ISSN 0022-202X

Le Saux, O., Urban, Z., Göring, H.H., Csiszar, K., Pope, F.M., Richards, A., Pasquali-Ronchetti, I., Terry, S., Bercovitch, L., Lebwohl, M.G., Breuning, M., van den Berg, P., Kornet, L., Doggett, N., Ott, J., de Jong, P.T., Bergen, A.A., & Boyd, C.D. (1999). Pseudoxanthoma elasticum maps to an 820-kb region of the p13.1 region of chromosome 16. *Genomics*, Vol. 62, No 1, pp. 1-10, ISSN 0888-7543

Le Saux, O., Urban, Z., Tschuch, C., Csiszar, K., Baccelli, B., Quaglino, D., Pasquali-Ronchetti, I., Pope, F.M., Richards, A., Terry, S., Bercovitch, L., de Paepe, A., & Boyd, C.D. (2000). Mutations in a gene encoding an ABC transporter cause pseudoxanthoma elasticum. *Nat Genet*, Vol. 25, No 2, pp. 223-227, ISSN 1061-4036

Le Saux, O., Beck, K., Sachsinger, C., Silvestri, C., Treiber, C., Göring, H.H., Johnson, E.W., De Paepe, A., Pope, F.M., Pasquali-Ronchetti, I., Bercovitch, L., Marais, A.S.,

Viljoen, D.L., Terry, S.F., & Boyd, C.D. (2001). A spectrum of ABCC6 mutations is responsible for pseudoxanthoma elasticum. *Am J Hum Genet*, Vol. 69, No 4, pp. 749-764, ISSN 0002-9297

Le Saux, O., Beck, K., Sachsinger, C., Treiber, C., Göring, H.H., Curry, K., Johnson, E.W., Bercovitch, L., Marais, A.S., Terry, S.F., Viljoen, D.L., & Boyd, C.D. (2002). Evidence for a founder effect for pseudoxanthoma elasticum in the Afrikaner population of South Africa. *Hum Genet*, Vol. 111, No 4-5, pp. 331-338, ISSN 0340-6717

Le Saux, O., Bunda, S., VanWart, C.M., Douet, V., Got, L., Martin, L., & Hinek, A. (2006). Serum factors from pseudoxanthoma elasticum patients alter elastic fiber formation in vitro. *J Invest Dermatol*, Vol. 126, No 7, pp. 1497-1505, ISSN 0022-202X

Lebwohl, M., Schwartz, E., Lemlich, G., Lovelace, O., Shaikh-Bahai, F., & Fleischmajer, R. (1993). Abnormalities of connective tissue components in lesional and non-lesional tissue of patients with pseudoxanthoma elasticum. *Arch Dermatol Res*, Vol. 285, No 3, pp. 121-126, ISSN 0003-987X

Lecerf, J.M., & Desmettre, T. (2010). Nutrition and age-related macular degeneration. *J Fr Ophtalmol*, Vol. 33, No 10, pp. 749-757, ISSN 0181-5512

Lewis, K.G., Lester, B.W., Pan, T.D., & Robinson-Bostom, L. (2006). Nephrogenic fibrosing dermopathy and calciphylaxis with pseudoxanthoma elasticum-like changes. *J Cutan Pathol*, Vol. 33, No 10, pp. 695-700, ISSN 0303-6987

Li, Q., Jiang, Q., Schurgers, L.J., & Uitto, J. (2007). Pseudoxanthoma elasticum: reduced gamma-glutamyl carboxylation of matrix gla protein in a mouse model (Abcc6-/-). *Biochem Biophys Res Commun*, Vol. 364, No 2, pp. 208-213, ISSN 0006-291X

Li, Q., Jiang, Q., Pfendner, E., Váradi, A., & Uitto, J. (2009). Pseudoxanthoma elasticum: clinical phenotypes, molecular genetics and putative pathomechanisms. *Exp Dermatol*, Vol. 18, No 1, pp. 1-11, ISSN 0906-6705

Li, T.H., Tseng, C.R., Hsiao, G.H., & Chiu, H.C. (1996). An unusual cutaneous manifestation of pseudoxanthoma elasticum mimicking reticulate pigmentary disorders. *Br J Dermatol*, Vol. 134, No 6, pp. 1157-1159, ISSN 0007-0963

Lund, H.Z., & Gilbert, C.F. (1976). Perforating pseudoxanthoma elasticum. Its distinction from elastosis perforans serpiginosa. *Arch Pathol Lab Med*, Vol. 100, No 10, pp. 544-546, ISSN 0003-9985

Maccari, F., Gheduzzi, D., & Volpi, N. (2003). Anomalous structure of urinary glycosaminoglycans in patients with pseudoxanthoma elasticum. *Clin Chem*, Vol. 49, No 3, pp. 380-388, ISSN 0009-9147

Maccari, F., & Volpi, N. (2008). Structural characterization of the skin glycosaminoglycans in patients with pseudoxanthoma elasticum. *Int J Dermatol*, Vol. 47, No 10, pp. 1024-1027, ISSN 0011-9059

Mainetti, C., Masouyé, I., & Saurat, J.H. (1991). Pseudoxanthoma elasticum-like lesions in the L-tryptophan-induced eosinophilia-myalgia syndrome. *J Am Acad Dermatol*, Vol. 24, No. 4, pp. 657-658, ISSN 0190-9622

Martin, L., Pissard, S., Blanc, P., Chassaing, N., Legac, E., Briault, S., Le Bert, M., & Le Saux, O. (2006). Increased haemoglobin A2 levels in pseudoxanthoma elasticum. *Ann Dermatol Venereol*, Vol. 133, No 8-9 Pt 1, pp. 645-651, ISSN 0151-9638

Martin, L., Douet, V., VanWart, C.M., Heller, M.B., & Le Saux, O. (2011). A mouse model of β-thalassemia shows a liver-specific down-regulation of Abcc6 expression. *Am J Pathol*, Vol. 178, No 2, pp. 774-783, ISSN 0002-9440

Matsuzaki, Y., Nakano, A., Jiang, Q.J., Pulkkinen, L., & Uitto, J. (2005). Tissue-specific expression of the ABCC6 gene. *J Invest Dermatol*, Vol. 125, No 5, pp. 900-905, ISSN 0022-202X

Mendelsohn, G., Bulkley, B.H., & Hutchins, G.M. (1978). Cardiovascular manifestations of Pseudoxanthoma elasticum. *Arch Pathol Lab Med*, Vol. 102, No 6, pp. 298-302, ISSN 0003-9985

Miksch, S., Lumsden, A., Guenther, U.P., Foernzler, D., Christen-Zäch, S., Daugherty, C., Ramesar R.K., Lebwohl, M., Hohl, D., Neldner, K.H., Lindpaintner, K., Richards, R.I., & Struk, B. (2005). Molecular genetics of pseudoxanthoma elasticum: type and frequency of mutations in ABCC6. *Hum Mutat*, Vol. 26, No 3, pp. 235-248, ISSN 1059-7794

Miller, D.M., Benz, M.S., Murray, T.G., & Dubovy, S.R. (2004). Intraretinal calcification and osseous metaplasia in coats disease. *Arch Ophthalmol*, Vol. 122, No 11, pp. 1710-1712, ISSN 0003-9950

Moe, S.M., & Chen, N.X. (2003). Calciphylaxis and vascular calcification: a continuum of extra-skeletal osteogenesis. *Pediatr Nephrol*, Vol. 18, No 10, pp. 969-975, ISSN 0931-041X

Muir, R.L. (2009). Peripheral arterial disease: Pathophysiology, risk factors, diagnosis, treatment, and prevention. *J Vasc Nurs*, Vol. 27, No 2, pp. 26-30, ISSN 1062-0303

Neldner, K.H., & Martinez-Hernandez, A. (1979). Localized acquired cutaneous pseudoxanthoma elasticum. *J Am Acad Dermatol*, Vol. 1, No 6, pp. 523-530, ISSN 0190-9622

Neldner, K.H. (1988). Pseudoxanthoma elasticum. *Int J Dermatol*, Vol. 27, No 2, pp. 98-100, ISSN 0011-9059

Neldner, K.H. & Struk, B. (2002). Pseudoxanthoma elasticum. In : *Connective Tissue and ist heritable disorders. Molecular, Genetic and medical aspects*, Royce, P.M., Steinmann, B., pp. 561-583, Wiley-Liss & Sons, ISBN 9780471251859, New York

Ng, A.B., O'Sullivan, S.T., & Sharpe, D.T. (1999). Plastic surgery and pseudoxanthoma elasticum. *Br J Plast Surg*, Vol. 52, No 7, pp. 594-596, ISSN 0007-1226

Nielsen, A.O., Christensen, O.B., Hentzer, B., Johnson, E., & Kobayasi, T. (1978). Salpeter-induced dermal changes electron-microscopically indistinguishable from pseudoxanthoma elasticum. *Acta Derm Venereol*, Vol. 58, No 4, pp. 323-327, ISSN 0001-5555

Noji, Y., Inazu, A., Higashikata, T., Nohara, A., Kawashiri, M.A., Yu, W., Todo, Y., Nozue, T., Uno, Y., Hifumi, S., & Mabuchi, H. (2004). Identification of two novel missense mutations (p.R1221C and p.R1357W) in the ABCC6 (MRP6) gene in a Japanese patient with pseudoxanthoma elasticum (PXE). *Intern Med*, Vol. 43, No 12, pp. 1171-1176, ISSN 1349-7235

Ohnishi, Y., Tajima, S., Ishibashi, A., Inazumi, T., Sasaki, T., & Sakamoto, H. (1998). Pseudoxanthoma elasticum-like papillary dermal elastolysis: report of four Japanese cases and an immunohistochemical study of elastin and fibrillin-1. *Br J Dermatol*, Vol. 139, No 1, pp. 141-144, ISSN 0007-0963

Oldenburg, J., von Brederlow, B., Fregin, A., Rost, S., Wolz, W., Eberl, W., Eber, S., Lenz, E., Schwaab, R., Brackmann, H.H., Effenberger, W., Harbrecht, U., Schurgers, L.J., Vermeer, C., & Müller, C.R. (2000). Congenital deficiency of vitamin K dependent coagulation factors in two families presents as a genetic defect of the vitamin K-epoxide-reductase-complex. *Thromb Haemost*, Vol. 84, No 6, pp. 937-941, ISSN 0340-6245

Olivieri, N.F. (1999). The beta-thalassemias. *N Engl J Med*, Vol. 341, No 2, pp. 99-109, ISSN 0028-4793

Palaniswamy, C., Sekhri, A., Aronow, W.S., Kalra, A., & Peterson, S.J. (2011). Association of warfarin use with valvular and vascular calcification: a review. *Clin Cardiol*, Vol. 34, No 2, pp. 74-81, ISSN 0160-9289

Pasquali-Ronchetti, I., Volpin, D., Baccarani-Contri, M., Castellani, I., & Peserico, A. (1981). Pseudoxanthoma elasticum. Biochemical and ultrastructural studies. *Dermatology*, Vol. 163, No 4, pp. 307-325, ISSN 1018-8665

Pasquali-Ronchetti, I., Garcia-Fernandez, M.I., Boraldi, F., Quaglino, D., Gheduzzi, D., De Vincenzi Paolinelli, C. Tiozzo, R., Bergamini, S., Ceccarelli, D., & Moscatello, U. (2006). Oxidative stress in fibroblasts from patients with pseudoxanthoma elasticum: possible role in the pathogenesis of clinical manifestations. *J Pathol*, Vol. 208, No 1, pp. 54-61, ISSN 0022-3417

Passi, A., Albertini, R., Baccarani Contri, M., de Luca, G., de Paepe, A., Pallavicini, G., Pasquali Ronchetti, I., & Tiozzo, R. (1996). Proteoglycan alterations in skin fibroblast cultures from patients affected with pseudoxanthoma elasticum. *Cell Biochem Funct*, Vol. 14, No 2, pp. 111-120, ISSN 0263-6484

Patel, D.V., Snead, M.P., & Satchi, K. (2002). Retinal arteriolar calcification in a patient with chronic renal failure. *Br J Ophthalmol*, Vol. 86, No 9, pp. 1063, ISSN 0007-1161

Pauli, R.M., Lian, J.B., Mosher, D.F., & Suttie, J.W. (1987). Association of congenital deficiency of multiple vitamin K-dependent coagulation factors and the phenotype of the warfarin embryopathy: clues to the mechanism of teratogenicity of coumarin derivatives. *Am J Hum Genet*, Vol. 41, No 4, pp. 566-583, ISSN 0002-9297

Pece, A., Avanza, P., Galli, L., & Brancato, R. (1997). Laser photocoagulation of choroidal neovascularization in angioid streaks. *Retina*, Vol. 17, No 1, pp. 12-16, ISSN 0275-004X

Pfendner, E.G., Vanakker, O.M., Terry, S.F., Vourthis, S., McAndrew, P.E., McClain, M.R., Fratta, S., Marais, A.S., Hariri, S., Coucke, P.J., Ramsay, M., Viljoen, D., Terry, P.F., De Paepe, A., Uitto, J., & Bercovitch, L.G. (2007). Mutation detection in the ABCC6 gene and genotype-phenotype analysis in a large international case series affected by pseudoxanthoma elasticum. *J Med Genet*, Vol. 44, No 10, pp. 621-628, ISSN 0022-2593

Phillips, J.E., Hutmacher, D.W., Guldberg, R.E., & García, A.J. (2006). Mineralization capacity of Runx2/Cbfa1-genetically engineered fibroblasts is scaffold dependent. *Biomaterials*, Vol. 27, No 32, pp. 5535-5545, ISSN 0142-9612

Plomp, A.S., Florijn, R.J., Ten Brink, J., Castle, B., Kingston, H., Martín-Santiago, A., Gorgels, T.G., de Jong, P.T., & Bergen, A.A. (2008). ABCC6 mutations in pseudoxanthoma elasticum: an update including eight novel ones. *Mol Vis*, Vol. 24, No 14, pp. 18-24, ISSN 1090-0535

Proudfoot, D., & Shanahan, C.M. (2001).Biology of calcification in vascular cells: intima versus media. *Herz*, Vol. 26, No 4, pp. 245-251, ISSN 0340-9937

Quaglino, D., Boraldi, F., Barbieri, D., Croce, A., Tiozzo, R., & Pasquali Ronchetti, I. (2000). Abnormal phenotype of in vitro dermal fibroblasts from patients with Pseudoxanthoma elasticum (PXE). *Biochim Biophys Acta*, Vol. 1501, No 1, pp. 51-62, ISSN 0925-4439

Quaglino, D., Sartor, L., Garbisa, S., Boraldi, F., Croce, A., Passi, A., De Luca, G., Tiozzo, R., & Pasquali-Ronchetti, I. (2005). Dermal fibroblasts from pseudoxanthoma elasticum patients have raised MMP-2 degradative potential. *Biochim Biophys Acta*, Vol. 1741, No 1-2, pp. 42-47, ISSN 0925-4439

Raybould, M.C., Birley, A.J., Moss, C., Hultén, M., & McKeown, C.M. (1994). Exclusion of an elastin gene (ELN) mutation as the cause of pseudoxanthoma elasticum (PXE) in one family. *Clin Genet*, Vol. 45, No 1, pp. 48-51, ISSN 0009-9163

Ringpfeil, F., Lebwohl, M.G., Christiano, A.M., & Uitto, J. (2000). Pseudoxanthoma elasticum: mutations in the MRP6 gene encoding a transmembrane ATP-binding cassette (ABC) transporter. *Proc Natl Acad Sci U S A*, Vol. 97, No 11, pp. 6001-6006, ISSN 0027-8424

Ringpfeil, F., McGuigan, K., Fuchsel, L., Kozic, H., Larralde, M., Lebwohl, M., & Uitto, J. (2006). Pseudoxanthoma elasticum is a recessive disease characterized by compound heterozygosity. *J Invest Dermatol*, Vol. 126, No 4, pp. 782-786, ISSN 0022-202X

Rosenzweig, B.P., Guarneri, E., & Kronzon, I. (1993). Echocardiographic manifestations in a patient with pseudoxanthoma elasticum. *Ann Intern Med*, Vol. 119, No 6, pp. 487-490, ISSN 0003-4819

Roth, D.B., Estafanous, M., & Lewis, H. (2005). Macular translocation for subfoveal choroidal neovascularization in angioid streaks. *Am J Ophthalmol*, Vol. 131, No 3, pp. 390-392, ISSN 0002-9394

Sakuraoka, K., Tajima, S., Nishikawa, T., & Seyama, Y. (1994). Biochemical analyses of macromolecular matrix components in patients with pseudoxanthoma elasticum. *J Dermatol*, Vol. 21, No 2, pp. 98-101, ISSN 0385-2407

Scheffer, G.L., Hu, X., Pijnenborg, A.C., Wijnholds, J., Bergen, A.A., & Scheper, R.J. (2002). MRP6 (ABCC6) detection in normal human tissues and tumors. *Lab Invest*, Vol. 82, No 4, pp. 515-518, ISSN 0023-6837

Schön, S., Schulz, V., Prante, C., Hendig, D., Szliska, C., Kuhn, J., Kleesiek, K., & Götting, C.(2006). Polymorphisms in the xylosyltransferase genes cause higher serum XT-I activity in patients with pseudoxanthoma elasticum (PXE) and are involved in a severe disease course. *J Med Genet*, Vol. 43, No 9, pp. 745-749, ISSN 0022-2593

Schulz, V., Hendig, D., Henjakovic, M., Szliska, C., Kleesiek, K., & Götting, C. (2006). Mutational analysis of the ABCC6 gene and the proximal ABCC6 gene promoter in German patients with pseudoxanthoma elasticum (PXE). *Hum Mutat*, Vol. 27, No 8, pp. 831, ISSN 1059-7794

Schurgers, L.J., Cranenburg, E.C., & Vermeer, C. (2008). Matrix Gla-protein: the calcification inhibitor in need of vitamin K. *Thromb Haemost*, Vol. 100, No 4, pp. 593-603, ISSN 0340-6245

Sepp, N., Pichler, E., Breathnach, S.M., Fritsch, P., & Hintner, H. (1990). Amyloid elastosis: analysis of the role of amyloid P component. *J Am Acad Dermatol*, Vol. 22, No 1, pp. 27-34, ISSN 0190-9622

Shepherd, R.F., & Rooke, T. (2003). Uncommon arteriopathies: what the vascular surgeon needs to know. *Semin Vasc Surg*, Vol. 16, No 3, pp. 240-251, ISSN 0895-7967

Sorrell, J.M., & Caplan, A.I. (2004). Fibroblast heterogeneity: more than skin deep. *J Cell Sci*, Vol. 117, No Pt 5, pp. 667-675, ISSN 0021-9533

Suarez, M.J., Garcia, J.B., Orense, M., Raimunde, E., Lopez, M.V., & Fernandez, O. (1991). Sonographic aspects of pseudoxanthoma elasticum. *Pediatr Radiol*, Vol. 21, No 7, pp. 538-539, ISSN 0301-0449

Taylor, N.E., Foster, W.C., Wick, M.R., & Patterson, J.W. (2004). Tumefactive lipedema with pseudoxanthoma elasticum-like microscopic changes. *J Cutan Pathol*, Vol. 31, No 2, pp. 205-209, ISSN 0303-6987

Tiozzo Costa, R., Baccarani Contri, M., Cingi, M.R., Pasquali Ronchetti, I., Salvini, R., Rindi, S., & De Luca, G. (1988). Pseudoxanthoma elasticum (PXE): ultrastructural and biochemical study on proteoglycan and proteoglycan-associated material produced by skin fibroblasts in vitro. *Coll Relat Res*, Vol. 8, No 1, pp. 49-64, ISSN 0174-173X

Tu, Y., Weiss, A.S. (2008). Glycosaminoglycan-mediated coacervation of tropoelastin abolishes the critical concentration, accelerates coacervate formation, and facilitates spherule fusion: implications for tropoelastin microassembly. *Biomacromolecules*, Vol. 9, No 7, pp. 1739-1744, ISSN 1525-7797

Uitto, J., Li, Q., & Jiang, Q. (2010). Pseudoxanthoma elasticum: molecular genetics and putative pathomechanisms. *J Invest Dermatol*, Vol. 130, No 3, pp. 661-670, ISSN 0022-202X

Vanakker, O.M., Voet, D., Petrovic, M., van Robaeys, F., Leroy, B.P., Coucke, P., & de Paepe, A. (2006). Visceral and testicular calcifications as part of the phenotype in pseudoxanthoma elasticum: ultrasound findings in Belgian patients and healthy carriers. *Br J Radiol*, Vol. 79, No 939, pp. 221-225, ISSN 0007-1285

Vanakker, O.M., Martin, L., Gheduzzi, D., Leroy, B.P., Loeys, B.L., Guerci, V.I., Matthys, D., Terry, S.F., Coucke, P.J., Pasquali-Ronchetti, I., & De Paepe, A. (2007). Pseudoxanthoma elasticum-like phenotype with cutis laxa and multiple coagulation factor deficiency represents a separate genetic entity. *J Invest Dermatol*, Vol. 127, No 3, pp. 581-587, ISSN 0022-202X

Vanakker, O.M., Leroy, B.P., Coucke, P., Bercovitch, L.G., Uitto, J., Viljoen, D., Terry, S.F., Van Acker, P., Matthys, D., Loeys, B., & De Paepe, A. (2008). Novel clinico-molecular insights in pseudoxanthoma elasticum provide an efficient molecular screening method and a comprehensive diagnostic flowchart. *Hum Mutat*. Vol. 29, No 1, pp. 205, ISSN 1059-7794

Vanakker, O.M., Martin, L., Schurgers, L.J., Quaglino, D., Costrop, L., Vermeer, C., Pasquali-Ronchetti, I., Coucke, P.J., & De Paepe, A. (2010). Low serum vitamin K in PXE results in defective carboxylation of mineralization inhibitors similar to the GGCX mutations in the PXE-like syndrome. *Lab Invest*, Vol. 90, No 6, pp. 895-905, ISSN 0023-6837

Verbraak, F.D. (2010). Antivascular endothelial growth factor treatment in pseudoxanthoma elasticum patients. *Dev Ophthalmol*, Vol. 46, pp. 96-106, ISSN 0250-3751

Wang, J., Near, S., Young, K., Connelly, P.W., & Hegele, R.A. (2001). ABCC6 gene polymorphism associated with variation in plasma lipoproteins. *J Hum Genet*, Vol. 46, No 12, pp. 699-705, ISSN 1434-5161

Wajih, N., Hutson, S.M., & Wallin, R. (2007). Disulfide-dependent protein folding is linked to operation of the vitamin K cycle in the endoplasmic reticulum. A protein disulfide isomerase-VKORC1 redox enzyme complex appears to be responsible for vitamin K1 2,3-epoxide reduction. *J Biol Chem*, Vol. 282, No 4, pp. 2626-2635, ISSN 0021-9258

Zarbock, R., Hendig, D., Szliska, C., Kleesiek, K., & Götting, C. (2007). Pseudoxanthoma elasticum: genetic variations in antioxidant genes are risk factors for early disease onset. *Clin Chem*, Vol. 53, No 10, pp.1734-1740, ISSN 0009-9147

Zarbock, R., Hendig, D., Szliska, C., Kleesiek, K., & Götting, C. (2009). Vascular endothelial growth factor gene polymorphisms as prognostic markers for ocular manifestations in pseudoxanthoma elasticum. *Hum Mol Genet*, Vol. 18, No 17, pp. 3344-3351, ISSN 0964-6906

Part 3

Multifactorial or Polygenic Disorder

16

Peroxisomal Biogenesis: Genetic Disorders Reveal the Mechanisms

Manuel J. Santos[1] and Alfonso González[2]
[1]*Departamento de Biología Celular y Molecular and Departamento de Pediatría, Facultad de Medicina,*
[2]*Departamento de Inmunología Clínica y Reumatología, Facultad de Medicina, y Centro de Envejecimiento y Regeneración (CARE), Facultad de Ciencias Biológicas, Pontificia Universidad Católica de Chile*
Chile

1. Introduction

Peroxisomes are small and abundant membrane-bound organelles that contain enzymes for a variety of metabolic functions, including ß-oxidation of fatty acids, synthesis of plasmalogens and bile acids, and H_2O_2 production (1, 2). A group of human genetic diseases involves peroxisomal disorders (3) derived from two type of alterations: i) defects in a single peroxisomal enzyme, as found in X-Linked Adrenoleukodystrophy and Acatalasemia; and ii) Peroxisome Biogenesis Disorders (PBDs), which include the Zellweger's Syndrome (ZS). Intense research has been devoted for decades to understand the mechanisms of biogenesis and maintenance of peroxisomes. Despite the paramount progress, there are still enigmatic aspects, specially regarding the pathways followed by peroxisomal membrane proteins and the origin of peroxisomal membrane precursors (2). Here we give an overview of the evidence that involves the endoplasmic reticulum (ER) from the most important genetic tools in the field: fibroblast cultures derived from Zellweger patients and yeast mutants.

2. Peroxisome biogenesis: challenging the paradigm

2.1 Zellweger's Syndrome (ZS) as the prototypic Peroxisome Biogenesis Disorder (PBD)

ZS is characterized by craniofacial dysmorphia, neurological impairment, severe metabolic disturbances and neonatal death, caused either by complete absence of peroxisomes or by defects in protein importation into peroxisomal membrane precursors (1, 4-8). From the clinical point of view, a severity spectrum of these disorders has been established (SZ spectrum), including Neonatal Adrenoleukodystrophy (NALD; MIM 202370), Infantile Refsum disease (IRD; MIM] 266510) and SZ (ZS; MIM 214100) as the most severe (8). Initial studies in liver biopsies of ZS patients failed to find evidence of peroxisomal components and thus led to the notion that ZS patients lack peroxisomes (9). Later studies in Zellweger fibroblasts detected membranes containing peroxisomal membrane proteins (PMPs) but that lack most of the matrix proteins and were called "peroxisomal membrane ghosts" (10-12). Since then, a defect in the peroxisomal importing machinery for matrix proteins became apparent as a crucial cause of ZS. The fibroblasts from these patients provided a genetic model system for studying the mechanisms of peroxisomal biogenesis (1), while the incorporation of genetic tools in yeast allowed complementary and more detailed approaches (13-15).

2.2 Peroxisome growth and division versus *de novo* synthesis

In 1985, Lazarow and Fujiki postulated that peroxisomes are autonomous organelles, like mitochondria and chloroplasts, that form by growth and division (16). This assumption was based on the findings that peroxisomal matrix and membrane proteins are synthesized on free ribosomes and are imported post-translationaly into pre-existing parenteral organelles. Kinetics assays measuring the peroxisomal incorporation of newly synthesized proteins (17), as well as the discovery of specific targeting sequences recognized by soluble receptors that direct import into the organelle, gave further support to this hypothesis (18). Furthermore, most of the complementation groups exhibit only peroxisomal ghosts as the result of defects in the importing machinery for peroxisomal matrix proteins (10, 11). However, the observation that *de novo* peroxisomal synthesis is possible, first demonstrated in yeast (13) and then in mammalian cells (19), challenges the "growth and division" model..

2.3 The biogenesis of new peroxisomes is orchestrated by Pex3p, Pex16p and Pex19p peroxins

The analysis of the genetic heterogeneity in ZS and disorders of peroxisome biogenesis in mammalian cells led to discover the peroxins and their encoding genes (PEX) as the source of alterations causing several phenotypes (20). To date 32 PEX genes encoding the peroxisomal biogenetic machinery have been identified and at least 12 different complementation groups have been described among ZS patients, most of them displaying peroxisomal ghosts (7, 8, 18, 20). However, three of these complementation groups, groups 9 (PEX16 gene defect), 12 (PEX3 gene defect) and 14 (PEX19 gene defect) lack peroxisomes, peroxisome ghosts and any peroxisomal membrane (5, 7, 14, 19-26). This phenotype is reproduced in yeast by PEX3 and PEX19 mutations (13, 27). Strikingly, the expression of exogenous wild type PEX genes in ZS cells and mutant yeasts reestablish the generation of functional peroxisomes (13, 14, 19, 22, 26-31), demonstrating that new peroxisomes can be generated without requiring a preexisting organelle.

These observations also indicate that early stages of peroxisome biogenesis are driven by peroxins Pex3p, Pex16p and Pex19p, respectively encoded by PEX3, PEX16 and PEX19 genes (18). Therefore, it became clear that elucidating the function of these peroxins should help to understand the biogenetic mechanisms of peroxisomes, from preexisting organelles or/and from newly made precursor membranes.

Both matrix and PMPs are synthesized on free polysomes and captured in the cytosol by soluble receptors that direct them to peroxisomes. However, the importing machinery for PMPs involving Pex3p, Pex16p and Pex19p is different from the importing machinery for matrix proteins, both in sorting signals and importing peroxins (15, 32-35). Matrix proteins contain at least two distinct sorting signals: a tripeptide Peroxisomal Targeting Signal type I (PTS-1) and a nonapeptide Peroxisomal Targeting Signal type 2 (PTS-2), which are recognized by their respective cytosolic receptors Pex5p and Pex7p. These complexes are translocated by membrane importers involving Pex14p and RING peroxins (18, 36, 37). Instead, import of most PMPs depends on Pex19p that recognizes peroxisomal membrane-targeting signals (mPTS) and acts as a cytoplasmic chaperone for nascent PMPs, stabilizing and targeting them to the peroxisomal membrane (18). Recent evidence indicates that Pex3p, which is an integral membrane protein initially considered the only PMP imported independently of Pex19p (33, 34), actually also interacts with Pex19p and is imported through a mechanism involving Pex16p as docking element (35). Pex16p is also an integral membrane protein and seems to act as a Pex3p receptor or as a membrane translocator component (34). In turn, Pex3p once integrated into the peroxisomal membrane constitutes a Pex19p docking element and recruits complexes of Pex19p and PMPs as part of the PMPs incoming mechanisms (18, 34).

Recent experiments using a peroxisome-targeting assay in semi-intact CHO-K1 cells strengthened the notion that PMPs are directly imported into the peroxisomal membranes (35). This work also proposed a new classification of the import pathways. Previous work suggested the existence of two distinct PMPs import pathways (33, 34): *(i)* a Pex19p and Pex3p-dependent class I pathway followed by most PMPs including Pex16p, and; *(ii)* a Pex19p- and Pex3p-independent class II pathway, which so far had included Pex3p as the only PMP cargo yet identified. However, the most recent work found that Pex3p follows a novel import pathway involving a complex with Pex19p in the cytosol and a subsequent docking at Pex16p in the peroxisomal membrane (35). Based on these observations, it was suggested that pathways that depend on Pex19p-mediated membrane docking be classified as follows: *(i)* a class I pathway involving Pex3p as the membrane receptor, and; *(ii)* a class II pathway where Pex16p provides the docking site.

Under this new scenery a problem arises regarding the initial stages of peroxisome membrane biogenesis. Pex16p is known to be imported by the Pex19p-dependent pathway mediated by Pex3p as membrane receptor for the Pex16p/Pex19p complex (33, 34, 38, 39). At the same time, in the new pathway the import of Pex3p is mediated by Pex16p acting as receptor of the Pex3p/Pex19p complex (35). This apparent "chicken-and egg" problem can be solved by considering an ER pathway in which Pex16p would use another membrane insertion mechanism than Pex3p (26, 30).

3. The endoplasmic reticulum in peroxisomal biogenesis

The absence or non-sense mutations of any of the PEX3; PEX19 and PEX16 genes preclude the generation of peroxisomes, which as mentioned above can be re-established by reintroducing the respective wild type genes (18). In yeast, the endoplasmic reticulum clearly emerged as the source of membrane involved in the initial biosynthetic event (40). Plants also contributed with evidence of an ER-to- peroxisome pathway (41-43). Although in mammalian cells such possibility has been more controversial, accumulated evidence (26, 30) prompts reconsidering its validity.

3.1 Experiments in yeast involve the endoplasmic reticulum as the origin of newly formed peroxisomes

Yeast model systems provided the first evidence involving the ER in peroxisome biogenesis (44-46). In *Yarrowa lipolytica*, the finding of N-glycosylation in Px16p and Pex2p indirectly revealed trafficking through the ER to peroxisomes (40, 44). In *Hansenula polymorpha*, Pex3p, Pex8p and Pex14p accumulate in the ER in the presence of presence of Brefeldin (BFA) and become targeted to peroxisomes after BFA removal (47). In *Saccharomyces cerevisiae*,

Hoepfner *et al.*, (14) showed direct evidence that Pex3p and Pex19p are synthesized in the ER and then move to peroxisomes. Complementation experiments in yeast lacking Pex3p, and thus lacking peroxisomes, demonstrated that certain structures growing out from the ER, and containing Pex3p-GFP, constitute peroxisomal precursors that delineate a subdomain of the ER (14, 31). Also in yeast, recombinant Pex3p bearing an attached signal sequence and, therefore, unequivocally addressed to the ER, ends up integrated into peroxisomes (22). More recently, work on *Saccaromyces* reported ER targeting of 16 PMPs mediated by Sec61p and Get13, both in proliferating wild-type cells and in mutant cells lacking peroxisomes (48). This work also showed that PMPs leave the ER in a Pex3-Pex19p-dependent manner, implying a new functional role for Pex3p and Pex19p, i.e. promoting exit from the ER. The recent isolation of vesicular carriers that buds from the ER through a mechanism requiring Pex19p and carrying Pex3p and Pex15p provided compelling evidence for the existence of an ER-to- peroxisome pathway, which is independent of the COPII mediated pathway characteristic of the exocytic route (49).

3.2 The ER-to-peroxisome pathway in plants

Plants have also provided evidence of an ER-to-peroxisome pathway. In germinating castor beans, early pulse chase experiments showed peroxisomal proteins appearing first in the ER while en route to glyoxisomes that are specialized peroxisomes (41, 42). Pex16p has been reported in the ER as well as in peroxisomes (43) and its distribution suggested that specific domains might exist in the ER, defined by the concentration of certain peroxisomal proteins.

3.3 The ER-to-peroxisome pathway in mammalian cells

The ER-to-peroxisome pathway has been more difficult to disclose in mammalian cells. Several observations initially argued against the possibility that such a pathway might even exist or play a physiologically relevant function. For instance, kinetics studies have shown that Pex3p is rapidly imported into preexisting peroxisomes in wild type cells, one or two order of magnitude faster than the process of *de novo* peroxisome biogenesis (28). Thus, the chance to mediating *de novo* peroxisome biogenesis while most Pex3p is being consumed by importation into preexisting organelles seemed remote. On the other hand, attempts to follow up the newly synthesized Pex3p *in vivo* failed to find evidence of traffic through the ER to peroxisomes, both in wild type cells and in cells that lack peroxisomes (28, 34). This failure suggested that previous observations in yeast might not be extensible to mammalian cells. Until recently, the lack of direct evidence involving the ER in peroxisomal biogenesis in mammalian cells contributed to maintain the original notion of fission of pre-existing peroxisomes as the only source of the organelles (17).

Early electron-microscopic observations revealed close associations of peroxisomes and the ER in intestinal cells (50). The functional relevance of such observations remained for a long time enigmatic. Suggestive evidence of an ER involvement in peroxisomal biogenesis includes the finding of synthesis of PMP50 in ER-bound ribosomes in rat liver (51) and lamellar structures containing Pex13 and PMP70 that are continuous with both the ER and peroxisomes in dendritic cells (52). The role of the ER so clearly shown in yeast, as a platform for the outgrowth of new peroxisomes, had to wait in mammalian cells for new experimental approaches. The most direct evidence of the ER in peroxisome biogenesis came from live cell imaging in synchronized transport systems. First, it was shown that Pex16p is addressed to the ER before its sorting to peroxisomes (30). Afterwards, a similar route was revealed for Pex3p in ZS fibroblasts (26), thus providing the elusive evidence of previous studies.

In wild type mammalian cells (Cos7 cells), experiments with a photoactivable Pex16p-GFP revealed a trafficking pathway initiated at the ER and leading to peroxisomes (30). These studies also showed that incorporation of Pex16p into the ER is independent of Pex19p and occurs cotranslationally (30), thus contrasting with the direct post-translational pathway that requires both Pex19p and Pex3p for import of Pex16p into the peroxisomal membrane (33, 34, 38, 39). Furthermore, overexpression of Pex16p in cells lacking peroxisomes due to a nonsense mutation of the PEX16 gene relocates Pex3p from mitochondria to the ER (30), suggesting that Pex16p is a Pex3p recruiting receptor at the ER, perhaps mimicking its recently proposed role in pre-existing peroxisomes (35). The evidence suggested that most peroxisomes derive from the ER pathway rather than from preexisting organelles.

Prompted by the refreshing results on Pex16p traffic in living mammalian cells (30) and the contrasting observations regarding Pex3p trafficking in yeast (14, 22, 31) and mammalian cells (28, 34), we decided to study the sorting behavior of Pex3p and Pex16p in a fibroblast cell line (called MR) derived from a Chilean patient with ZS (26). In this new MR cell line we found complete lack of peroxisomes, including peroxisomal membrane ghosts, due to nonsense mutation in the PEX3 gene. An inactivating nonsense mutation generated a stop codon at position 53, previously reported in PEX3 deficient human cells (28). Cell fractionation and immunofluorescence showed peroxisomal matrix enzymes such as catalase and thiolase in the cytosol of these cells. Exogenous expression of Pex3p (tagged with GFP) restored the peroxisomal biogenesis. The newly generated peroxisomes imported catalase and thiolase. Therefore, the MR cells show the expected phenotype for the lack of function of Pex3p and for the reestablishment of Pex3p expression.

Unexpectedly, we detected an important phenotypic feature previously unnoticed in ZS. Cells with PEX3 or PEX19 mutations usually mistarget endogenous PMPs to mitochondria, perhaps due to the presence of a cryptic and weak mitochondrial signal (24, 53). In congruency, by using a reported serum that specifically recognizes several human PMPs (11), we detected the majority of PMPs distributed in mitochondrial membranes in both MR and GM6231 cell lines (26). However, we also detected a small pool of endogenous PMPs distributed in ER membranes and small cytoplasmic vesicles (26). An early study in rat liver using cell fractionation methods described data suggesting the presence of PMP50 and PMP36 in ER membrane fractions (51). Only very recently a targeting of a variety of PMPs to the ER has been reported in yeast (48). However, this is a previously unknown feature of ZS cells, which not only entails great interest regarding the role of the ER in peroxisomal biogenesis but also suggests a new role of Pex3p and Pex16p dealing with the traffic of PMPs from the ER to peroxisomes.

The interrelated functions of Pex16p and Pex3p (34, 35) suggest that these peroxins should act in concert. Thus, we analyzed the sorting behaviour of newly synthesized Pex3p and Pex16p in their respective mutant ZS as well as in the counterpart mutations. Microinjection expression experiments of GFP-coupled versions of these peroxins allowed the study of early stages of their transport. Previous studies in mammalian cells lacking PEX3 have shown that nuclear microinjection of PEX3 gene re-establishes peroxisomes within 3 h (28), but did not report an analysis of Pex3p distribution at shorter time periods. Strikingly, we found Pex3p-GFP localizing first to the ER and subsequently to peroxisomes in MR cells. Within the first hour of expression we detected almost 70% of the Pex3p-GFP mainly in the

ER. After 4 h Pex3p-GFP became clearly detectable in newly formed peroxisomes. These results contrast with those that failed to detect Pex3p sorted into an ER-to- peroxisome pathway in mammalian cells (28, 34). Our evidence that Pex3p follows the same pathway of Pex16p (26), strengthen the notion that mammalian cells share with yeast an ER involvement in peroxisomal biogenesis.

In agreement with previous studies (30), we also found that Pex16p-GFP exogenously expressed in ZS cells GM6231, which carry a well characterized mutation of PEX16 and lack peroxisomes, follows an ER-to- peroxisome pathway and reestablishes peroxisomal biogenesis. In these GM6231 cells, Pex16p-GFP expressed by microinjection distributed in bright dots or vesicles likely corresponding to peroxisome precursors (26). Interestingly, we observed that MR fibroblasts lacking Pex3p distributed Pex16p-GFP mainly to the ER (26). Previous studies in mammalian cells lacking Pex19p have shown that exogenously expressed Pex16p-GFP is targeted to the ER and accumulates there without promoting newly synthesis of peroxisomes (30). There are also studies in yeast lacking Pex3p or Pex19p that show PMPs arrested in the ER (48), and more recently, that Pex19p is part of the mechanism which produces membrane carriers containing Pex3p from the ER (49). Taken together with our results, the overall evidence indicates that Pex16p does not require Pex3p for its insertion into the ER membrane, in agreement with its previously reported cotranslational incorporation (30), but seemingly does require Pex3p and Pex19p for exiting the ER in peroxisomal membrane precursors. Because Pex3p is a docking factor for Pex19p in peroxisomes (34), a likely explanation is that a Pex3p/Pex19p complex formed at the ER membrane promotes the formation of membrane carriers for Pex16p and presumably other PMPs.

With regard to the role of Pex16p, GM6231 cells lacking Pex16p distributed Pex3p-GFP to mitochondria, indicating that Pex16p is crucial for the ER incorporation of Pex3p (26). Pex16p seems to act at earlier stages of peroxisomal membrane biogenesis than Pex3p (25). Actually, there is evidence that Pex16p is cotranslationally inserted into the ER and its overexpression leads to Pex3p recruitment to the ER (30). It is very likely that Pex16p once inserted into the ER membranes acts as receptor for Pex3p in the process leading to ER derived peroxisomal precursors. A requirement of Pex16p for ER targeting of Pex3p marks a big difference with most yeast strains, which do not express Pex16p. On the other hand, Pex3p could provide a docking site for Pex19p coupled to PMPs, as described in pre-existing peroxisomes (54). Pex19p-dependent recruitment of PMPs could then drive further progression of peroxisomal biogenesis.

The mechanism of Pex3p incorporation into the ER remains unknown, but likely involves Pex16p cotranslationally inserted in the ER membrane (30). Other PMPs might be inserted into the ER following a Sec61-translocon mediated mechanism similar to that described for a number of PMPs in yeast (48). The process might include maturation of incipient peroxisomal membrane at certain regions of the ER or homotypic fusion with other peroxisomal precursor vesicles.

Evidence in yeast indicates that new peroxisomes form by budding from ER in a COPI- and COPII- independent manner using a new branch of the secretory pathway (45). Definitive evidence of a COPII independent pathway has been recently reported in a reconstituted *in vitro* transport system in yeast (49). These observations in yeast agree with previous observations in mammalian cells (28, 55, 56) and with our recent results in MR and GM6231 cells (26). Inhibition of either the COPI vesicular pathway with Brefaldin A or the COPII

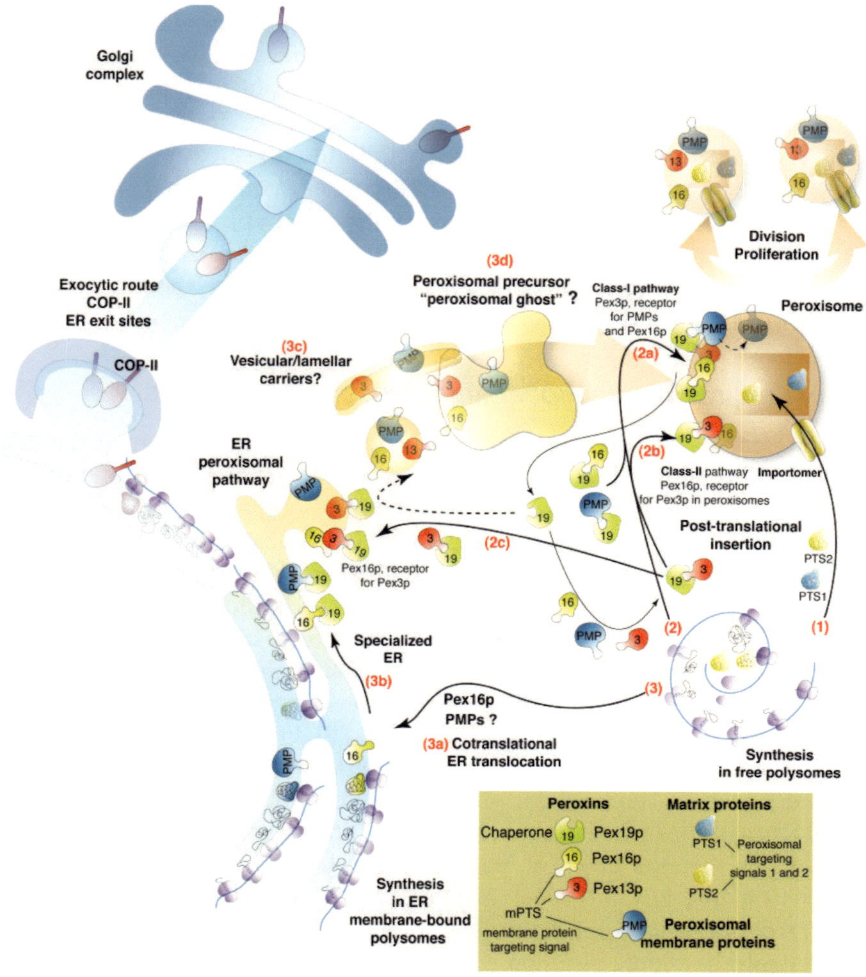

Fig. 1. Integrated model of peroxisome biogenesis pathways. As previous models established, matrix and PMPs are synthesized in free polysomes and are post-translationally imported into pre-existent peroxisomes. Routes followed by these proteins are depicted as routes: (1) for matrix proteins bearing PTS1 or PTS2 that are incorporated into mature peroxisomes by importomer complex (18, 36, 37); (2) PMPs, including Pex16p and Pex3p, forming a complex with Pex19p follow either a subroute (2a) in which Pex3p acts as a docking site for Pex19p-PMPs complexes (18, 34), or subroute (2b) mediated by Pex16p acting as docking site for Pex3p (34, 35). An additional subroute (2c) is followed by Pex3p targeted to the ER, presumably also in complex with Pex19p and requiring Pex16p as docking site (26). The ER-to-peroxisome route (3) includes the following steps: (3a) direct co-translational insertion of Pex16p (30), and likely other PMPs, as described in yeast (48); (3b) segregation of these proteins into specialized ER areas lacking ribosomes and other ER components, as suggested by the studies in dendritic cells (53); (3c) generation of hypothetical vesicular carriers, similar to those described in yeast (49), and/or lamellar carriers based on observations in dendritic cells (50). The ER-to-peroxisome transport requires Pex19p (30, 49); (3d) formation of peroxisomal precursors, still lacking matrix proteins, which might be equivalent to the peroxisomal ghosts described in most ZS cells (10-12). Mature peroxisomes proliferate by growth and division (16)

vesicular pathway by a Sar1 mutant in PEX3 or PEX16 mutant fibroblasts do not affect the recovery of peroxisome biogenesis (28). Our experiments in PEX3 and PEX16 mutant fibroblasts (MR and GM6231) indicates that PMPs are incapable of leaving the ER, causing an enlargement of ER cisternae (26), while the biosynthetic traffic of the temperature sensitive VSVG-tsO45 seem to function normally (unpublished results). At the non-permissive temperature of 40°C, VSVG-tsO45 accumulates at the ER, but after shifting to the permissive temperature it becomes transported to the Golgi apparatus and then to the cell surface in both MR and GM6231 cells, at similar kinetics as in wild type cells. This observation provides the first evidence of a normal traffic between the ER, Golgi apparatus and plasma membrane in ZS lines.

4. Summary and integrative model of peroxisome biogenesis

We reviewed here the evidence supporting a role of the ER as a platform for the function of PMPs (Pex3p and Pex16p) in the initial stages of peroxisomal biogenesis and integrated all data in the model depicted in Figure 1. Our recently published data suggested that other PMPs are addressed to the ER and accumulate there in the absence of Pex3p or P16p (26), in agreement with the most recent results in yeast (48). There is no doubt that peroxisomes can be originated *de novo* and that peroxins crucially involved in the initial steps of peroxisome biogenesis can be sorted first to the ER and from there to nascent peroxisomes following a COP-II-independent route (45, 49). However, in mammalian cells there is also strong evidence of a direct pathway from the cytosol to pre-existing peroxisomes, which under normal circumstances seems to be a mayor route (28, 35). Even though only a small fraction of Pex3p might be targeted to the ER, this could be enough for providing new peroxisomal membrane precursors as required for sustaining a continuous peroxisomal growth and proliferation. Peroxisomes possess a machinery for direct import of Pex3 in a Pex19p- and Pex16p dependent manner (35). On the other hand, peroxisomal targeting of Pex16p depends on Pex19p and Pex3p (33, 34). This apparent "chicken-and-egg" problem (35) can be solved considering a Pex3p-independent source of Pex16p in peroxisomal precursors, generated after cotranslational insertion into ER membranes (26, 30). ER targeting of Pex16p would conform the platform for *de novo* peroxisome biogenesis, offering a docking site for Pex3p at the ER, as it does at the peroxisomal membrane. Once inserted in the ER membrane, Pex3p would offer a docking site for Pex19p complexes with other PMPs. This pathway would generate pre-peroxisomes that mature towards complete and functional entities in concert with the direct import route. Co-existing with the ER-to- peroxisome pathway, both Pex16p and Pex3p peroxins would become directly targeted to pre-existing peroxisomes in the described "mutual-dependent targeting" manner (35). In this way, the classical "growth and division" model of peroxisome biogenesis is complemented with an ER-dependent mechanism responsible for *de novo* renewal of peroxisomal membranes. These cellular mechanisms are important to consider when evaluating the pathogenesis of Human Peroxisomal Genetic Disorders.

5. Acknowledgments

This work was supported by FONDECYT grant # 1040792, Fondo Nacional de Areas Prioritarias (FONDAP) grant #: 13980001 and Basal Financial Program/CONICYT (PFB 12/2007).

6. References

[1] Wanders RJ (2004) Metabolic and molecular basis of peroxisomal disorders: a review. *Am J Med Genet A* 126A(4):355-375

[2] Schrader M & Fahimi HD (2008) The peroxisome: still a mysterious organelle. *Histochem Cell Biol* 129(4):421-440

[3] Fidaleo M (Peroxisomes and peroxisomal disorders: the main facts. *Exp Toxicol Pathol* 62(6):615-625

[4] Gould SJ & Valle D (2000) Peroxisome biogenesis disorders: genetics and cell biology. *Trends Genet* 16(8):340-345

[5] Sacksteder KA & Gould SJ (2000) The genetics of peroxisome biogenesis. *Annu Rev Genet* 34:623-652

[6] Brosius U & Gartner J (2002) Cellular and molecular aspects of Zellweger syndrome and other peroxisome biogenesis disorders. *Cell Mol Life Sci* 59(6):1058-1069

[7] Oglesbee D (2005) An overview of peroxisomal biogenesis disorders. *Mol Genet Metab* 84(4):299-301

[8] Ebberink MS, *et al.* (2011) Genetic classification and mutational spectrum of more than 600 patients with a Zellweger syndrome spectrum disorder. *Hum Mutat* 32(1):59-69

[9] Goldfischer S, *et al.* (1973) Peroxisomal and mitochondrial defects in the cerebro-hepato-renal syndrome. *Science* 182(107):62-64

[10] Santos MJ, Henderson SC, Moser AB, Moser HW, & Lazarow PB (2000) Peroxisomal ghosts are intracellular structures distinct from lysosomal compartments in Zellweger syndrome: a confocal laser scanning microscopy study. *Biol Cell* 92(2):85-94

[11] Santos MJ, Imanaka T, Shio H, & Lazarow PB (1988) Peroxisomal integral membrane proteins in control and Zellweger fibroblasts. *J Biol Chem* 263(21):10502-10509

[12] Santos MJ, Imanaka T, Shio H, Small GM, & Lazarow PB (1988) Peroxisomal membrane ghosts in Zellweger syndrome--aberrant organelle assembly. *Science* 239(4847):1536-1538

[13] Hohfeld J, Veenhuis M, & Kunau WH (1991) PAS3, a *Saccharomyces cerevisiae* gene encoding a peroxisomal integral membrane protein essential for peroxisome biogenesis. *J Cell Biol* 114(6):1167-1178

[14] Hoepfner D, Schildknegt D, Braakman I, Philippsen P, & Tabak HF (2005) Contribution of the endoplasmic reticulum to peroxisome formation. *Cell* 122(1):85-95

[15] Hettema EH, Girzalsky W, van Den Berg M, Erdmann R, & Distel B (2000) Saccharomyces cerevisiae pex3p and pex19p are required for proper localization and stability of peroxisomal membrane proteins. *EMBO J* 19(2):223-233

[16] Lazarow PB & Fujiki Y (1985) Biogenesis of peroxisomes. *Annu Rev Cell Biol* 1:489-530

[17] Lazarow PB (2003) Peroxisome biogenesis: advances and conundrums. *Curr Opin Cell Biol* 15(4):489-497

[18] Heiland I & Erdmann R (2005) Biogenesis of peroxisomes. Topogenesis of the peroxisomal membrane and matrix proteins. *FEBS J* 272(10):2362-2372

[19] South ST & Gould SJ (1999) Peroxisome synthesis in the absence of preexisting peroxisomes. *J Cell Biol* 144(2):255-266

[20] Wanders RJ & Waterham HR (2006) Biochemistry of mammalian peroxisomes revisited. *Annu Rev Biochem* 75:295-332

[21] Shimozawa N, *et al.* (2000) Identification of PEX3 as the gene mutated in a Zellweger syndrome patient lacking peroxisomal remnant structures. *Hum Mol Genet* 9(13):1995-1999
[22] Kragt A, Voorn-Brouwer T, van den Berg M, & Distel B (2005) Endoplasmic reticulum-directed Pex3p routes to peroxisomes and restores peroxisome formation in a Saccharomyces cerevisiae pex3Delta strain. *J Biol Chem* 280(40):34350-34357
[23] Ghaedi K, *et al.* (2000) PEX3 is the causal gene responsible for peroxisome membrane assembly-defective Zellweger syndrome of complementation group G. *Am J Hum Genet* 67(4):976-981
[24] Muntau AC, Mayerhofer PU, Paton BC, Kammerer S, & Roscher AA (2000) Defective peroxisome membrane synthesis due to mutations in human PEX3 causes Zellweger syndrome, complementation group G. *Am J Hum Genet* 67(4):967-975
[25] Honsho M, Hiroshige T, & Fujiki Y (2002) The membrane biogenesis peroxin Pex16p. Topogenesis and functional roles in peroxisomal membrane assembly. *J Biol Chem* 277(46):44513-44524
[26] Toro AA, *et al.* (2009) Pex3p-dependent peroxisomal biogenesis initiates in the endoplasmic reticulum of human fibroblasts. *J Cell Biochem* 107(6):1083-1096
[27] Gotte K, *et al.* (1998) Pex19p, a farnesylated protein essential for peroxisome biogenesis. *Mol Cell Biol* 18(1):616-628
[28] South ST, Sacksteder KA, Li X, Liu Y, & Gould SJ (2000) Inhibitors of COPI and COPII do not block PEX3-mediated peroxisome synthesis. *J Cell Biol* 149(7):1345-1360
[29] Matsuzono Y, *et al.* (1999) Human PEX19: cDNA cloning by functional complementation, mutation analysis in a patient with Zellweger syndrome, and potential role in peroxisomal membrane assembly. *Proc Natl Acad Sci U S A* 96(5):2116-2121
[30] Kim PK, Mullen RT, Schumann U, & Lippincott-Schwartz J (2006) The origin and maintenance of mammalian peroxisomes involves a de novo PEX16-dependent pathway from the ER. *J Cell Biol* 173(4):521-532
[31] Tam YY, Fagarasanu A, Fagarasanu M, & Rachubinski RA (2005) Pex3p initiates the formation of a preperoxisomal compartment from a subdomain of the endoplasmic reticulum in Saccharomyces cerevisiae. *J Biol Chem* 280(41):34933-34939
[32] Chang CC, Warren DS, Sacksteder KA, & Gould SJ (1999) PEX12 interacts with PEX5 and PEX10 and acts downstream of receptor docking in peroxisomal matrix protein import. *J Cell Biol* 147(4):761-774
[33] Jones JM, Morrell JC, & Gould SJ (2004) PEX19 is a predominantly cytosolic chaperone and import receptor for class 1 peroxisomal membrane proteins. *J Cell Biol* 164(1):57-67
[34] Fang Y, Morrell JC, Jones JM, & Gould SJ (2004) PEX3 functions as a PEX19 docking factor in the import of class I peroxisomal membrane proteins. *J Cell Biol* 164(6):863-875
[35] Matsuzaki T & Fujiki Y (2008) The peroxisomal membrane protein import receptor Pex3p is directly transported to peroxisomes by a novel Pex19p- and Pex16p-dependent pathway. *J Cell Biol* 183(7):1275-1286

[36] Miyata N & Fujiki Y (2005) Shuttling mechanism of peroxisome targeting signal type 1 receptor Pex5: ATP-independent import and ATP-dependent export. *Mol Cell Biol* 25(24):10822-10832
[37] Fujiki Y, Okumoto K, Kinoshita N, & Ghaedi K (2006) Lessons from peroxisome-deficient Chinese hamster ovary (CHO) cell mutants. *Biochim Biophys Acta* 1763(12):1374-1381
[38] Matsuzono Y & Fujiki Y (2006) In vitro transport of membrane proteins to peroxisomes by shuttling receptor Pex19p. *J Biol Chem* 281(1):36-42
[39] Matsuzono Y, Matsuzaki T, & Fujiki Y (2006) Functional domain mapping of peroxin Pex19p: interaction with Pex3p is essential for function and translocation. *J Cell Sci* 119(Pt 17):3539-3550
[40] Titorenko VI & Rachubinski RA (1998) The endoplasmic reticulum plays an essential role in peroxisome biogenesis. *Trends Biochem Sci* 23(7):231-233
[41] Gonzalez E (1986) Glycoproteins in the matrix of glyoxysomes in endosperm of castor bean seedlings. *Plant Physiol* 80(4):950-955
[42] Gonzalez E & Beevers H (1976) Role of the endoplasmic reticulum in glyoxysome formation in castor bean endosperm. *Plant Physiol* 57(3):406-409
[43] Mullen RT & Trelease RN (2006) The ER-peroxisome connection in plants: development of the "ER semi-autonomous peroxisome maturation and replication" model for plant peroxisome biogenesis. *Biochim Biophys Acta* 1763(12):1655-1668
[44] Titorenko VI & Rachubinski RA (1998) Mutants of the yeast Yarrowia lipolytica defective in protein exit from the endoplasmic reticulum are also defective in peroxisome biogenesis. *Mol Cell Biol* 18(5):2789-2803
[45] Schekman R (2005) Peroxisomes: another branch of the secretory pathway? *Cell* 122(1):1-2
[46] Kunau WH & Erdmann R (1998) Peroxisome biogenesis: back to the endoplasmic reticulum? *Curr Biol* 8(9):R299-302
[47] Salomons FA, van der Klei IJ, Kram AM, Harder W, & Veenhuis M (1997) Brefeldin A interferes with peroxisomal protein sorting in the yeast *Hansenula polymorpha*. *FEBS Lett* 411(1):133-139
[48] van der Zand A, Braakman I, & Tabak HF (2010) Peroxisomal membrane proteins insert into the endoplasmic reticulum. *Mol Biol Cell* 21(12):2057-2065
[49] Lam SK, Yoda N, & Schekman R (2010) A vesicle carrier that mediates peroxisome protein traffic from the endoplasmic reticulum. *Proc Natl Acad Sci* USA: 107(50):21523-21528
[50] Novikoff PM & Novikoff AB (1972) Peroxisomes in absorptive cells of mammalian small intestine. *J Cell Biol* 53(2):532-560
[51] Bodnar AG & Rachubinski RA (1991) Characterization of the integral membrane polypeptides of rat liver peroxisomes isolated from untreated and clofibrate-treated rats. *Biochem Cell Biol* 69(8):499-508
[52] Geuze HJ, *et al.* (2003) Involvement of the endoplasmic reticulum in peroxisome formation. *Mol Biol Cell* 14(7):2900-2907
[53] Sacksteder KA, *et al.* (2000) PEX19 binds multiple peroxisomal membrane proteins, is predominantly cytoplasmic, and is required for peroxisome membrane synthesis. *J Cell Biol* 148(5):931-944

[54] Fujiki Y, Matsuzono Y, Matsuzaki T, & Fransen M (2006) Import of peroxisomal membrane proteins: the interplay of Pex3p- and Pex19p-mediated interactions. *Biochim Biophys Acta* 1763(12):1639-1646

[55] Voorn-Brouwer T, Kragt A, Tabak HF, & Distel B (2001) Peroxisomal membrane proteins are properly targeted to peroxisomes in the absence of COPI- and COPII-mediated vesicular transport. *J Cell Sci* 114(Pt 11):2199-2204

[56] Toro A et al. (2007) Evaluation of the role of the Endoplasmic Reticulum-Golgi transit in the biogénesis of peroxisomal membrane proteins in wild type and peroxisome biogenesis mutante CHO cells. *Biol Res* 40:231-241.

17

Repair of Impaired Host Peroxisomal Properties Cropped Up Due to Visceral Leishmaniasis May Lead to Overcome Peroxisome Related Genetic Disorder Which May Develop Later After Treatment

Salil C. Datta[1,2], Shreedhara Gupta[3] and Bikramjit Raychaudhury[1,2]
[1]*School of Biotechnology and Biological Sciences, West Bengal University of Technology, Kolkata,*
[2]*Indian Institute of Chemical Biology, Kolkata*
[3]*Department of Chemistry, Heritage Institute of Technology, Anadapur, Kolkata*
India

1. Introduction

The leishmaniasis is a group of diseases caused by protozoan haemoflagelates of the genus *Leishmania*[1,2]. These parasites belong to the family of the *Trypanosomatidae* (order *Kinetoplastida*) and are closely related to the Trypanosomes[3]. Despite enormous efforts, it has proved difficult to predict the exact scale of the impact of leishmaniasis on public health, since many cases remain unreported or misdiagnosed[4]. It is estimated that approximately 12 million people are currently infected and a further 367 million are at risk of acquiring leishmaniasis in 88 countries, 72 of which are developing countries and 13 of them are among the least developed in the world[1, 4]. Hence we can link leishmaniasis to poverty, economic development and various environmental changes such as deforestation, urbanization, migration of people into endemic areas and building of damns etc[5]. The annual incidence rate is estimated to be 1 to 1.5 million cases of cutaneous leishmaniasis (CL) and 5,00,000 cases of visceral leishmaniasis (VL); these are the two major clinical types of leishmaniasis[6]. The only proven vector of the *Leishmania* parasite is the blood-sucking female sandfly[1, 7] of the genus *Phlebotomus* in the old world and *Lutzomyia* in the new world[8]. The insects are 2-3 mm long (one-third the size of typical mosquitoes) and are found throughout the tropical and temperate parts of the world. The sandfly larvae require organic matter, heat and humidity for development and so are commonly found in house-hold rubbish, burrows of old trees and in cracks in house walls[9]. The sand flies usually feed at night while the host is asleep[10]. There are five most important *Leishmania* species namely *L. tropica, L. major, L. donovani, L. braziliensis braszliensis, L. b. peruviensis and L. mexicana* which cause the three forms of the disease dermal CL (oriental sore), VL and mucocutaneous leishmaniasis (Chiclero's diseases and Espundi)[11, 12, 13]. *Leishmania* exhibits a dimorphic life cycle[14] involving two life-cycle stages, the elongated promastigote with free flagellum present in the insect and the intracellular amastigote form[15].

VL, commonly known as kala azar, is characterized by irregular bouts of fever, substantial weight loss, swelling of the spleen and liver, and anaemia (occasionally serious)[16]. VL was first described in 1903, by Dr. William Boog Leishman[17, 18, 19], an English military surgeon and Dr. Charles Donovan[17, 20], an Irish physician by identifying the parasites in spleen smears of a patient died of "Dum-Dum fever" i.e. a low degree of fever with hepatosplenomegaly and severe progressive cachexia (wasting), swollen lymph glands, leucopeania, thrombocytopaenia with relative monocytosis and loss of hair[18, 20]. These physicians reported the existence of the parasite for visceral leishmaniasis and so the causative agent acquired the name as *Leishmania donovani*[21]. This is not to say that leishmaniasis did not exist before 1903, on the contrary. Archibadi in 1922 described an epidemic of Kala-azar, which occurred in the Garo hills of Assam[22] and in Saudi Arabia[23, 24] as far back as 1870. Cunningham recorded a similar disease that occurred in 1885, caused by a parasite[25], which was later named *Leishmania tropica,* the causative agent of CL[26]. Nicolle in 1908 reported that mammals including dogs could act as reservoir hosts for the *Leishmania* parasite[27]. Swaminath *et al* in 1942, proved using human volunteers that the *Leishmania* parasite could be transmitted by the phlebotomus sandflies[28].

If left untreated, the fatality rate of VL in developing countries can be as high as 100% within 2 years. The recommended drugs for VL are the pentavalent antimonials sodium stibogluconate (Pentostam) and Meglumine Antimoniate (Glucantime)[29]. Both drugs have been used for over 50 years, and they require long courses of parenteral administration. The treatment has traditionally been unsatisfactory because of drug toxicities, poor responses, multiple disease syndromes and other factors including the recent emergence of antimony-resistant strains[30]. Side effects of sodium stibo gluconate (SAG) include changes in liver function, biochemical pancreatitis, electrocardiogram (EKG) changes, musculoskeletal symptoms, thromboctopenia etc. Alternative treatments for VL include the polyene antibiotic amphotericin B[31] that constitute highly effective, less toxic lipid formulations[32, 33]. In regions of India where there is a high frequency of resistance to antimony, amphotericin B in a dose of 15-20 mg/kg, body wt is administered intravenously (IV) over a period of 30-40 days[34]. Recently several compounds of herbal origin have been reported to have potency against VL[35, 36, 37].

Post Kala azar dermal leishmaniasis (PKDL) occurs in India and mainly in Sudan and Kenya in Africa[38]. Reports of PKDL in China, Iraq and Nepal have also been documented [39,40]. In the new world PKDL is extremely rare[41]. Usually PKDL follows recovery from a Kala azar infection, though less commonly, it has been known to occur in patients who have not suffered previously from Kala azar[42]. Both the Indian and the African PKDL display similar symptoms. The disease begins with small measles-like lesions (hypopigmented macules, papules or nodules) appearing on the face, and gradually increase in size. Eventually the lesions spread to the upper trunk, arms, forearms, thighs, legs, abdomen, the neck and the back. The multiple lesions can coalesce to form larger lesions and can lead to the gross enlargement of facial features such as the nose and lips, giving an appearance similar to leprosy. The disease is particularly severe if the lesions spread to the mucosal surfaces of the nasal septum, hard and soft palate, oropharynx, larynx or the eye lids and the cornea leading to blindness[43, 44]. Potentially the lesions can appear on any part of the body. There have been reports of lesions occurring on the glands of the penis and genital mucosa hence the possibility of PKDL being transmitted sexually. In addition to the disease being confused with leprosy, PKDL can also resemble cutaneous leishmaniasis, secondary syphillis and sarcoidosis[44]. The lesions are usually self-limiting, however those that do not heal spontaneously within six months have to be treated[45]. Pentavalent antimonials remain the drugs of choice for treating PKDL. SAG at a dose of 20 mg/Kg of body weight administered intramuscularly for 4-5 months is recommended. In addition Ketoconazole and allopurinol can be given orally to improve response. In antimony resistant cases amphotericin B is an effective replacement[44, 46]. The reason for incidence of PKDL is still not clear and the evidence is yet to be explored. Several studies indicate that PKDL may develop as a result of genetic disorder during the parasitic disease kala azar. Indian PKDL appears anything between 1-7 years after apparent cure of Kala azar, although longer periods of upto 20-30 years have been reported[47] The African form of the disease usually appears within a few months after cure, in most cases within 6 months, on average within 56 days. However it can develop during the treatment Kala azar, in which case the term Para Kala azar dermal leishmaniasis would seem more fitting[48]. The choice available drug is limited and inadequate[49].

Although the geographical distribution of *Leishmania* infection is restricted to the area of distribution of *Phlebotomus* sandflies, Human immunodeficiency virus (HIV) infection may modify the traditional anthroponotic pattern of VL transmission. Very rarely *Leishmania* transmission has been described by alternative means that are also shared by HIV transmission, including blood transfusion[50] congenital transmissions[51, 52, 53] and laboratory acquired[54]. Worldwide, VL mainly occurs in HIV negative individuals more so in paediatric patients[55]. The association of *Leishmania* with HIV[56] has lead to a significant shift in the age of people at risk[57, 58, 59].

In South West Europe, 75 per cent of HIV sero negative and 80-83 per cent of HIV positive patients seen with VL were men[59, 60].

Leishmania/HIV co-infection is emerging as a serious new disease pattern and is becoming increasingly frequent. Of the 1700 cases of co-infection reported to the World Health Organization from 33 countries worldwide up to 1998, 1440 cases were from South-West Europe: Spain (835), Italy (229), France (259) and Portugal (117). Of 965 cases retrospectively analyzed, 83.2 per cent were males, 85.7 per cent were young adults (20-40 yr) and 71.1 per cent were intravenous drug users[61].

Most co-infections in the Americas are reported from Brazil where the incidence of HIV has risen from 0.8 cases per 100,000 inhabitants in 1986 to 10.5 cases per 100,000 inhabitants in 1997[62]. In India, the HIV/*Leishmania* co-infection has not been extensively studied. The risk of visceralization for HIV positive person, infected with *Leishmania* species typically associated with cutaneous disease, is not much of a problem, since VL is several thousand times more common than CL in India. However, this may be a very serious issue in the Mediterranean countries where CL is very common[63].

A majority of HIV/*Leishmania* co-infected cases show classical features of VL. These co-infected patients may also have other features, viz., atypical location due to decreased cell mediated immunity (CMI) [64,65], parasitic dissemination to skin, cutaneous and reticulo-endothelial system (RES), a chronic and a relapsing course, poor drug response and lack of anti-leishmanial antibodies.

The incubation period is variable and may be age related[66, 67]. Other concomitant opportunistic infections are diagnosed in 42-68 per cent of HIV-positive patients[68]. Fever, pancytopenia, hepatosplenolmegaly are common. Classically, splenomegaly may be less in HIV positive patients[69]. Constitutional symptoms (asthenia, anorexia, weight loss etc.) are seen in 50-70 per cent of patients and lymphadenopathy in 15-60 per cent of patients. VL with HIV infection may present as pyrexia of unknown origin (PUO). Other opportunistic infections like mycobacterial infection, cytomegalovirus (CMV), pneumonias and Acquired immune deficiency syndrome (AIDS) related neoplasms may also occur[70, 71].

Gastrointestinal (GI) symptoms are among the most frequent complaints[72, 73, 74]. Leishman-Donovan (LD) bodies have been identified in up to 50 per cent of such patients. The commonest site of involvement is the jejunum[75, 76]. Endoscopy and routine biopsy are important tools in the diagnosis. The symptoms may include diarrhoea, malabsorption, and hypoalbuminaemia and weight loss. There may be erosive gastro-duodenitis, ulcers and colony lesions.

Cutaneous involvement[77] may appear in the skin with Karposi sarcoma, Herpes simplex or Zoster. *Leishmania* may be associated with dermatofibroma, psoriasis, Reiter's syndrome, bacillary angiomatosis, cryptococcosis and oral aphthous ulceration. It may also present as dermatomyositis like eruption[78, 79].

Respiratory tract involvement occurs in alveoli and pulmonary septa in 75 per cent of patients with VL[80]. They could present with pulmonary tuberculosis and pneumonia, more commonly Pneumocystis carinii pneumonia (PCP). The symptoms could be cough, breathlessness, haemoptysis and excessive sputum production. Renal involvement can occur. Glomerulonephritis with mild proteinuria, haematuria and even acute renal failure have been reported. Tubulointerstitial damage can also occur[81].

Central nervous system (CNS) involvement is very common in the late stages. Pandey et al[82] reported cases in which HIV-*Leishmania* co-infection was associated with pulmonary tuberculosis and tuberculoma in the brain neurocysticercosis and tuberculous meningitis. AIDS dementia complex occurs in the late stages and may lead to early death. In such cases, cluster of differentiation 4 (CD4) count has been reported to be as low as <50 cells/mm^3. Pancreatic, pulmonary, pleural, laryngeal, adrenal, pericardial, myocardial and lingual leishmaniasis have also been reported. Mucocutaneous leishmaniasis appears in 2-3 per cent of VL-HIV co-infected patients[83-89].

Diagnosis is quite difficult as only 40-50 per cent of VL/HIV co-infected cases have a positive *Leishmania* serology[90]. This percentage is inversely proportional to CD4 cell depletion. Anti-*Leishmania* antibodies in HIV-positive patients are 50 times less than those in HIV-negative patients[91]. Therefore, there may be many false negative tests. The direct examination of amastigotes in the splenic and bone marrow aspiration has been the gold standard. Detection of *Leishmania* antigens by Western blot in the urine samples is being tried. Polymerase chain reaction (PCR) techniques requiring blood and tissue samples are very time consuming[92, 93]. However, when used in combination with Enzyme-linked immunosorbent assay (ELISA) and Direct Agglutination Test (DAT) the results are very encouraging. Nested PCR assay has a sensitivity of 95 per cent in the peripheral blood and 100 per cent in bone marrow/ splenic aspirates[94, 95].

Certain issues are significant in the management of HIV/*Leishmania* co-infected patients. Firstly, optimal duration of treatment is to be given. Secondly, the dose has to be monitored and thirdly, there is frequent relapse.

Sodium antimony gluconate (SAG) has developed resistance and low cure rates of 30-50 per cent have been reported[32]. In such patients, the treatment with SAG has to be given for a longer period[96]. However, the longer duration of therapy may lead to cardiotoxicity. With SAG, there are frequent relapses as seen often in Bihar, India[97]. Amphotericin B has also been tried and response rate of 60 per cent has been observed but 25-60 per cent of the patients treated with amphotercin B, are likely to have relapse during the first year after completion of treatment[98]. HIV infected individuals are more likely to suffer from drug related adverse events. In almost all the patients, depending on the CD4 counts (<200/ml) Highly Active Antiretoviral Therapy (HAART) can be given[99]. Amphotericin B can be given at a dose of 1 mg/kg for 15 days. Although lipid formulations are less toxic, they are very costly [99]. Pentamidine is usually not effective and should not be used due to its toxic effects. Oral miltefosine[100, 101] is a promising alternative at a dose of 2.5 mg/kg for 28 days and has been tried by Thakur et al[102] in six co-infected patients with good results. Besides treatment of VL and administration of HAART, other secondary infections like tuberculosis of the chest, oral cadidiasis, CMV infections, Pneumocystis carinii pneumonia (PCP), toxoplasmosis, Karposi sarcoma also need to be treated[103].

Peroxisomes[104, 105] are the single-membrane bound, catalase containing cytoplasmic organelles that contain a fine granular matrix, present in all eukaryotic cells (except the red blood cells), including the mammalian host. No such catalase containing subcellular organelle is present in the parasitic protozoa *Leishmania*[106]

Peroxisomes were first detected morphologically; their biochemical functions were characterized sometimes later. Johannes Rhodin, in 1954, described small organelles (0.5 μm in diameter) in mouse kidney cells and identified them as microbodies. Later in 1965, Christian de Duve[107] proposed the name peroxisomes (as they are peroxide-metabolizing organelles), for the distinct organelles isolated by density-gradient centrifugation. These organelles contained enzymes for both the production and disposal of hydrogen peroxide (H_2O_2). H_2O_2 generates reactive oxygen species, which are fatal in all respects. They interact with a variety of cellular macromolecules and lead to variety adverse effects like, membrane damage (lipid peroxidation), DNA damage (strand breakage), alteration in the protein structure (thiol oxidation) and the ultimate consequence may be the loss of cell viability (cytotoxicity and cell death) [108].

Catalase is the marker enzyme for peroxisome as it is the most abundant enzyme within the structure[109]. Active catalase is a heme- containing protein with four identical subunits (tetramer). In mammalian liver and kidney cells, peroxisomes are roughly spherical and relatively large (0.5 to 1.5 μm in diameter). In other tissues, they are smaller (0.1 μm) and known as micro-peroxisomes. In mammalian cell, the average number of peroxisomes is approximately 400 that occupy 1% of the total volume of the cell. However, their size, number, and enzyme profile vary between different tissues[110]. In most cases, peroxisomes contain dense or granular matrix containing catalase (About 40% of the total peroxisomal protein is catalase) and a crystalline core composed of enzyme urate oxidase. Peroxisomes have a half-life of about 36 hrs and they divide by fission[111].

The process of formation of peroxisome involves multiple pathways. Lipids must be recruited to form the membrane. Lipid composition of the peroxisomal membrane differs from that of the total cellular profile[112]. Peroxisomal proteins (not glycosylated) are synthesized in the cytosolic free polyribosomes[113] and transported to pre-existing peroxisomes. These include both the peroxisomal membrane proteins (PMP) and peroxisomal enzymes[114]

The multifunctional structures begin through orchestrated reactions of some proteins, called peroxins[115]. These are the critical processes as their defects leave the cells either devoid of peroxisomes or with organelles rendered unable to carry out numerous biochemical and metabolic functions attributed to them; such failings often cause a disease[116].

Approximately fifty different biochemical processes occur exclusively within a peroxisome. Some of the reactions are anabolic i.e. constructive, resulting in the synthesis of essential biochemical compounds including bile acids, cholesterol, plasmalogens (phospholipid analogues), and docosahexanoic acid (DHA), which is a long chain fatty acid that is a component of complex lipids, including the membranes of central nervous system. Other reactions are catabolic i.e. destructive and lead to the lysis of some fatty acids, via β-oxidation including very long chain fatty acids[117-119].

Peroxisomes contain several oxidative enzymes, which generate H_2O_2 as a by-product of their reactions. This highly poisonous reactive oxygen species (ROS) is rapidly converted to H_2O through the action of peroxisomal catalase, at least under most circumstances. A number of degenerative diseases are linked to ROS induced alternation in cellular functions[120]. The reactions are catalyzed by appropriate FAD-linked enzyme: a) urate oxidase, b) xanthine oxidase, and c) L- and D- amino acid oxidases. Flavin oxidases reduce oxygen to H_2O_2, which is then decomposed by catalase[121]. However the peroxisomal pathway differs from that of the mitochondria in several important respects[122].

β -oxidation pathway similar to that of mitochondria is present in peroxisomes and the process is carried out by two distinct groups of enzymes. The classical first group utilizes straight chain saturated fatty acyl-CoA as substrates, whereas the second group acts on the branched chain acyl-CoA[119, 124].

Severe effects of peroxisomal dysfunction, which secondarily leads to several human and animal diseases, emphasize the importance of peroxisomes for survival. Depending on the specific defect, clinical manifestations range from the mild to the fatal.

There are about 25 peroxisomal disorders known, although the number of diseases that are considered to be separate, distinct peroxisomal disorder varies among the researchers and health practitioners[125, 126]. Peroxisomal disorders are subdivided into two major categories.

The first category is the disorders resulting from a defect in a single peroxisomal enzyme[127]. These disorders include hyperoxaluria type I (alanine: glyoxylate aminotransferase), Refsum's disease (phytanoyl-CoA hydroxylase), X-linked adreno-leukodystrophy (ALDP), rhizomelic condrodysplasia punctata (RCDP) types II and III (dihydroxyacetone phosphate acyl transferase), and the β-oxidation disorders (acyl CoA-oxidase, bifunctional protein, and thiolase). These disorders result from a deficiency in only a single enzyme of the peroxisome, and therefore generally only affect a single peroxisomal metabolic pathway.

Conversely, there is also a set of disorders which results from a malfunction to form intact, normal peroxisomes, resulting in multiple metabolic abnormalities, which are referred to as peroxisome biogenesis disorders (PBD) or as generalized peroxisomal disorders[128] and include the Zellweger syndrome (ZS), Neonatal adrenoleukodystrophy (NALD), Infantile Refsum disease (IRD). Rhizomelic chondrodysplasia punctata (RCPD) type I.

Several proteins have been identified which play a role in the degradation of peroxisomes[129-133]. There are a number of reports in the literature describing the histology of the liver, spleen. and lymphoid organs of VL, during human disease and experimental infection[134-136]. In an experimental model of VL in golden hamsters, histopathological analysis showed[137] dissemination of the parasite mainly to liver & spleen. The former organ showed hypertrophy and hyperplasia of Kupffer cells with focal areas of inflammatory infiltration in nodular pattern. Gross examination of the liver indicated hepatomegaly. The spleen disclosed intense proliferation and enlargement of mononuclear phagocytic cells, revealing nodular configuration.

Both biochemical and morphological changes that take place in host peroxisomes during *Leishmania* infection, was detected [138, 139] pointing to the occurrence of a peroxisomal disorder during this parasitic disease. Liver peroxisomes were found to be functionally defective when purified after *L. donovani* infection. The activities of key enzymes catalase, urate oxidase, dihydroxy acetyl phosphate acyl transferase (DHAPAT) and superoxide dismutase (SOD) were either deficient or could not be detected after parasite infection. H_2O_2 producing peroxisomal β-oxidation was significantly elevated after 90 days of infection, with concomitant induction of superoxide radical production. Proteolytic activity in infected liver peroxisome was found to be inhibited, pointing to possible uneven processing of peroxisomal proteins. The morphology of peroxisomes after *Leishmania* infection was impaired. The evidence obtained for *Leishmania*-induced peroxisomal dysfunction may provide clues to develop new drugs against this parasite, capable of protecting normal function of this ubiquitous host organelle for successful treatment. Calcium is known to be stored in mitochondria and endoplasmic reticulum and is mobilized by second messengers[140, 141]. As one of the vital organelles of eukaryotic system, role of peroxisomes in mobilizing calcium has recently been explored in which peroxisome was identified as a calcium-containing intracellular organelle for its possible candidacy as one of the mediators towards cell signaling[142].

Immense interest has recently been developed to study peroxisomal properties in more details due to involvement of this mammalian microbody in normal cellular function[140]. It has already been reported that infection due to *Leishmania* pathogen leads to host peroxosomal damage[108]. As peroxisome is known to be involved in various metabolic pathways to monitor normal function of the host cells[109], it is essential that *Leishmania*-induced dysfunction of this organelle should totally be repaired during treatment of VL. Moreover, a group of human diseases can occur when peroxisomal properties are impaired[7]. It may lead to genetic disorder resulting in various other complications[143, 144]. It is thus logical to investigate whether treatment of this parasite-borne disease with the existing drugs can reverse peroxisomal defects developed due to *Leishmania* infection to avoid post therapeutic problems[111] which may occur due to unavailability of specific non toxic drugs against this pathogenic disease. In the present work it has been clearly shown that resumption of normal peroxisomal function could not be attained when one of the existing drugs SAG [112] was used for chemotherapy against VL.

2. Materials and methods

2.1 Materials

All the reagents except fetal calf serum (FCS), Medium-199 and sodium antimony gluconate (SAG) were purchased from Sigma Chemicals, USA. Fetal calf serum and Medium-199 were obtained from Gibco BRL, USA. SAG was procured from GlaxoSmithKline, UK.

L. donovani strain MHOM/IN/AG/83 was obtained from Indian kala-azar patient[145] and maintained by intracardial passage every 8 weeks in Syrian golden hamsters. Promastigotes were obtained by transforming amastigotes isolated from infected spleen[146] and maintained in medium- 199 supplemented with 10% fetal calf serum in vitro.

2.2 In vivo study with SAG in *L. donovani* infected hamsters

Syrian Golden hamsters (4 weeks old weighing 50-65 gm) were infected individually with freshly purified *L. donovani* amastigotes through cardiac route. After 30 days of infection the animals were treated with SAG (30 mg/kg body weight). Each hamster received intramuscular injections of the drugs every alternate date for 15 days. The compound was dissolved in DMSO. The final concentration of DMSO was $\leq 0.1\%$ (v/v). Infected hamsters in the control group received 200ml of 0.1% DMSO per animal intramuscularly. Animals of all groups were sacrificed two month after administration of last treatment. The splenic parasite burden was determined from impressions smears after Giemsa staining[147]. Total parasite burden was calculated from the following formula—organ weight (mg) x number of amastigotes per cell nucleus x (2 x 10^5) All animal experiments were approved by the local body of our institute's animal ethics committee.

2.3 Isolation of Hamster liver peroxisomes

Peroxisomes from normal and infected liver were purified according to the procedure already reported[148]. Hamster liver was dissected out to homogenize with buffer at 4 °C containing 0.25 M sucrose, 10 mM TES of pH 7.5, 1 mM EDTA, 0.4 mM phenylmethylsulfonyl fluoride, 0.2 mM leupeptin and 0.1% ethanol. Light mitochondrial fraction from the homogenate was separated by differential centrifugation and then suspended in the same TES-EDTA buffer mentioned above at the 1:1 ratio of liver weight to buffer. 30% Nycodenz (w/v) was prepared in a buffer of pH 7.5 that contained 10 mM TES and 1 mM EDTA. 2 ml of the light mitochondrial suspension was layered over 10 ml of freshly prepared nycodenz solution and centrifuged at 105000×g for 50 min in a Sorvall-ultra 80 ultracentrifuge using T-865 fixed angle rotor. After centrifugation the interfacial materials were aspirated off to obtain pelleted peroxisome which was separated at the bottom of the centrifuge tube. Purified peroxisomes were then suspended in a minimum volume of homogenizing buffer to store at -20 °C.

2.4 Western blot analysis

Peroxisomal proteins were separated by a 10% SDS–PAGE[149] followed by affinity transfer blotting using nitrocellulose paper[150] .

2.5 Activity staining for SOD

Peroxisomal SOD was separated on a 10% nondenaturing polyacrylamide gel[149] for activity staining[151]. Gels were incubated in solution A (20 mg Nitro Blue Tetrazolium in 10 ml glass distilled water) for 20 min, then in solution B (4mg Riboflavin, 0.4 gm K_2HPO_4 and 600 μl TEMED in 50 ml glass distilled water, pH 7.8) for another 20 min and finally illuminated until white bands appeared on a blue background

2.6 Assay of enzymes

Catalase activity was determined by monitoring the decomposition of H_2O_2 at 240 nm[152]. SOD activity was assayed by determining ability of this enzyme to inhibit pyrogallol autoxidation rate[153]. The assay mixture contained 0.2mMpyrogallol in air-equilibrated 50mMTris–cacodylic acid buffer, pH 8.2, and 1mM ethylenediaminetetraacetic acid. Rate of autoxidation was obtained by monitoring the increase in absorbance at 420 nm in a Hitachi spectrophotometer, No U2000. SOD has the ability to inhibit autoxidation and the extent of inhibition is taken as the measure of enzymic activity. Protein was determined using Folin and Ciocalteu's phenol reagent[154] .

2.7 Electron microscopy

Peroxisomes were fixed, processed to embed in Spur medium[155] to cut thin sections, and then stained to examine under an electron microscope (Hitachi-H600) at 75KV.

2.8 Immunofluorescence

Peroxisomess were fixed with formaldehyde in PBS for 15min, permeabilized 0.3% Triton X-100 in PBS for 5min, and then blocked with 3% bovine serum albumin in PBS for 30min.

were first incubated with appropriate primary antibodies (1: 100) for 30min followed by Alexa 633 coupled secondary antibody (1:100) for another 30min and then examined under TCS-SP Leica confocal microscope having krypton–argon mixed-laser facility.

2.9 Statistical analysis
Statistical analyses were conducted through Student's *t*-test as described[156]

3. Results

3.1 Effect of SAG on Leishmania infected hamsters macrophages
Following 30 days of *L. donovani* infection the animals were treated SAG at a dose of 30 mg/kg body weight, dissolved in DMSO, and the splenic parasite burden was determined after two months of the last dose given as described in materials and methods. In case of the SAG treated animals, no parasite was detected (data not shown).

3.2 Electron microscopic study of Peroxisomes after SAG treatment
Peroxisomes were isolated from normal, *Leishmania* infected as well as cured SAG treated hamster livers and processed for electron microscopic studies. In case of normal peroxisomes, electron dense core was observed inside the matrix and the average diameter was found to be 0.37 μm (Figure 1A). But peroxisomes isolated after infection were found to be swollen with severe membrane distortion, and the electron core became scattered, and a few of them had no core inside. The average diameter of the swollen organelle was determined to be 0.82 μm (Figure 1B). Peroxisomes obtained after SAG treatment showed interesting results. The membranes were no more distorted and the organelles were reduced almost to their normal size. The average diameter was found to be 0.4 μm (Figure 1C). But in most of the organelles, the dense electron core inside the matrix was not detected.

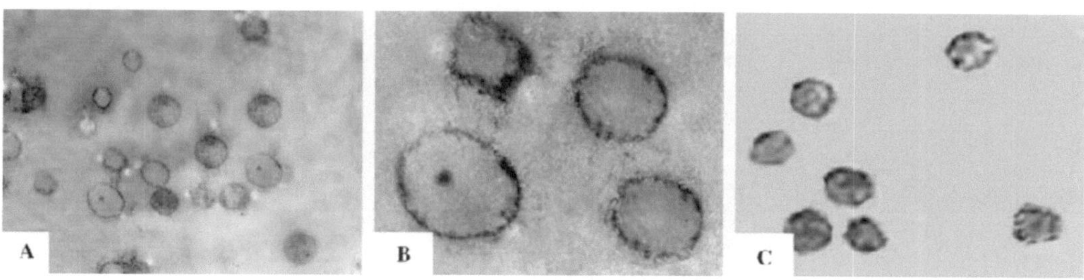

Fig. 1. Electron micrograph of hamster liver peroxisomes (x 50,000). Peroxisomes after pre- and post-fixation with 6% gluteraldehyde and 1% osmium tetroxide were examined under Hitachi electron microscope at 75 KV. A. Normal Peroxisomes, B. Peroxisomes post 90 days infection, C. post SAG treatment

3.3 Assay of peroxisomal enzymes before and after SAG treatment
Peroxisomal marker enzyme catalase was assayed in peroxisomes isolated from normal, *L. donovani* infected as well as cured animal livers after SAG treatment. Specific activity of Catalase is known to be diminished during *Leishmania* infection[157] and the same was obtaiuned in this case (Table 1), but catalase activity was not restored back in peroxisomes obtained from SAG treated cured hamsters (Table 1). Activity of another important peroxisomal enzyme SOD was also not detected in case of peroxisomes isolated after SAG treatment (Table 1).

Enzyme Specific Activity (unit/mg protein)	Normal	Infected	SAG Treated
Catalase	3373	1884	1763
SOD	3.2	ND	ND

Table 1. Enzyme activities in normal peroxisome, peroxisome after 90 days infection and peroxisomes after post SAG treatment. Results are in mean ± S.D. for three different experiments

3.4 Protein profiles of peroxisomes

Figure 2 indicates that the peroxisomal protein profiles of normal, infected and SAG treated cured hamsters livers were different when subjected to SDS-PAGE. Densitometric scanning pointed to three distinct protein bands of Mr 104.5, 80.6 and 50.4, although when found to be present in peroxisomes after infection and after SAG treatment, they could not be detected in normal peroxisomes. Significant differences were also observed for the protein bands of Mr 30.2, 28.0, 20.9, 10.3 and 9.7 (Figure 2).

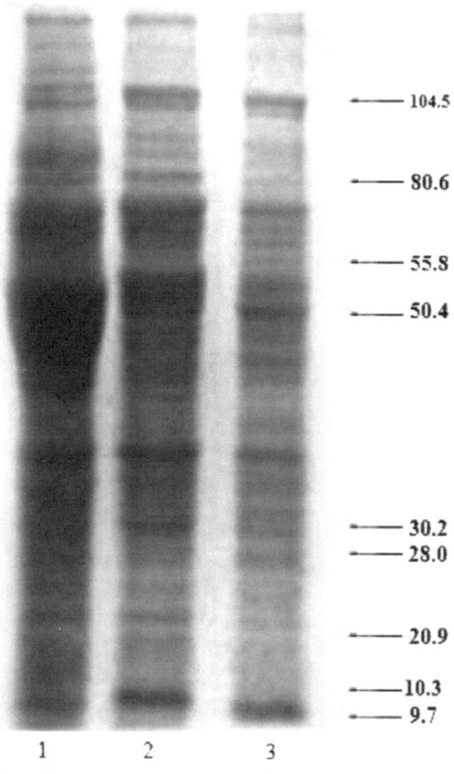

Fig. 2. SDS-PAGE analysis of peroxisome prepared from normal hamster liver (Lane 1), hamster liver infected with *Leishmania* parasite for 90 days (Lane 2), post SAG treatment (Lane 3). 40 µg protein samples were run on 10% polyacrylamide gel

The same PAGE when subjected to Western Blotting and probed with anti Cu-Zn SOD to find out the presence of SOD in the organelles isolated at various conditions, showed that SOD was not detected in peroxisomes obtained infected as well as SAG treated cured hamsters (Figure 3).

33.4 →

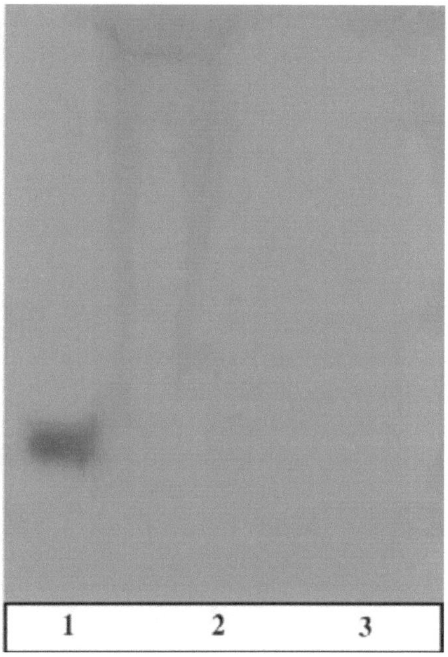

Fig. 3. Western blot analysis of glycosomal proteins. Peroxisomes were subjected to SDS PAGE for separation of proteins, transferred to nitrocellulose, and then incubated With antibody against Cu- Zn SOD. Normal peroxisomes (Lane 1), peroxisomes post 90 days infection (Lane 2), peroxisomes post SAG treatment

3.5 Impact on SOD activity

Activity staining of native polyacrylamide gels clearly showed that SOD activity of infected and SAG treated peroxisomes was totally lost (Figure 4).

In a separate experiment, presence of SOD was examined using anti Cu-Zn SOD under confocal microscope. SOD was not detected in infected (Figure 5B) as well as in SAG treated (Figure 5C) hamster liver peroxisomes. Normal peroxisomes were used as positive controls (Figure 5A).

4. Discussion

Peroxisomes are abundant in host reticuloendothelial cells[158]. The role and importance of peroxisomes in a wide variety of metabolic pathways, including longchain fatty acid β-oxidation, ether-linked glycerolipid biosynthesis, and H_2O_2-based respiration, have been thoroughly studied[159-161]. The importance of fatty acid β-oxidation for the survival of microorganisms in other parasitic and fungal diseases has already been documented[162-164].

Hamster liver peroxisomes are found to be severely damaged, both morphologically and bichemically, during *Leishmania* infection[157]. The structure and function of this host organelle are reported to be highly affected by the parasitic attack. The pentavalent antimonial compound SAG are widely used as first-line chemotherapeutic[165, 166] agents against all forms of leishmaniasis including visceral leishmaniasis[167, 168]. In this work, we have assessed the status of host liver peroxisomes after the complete treatment of the *L. donovani* infected animals with standard dose of SAG.

Fig. 4. Activity staining of SOD after conducting non denaturing PAGE. Staining was carried out according to the procedure described under Materials and methods Normal peroxisomes (Lane 1), peroxisomes post 90 days infection (Lane 2), peroxisomes post SAG treatment (Lane 3)

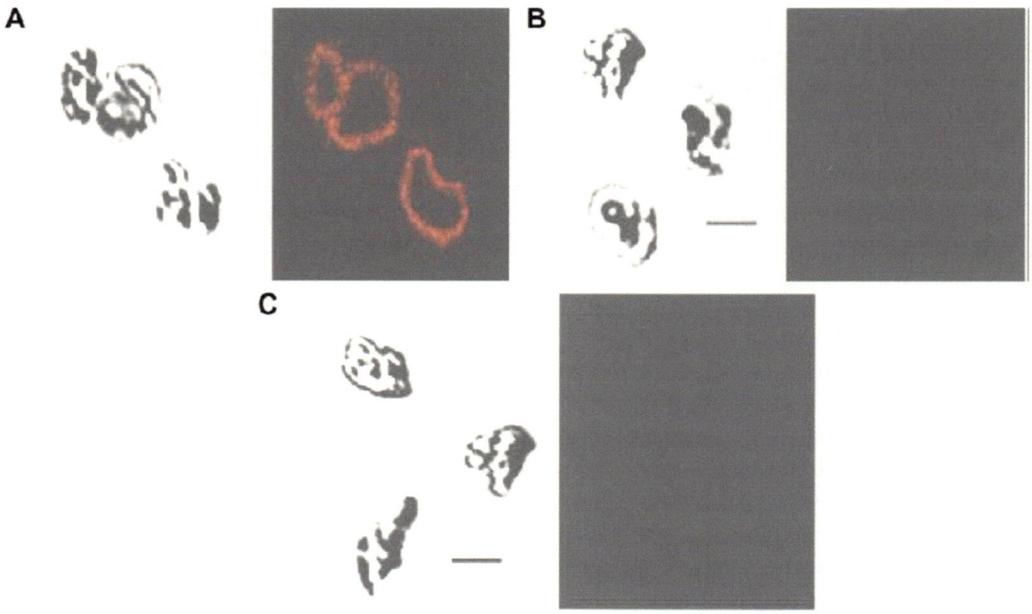

Fig. 5. Confocal microscopy of Normal Peroxisomes After treatment anti Cu-Zn SOD peroxisomes were examined under a Leica DM IRB inverted microscope. Normal peroxisomes (Set A), peroxisomes post 90 days infection (Set B), peroxisomes post SAG treatment (Set C)

Peroxisomes were isolated by standard procedure[148] from normal hamters, also from animals after *Leishmania* infection and from hosts after complete cure of the parasitic disease using conventional SAG treatment[169,170]. When parasite burden was measured two months after administration of the last dose, no parasite was detected in hamster spleen or liver, and that gave indication towards the complete cure of the disease.
The diameter of normal peroxisome is known to vary between 0.5 to 1.0 µm in animal tissues[171, 172]. However, the average diameter of hamster liver peroxisome was found to be 0.37 µm. As evidenced by electron microscopic examination the morphology of the peroxisomes after parasite infection was found to be different. Membrane structure was damaged and the dense electron matrix[172] was unevenly distributed, with the appearance of dark patches having an average diameter of 0.82 µm. The presence of large peroxisomes suggests the swelling of these organelles during infection. But the average diameter of peroxisomes isolated from hamsters after SAG treatment was determined to be 0.4 µm, which is quite similar to that of the normal organelles, indication that damaged peroxisomes are morphologically repaired after SAG treatment.
On the other hand, the key peroxisomal enzyme catalase[173, 174, 175] was found to be less active after host-parasite interaction. But when catalase activity was examined in SAG treated hamster liver peroxisomes, it was found that the enzyme activity was not restored back, even after complete cure of the parasitic disease, indicating that the peroxisomes are biochemically not repaired after SAG treatment.
SOD is one of the key enzymes of oxygen defense system. It is known to be an essential factor in mediating normal cellular functions[176, 177]. It is already reported that peroxisomal SOD activity is not detected after *Leishmania* infection[157]. In this study, the results clearly revealed that this essential enzyme is absent even in the peroxisomes isolated from hamster livers, after SAG treatment. In a separate experiment, Western Blot analysis showed no band for SOD in case SAG treated host liver peroxisomes. Activity staining of native polyacrylamide gels also showed that activity of peroxisomal SOD, was lost completely after parasitic disease, and could not be detected after SAG treatment. Confocal microscopic studies also revealed the same results, indicating that peroxisomal SOD activity was not restored back post SAG therapy.
Difference in protein profile in peroxisomes isolated from normal, infected as well as SAG treated hamster livers also indicate towards the status of peroxisomes. Some distinct bands were found in the infected and SAG treated peroxisomes, but were absent in normal peroxisomes. During *Leishmania* infection, some proteins get damaged and also proteolytic cleavage takes place, as result, more bands were obtained in infected peroxisomes[157]. The similarity in protein profiles between infected and SAG treated peroxisomes reveled that the biochemical properties of peroxisomes are not restored properly after SAG treatment.
Considering the knowledge we have gathered from the present work, it is clearly established that the peroxisomes, that get damaged during *Leishmania* infection are morphologically repaired after treatment with a common antileishmanial afent SAG, but the biochemical properties are not restored back.
PKDL is a common problem[178, 179] in kala azar patients but the actual reason behind the occurence of this disease is not yet known. Several peroxiomal disordes like ZS, IRD etc are also reported. Treatment with a common drug SAG, could repair the morphology of the distorted peroxisomes but the biochemical properties are not restored[180].
We propose that the peroxisomal defects caused by infection of the parasite *Leishmania donovani* lead to induce symptoms similar to genetic defects in the biogenesis of

peroxisomes. Although there is no authentic evidence available at this time, defective peroxisomes may also be the root to crop up PKDL in post kala-azar patients. Extensive investigations are still needed to sort out various unresolved problems in these areas to provide clues for new drug development against leishmaniasis. Present research in our laboratory is oriented towards this direction.

5. Conclusion

VL is a deadly disease of viscera caused by the parasite *Leishmania donovani* and also known as kaka-azar. The internal organs particularly liver, spleen, bone marrow and lymph nodes are attacked when the parasitic protozoa is transmitted to humans by infected female sand fly bites. People of Mediterranean and adjacent countries are attacked with this pathogen in the form of flagellated promastigotes. However, aflagellated amastigotes are found inside and outside of the affected reticuloendothelial cells.

At this time there is no definite antileishmania agent which may be used confidently to treat VL for a permanent cure. Drugs of choice available in the market, are being taken up selectively by trial and error methods. Most of them are too toxic to cause severe secondary infections and at the same time very costly to afford. Moreover, drug resistance is one of the acute problems to provide guarantee for a complete cure of VL. As a result there is an urgent need to explore for new drug development against this parasitic disease which is lethal, if untreated.

While exploring our attempts to identify an authentic chemotherapeutic agent against VL we also took into account the occurrence of PKDL. There are reports to believe that cured kala-azar patients as certified by the physicians, are susceptible to return for the treatment of PKDL.

Cause of PKDL is still not known. It is possible that the said pathogenic disease is occurred due to continued impaired function of the internal host organs even after treatment with commonly found drugs. We have shown that host liver peroxisomal properties are impaired due to the attack by *Leishmania* pathogen. We have also reported that the affected peroxisomes are not repaired after adequate treatment with the existing drugs. Treated animals with deficiency in peroxisomal properties also do not survive for a long time.

It is known that that peroxisomal defects lead to various genetic disorders. It is still not known whether in treated patients of VL who are likely to carry peroxisomal deficiencies even after traditional treatments, symptoms similar to genetic defects in the biogenesis of peroxisomes are developed.

A novel chemotherapeutic agent has been discovered in our laboratory to prove that this antileishmania agent has the ability to repair peroxisomal damage which takes place due to attack by VL. This finding may lead to provide effective clues to develop new and more potent drugs to stop recurrence of this pathogenic disease in other forms including chance to trigger symptoms develop due to peroxisomal disorder.

6. References

[1] Piscopo, T. V. and Mallia, A. C. Leishmaniasis. Postgrad Med J. 2006 82(972): 649-57. Review

[2] Soares, R. P., Turco, S. J. *Lutzomyia longipalpis* (Diptera: Psychodidae: *Phlebotominae*): a review. An. Acad. Bras. Cienc. 2003 75 (3): 301-30

[3] Opperdoes, F. 1997 8 October. Web Article and Desjeux, P. Human leishmaniases: epidemiology and public health aspects. World Health Stat Q 1992 45: 267-75
[4] The World Health Report: WHO 1996, Geneva: Switzerland.
[5] World Health Organization (WHO). Annex 3: Burden of disease in DALYs by cause, sex and mortality stratum in WHO regions, estimates for 2001. In: The world health report. Geneva: WHO, 2002 192-7
[6] WHO website (www.who.int) 1997
[7] Wenyon, C. The transmission of *Leishmania* infections. Trans R. Soc. Trop Med Hyg 1932 25: 319
[8] Killick-Kendrick, R. *Phlebotomine* vectors of the leishmaniasis: a review. Med Vet Entomol 1990 4: 1
[9] Hawkey, P. M and Gillespie, S. H in Medical Parasitology: A Practical Approach by - published by Oxford University Press1995 pp 151
[10] Arias, J.R., Monteiro, P.S. and Zicker, F. The reemergence of visceral leishmaniasis in Brazil. Emerg Infect Dis. 1996 2(2): 145-6
[11] Grevelink, S.A. and Lerner, E. A. Leishmaniasis. J Am Acad Dermatol. 1996 34(2 Pt 1): 257-72. Review
[12] Opperdoes, F. 1997 8 October and Kane, M. M., and Mosser, D.M. *Leishmania* parasites and their ploys? To disrupt macrophage activation. Curr. Opin. Hematol. 2000 7: 26-31
[13] Chang, K. P., Fong, D. and Bray, R. S. Leishmaniasis, in: K. P. Chang, R. S. Bray (Eds.), Elsevier, New York, 1985 pp. 1–30
[14] Kamhawi, S. *Phlebotomine* sand flies and *Leishmania* parasites: friends or foes? Trends Parasitol. 2006 22(9): 439-45. Review
[15] Zhang, W. W., Charest, H., Ghedin, E. and Matlashewski, G. Identification and over expression of the A2 amastigote-specfic protein in *Leishmania donovani*, Mol. Biochem. Parasitol. 1996 78: 79–90.
[16] Cunnigham, C. A. Parasite Adaptive Mechanisms in Infection by *Leishmania;* Experimental and Molecular Pathology. 2002 72: 132-41
[17] Herwaldt, B. L. Leishmaniasis. The Lancet. 1999 354(9185): 1191-9. Review
[18] Leishman, W. B. On the possibility of the occurrence of trypanosomiasis in India. 1903. Natl Med J India. 1994 7(4): 196-200.
[19] Leishman, W. B. On the possibility of the occurrence of trypanosomiasis in India. 1903. Indian J Med Res. 2006 123(3): 1252-4
[20] Donovan, C. On the possibility of the occurrence of trypanosomiasis in India. 1903.Natl Med J India. 1994 7(4): 196, 201-2
[21] Sengupta, P.C., Bhattacharjee, B. and Ray, H. N. The cytology of Leishmania donovani (Laveran & Mesnil, 1903) Ross, 1903, J. Indiana State Med Assoc. 1953 22(8): 305-8
[22] Sengupta, P. C. A report on kala-azar in Assam. Ind Med Gaz. 1951 86(6): 266-71 and A report on kala-azar in Assam (concld.). Ind Med Gaz. 1951 86(7): 312-7
[23] al-Zahrani, M. A., Peters, W. and Evans, D. A. Visceral leishmaniasis in man and dogs in southwest Saudi Arabia. Trans R Soc Trop Med Hyg. 1988 82(6): 857
[24] el Sebai, M.M. A case of kala azar in Saudi Arabia. J Egypt Soc Parasitol. 1987 17(1): 411
[25] Cunnigham, C. A. Parasite Adaptive Mechanisms in Infection by *Leishmania;* Experimental and Molecular Pathology. 2002 72: 132-41

[26] Alder, S. The transmission of *Leishmania tropica* by the bite of Phlebotomus papatasii. Indian J Med Res 1941 29: 803

[27] Ashford, R.W. The leishmaniasis as model zoonoses. Ann. Trop. Med. Parasitol. 1997 91: 693-701

[28] Swaminath, C., Shortt, H. and Anderson, L. Transmission of Indian kala-azar to man by he bites of *Phlebotomus argentipes*, ann. and burn. Indian Med Res 1942 30: 473

[29] Sundar, S. and Chatterjee, M. Visceral leishmaniasis - current therapeutic modalities. Indian J Med Res. 2006 123: 345-352.

[30] Brochu, C., Wang, J., Roy, G., Messier, N., Wang, X. Y., Saravia, N.G. and Ouellette, M. Antimony uptake systems in the protozoan parasite *Leishmania* and accumulation differences in antimony-resistant parasites. Antimicrob Agents Chemother. 2003 47(10): 3073-9

[31] Thakur, C. P., Singh, R. K. Hazar, S. M. Kumar, R., Narain, S. and Kumar, A. Amphotericin B deoxycholate treatment of visceral leishmaniasis with newer modes of administration and precautions: a study of 938 cases. Trans. R. Soc Trop Med Hyg. 1999 93(3): 319-27

[32] Sundar, S. Drug resistance in Indian visceral leishmaniasis. Tropical Medicine and International Health. 2001 6(II): 849-54

[33] Bern, C., Adler-Moore, J., Berenguer, J., Boelaert, M., den Boer, M., Davidson, R. N., Figueras, C., Gradoni, L., Kafetzis. D. A., Ritmeijer, K., Rosenthal, E., Royce, C., Russo, R., Sundar, S. and Alvar, J. Liposomal amphotericin B for the treatment of visceral leishmaniasis. Clin Infect Dis. 2006 43(7): 917-24

[34] Sudar, S., Jha, T, K. and Thakur, C. P. Oral Miltefosine for Indian visceral leishmaniasis. N. Engl. J. Med. 2002 347: 1739-46

[35] Rocha LG, Almeida JR, Macedo RO, Barbosa-Filho JM. A review of natural products with antileishmanial activity. Phytomedicine 2005;12:514–35.

[36] Bhattacharjee S, Gupta G, Bhattacharya P, Mukherjee A, Majumdar SB, Pal A, et al. Quassin alters the immunological patterns of murine macrophages through generation of nitric oxide to exert antileishmanial activity. J Antimicrob Chemother

[37] Gupta. S, Datta, S.C et al. Momordicatin purified from fruits of *Momordica charantia* is effective to act as a potent antileishmania agent. Parasitology International. 2010 59: 192-197

[38] Zijlstra, E. E, Musa, A.M. and Khalil, A. M. Post kala-azar dermal leishmaniasis. Lancet Infect Dis. 2003 3(2): 87-98

[39] Ramesh, V. and Mukherjee, A. Post kala azar dermal leishmaniasis. Int. J. Dermatol. 1995 34(2): 85-91

[40] Gang, U.K., Agrawal, S. and Rani, S. Post-kala-azar dermal leishmaniasis in Nepal. Int J Derm 2001 40:179-84

[41] WHO expert committee report: Control of the leishmaniasis. 1991 Technical report series 793

[42] Hashim, F. A., Ali, M. S., Satti, M., El-Hassan, A.M., Ghalib, H. W., El-Safi, S. and El-Hag, I. A. An outbreak of acute kala azar in a nomadic tribe in western Sudan: features of the disease in a previously non-immune population. Trans. R. Soc. Trop. Med. Hyg. 1995 88(4): 431-2

[43] Hashim, F, A., Ahmed, A. E., El-Hassan, M., El-Mubarak, M. H., Yagi, H., Ibrahim, E. N. and Ali, M. S. Neurologic changes in visceral leishmaniasis. Am. J. Trop. Med. Hyg. 1995 52(2): 149-54

[44] Ramesh, V. and Mukherjee, A. Post kala azar dermal leishmaniasis. Int. J. Dermatol. 1995 34(2): 85-91

[45] Hashim, F. A., Khalil, E. A., Ismail, A. and El-Hassan, A. M. Apparently successful treatment of two cases of post kala azar dermal leishmaniasis with liposomal amphotericin B. Trans. R. Soc. Trop. Med. Hyg. 1995 89(4): 440

[46] Gang, U.K., Agrawal, S. and Rani, S. Post-kala-azar dermal leishmaniasis in Nepal. Int J Derm 2001 40:179-84

[47] Zijlstra, E. E., El-Hassan, A. M., Ismael, A., Ghalib, H. W. Endemic kala-azar in eastern Sudan: a longitudinal study on the incidence of clinical and subclinical infection and post kala azar dermal leishmaniasis. Am. J. Trop. Med. Hyg. 1994 51(6): 826-36

[48] Salotra, P. and Singh, R. Challenges in the diagnosis of post kala-azar dermal leishmaniasis. Indian J Med Res. 2006 123(3): 295-310. Review

[49] Tripathy, K, Rath, J et al. A Case of Post Kala-Azar Dermal Leishmaniasis in India. Korean J Parasitol.2010 48: 245-246. DOI: 10.3347/kjp.2010.48.3.245

[50] Kostman, R., Barr, M., Bengtsson, E., Garnham, P. C. C. and Hult, G. Kala-azar transferred by exchange blood transfusion in two Swedish infants. In: Proceedings of the 7th International Congress of Tropical Medicine and Malaria. Geneva: Switzerland: World Health Organization; 1963 p. 384

[51] Loke, Y. Transmission of parasites across the placenta. Advances in Parasitology, New York: Academic Press 1982 21: 155

[52] Nuwayri-Salti, N. and Khansa, H. Direct non-infect vector transmission of *Leishmania* parasite in mice. Int J Parasitol 1985 15: 497

[53] Napier, L. and Gupta, C. D. Indian Kala-azar in a new borne. Indian Med Gaz 1928 62: 199

[54] Rosethal, P. J., Chaisson, R. E., Hadley, W.K. and Leech, J. H. Rectal leishmaniasis in a patient with acquired immuno deficiency syndrome. Am J Med 1988 84: 307-9

[55] Cascio, A., Colomba, C., Antinori, S., Orobello, M., Paterson, D. and Titone, L. Paediatric Visceral leishmaniasis in Western Sisily, Italy: A retrospective analysis of 111 cases. Eur J Clin Microbiol Infect Dis 2002 21: 277-82

[56] Berhe, N., Hailu, A., Wolday, D., Negesse, Y., Cenini, P. and Frommel, D. Ethiopian visceral leishmaniasis patients co-infected with human immunodeficiency virus. Trans. R. Soc. Trop. Med. Hyg. 1995 89(2): 205-7

[57] Belazzoug, S. Leishmaniasis in Mediterranean countries. Vet Parasitol 1992 44: 15-9

[58] Aggarwal, P. and Prakash Wali, J. P. Profile of kala-azar in north India. Asia Pacific J Public Health 1991 5: 90-3

[59] Pintado, V., Martin Rabadan, P., Rivera, M. L., Morino, S. and Bauza, E. Visceral leishmaniasis in human immunodeficiency virus infected and non-HIV infected patients- A comparative study. Medicine 2001 80: 54-73

[60] The World Health Report, Geneva: World Health Organization. 2001

[61] Desjeux, P., Meert, J.P., Piot, B., Alwar, J., Medrano, F.J. and Portus, M. *Leishmania*/ HIV co-infection, South Western Europe 1990-98. Document WHO/LEISH/2000. 42 Geneva: World Health Organization

[62] Rabello, A., Orsini, M. and Disch, J. *Leishmania*/ HIV coinfection in Brazil: an appraisal. Ann Trop Med Parasitol 2002 97: 17-28
[63] Sinha, P. K., Pandey, K. and Bhattacharya, S. K. Diagnosis & management of *Leishmania*/HIV co-infection. Indian J Med Res 2005 121: 407-14
[64] Montalban, C., Martinez Fernandez, R., Calleza, Z. L., Garcia- Diaz, Z. E., Rubio, R. and Dronda, F. Visceral leishmaniasis (Kala-azar) as an opportunistic infection in patients infected with human immunodeficiency virus in Spain. Rev Infect Dis 1989 11: 655-60
[65] del Mar Sanz, M., Rubio, R., Casillas, A., Guijarro, C., Costa, J. R., Martinez, R. and de Dios Garcia, J. Visceral leishmaniasis in HIV infected patients. AIDS 1991 5: 1272-4
[66] Evanas, T. G. Leishmaniasis. Infect Dis Clin North Am 1993 7: 527-46
[67] Alvar, J., Canavate, C., Gutierrez-Solar, B., Jimen, E. Z. M., Laguna, F. and Lopez-Velez, R. *Leishmania* and human immunodeficiency virus co-infection: The first 10 years. Clin Microbiol Rev 1997 10: 298-319
[68] De-Gorgolas, M. and Miles, M. A. Visceral leishmaniasis and AIDS. Nature. 1994 372(6508): 734
[69] Montalban, C., Calleja, J. L., Erice, A., Laguna, F., Clotet, B. and Podzamczer, D. Visceral leishmaniasis in patients infected with human immunodeficiency virus-Co-operative group for the study of Leishmaniasis in AIDS. J Infect 1990 21: 261-70
[70] Alvar, J., Gutierrez-Solar, B. and Molina, R. Prevalence of *Leishmania* infection among AIDS patients. Lancet 1992 339: 264-65
[71] Miralles, P., Moreno, S., Perez-Tascon, M., Cosin, J., Diaz, M. D. and Bouza, E. Fever of uncertain origin in patients infected with the human immunodeficiency virus. Clin Infect Dis 1995 20: 872-5
[72] Janoff, E.N. and Smith, P. D. Perspectives on gastro-intestinal infections in AIDS. Gastrointerol Clin North Am 1988 17: 451-63
[73] Malebranche, R., Arnoux, E., Guerin, J. M., Pierre, G. D., Laroche, S. E. and Pean-Guichard, C. Acquired immunodeficiency syndrome with severe gastrointestinal manifestations in Haiti. Lancet 1983 2: 873-8
[74] Laguna, F., Garcia-Samaniego, J., Sorianao, V., Valencia, E., Redondo, C. and Alonso, M. J. Gastro-intestinal leishmaniasis in human immunodeficiency virus infected patients: Report of 5 cases and review. Clin Infect Dis 1994 19: 48-53
[75] Muigai, R., Gatei, D. and Shaunak, S. Jejunal function and pathology in visceral leishmaniasis. Lancet 1983 27: 476-9
[76] Villanueva, J. L., Torre-Cisneros, J. and Jurado, R. *Leishmania* esophagitis in an AIDS patient: an unusual form of visceral leishmaniasis. Am J Gastroenterol. 1994 89: 273-5
[77] Perrin, C., Taillan, B., Hofman, P., Mondain, V., Lefichoux, Y. and Michiels, J. F. Atypical cutaneous histological features of visceral leishmaniasis in acquired immunodeficiency syndrome. Am. J Dermatopathol 1995 17: 145-50
[78] Romeu, J., Milla, F., Batlle, M., Sirera, G., Ferrendiz, C., Carreres, A., Condom, M. J. and Clotet, B. Visceral leishmaniasis involving lungs and a cutaneous Kaposi's sarcoma lesions. AIDS 1991 5: 1272
[79] Lahdevirta, J., Maury, C. P., Teppo, A. M. and Repo, H. Elevated levels of circulating cachectin / TNF in patients with AIDS. Am J Med 1988 85: 289-91

[80] Duarte, M. I. S., da Matta, V. L. R., Corbett, C. E. P, Laurenti, M. D, Chebabo, R. and Goto, H. Interstitial pneumonitis in human visceral leishmaniasis. Trans R Soc Trop Med Hyg 1989 83: 73-6

[81] Clevenbergh, P., Okome, M. N. and Benoit, S. Acute renal failure as initial presentation of visceral leishmaniasis in an HIV 1 infected patient. Scand J Infect Dis 2002 100: 71-4

[82] Pandey, K., Sinha, P. K., Ravidas, V. N. R., Kumar, N., Verma, N. and Lal, C. S. Nexus of infection with human immunodeficiency virus, pulmonary tuberculosis and visceral leishmaniasis: A case report from Bihar, India. Am J Trop Med Hyg 2005 72: 30-2

[83] Berenguer, J., Moreno, S., Cercenado, E., Bernaldo de Quiros, J. C. and Garcia de la, Fuente A, Visceral leishmaniasis in patients infected with human deficiency virus (HIV). Ann Intern Med 1989 111: 129-32

[84] Greder, A., Malet, M. and Gautier, P. Pleurisy revealing leishmaniasis in acquired immunodeficiency syndrome. Presse Med 1989 18: 1390-1

[85] Gonzalez-Anglada, M. I., Pena, J. M., Barbado, F. J., Gonzalez, J.J., Redondo, C. and Galera, C. Two cases of laryngeal leishmaniasis in patients infected with HIV. Eur J Clin Microbiol Infect Dis 1994 13: 509-11

[86] Mondain-Miton, V., Toussaint-Gari, M., Hofman, P., Marty, P. Carles, M. and Desalvoldor, F. A typical leishmaniasis in a patient infected with human immunodeficiency virus. Clin Infect Dis 1995 21: 663-5

[87] Mofredj, A., Guerin, M. J., Leibinger, F. and Masmoudi, R. Visceral leishmaniasis with pericarditis in an HIV infected patient. Scand J. Infect Dis 2002 34: 151-3

[88] Vazquez-Pineiro, T., Fernandez-Alvarez, J. M., Gonzalo Lafuente, J. C., Cano, J., Gimeno, M. and Berenger, J. Visceral leishmaniasis: a lingual presentation in a patient with HIV infection. Oral Surg Oral Med Oral Pathol Oral Radiol Endod 1998 86: 179-82

[89] Miralles, E. S., Nunez, M., Hilara, Y., Harto, A., Moreno, R. and Ledo, A. Mucocutaneous leishmaniasis and HIV. Dermatology 1994 189: 275-7

[90] Manfredi, R., Mazzoni, A., Pileri, S., Marinacci, G., Nanetti, A., Poggi, S. and Chiodo, F. Simultaneous occurrence of visceral leishmaniasis and disseminated histoplasmosis in an Italian patient with HIV infection. Infection. 1994 22(3): 224-5

[91] Mary, C., Lamouroux, D., Dunan, S. and Quilici, M. Western blot analysis of antibodies to *Leishmania infantum* antigens: potential of the 14-kD and 16-kD antigens for diagnosis and epidemiologic purposes. Am J Trop Med Hyg 1992 47: 764-71

[92] Lopez, M., Inga, R., Cangalaya, M., Echevarria, J., Llanos- Cuentas, A. and Orrego, C. Diagnosis of Leishmania using the polymerase chain reaction: a simplified procedure for field work. Am J Trop Med Hyg 1993 49: 348-56

[93] de Brujin, M. H., Labrada, L. A., Smyth, A. J., Santrich, C. and Barker, D.C. A comparative study of diagnosis by the polymerase chin reaction and by current clinical methods using biopsies from Colombian patients with suspected lesihmaniasis. Trop Med Parasitol 1993 44: 201-7

[94] Cruz, I., Canavate, C. and Rubio, J. M. A nested polymerase chain reaction (Ln-PCR) for diagnosing and monitoring *Leishmania infantum* infection in patients co-infected with human immunodeficiency virus. Trans R Soc Trop Med Hyg 2002 96(Suppl 1): S185-9

[95] Fisa, R., Riera, C., Ribera, E., Gallego, M. and Portus, M. A nested polymerase chain reaction for diagnosis and follow up of human visceral leishmaniasis patients using blood samples. Trans R Soc Trop Med Hyg 2002 96 (Suppl 1): S191-4
[96] Ritmeijer, K., Veeken, H, Melaku Y, Leal G, Amsalu R, Seaman J, Ethiopian visceral leishmaniasis: Generic and proprietary sodium stibogluconate are equivalent: HIV co-infected patients have a poor outcome. Trans R Soc Trop Med Hyg 2001 95: 668-72
[97] Laguna, F., Lopez-Velez, R. and Pulido, F. Treatment of Visceral Leishmanisis in HIV infected patients: a randomized trial comparing meglumine antimoniate with amphotericin B. Spanish HIV-*Leishmania* Study Group. AIDS 1999 13: 1063-9
[98] Autran, B., Crxelain, G. and Li, T.S. Positive effects of combined antiretroviral therapy on CD4+ T-cell Homeostasis and function in advanced HIV disease. Science. 1997 277: 112-6
[99] McBride, M., Linney, M., Calydon, E.J. and Weber, J. Visceral leishmaniasis following treatment with liposomal amphotericin B. Clin Infect Dis 1994 19: 362
[100] Sundar, S., Jha, T. K., Thakur, C. P., Engel, J., Sindermann, H., Fischer, C., Junge, K., Bryceson, A. and Berman, J., Oral miltefosine for Indian visceral leishmaniasis. New England Journal of medicine. 2002 347(22): 1739-46
[101] Jha, T. K., Sundar, S. and Thakur, C. P. Miltefosine as oral agent for the treatment of Indian visceral leishmaniasis. N. Engl. J. Med. 1999 341: 1795-800
[102] Thakur, C.P., Sinha, P.K., Singh, R.K., Hassan, S.M. and Narain, S. Miltefosine in case of visceral leishmaniasis with HIV coinfection and rising incidence of this disease in India. Trans R Soc Trop Med Hyg 2000 94: 696-7
[103] Matherson, S., Cabie, A., Parquin, F., Mayaud, C., Roux, P. and Antoine, M. Visceral leishmaniasis and HIV infection: unusual presentation with pleuropulmonary involvement, and effect of secondary prophylaxis. AIDS 1992 6: 238-40
[104] Mannaerts, G.P. and Van Veldhoven, P.P. Metabolic pathways in mammalian peroxisomes; Biochimie. 1993 75: 147-58
[105] Tolbert, N.E. Metabolic pathways in peroxisomes and glyoxysomes. Annu Rev Biochem, 1981 50: 133-57
[106] Chang, K.P., Fong, D. and Bray, R.S. Leishmaniasis. New York: Elsevier, 1985
[107] de Duve, Ch. The separation and characterization of subcellular particles. Harvey Lect. 1965 59: 49-87
[108] Mahmoud, S.S., Michael, L.C., Jason, D.M., Roberts, L. J. and Mostafa, Z.B. Evidence against peroxisome proliferation - induced hepatic oxidative damage; Biochemical Pharmacology, 1997 53: 1369-74
[109] Van-Den Bosch, H., Schutgens, R.B., Wanders, R.J. and Tager, J.M. Biochemistry of peroxisomes. Ann Rev Biochem 1992 61: 157-97
[110] de Duve, C. Microbodies in the living cell. Sci Am. 1983 248(5): 74-84
[111] Perdue, P.E. & Lazarow, P.B. Peroxisome biogenesis; Annu Rev. Cell Dev. Biol. 2001 17: 701-52
[112] Opperdoes, F. R., Baudhuin, P., Coppens, I, De Roe C., Edwards, S. W., Weijers, P. J. and Misset, O. Purification, morphometric analysis, and characterization of the glycosomes (microbodies) of the protozoan hemoflagellate *Trypanosoma brucei.* J Cell Biol. 1984 98: 1178-84

[113] Lazarow, P.B. and Fujiki, Y. Biogenesis of peroxisome. Annu Rev. Cell Dev Biol 1985 1: 459-530

[114] Girzalsky, W., Rehling, P., Stein, K., Kipper, J., Blank, L., Kunau, W.H. and Erdmann, R. Involvement of Pex13p in Pex14p localization and peroxisomal targeting signal 2-dependent protein import into peroxisomes. J Cell Biol. 1999 144(6): 1151-62

[115] Terlecky, S.R. and Fransen, M. How peroxisomes arise. Traffic 2000 1: 465-73.

[116] Gould, S.J. and Valle, D. Peroxisome biogenesis disorders: genetics and cell biology. Trends Genet. 2000 16: 340-45

[117] Lazarow, P.B. and de Duve, C. A fatty acyl-CoA oxidizing system in rat liver peroxisomes; enhancement by clofibrate, a hypolipidemic drug. Proc Natl Acad Sci USA.1976 73: 2043-60

[118] Demoz, A., Daniel, K., Lie, A.O. and Berge, R. K. Modulation of plasma and hepatic oxidative status and changes in plasma lipid profile by n-3 (EPA and DHA), n-6 (corn oil) and a 3-thia fatty acids in rats. Biochimica et Biophysica Acta. 1994 1199(3): 238-244

[119] Henk, F., Tabak, B.I. and Distel, B. Peroxisomes: simple in function but complex in maintenance. Trends in Cell Biology. 1999 9(11): 447-453

[120] Henk, F., Tabak, B.I. and Distel, B. Peroxisomes: simple in function but complex in maintenance. Trends in Cell Biology. 1999 9(11): 447-453

[121] Masters, C.J. and Crane, D. I. On the role of the peroxisome in the ontogeny, ageing and degenerative disease. Mech. Ageing Dev. 1995 80: 69-83.

[122] Singh, I. Mammalian Peroxisomes: metabolism of oxygen and reactive oxygen species. In: Peroxisomes: Biology and Role in Toxicology and Disease, ed. Reddy, J.K., Suga, T, Mannaerts, G.P., Lazarow, P.B., and Subramoni, S., eds. New York: Annals of the New York Academy of Sciences. 1996 804: 612-27.

[123] Kondrup, J. and Lazarow, P.B. Flux of palmitate through the peroxisomal and mitochondrial beta-oxidation systems in isolated rat hepatocytes. Biochim Biophys Acta. 1985 835(1): 147-53

[124] Baumgart, E., Vanhooren, J.C., Fransen, M., van Veldhoven, P.P. et al. Molecular characterization of the human peroxisomal branched-chain acyl-CoA oxidase: cDNA cloning, chromosomal assignment, tissue distribution, and evidence for the absence of the protein in Zellweger syndrome. Proc Natl Acad Sci U S A 1996 93(24): 13748-53

[125] Raymond, G.V. Peroxisomal Disorders, Current Opinions in pediatrics, 1999 11: 572-76

[126] Reddy, C., Janardan, K., Tetsuya Suga, and Guy P. Mannaerts, eds. Peroxisomes: Biology and Role in Toxicology and Disease, Annals of New York, Academy of Sciences. New York: New York Academy of Sciences. 1996 804

[127] Schmitt, K., Molzer, B., Stockler, S., Tulzer, G. and Tulzer, W. Zellweger syndrome, neonatal adrenoleukodystrophy or infantile Refsum's disease in a case with generalized peroxisome defect. Wien Klin Wochenschr.1993 105(11): 320-2

[128] Weller, S., Gould, S.J. and Valle, D. Peroxisome biogenesis disorders. Annu Rev Genomics Hum Genet. 2003 4: 165-211

[129] Schu, P.V., Takegawa, K., Fry, M.J., Stack, J.H., Waterfield, M.D. and Emr, S.D. Phosphatidylinositol 3-kinase encoded by yeast VPS34 gene essential for protein sorting. Science. 1993 260(5104): 88-91

[130] Kiel, J.A., Rechinger, K.B., van der Klei, I.J., Salomons, F.A., Titorenko, V.I. and Veenhuis, M. The Hansenula polymorpha PDD1 gene product, essential for the selective degradation of peroxisomes, is a homologue of *Saccharomyces cerevisiae* Vps34p. Yeast. 1999 15(9): 741-54

[131] Kim, J., Dalton, V.M., Eggerton, K.P., Scott, S.V. and Klionsky, D.J. Apg7p/Cvt2p is required for the cytoplasm-to-vacuole targeting, macroautophagy, and peroxisome degradation pathways. Mol Biol Cell. 1999 10(5): 1337-51

[132] Tanida, I., Mizushima, N., Kiyooka, M., Ohsumi, M., Ueno, T., Ohsumi, Y. and Kominami, E. Apg7p/Cvt2p: A novel protein-activating enzyme essential for autophagy. Mol Biol Cell. 1999 10(5): 1367-79

[133] Yuan, W., Stromhaug, P.E. and Dunn, W.A. Jr. Glucose-induced autophagy of peroxisomes in Pichia pastoris requires a unique E1-like protein. Mol Biol Cell. 1999 10(5): 1353-66

[134] Singh, A.K., Tekwani, B.L., Guru, P.Y., Rastogi, A.K. and Pandey, V.C. Suppression of the hepatic microsomal cytochrome P-450 dependent mixed function oxidase activities in golden hamster during *Leishmania donovani* infection. Pharmacol Res. 1989 21(5): 507-12

[135] Corbett, C. E. Histopathology of lymphoid organs in the experimental leishmaniasis. Int J Exp Pathol. 1992 73(4): 417-33

[136] Leite, V.H., Croft. SL. Hepatic extracellular matrix in BALB/c mice infected with *Leishmania donovani*: Int J Exp. Pathol, 1996 77(4): 181-90

[137] Goto, H. Immunological Parameters of visceral leishmaniasis of *Leishmania major*-infected golden hamsters; Allergol Immunopathol (Madr). 1987 15(6): 349-53

[138] Raychaudhury, B., Banerjee, S. and Datta, S.C. Peroxisomal function is altered during *Leishmania* infection, Med. Sci. Monit 2003 9: 125–129.

[139] Vianna, V.L.P., Takiya, C.M. and de Brito-Gitirana, L. Histopathologic analysis of hamster hepatocytes submitted to experimental infection with *Leishmania donovani*, Parasitol. Res. 2002 88: 829–836

[140] Titorenko, V.I. and Rachubinski, R.A. Dynamics of peroxisome assembly and function, Trends Cell Biol. 2001 1122–29

[141] McCormack, J.G. and Denton, R.M. The role of mitochondrial Ca^{2+} transport and matrix Ca^{2+} in signal transduction in mammalian tissue, Biochim. Biophys. Acta 1990 1018: 287–291

[142] Raychaudhury, B, Gupta, S and Datta. Peroxisome is a reservoir of intracellular calcium. Biochim. Biophy. Acta 2006 1760: 989-992

[143] Fidaleo M. Peroxisomes and peroxisomal disorders: The main facts. Experimental and Toxicologic Pathology.2010 62: 615-625

[144] Wanders RJA, J.M. Tager et al Peroxisomal disorders in nerulogy. J. Neurol. Sciences. 1988 88: 1-39

[145] Ghosh, A.K., Bhattacharya, F..K. and Ghosh, D..K. *Leishmania donovani*: amastigote inhibition and mode of action of berberine. Exp. Parasitol 198560, 404–13.

[146] Jaffe, C.L., Grimaldi, G. and McMahon-Pratt, D.. In: Morel, C.M.(Ed.), Genes and Antigens of Parasites: A Laboratory Manual. Fundaao Oswaldo Cruz, Rio de Janeiro. 1984 pp. 47.

[147] Stauber, L.A., Franchino, E.M. and Grun, J.. An eight-day method of screening compounds against *Leishmania donovani* in the golden hamster. J. Protozool. 1958; 5, 269–73.

[148] Datta, S.C., Ghosh, M. K. and Hajra A.K., Purification and properties of acyl/ alkyl dihydroxyacetonephosphate from guinea pig liver. J. Biol. Chem. 1990. 265, 8268–74.

[149] Laemmli, U.K., Cleavage of structural proteins during the assembly of the head of bacteriophage T4. Nature 1970. 227, 680–85.

[150] Towbin, H., Staehelin, T. and Gordon, J., Electrophoretic transfer of proteins from polyacrylamide gels to nitrocellulose sheets: procedure and some applications. Proc. Natl. Acad. Sci. USA 1979. 76, 4350–54.

[151] Beauchamp, C., and Fridovich, I., Superoxide dismutase: improvedassays and an assay applicable to acrylamide gels. Anal. Biochem 1971. 44, 276–87.

[152] Leighton, F., Pool, B., Beaufy, H., Baudhuin, P., Coffey, J.W., Fouler, S. and de Duve C., The large-scale separation of peroxisomes, mitochondria and lysosomes from the livers of rats injected with Triton WR-1339. J. Cell Biol. 1968. 37, 482–513.

[153] Markland, S. Markland, G.,. Involvement of superoxide anion radical in the autoxidation of pyrogallol and a convenient assay for superoxide dismutase. Eur. J. Biochem. 1974 47, 469–74.

[154] Lowry, O. H., Rosebrough, N.J., Farr, A.L. and Randall, R. J.,. Protein estimation with the Folin-phenol reagent. J. Biol. Chem. 1951 193, 265–75.

[155] Majumdar, S., Dey, S.N., Chaudhury, R. and Das, J., Intracellular development of choleraphage phi 149 under permissive and nonpermissive conditions: an electron microscopic study. Intervirology. 1988. 29, 27–38.

[156] Mishra, B.N. and Mishra, M. K. Introductory Practical Biostatistics. Naya Prakash. 1983. p. 89.

[157] Raychaudhury, B., Banerjee, S., Datta, S. C.,. Peroxisomal function is altered during *Leishmania* infection. Med. Sci. Monit 2003. 9, 125-29.

[158] Wanders, R.J.A., Peroxisomes, lipid metabolism, and peroxisomal disorders. Mol. Genet. Metab. 2004. 83, 16–27.

[159] Nguyen, S.D., Baes, M. and Veldhoven, P.P.V., Degradation of very long chain dicarboxylic polyunsaturated fatty acids in mouse hepatocytes, a peroxisomal process. Biochimica et Biophysica Acta. - Molecular and Cell Biology of Lipids 2008 1781: 400-5.

[160] Van-Den Bosch, H., Schutgens, R.B., Wanders, R.J. and Tager, J.M.,.Biochemistry of peroxisomes. Ann Rev Biochem. 1992 61, 157-97

[161] Lazarow, P.B., Moser, H.W.,. The metabolic basis of inherited diseases. vol II. New York: McGraw-Hill, 1995 2287-2324.

[162] Goepfert, S. and Poirier, Y.,. β-Oxidation in fatty acid degradation and beyond. Current Opinion in Plant Biology, 2007 10, 245-51

[163] Duran, E, Walker, D.J., Johnson, K. R.,. Developmental and tissue specific expression of 2-methyl branched –chain enoyl Co-A reductase isoforms in the parasitic nematode. Ascaris suum Mol Biochem Parasitol. 1998 91, 307-18

[164] Hamberg, M, Stereochemical aspects of fatty acid oxidation: hydroperoxide isomerases. Acta Chem Scand. 1996 50, 219-24.

[165] Fricker, S.P., Mosi, R.M., Cameron, B.R., Baird, I., Zhu, Y., Anastassov, V., Cox, J., Doyle, P.S., Hansell, E., Lau, G., Langille, J., Olsen, M., Qin, L., Skerlj, R., Wong, R.S.Y., Santucci, Z.. and McKerrow, J.H.,. Metal compounds for the treatment of parasitic diseases. Journal of Inorganic Biochemistry 2008. 102, 1839-45

[166] Murray, H.W.,.Clinical and experimental advances in treatment of visceral leishmaniasis. Antimicrob. Agents Chemother. 2001 45, 2185–97.

[167] Sinha,P.K., Ranjan, A., Singh, V.P., Das, V.N.R. , Pandey, K., Kumar, N. , Verma, N., Lal, C.S., Sur, D., Manna, B. and Bhattacharya,S.K.,. Visceral leishmaniasis (kala-azar)—the Bihar (India) perspective. Journal of Infection. 2006 53, 60-64

[168] Werbozetv, K.,. Diamidines as antitrypanosomal, antileishmanial and antimalarial agents. Curr Opin Investig Drugs. 2006 7, 147-57.

[169] Fricker, S.P., Mosi, R.M., Cameron, B.R., Baird, I., Zhu, Y., Anastassov, V., Cox, J., Doyle, P.S., Hansell, E., Lau, G., Langille, J., Olsen, M., Qin, L., Skerlj, R., Wong, R.S.Y., Santucci, Z. and McKerrow, J.H.,. Metal compounds for the treatment of parasitic diseases. Journal of Inorganic Biochemistry. 2008 102, 1839-45

[170] Sundar, S, and Chatterjee, M. Visceral leishmaniasis - current therapeutic modalities. Indian J Med Res. 2006 123, 345-352.

[171] Novikoff, A.B., and Novikoff, P.M.,.Microperoxisomes. J Histochem Cytochem. 1973 21, 963-66.

[172] Wilcke, M, Hultenby, K, Alexon S.H.E.,. Novel peroxisomal populations in subcellular fractions from rat liver. Implication for peroxisome structure and biogenesis. J Biol Chem. 1995 270, 6949-58

[173] Baudhuin, P., Beaufy H, deDuve C.,. Combined biochemical and morphological study of particulate fraction from rat liver. Analysis of preparations enriched in lysosomes or in particles containing urate oxidase, D-amino acid oxidase, and catalase. J Cell Biol. 1965 26, 219-43.

[174] Koepke, J.I., Wood, C.S., Terlecky, L.J., Walton, P.A. and Terlecky, S.R.,. Progeric effects of catalase inactivation in human cells. Toxicology and Applied Pharmacology. 2008 232, 99-108.

[175] Schrader, M. and Fahimi, H.D.,. Peroxisomes and oxidative stress. Biochim Biophys Acta 2006 1763, 1755-66.

[176] Herrero, E., Ros, J., Bellí, G. and Cabiscol, E.,. Redox control and oxidative stress in yeast cells. Biochimica et Biophysica Acta 2008 1780, 1217-35

[177] Fattman, C.L., Schaefer, L.M., and Oury, T.D.,. Extracellular superoxide dismutase in biology and medicine. Free Radic. Biol. Med. 2003 35: 236–56.

[178] Dey, A. and Singh, S., Genetic heterogeneity among visceral and post kala azar dermal leishmaniasis strains from eastern India Infection, Genetics and Evolution, 2007. 7, 219-22

[179] Zijlstra, E.E., Musa, A.M. and Khalil, A.M.,. Post kala-azar dermal leishmaniasis. Laneet Infect Dis. 2003 3, 87-98.

[180] Gupta S, Raychaudhury B and Datta S.C Host peroxisomal properties are not restored to normal after treatment of visceral leishmaniasis with sodium antimony gluconate. Exp. Parasitology 2009 123 140–145.

18

Genetic Basis of Inherited Bone Marrow Failure Syndromes

Yigal Dror
The Hospital for Sick Children and The University of Toronto, Toronto Canada

1. Introduction

Inherited bone marrow failure syndromes (IBMFSs) are multi-system disorders with varying degrees of defective production of erythrocytes, granulocytes and platelets in the bone marrow, leading to single-lineage or multilineage cytopenia (Table 1).(Dror 2006) The term IBMFSs is reserved for disorders that are caused by mutations, which are either inherited from the parents or occurred de-novo.(Alter 2003; Dokal and Vulliamy 2008) Based on the transmission patterns of the diseases (e.g. dominant or recessive autosomal or X-linked) and the segregation of known IBMFSs genes within multiplex families, the IBMFSs are considered as monogenic (Mendelian) diseases.(Alter 2003; Shimamura 2006; Dokal and Vulliamy 2008) The incidence of establishing a diagnosis of IBMFSs is about two new cases per a general population of million people per year and 65 cases per 10^6 child births.(Tsangaris, Klaassen et al. 2011)

In some IBMFSs (e.g. Fanconi anemia) pancytopenia ($\geq$2 lineages affected) usually evolves. In others, one lineage is predominantly affected (e.g. neutropenia in Kostmann/severe congenital neutropenia, anemia in Diamond Blackfan anemia or thrombocytopenia in thrombocytopenia absent radii).

The bone marrow failure often causes substantial morbidity and mortality, and many patients require life-long blood transfusions, treatment for infections, growth factors and hematopoietic stem cell transplantation (HSCT). Due to hematological and non-hematological problems, high risk of cancer and major treatment-related toxicity, the life expectancy of the patients is substantially reduced.(Dror 2006; Alter 2007)

IBMFSs have both unique and common features. The clinical manifestations could not always discriminate between the various IBMFSs or between IBMFSs from acquired bone marrow failure syndromes. The associations of bone marrow failure with either congenital malformations or presentation during the first year of life or an affected first-degree relative are important diagnostic features.(Teo, Klaassen et al. 2008) A wide range of physical anomalies (e.g. craniofacial, skeletal, cardiovascular, gastrointestinal, renal, neurological and dermatological) are associated with IBMFSs and may help to establish a diagnosis. However, substantial phenotypic overlap exists among the disorders, which frequently limits the ability to establish a diagnosis based solely on clinical manifestations. Further, some of the disorders are not associated with physical anomalies, or the malformations develop later in life; for example, nail dystrophy in dyskeratosis congenita and metaphyseal dysplasia in Shwachman-Diamond syndrome. Therefore, genetic testing is critical for establishing a diagnosis and provides family counseling and management.

Disorder	Gene	Protein	Gene Locus	Inheritance	Reference
Fanconi anemia	*FANCA*	FANCA	16q24.3	AR	(Lo Ten Foe, Rooimans et al. 1996)
	FANCB	FANCB	Xp22.31	XLR	(Meetei, Levitus et al. 2004)
	FANCC	FANCC	9q22.3	AR	(Strathdee, Gavish et al. 1992)
	FANCD1/ BRCA2	FANCD1/ BRCA2	13q12.3	AR	(Howlett, Taniguchi et al. 2002)
	FANCD2	FANCD2	3p25.3	AR	(Timmers, Taniguchi et al. 2001)
	FANCE	FANCE	6p21.3	AR	(de Winter, Leveille et al. 2000)
	FANCF	FANCF	11p15	AR	(de Winter, Rooimans et al. 2000)
	FANCG/ XRCC9	FANCG	9p13	AR	(de Winter, Waisfisz et al. 1998)
	FANCI	FANCI	15q25-q26	AR	(Levitus, Rooimans et al. 2004)
	FANCJ/ BRIP1	FANCJ/ BRIP1	17q22	AR	(Levitus, Rooimans et al. 2004)
	FANCL/ PHF9	FANCL/ PHF9	2p16.1	AR	(Meetei, de Winter et al. 2003)
	FANCM	FANCM	14q21.3	AR	(Meetei, Medhurst et al. 2005)
	FANCN/ PALB2	FANCN/ PALB2	16p12	AR	(Reid, Schindler et al. 2007)
	FANCP/ SLX4	FANCP/ SLX4	16p13.3	AR	(Stoepker, Hain et al.)
	FANCO/ RAD51C	FANCO/ RAD51C	17q22	AR	(Vaz, Hanenberg et al.)

Disorder	**Gene**	**Protein**	**Gene Locus**	**Inheritance**	**Reference**
	Mono-somy 21q22.11-q22.13	UK	UK	UK	(Byrd, Zwerdling et al.)
Shwachman-Diamond syndrome	*SBDS*	7q11.2	7q11	AR	(Boocock, Morrison et al. 2003)
Dyskeratosis congenita	*DKC1*	Dyskerin	Xq28	XLR	(Heiss, Knight et al. 1998)
	TINF2	TIN2	14q12	AD	(Savage, Giri et al. 2008)
	TERC	TERC	3q21-q28	AD	(Vulliamy, Marrone et al. 2001)
	TERT	Telomerase	5p15.33	AD	(Vulliamy, Walne et al. 2005)
	NOP10	NOP10	15q14-q15	AR	(Walne, Vulliamy et al. 2007)
	NHP2	NHP2	5q35.3	AR	(Vulliamy, Beswick et al. 2008)
	TCAB1	*TCAB1*	17p13	AR	(Zhong, Savage et al. 2011)
Congenital amegakaryocytic thrombocytopenia	*MPL*	Thrombo-poietin receptor	1p34	AR	(van den Oudenrijn, Bruin et al. 2000)
Reticular dysgenesis	*AK2*	Adenylate kinase 2	1p34	AR	(Lagresle-Peyrou, Six et al. 2009; Pannicke, Honig et al. 2009)
Pearson's syndrome	*mDNA*	Variable	Mito-chondrial DNA	Maternal	(Rotig, Cormier et al. 1990)
Lig4-associated aplastic anemia	*LIG4*	DNA Ligase IV	1q22-q34		(O'Driscoll, Cerosaletti et al. 2001)

Disorder	Gene	Protein	Gene Locus	Inheritance	Reference
Diamond-Blackfan anemia	*RPS19*	RPS19	19q13.3	AD	(Draptchinskaia, Gustavsson et al. 1999)
	RPL5	RPL5	1p22.1	AD	(Gazda, Sheen et al. 2008)
	RPS26	RPS26	12q	AD	(Doherty, Sheen et al. 2010)
	RPL11	RPL11	1p35-p36.1	AD	(Gazda, Sheen et al. 2008)
	RPS24	RPS24	10q22-q23	AD	(Gazda, Grabowska et al. 2006)
	RPL35a	RPL35a	3q29	AD	(Farrar, Nater et al. 2008)
	RPS7	RPS7	15q	AD	(Doherty, Sheen et al. 2010)
	RPS17	RPS17	15q	AD	(Doherty, Sheen et al. 2010)
	RPS10	RPS10	6p	AD	(Doherty, Sheen et al. 2010)
Inherited sideroblastic anemia	*ALAS2*	ALAS	Xp11.21	XL	(Cotter, Baumann et al. 1992)
	ABC7	ATP-binding cassette transporter 7	Xq13.1-q13.3	XL	(Allikmets, Raskind et al. 1999)
	SLC19A2	thiamine transporter 2	1q23.3	AR	(Fleming, Tartaglini et al. 1999)
	PUS1	Pseudo-uridine synthase 1	2p16.1	AR	(Zeharia, Fischel-Ghodsian et al. 2005)
	SLC25A38	SLC25A38	3p22.1	AR	(Guernsey, Jiang et al. 2009)

Disorder	Gene	Protein	Gene Locus	Inheritance	Reference
Congenital dyserythropoietic anemia type I	*CDAN1*	Codanin-1	15q15	AR	(Dgany, Avidan et al. 2002)
Congenital dyserythropoietic anemia type II	*SEC23B*	SEC23B	20p11.2	AR	(Bianchi, Fermo et al. 2009; Schwarz, Iolascon et al. 2009)
Congenital dyserythropoietic anemia type III	*UK*	UK	UN	AR	
Congenital dyserythropoietic anemia - unclassified	*KLF1*	KLF1	19p13.12-p13.13	AR	(Arnaud, Saison et al.)
Kostmann/Severe congenital neutropenia	*ELA2*	Neutrophil Elastase	19p13.3	AD	(Dale, Person et al. 2000)
	HAX1	HAX1	1q21.3	AR	(Klein, Grudzien et al. 2007)
	GLI1	GFI1	1p22	AD	(Person, Li et al. 2003)
	WASP	WASP	Xp11.23-p11.22	XLR	(Devriendt, Kim et al. 2001)
Dursun syndrome	*G6PC3*	Glucose-6-phosphatase catalytic unit 3	17q21		(Banka, Newman et al. ; Boztug, Appaswamy et al. 2009)
Cyclic neutropenia	*ELA2*	Neutrophil Elastase	19p13.3	AD	(Horowitz, Benson et al. 1999)
WHIM syndrome	*CXCR4*	CXCR4	2q21	AD	(Hernandez, Gorlin et al. 2003)
Glycogen storage diseases Ib	*G6PT*	G6PT	11q23	AR	(Annabi, Hiraiwa et al. 1998)
Barth syndrome	*TAZ*	Taffazin	Xq28	XL	(Bione, D'Adamo et al. 1996)

Disorder	Gene	Protein	Gene Locus	Inheritance	Reference
Poikiloderma with neutropenia	*C16orf57*	Not-determined	16q13	AR	(Volpi, Roversi et al.)
Thrombocytopenia absent radii	*UK*	UK	UK	AR	
Epstein/Fechtner/Sebastian/May-Hegglin/ Alport syndrome	*MYH9*	nonmuscle myosin heavy chain IIA	22q11-q13	AD	(Seri, Pecci et al. 2003)
Mediterranean platelet disorder	*GPIBA*	GPIb	17pter-p12	AD	(Savoia, Balduini et al. 2001)
Familial autosomal dominant non-syndromic thrombocytopenia	*MASTL*	microtubule-associated serine/threonine-like kinase	10p11-12	AD	(Gandhi, Cummings et al. 2003)
	ACBD5	ACBD5	10p12.1	AD	(Punzo, Mientjes et al. 2010)
	ANKRD26	ANKRD26	10q22.1	AD	(Pippucci, Savoia et al.)
Thrombocytopenia with dyserythropoiesis	*GATA1*	GATA1	Xp11.23	XL	(Nichols, Crispino et al. 2000)
Thrombocytopenia with associated myeloid malignancies	*CBFA2*	CBFA2	21q22.1-22.2	AD	(Song, Sullivan et al. 1999)
X-linked thrombocytopenia	*WASP*	WASP	Xp11.23	XL	(Devriendt, Kim et al. 2001)
Thrombocytopenia with radio-ulnar synostosis	*HOXA11*	HOXA11	7p15-p14.2	AD	(Thompson and Nguyen 2000)

Table 1. The inherited bone marrow failure syndromes

2. The inherited bone marrow failure syndromes and genes

Mutations in IBMFS genes result in high-penetrance alleles; namely alleles that cause Mendelian (monogenic) diseases transmitted in a autosomal dominant, autosomal recessive autosomal or X-linked recessive patterns.(Balmain, Gray et al. 2003) The IBMFS genes are crucial for fundamental cellular processes such as DNA repair,(Cohn and D'Andrea 2008) telomere maintenance,(Vulliamy and Dokal 2008) ribosome biogenesis(Choesmel, Bacqueville et al. 2007; Ganapathi, Austin et al. 2007; Menne, Goyenechea et al. 2007) microtubule stabilization,(Austin, Gupta et al. 2008) chemotaxis,(Wessels, Srikantha et al. 2006) signaling from hematopoietic growth factor,(Ihara, Ishii et al. 1999) signal transduction related to hematopoietic cell differentiation,(Song, Sullivan et al. 1999; Nichols, Crispino et al. 2000) granulocytic enzymes,(Dale, Person et al. 2000) and cell survival.(Cumming, Lightfoot et al. 2001; Miyake, Flygare et al. 2005; Klein, Grudzien et al. 2007; Rujkijyanont, Watanabe et al. 2008; Watanabe, Ambekar et al. 2009) Although rare, the study of IBMFSs genes made critical contributions to the understanding of not only the pathogenesis of the individual disorders, but also to common health problems such as cancer(Friedenson 2007; Londono-Vallejo 2008) and aging.(Aubert and Lansdorp 2008)

2.1 Fanconi anemia

2.1.1 Clinical features of Fanconi anemia

Fanconi anemia (FA) is an IBMFS with increased chromosome breakage. It has the highest child birth incidence among the IBMFSs.(Tsangaris, Klaassen et al. 2011) It was first described by Professor Fanconi in 1927. (Fanconi 1927) It is a multisystem disorder which commonly affects the bone marrow and the development of other organs.(Auerbach, Rogatko et al. 1989) Hematologically the patients suffer from aplastic anemia, which is characterized by various degrees of single or multilineage cytopenia, red blood cell macrocytosis, high fetal hemoglobin levels and reduced bone marrow cellularity. Common malformations include cafe-au-lait spots, hypopigmented skin patches, hypoplasia/absence of the thumbs, dysplastic/absence kidneys, characteristic delicate faces, microcephaly, developmental delay and various heart defects. Also, the patients have a high predisposition for myelodysplastic syndrome (MDS), leukemia (particularly acute myeloid leukemia, AML) and solid cancer. The cumulative incidence of developing bone marrow failure, MDS/AML and solid neoplasms were estimated at 90%, 33%, and 28% by 40 years of age.(Kutler, Singh et al. 2003) At presentation patients may have an either classic phenotype comprised of both physical anomalies and abnormal hematology, or typical physical anomalies but normal hematology, or normal physical features but abnormal hematology. The disease occurs in all racial and ethnic groups. The treatment for the bone marrow failure includes androgens or hematopoietic stem cell transplantation (HSCT). The later is the only curative therapy for the bone marrow failure. Surgical interventions may be required for some organ malformations or cancer.

2.1.2 Fanconi anemia genes

FA is a genetically heterogeneous disease with 15 genes currently identified (Table 1). Most genetic groups are inherited in an autosomal recessive manner with an estimated overall FA heterozygote frequency of about 1 in 200. This was confirmed with the identification of the FA genes. However, a XL-recessive inheritance characterizes the rare FA group B. The most commonly mutated FA genes are *FANCA, FANCC* and *FANCG*. Based on the ability to correct the chromosome fragility phenotype by forming hybrid cells with another genetic group cells(Yoshida 1980; Duckworth-Rysiecki, Cornish et al. 1985) or by vector-mediated gene transduction,(Antonio Casado, Callen et al. 2007) each genetic group is also called complementation group.

DNA Repair

A major finding in FA is abnormal chromosome fragility; this is seen in metaphase preparations of peripheral blood lymphocytes or cultured skin fibroblasts either spontaneously or after treating the cells with DNA cross linking agents such as mitomycin C, di-epoxybutane and cisplatinum (Fig 1). The FA cellular karyotype shows chromatid breaks, rearrangements, gaps, endoreduplications, and chromatid exchanges. Spontaneous chromosomal breaks are occasionally absent in FA,(Auerbach, Rogatko et al. 1989) but is strikingly enhanced if cross linking agents are added to the cell culture.(Auerbach, Rogatko et al. 1989) It is postulated that the increased chromosomal fragility is caused by a defects in DNA repair. Indeed, some of the FA genes have been previously shown to be tumor suppressor genes related to DNA repair.(Mavaddat, Pharoah et al. 2010) *FANCD1* is *BRCA2*, which is mutated in the germline of 12% of patients with familial breast cancer and also contributes to a risk of ovarian and pancreatic cancer. *FANCJ* was identified as BRIP1 or BACH1, which is mutated in 1-2% of familial breast cancer. *FANCN* is *PALB2* which is mutated 1-2% of familial breast cancer.

The FA genes might have variety of functions, but all belong to the FA homologous recombination DNA repair pathway (Reviewed by de Winter & Joenje(de Winter and Joenje 2008)) (Fig 2). During S phase, the replication forks are stalled in areas of DNA interstrand crosslinks. FANCM associates with FAAP24, which senses the stalled replication forks. FANCM then recruits the FA core complex to chromatin at the site of DNA damage.(Huang 2010) The core FA complex is composed of FANCA,B,C,E,F,G,L,M, which associate with each other in a stepwise manner. Activation of the FA core complex via phosphorylation of FANCA, FANCE, FANCD2 and FNACI occurs in response to DNA damage in an ATR dependent manner. The complex is required for monoubiquination of two downstream FA proteins, FANCD2 and FANCI, through the E3 ubiquiten ligase domain of FANCL and by the E2 conjugating enzyme UBE2T. There is evidence that FANCI phosphorylation promotes FAND2 monoubiquination in an ATR-dependent manner and functions as a molecular switch to turn on the FA pathway.(Ishiai, Katao et al. 2008) Once ubiquinated, FANCD2 and FANCI bind to chromatin at DNA damage foci. Other DNA repair proteins that are recruited to these foci are FANCD1, BRCA1, RAD51, NSB1, BLM and PCNA. The recruitment of FANCD2 and FANCI to DNA damage foci likely facilitates DNA repair through homologous recombination, nucleotide excision repair and translesion synthesis; however, the exact biochemical functions are still unclear. FANCO (RAD51C) protein is critical for formation of RAD51 foci in response to DNA damage.(Godthelp, Artwert et al. 2002; Smeenk, de Groot et al. 2010) FANCP (SLX4) is a regulator of structure-specific endonucleases that repair DNA interstrand crosslinks. (Fekairi, Scaglione et al. 2009) The FA protein-related DNA damage foci are thought to be assembled during S phase and mostly disassembled once the damage is repaired, before the exit from S phase.

Mutations in any member of the core FA protein complex reduces FANCD2 ubiquitinylation and its recruitment to DNA damage foci.(Garcia-Higuera, Taniguchi et al. 2001) Mutations in downstream FANC proteins such as FANCD1 prevent localization of DNA repair proteins such as RAD51 in damage-induced nuclear foci,(Godthelp, Artwert et al. 2002; Howlett, Taniguchi et al. 2002) but do not affect FAND2 monoubiquination.

Apoptosis

The FA proteins might also be directly involved in protecting cells from apoptosis. Enhanced apoptosis of hematopoietic stem cells progenitors is probably a key cellular mechanism promoting bone marrow failure in FA. Most of apoptosis-related work was done on the FANCC subgroup. First, *FANCC* associates with HSP70, upon exposure to either combinations of tumor necrosis factor and interferon-gamma or double-stranded

RNA and interferon-gamma. This interaction facilitates HSP70 binding to and inactivation of double-stranded RNA-dependent protein kinase, thereby protecting from apoptosis.(Pang, Keeble et al. 2001) Mutations in the *FANCA*, *FANCC*, and *FANCG* genes markedly increase the amount of RNA-dependent protein kinase, leading to hypersensitivity of hematopoietic progenitor cells to growth inhibition by interferon-γ and tumor necrosis factor-α.(Zhang, Li et al. 2004) Second, it has been shown that FANCC interacts with and enhances the function of GSTP1, which detoxifies by-products of redox stress and xenobiotics, whereby it might protect cells from inducers of apoptosis.(Cumming, Lightfoot et al. 2001) Third, it has also been shown that oxidative stress through excess inflammatory cytokines such as tumor necrosis factor-α may contribute to the loss of FA hematopoietic stem cells/early progenitors. High production of inflammatory cytokines including tumor necrosis factor-α was observed in FA patients(Dufour, Corcione et al. 2003) and in *Fancc*$^{-/-}$ mice challenged with lipopolysaccharide.(Sejas, Rani et al. 2007) *Fancc*$^{-/-}$ hematopoietic progenitors are hypersensitive inflammatory mediators such as interferon-γ and lipopolysaccharide with a concomitant increase in tumor necrosis factor-α-dependent apoptosis.(Sejas, Rani et al. 2007) Importantly, the inflammatory-related apoptosis in FA requires the production of reactive oxygen species. It has been shown that enhanced oxidant and tumor necrosis factor- α–induced apoptosis in *Fancc*$^{-/-}$ murine hematopoietic progenitors is dependent on apoptosis signal-regulating kinase 1.(Bijangi-Vishehsaraei, Saadatzadeh et al. 2005) Abnormal p38 MAPK and JNK activation was shown to partially contribute to lipopolysaccaride-induced *Fancc*$^{-/-}$ hematopoietic suppression. Saadatzadeh et al(Saadatzadeh, Bijangi-Vishehsaraei et al. 2009) showed that p38 MAPK and JNK inhibition protected c-kit^{+} bone marrow cells from tumor necrosis factor-α-induced apoptosis and enhanced *Fancc*$^{-/-}$ hematopoietic colony formation in the presence of tumor necrosis factor-α. However, engraftment and in-vivo hematopoietic reconstitution might be inhibited by p38MAPK rather than JNK.

Replication fork progression

FANCM has been proposed to directly function in DNA replication and repair. It contains ATP-dependent translocase activity, which promotes replication fork reversal(Gari, Decaillet et al. 2008) and has been proven to control replication fork.(Luke-Glaser, Luke et al. 2010)

Cytokinesis

FA cells demonstrate G_2-phase cell cycle arrest.(Sabatier and Dutrillaux 1988) A small number of monoubiquinated FANCD2/FANCI foci localize to DNA fragile sites, persist into mitosis(Chan, Palmai-Pallag et al. 2009; Naim and Rosselli 2009) and mark the extremities of ultrafine DNA bridges;(Chan, Palmai-Pallag et al. 2009) ssDNA which link the centromeres of sister chromatids during mitosis.(Chan, North et al. 2007) The ultrafine DNA bridges are naturally coated by BLM and Plk-interacting checkpoint helicase (PICH) (Baumann, Korner et al. 2007; Chan, North et al. 2007) The ultrafine DNA bridges which contain PICH and BLM also display FANCD2/FANCI foci at their extremities. They are generated when replication is incomplete, particularly at fragile loci under replication stress, but also in between two replication forks. BLM participates in the resolution of these bridges during mitosis and persistent DNA bridges may lead to micronucleation.(Chan, Palmai-Pallag et al. 2009) Vinciguerra et al.(Vinciguerra, Godinho et al. 2010) demonstrated abnormally high number of ultrafine DNA bridges in cellular models of FA, which was correlated with a higher rate of cytokinesis failure and formation of binucleated cells.

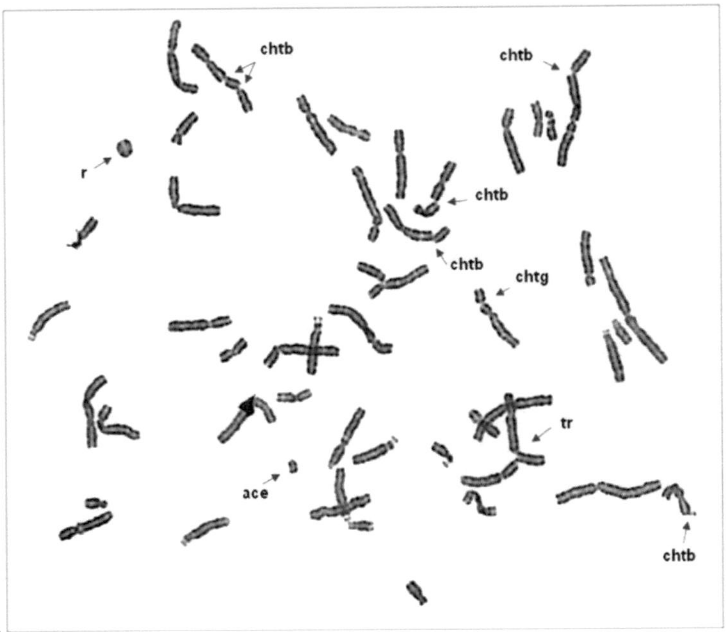

Fig. 1. Characteristic chromosome fragility seen in Fanconi anemia (chtb, chromatid break; chtg, chromatid gap; r, ring; ace, acentric fragment; tr, tri-radial figure)

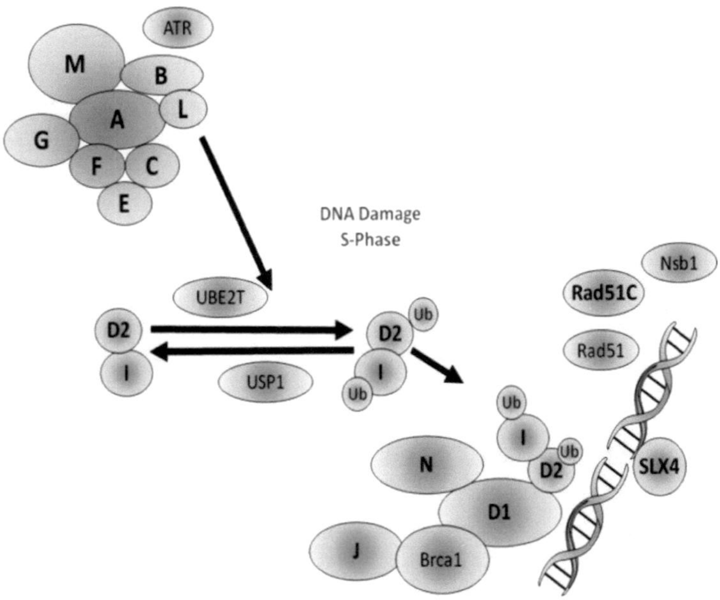

Fig. 2. The Fanconi anemia gene pathway and its reaction to DNA damage. The genes encoding for the proteins in bold are mutated in Fanconi anemia

2.1.3 Genotype phenotype correlation

The abnormal chromosome pattern, number of breaks/cell and variations in proportion of abnormal cells have no direct correlation with the severity of the hematological defects or clinical course of individual patients. (Gillio, Verlander et al. 1997) However, sensitivity to interstrand linking inducing agents may correlate with increased physical malformations. (Castella, Pujol et al. 2011)

A certain degree of correlation exists between genotype and phenotype. FA group A patients with homozygous for null mutations tend to have an earlier onset of anemia and a higher incidence of leukemia than those with mutations producing an altered protein. (Faivre, Guardiola et al. 2000) Also, FA group C patients with IVS4+4A>T or exon 14 mutations usually, (Gillio, Verlander et al. 1997; Faivre, Guardiola et al. 2000) but not always, (Futaki, Yamashita et al. 2000) have more somatic abnormalities and earlier onset of hematological abnormalities and poorer survival compared to patients with other *FANCC* 1 mutation. FA group G patients have severe cytopenia and a higher incidence of leukemia. FA group D1 and N patients may present with solid cancer without apparent bone marrow failure or physical anomalies. Common types of cancer in these groups include medulloblastoma, Wilm's tumor and AML.

2.2 Shwachman-Diamond syndrome

2.2.1 Clinical features of Shwachman-Diamond syndrome

SDS is an autosomal recessive multi-system disorder.(Shwachman 1964) It usually presents in childhood and commonly includes bone marrow failure, exocrine pancreatic insufficiency and bony metaphyseal syaplasia.(Aggett, Cavanagh et al. 1980) The patients have a high risk of leukemia, particularly AML.(Donadieu, Leblanc et al. 2005) The clinical diagnosis of SDS relies on having an evidence of bone marrow dysfunction and exocrine pancreatic dysfunction.

Neutropenia is the most common hematological abnormality, occurring in virtually all patients, followed by reticulocytopenic anemia and thrombocytopenia. Trilineage cytopenias occur in up to 65% of patients. Severe aplastic pancytopenia has occasionally been reported.(Aggett, Cavanagh et al. 1980; Tsai, Sahdev et al. 1990; Barrios, Kirkpatrick et al. 1991) Various degrees of abnormalities in B and T-cell lymphocytes as well as natural killer cells have also been reported in SDS.(Hudson and Aldor 1970; Aggett, Cavanagh et al. 1980; Dror, Ginzberg et al. 2001) Bone marrow biopsy usually shows a hypoplastic specimen.(Aggett, Cavanagh et al. 1980; Dror and Freedman 1999) The only curative therapy for the hematological complications in SDS is HSCT.(Donadieu, Michel et al. 2005)

2.2.2 The Shwachman-Diamond syndrome gene

SBDS is the only gene currently known to be associated with SDS. Mutations in *SBDS* can be identified in 90% of the patients.(Boocock, Morrison et al. 2003) *SBDS* was originally identified by Lai and colleagues(Lai, Chou et al. 2000) in 2000. The protein is 250 amino acids-long, and is highly conserved in evolution. Three structural/functional domains were predicted for the human(de Oliveira, Sforca et al.) and archael(Shammas, Menne et al. 2005) orthologues. The SBDS N-terminal domain was postulated to play a role in protein-protein interaction, the central domain is predicted to bind DNA,(Luscombe, Austin et al. 2000) and the C-terminus to bind RNA.(Birney, Kumar et al. 1993)

Data from the Canadian registry showed that *SBDS* is the most commonly mutated gene among the IBMFSs. This is probably because SDS is a common IBMFS and genetically homogenous.(Tsangaris, Klaassen et al. 2011) *SBDS* was mutated in 85%-90% of the SDS

patients.(Boocock, Morrison et al. 2003) The other 10-15% of the patients were diagnosed based on clinical characteristics, and are likely to have mutations in an additional, yet unknown, SDS gene(s).
Ninety six percent of the SBDS mutations are in exon 2.(Boocock, Morrison et al. 2003) The type of mutations include nonsense, splice site mutation, frameshift, missense and complex rearrangements comprising of deletion/insertion. The two common mutations are 183-184TA>CT (nonsense) and 258+2T>C (intronic with predicted alternative splicing & frameshift reading). The mutations are mostly in the N-terminal domain of the protein and cause markedly reduced protein levels.(Woloszynek, Rothbaum et al. 2004)
SBDS mRNA is ubiquitously expressed.(Boocock, Morrison et al. 2003) The protein is essential as no patients with homozygous null mutations have been reported, and residual protein levels can usually be detected in SDS patients.(Woloszynek, Rothbaum et al. 2004; Austin, Leary et al. 2005) Further, a complete loss of the protein in mice causes developmental arrest prior to embryonic day 6.5 and early lethality.(Zhang, Shi et al. 2006) SBDS seems to be multifunctional and play a role in several cellular pathways.

Ribosomal biogenesis

SBDS was found by one group to concentrate in the nucleolus during G1 and G2,(Austin, Leary et al. 2005) and is associated with rRNA.(Ganapathi, Austin et al. 2007) Synthetic genetic arrays of YHR087W, a yeast homolog of the N-terminal domain of SBDS, suggested interactions with several genes involved in RNA and rRNA processing.(Savchenko, Krogan et al. 2005) The loss of the protein in yeast results in a defect in maturation of the 60S ribosomal subunit due to defect in release and recycling of the nucleolar shuttling factor TIF6 from pre-60S ribosomes (Fig 3).(Menne, Goyenechea et al. 2007)

Apoptosis

Bone marrow cells from patients with SDS are characterized by decreased frequency of CD34+ progenitors,(Dror and Freedman 1999) and a reduced ability to generate hematopoietic colonies of all lineages *in vitro*.(Dror and Freedman 1999) Marrow cells(Dror and Freedman 2001) as well as *SBDS*-knockdown HeLa cells(Rujkijyanont, Watanabe et al. 2008) are characterized by accelerated apoptosis.(Dror and Freedman 2001) The accelerated apoptosis in marrow cells and *SBDS*-knockdown cells seems to be through the FAS pathway and not through the BAX/BCL-2/BCL-XL pathway.(Dror and Freedman 2001; Rujkijyanont, Watanabe et al. 2008) Depletion of SBDS results in accumulation of FAS at the plasma membrane level and specific overexpression of FAS transcript 1; the main FAS transcript which contains both the transmembrane domain and the death domain.

Chemotaxis

SDS patients have a defect in leukocyte chemotaxis.(Dror, Ginzberg et al. 2001; Stepanovic, Wessels et al. 2004) Consistent with this observation, the SBDS homologue in ameba was found to localize to the pseudopods during chemotaxis.(Wessels, Srikantha et al. 2006) These observations suggest that the SBDS-deficiency in SDS causes the chemotaxis defects in patients.

Mitotic spindle formation

SBDS has been shown to localize to the mitotic spindle, binds microtubles and stabilize them.(Austin, Gupta et al. 2008) Its deficiency results in centrosomal amplification and multipolar spindles.

Bone marrow stromal function

SDS bone marrows are also characterized by a defect in the ability of the stroma to support normal hematopoiesis in cross over experiments of normal CD34+ cells over SDS stroma.(Dror and Freedman 1999)

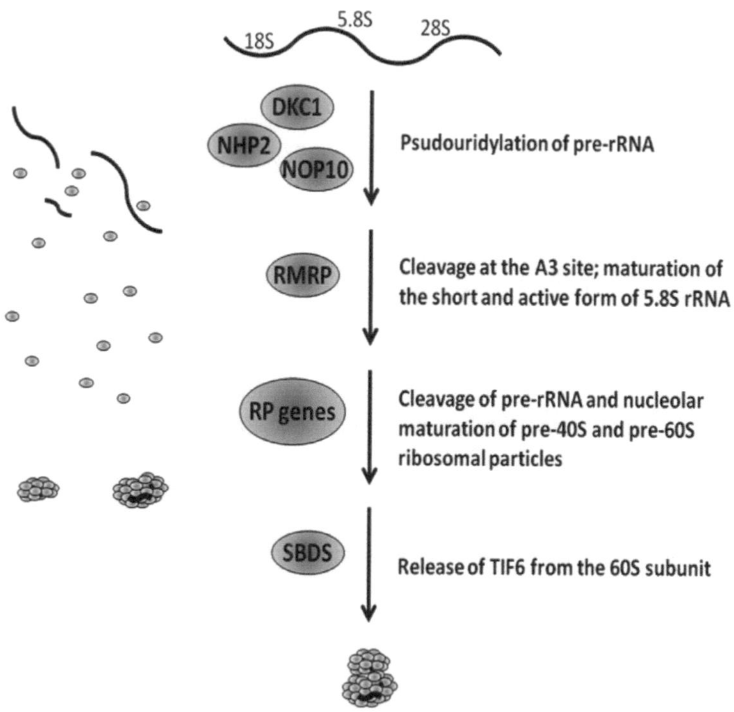

Fig. 3. Ribosome biogenesis and the steps where the inherited bone marrow failure syndrome proteins that are known or hypothesized to function

2.2.3 Genotype phenotype correlation

The study of genotype-phenotype correlation in SDS is difficult since most patients have at least one of the two common mutations. Nevertheless, with regard to the common mutations, patients with severe phenotype including major skeletal abnormalities (Makitie, Ellis et al. 2004) or AML(Majeed, Jadko et al. 2005) have been found to have common mutations.

Based on relatively small numbers is was suggested that SDS patients without mutations in the *SBDS* coding region or flanking intronic regions had more severe hematological disease (lower hemoglobin levels and higher incidence of severe bone marrow failure) but milder pancreatic disease compared to patients with biallelic *SBDS* mutations.(Hashmi, Allen et al. 2010)

2.3 Dyskeratosis Congenita

2.3.1 Clinical features of Dyskeratosis Congenita

Dyskeratosis congenital (DC) is characterized by mucocutaneous abnormalities,(Zinnsser 1906; Cole, Rauschkolb et al. 1920) bone marrow failure,(Dokal 2000) cancer predisposition(Dokal 2000) and extreme telomere shortening.(Vulliamy, Knight et al. 2001) With the recent advances in understanding the molecular basis of the disease, patients with hematological abnormalities without dermatological anomalies have been identified, which changed dramatically the historical definition of the disease.(Vulliamy, Marrone et al. 2002) The original diagnostic triad included oral leukoplakia, nail dystrophy and skin hyperpigmentation. Patients may have many other manifestations including immunodeficiency, dacryostenosis, urethral meatal stenosis, pulmonary fibrosis, hepatic fibrosis and gastrointestingal bleeding due to vascular anomalies. The treatment for the bone marrow failure includes androgens or HSCT. Surgical interventions may be required for some organ malformations or solid cancer.

2.3.2 Dyskeratosis Congenita genes

Multiple genes have been associated with DC.(Heiss, Knight et al. 1998; Vulliamy, Marrone et al. 2001; Vulliamy, Walne et al. 2005; Marrone, Walne et al. 2007; Walne, Vulliamy et al. 2007; Savage, Giri et al. 2008; Vulliamy, Beswick et al. 2008) All are components of the telomerase complex or shelterin (Fig 4). The X-linked recessive disease is a common form of DC. It was originally estimated as more than 50%, but with the identification of more DC genes and more patients with autosomal dominant inheritance, the true incidence seems lower at approximately 30%. The X-linked disease is caused by mutations in *DKC1* on chromosome Xq28.(Heiss, Knight et al. 1998) *DKC1*, encodes for the protein dyskerin. Dyskerin associates with the H/ACA class of RNA. Dyskerin binds to the 3' H/ACA small nucleolar RNA-like domain of the *TERC* component of telomerase. This stimulates telomerase to synthesize telomeric repeats during DNA replication. Dyskerin is also involved in maturation of nascent rRNA. It binds to small nucleolar RNA through their 3' H/ACA domain and catalyzes the isomerization of uridine to pseudouridine through its peudouridine synthase homology domain. This might be the mechanism for impaired translation from internal ribosome entry sites seen in mice and human DC cells.

There are several genes which are mutated in families with autosomal dominant inheritance. *TINF2* is probably the most commonly mutated gene in this group and accounts for approximately 11-25% of the DC families.(Walne, Vulliamy et al. 2008) TINF2 protein is part of the shelterin protein complex, which binds to telomeres and prevent their recognition as DNA breaks by DNA repair proteins. In the complex, TIN2 binds to TRF1, TRF2, POT1, TPP1 and RAP1.

Heterozygous mutations in *TERT* results in autosomal dominant disease. *TERT* encodes for the enzyme component of telomerase. Telomerase is a ribonucleoprotein polymerase that maintains telomere ends by synthesis and addition of the telomere repeat TTAGGG at the 3'-hydroxy DNA terminus using the *TERC* RNA as a template.

Heterozygous mutations in the *TERC* gene are another cause an autosomal dominant form of DC.(Vulliamy, Marrone et al. 2001) *TERC*, encodes for the RNA component of telomerase and has a 3' H/ACA small nucleolar RNA -like domain.

The autosomal recessive forms of DC are caused by biallelic mutations in *NOP10*, *NHP2*, *TERT* or *TCAB1*. In the telomerase complex, the H/ACA domain of nascent human telomerase RNA forms a pre-ribonucleoprotein with NAF1, dyskerin, NOP10, and NHP2. Initially the core trimer dyskerin-NOP10-NHP2 is forms to enable incorporation of NAF1,(Trahan and Dragon 2009; Trahan, Martel et al. 2010) and efficient reverse transcription of telomere repeats. NOP10 and NHP2 also play an essential role in the assembly and activity of the H/ACA class of small nucleolar ribonucleoproteins, which catalyze the isomerization of uridine to pseudouridine in rRNAs.

TCAB1 facilitates trafficking of telomerase to Cajal bodies. Mutations in this gene lead to misdirection of telomerase RNA to nucleoli and prevent elongation of telomeres by telomerase.(Zhong, Savage et al. 2011)

DC cells are characterized by very short telomeres. In several acquired and inherited marrow failure syndromes, telomere length is reduced. However, since the telomerase function is profoundly impaired in DC, the telomeres in this disease are very short (<1% of the median range for normal). Shortening of telomeres results in senescence, apoptosis ("cellular crisis") or chromosome instability. However, some cells may survive the crisis by harboring compensatory genetic mutations which confer proliferative advantage and neoplastic potential.

DC is a chromosome 'instability' disorder of a different type than Fanconi anemia.(Dokal 2000) Clastogenic stress studies of DC cells are normal.(Pai, Yan et al. 1989; Dokal 2000) However, probably due to the short telomeres, in some patients metaphases in peripheral blood cells, marrow cells and fibroblasts in culture showed numerous spontaneous unbalanced chromosome rearrangements such as dicentric, tricentric and translocations. Clonogenic assays of marrow cells showed a marked reduction or absence of CFU-GEMM, BFU-E, CFU-E and CFU-GM progenitors.(Saunders and Freedman 1978; Marsh, Will et al. 1992)

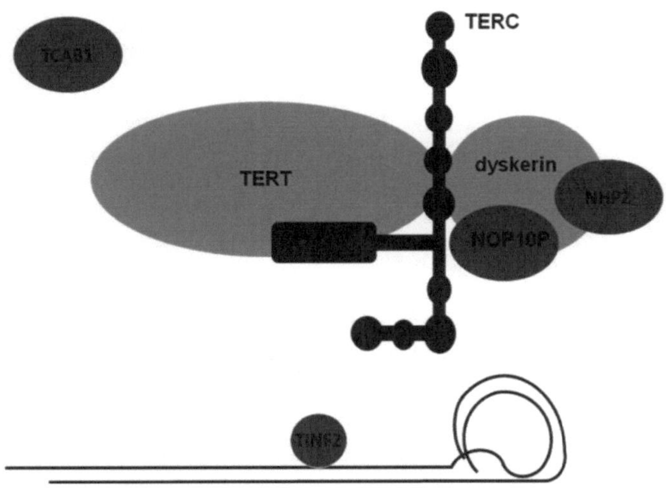

Fig. 4. Telomeres and the dyskeratosis congenita proteins

2.3.3 Genotype phenotype correlation

DC with mutations in the *DKC1, TINF2* can result in a severe form of DC called Hoyeraal Hreidarsson syndrome. It is characterized by hematological and dermatological manifestations of dyskeratosis congenita in addition to cerebellar hypoplasia. Immune deficiency is common when the syndrome is caused by *DKC1* mutations. Revez syndrome is a combination of classical manifestations of DC and exudative retinopathy. It is caused by mutations in *TINF2*. Biallelic mutations in *TERT* are also associated with a severe form of DC. However, heterozygosity for mutations in *TERT* is associated with milder phenotype,(Song, Sullivan et al. 1999) late presentation, severe aplastic anemia without physical malformations, pulmonary fibrosis and hepatic fibrosis. Heterozygosity for mutations in *TERC* is associated milder phenotype, late presentation and severe aplastic anemia without physical malformations. (Song, Sullivan et al. 1999)

2.4 Diamond Blackfan anemia

2.4.1 Clinical features of Diamond Blackfan anemia

Diamond–Blackfan anemia (DBA) is an inherited form of pure red cell aplasia. (Diamond and Blackfan 1938) It is the second most common IBMFSs with incidence of approximately 10 cases/million live births. (Tsangaris, Klaassen et al. (Under Revision)) DBA was first reported in 1936 and later described by Diamond and Blackfan in 1938. It is characterized by varying degrees of red cell aplasia. (Lipton, Atsidaftos et al. 2006; Vlachos, Ball et al. 2008; Lipton and Ellis 2009) Patients may present at birth or become symptomatic after birth with pallor, weakness and cardiac failure. Physical anomalies including short stature, craniofacial dysmorphism, thumb anomalies, among others. (Lipton, Atsidaftos et al. 2006; Vlachos, Ball et al. 2008; Lipton and Ellis 2009) Additionally, patients with DBA carry a high risk of developing malignancies including MDS/AML, osteosarcoma and Hodgkin lymphoma. (Lipton, Atsidaftos et al. 2006; Vlachos, Ball et al. 2008)

Many patients can be diagnosed clinically based on having anemia, low reticulocytes, reduced marrow erythroid progenitors, characteristic physical malformations and high adenosine deaminase levels. (Vlachos, Ball et al. 2008) However, mutations in several genes encoding ribosome proteins have been found mutated in DBA,(Draptchinskaia, Gustavsson et al. 1999; Gazda, Grabowska et al. 2006; Farrar, Nater et al. 2008; Gazda, Sheen et al. 2008; Cmejla, Cmejlova et al. 2009) and can help to establish a diagnosis in many cases when the diagnosis is unclear. (Lipton and Ellis 2009) Standard treatment options include chronic administration of low-dose prednisone (after induction with 2mg/kg/day), chronic red blood cell transfusions and HSCT from a related donor.

2.4.2 Diamond Blackfan anemia genes

About 80% of DBA cases are sporadic.(Halperin and Freedman 1989) The discovery of 11 DBA genes demonstrated heterozygosity for mutations in the respective genes; consistent with autosomal dominant inheritance in all currently known genetic groups. All known DBA proteins are structural components of either the small or large ribosomal subunits.(Doherty, Sheen et al. ; Draptchinskaia, Gustavsson et al. 1999; Farrar, Nater et al. 2008; Gazda, Sheen et al. 2008) The most common mutated DBA gene is *RPS19*. It is mutated in about 25% of the patients.(Gazda, Sheen et al. 2008; Cmejla, Cmejlova et al. 2009) *RPS19* encodes for the ribosomal protein S19, which is associated with the ribosomal subunit 40S.(Da Costa, Tchernia et al. 2003) Deficiency in RPS19 causes defective cleavage of the pre-rRNA at the ITS1 sequence and abnormal maturation of the 40S subunit (Fig 3).(Flygare, Aspesi et al. 2007) Its deficiency leads to apoptosis of erythroid progenitors,(Miyake, Utsugisawa et al. 2008) possible in a p53 dependent manner. (McGowan, Li et al. 2008)

Other ribosomal protein genes that are mutated in DBA are *RPL5* (12-21%),(Doherty, Sheen et al. ; Gazda, Sheen et al. 2008; Cmejla, Cmejlova et al. 2009) *RPL11* (7-9%),(Gazda, Sheen et al. 2008; Cmejla, Cmejlova et al. 2009) *RPS24* (2%),(Gazda, Grabowska et al. 2006; Gazda, Sheen et al. 2008; Cmejla, Cmejlova et al. 2009) *RPL35a*(Farrar, Nater et al. 2008) and other more rarely mutated (Table 1). Despite the identification of multiple genes, only about 50% of the patients with DBA can now be genotyped,(Gazda, Sheen et al. 2008; Cmejla, Cmejlova et al. 2009) and new DBA genes are still to be discovered.

DBA marrows are characterized by complete or nearly complete absence of erythroid precursors in 90% of the patients. The defect in DBA is intrinsic to the hematopoietic stem cells and selectively limits their ability to differentiate into and expand the erythroid compartment. DBA erythroid progenitors demonstrate subnormal colony growth in response to erythropoietin.(Tsai, Arkin et al. 1989) Clonogenic assays of marrow cells or CD34+ cells typically show absent BFU-E and CFU-E progenitors. Some patients show normal or even increased numbers of both progenitors or a block at the BFU-E stage. The colony growth can be improved *in vitro* by the addition of combinations of glucocorticoids and erythropoietin. (Chan, Saunders et al. 1982) DBA CD34+ cells had impaired ability also to undergo granulocytic-monocytic differentiation in addition to their erythroid differentiation defect.(Santucci, Bagnara et al. 1999) These results underscore a stem cell defect in DBA rather than an isolated erythroid defect. This is in keeping with the clinical observation that in addition to anemia patients can have neutropenia and thrombocytopenia.(Schofield and Evans 1991; Giri, Kang et al. 2000) The exact role of the RP genes such as *RPS19* in erythropoiesis is unclear. *RPS19* expression is highest at the earlier stages of erythropoiesis and decreases with differentiation.(Da Costa, Narla et al. 2003) Gene transfer of the wild type *RPS19* into CD34+ cells from DBA patients with *RPS19* mutations improves erythroid colony growth,(Hamaguchi, Ooka et al. 2002) proving the causative role of mutations in the gene in the pathogenesis of DBA. Studies of CD34+ cells from DBA patients and CD34+ cells in which RPS19 expression was reduced by approximately 50% showed that RPS19 promotes cell proliferation as well as differentiation into CFU-E progenitors.(Miyake, Flygare et al. 2005) Intermediate levels of RPS19 to approximately haploinsufficiency levels does not affect myeloid progenitors(Bagnara, Zauli et al. 1991; Olivieri, Grunberger et al. 1991) or megakaryocytic progenitors.(Bagnara, Zauli et al. 1991) It is likely that the genetic defects in the DBA gene/s accelerates apoptosis of erythroid progenitor cells(Perdahl, Naprstek et al. 1994; Flygare, Kiefer et al. 2005)

2.4.3 Genotype phenotype correlation

Patients with mutations in *RPL5* and *RPL11* are more likely to have multiple physical malformations.(Gazda, Sheen et al. 2008; Boria, Garelli et al. 2010) For example, thumb anomalies are seen in 56% and 39% of the patients with *RPL5* and *RPL11* mutations, respectively compared to 7% in patients who have *RPS19* gene mutations. Interestingly, cleft lip and/or palate were reported in 42% of the patients with *RPL5* mutations compared to 6% and 0% among the patients with *RPL11* and *RPS19* gene mutations.

2.5 Kostmann/Severe congenital neutropenia

2.5.1 Clinical features of Kostmann/severe congenital neutropenia

Kostmann neutropenia and severe congenital neutropenia (K/SCN) comprise a heterogeneous group of disorders. Herein, we will refer to K/SCN as disorders that are characterized by severe subtype of inherited neutropenia with typical onset at early childhood, profound neutropenia (absolute neutrophil count < 200/ml), recurrent life-threatening infections and a maturation arrest of myeloid precursors at the promyelocyte-myelocyte stage of differentiation. The mainstay of treatment is life-long daily injection with granulocyte-colony stimulating factor (G-CSF).

2.5.2 Kostmann/Severe congenital neutropenia genes

The original families described by Dr. Kostmann showed an inheritance typical of an autosomal recessive disorder.(Kostmann 1956) However, patients with severe congenital neutropenia with an autosomal dominant inheritance mode usually have exactly the same clinical phenotype.

The most common K/SCN gene is *ELA2*, which is associated with an autosomal dominant K/SCN.(Dale, Person et al. 2000) The prevalence of *ELA2* mutations seems to be higher in North America than in Europe, and was reported in about 40-80% of the K/SCN patients. (Horwitz, Benson et al. 1999; Xia, Bolyard et al. 2009) Although some healthy family members have been reported to have the same *ELA2* Genotype as their affected family members, (Germeshausen, Schulze et al. 2001) and although there is a lack of neutropenia in homozygous and heterozygous knock-out mice,(Belaaouaj, McCarthy et al. 1998) it is now widely accepted that *ELA2* mutations are causative. (Ancliff, Gale et al. 2002; Horwitz, Benson et al. 2003)

ELA2 encodes for neutrophil elastase, a glycoprotein synthesized in the promyelocyte/ myelocyte stages,(Fouret, du Bois et al. 1989) is packed in the azurophilic cytoplasmic granules, and released in response to infection and inflammation.(Cowland and Borregaard 1999) Computerized modeling of neutrophil elastase showed that *ELA2* mutations in K/SCN tend to cluster on the opposite face of the active site of the enzyme in contrast to cyclic neutropenia, where the mutations tend to cluster near the active site. (Dale, Person et al. 2000)

Neutrophil elastase normally localizes diffusely throughout the cytoplasm.(Benson, Li et al. 2003; Massullo, Druhan et al. 2005) The mutations in the protein are predicted to disrupt its AP3 protein recognition sequence, resulting in excessive membrane accumulation of elastase,(Benson, Li et al. 2003; Massullo, Druhan et al. 2005) leading to premature apoptosis of differentiating (myeloblasts and promyelocytes) but not proliferating myeloid progenitor cells.(Aprikyan, Kutyavin et al. 2003; Massullo, Druhan et al. 2005) Also, there is evidence that unfolded protein response occurs in primary granulocytic precursors from K/SCN patients and that expression of mutant neutrophil elastase induces unfolded protein response and apoptosis.(Grenda, Murakami et al. 2007)

HAX1 was reported to be mutated in 40% of patients with K/SCN in a European study,(Klein, Grudzien et al. 2007) but in none of the patients in the American studies, (Xia, Bolyard et al. 2009) and in none of the patients on the Canadian Inherited Marrow Failure Study.(Tsangaris, Klaassen et al. 2011) HAX1 localizes to the mitochondria. It contains two domains reminiscent of a BH1 and BH2 of the BCL-2 family. It promotes normal potential of the inner mitochondrial membrane and protects myeloid cells from apoptosis.

Mutations in the gene encoding the transcriptional repressor *GFI1* were also identified in severe congenital neutropenia.(Person, Li et al. 2003) The mutated protein appears to cause overexpression of *ELA2*, and higher neutrophil elastase levels in all subcellular compartments. *GFI1*-deficient mice also exhibit severe neutropenia. (Karsunky, Zeng et al. 2002)

Activating *WASP* gene mutations are another cause of severe congenital neutropenia. (Devriendt, Kim et al. 2001) The mutant protein is constitutively activated due to disruption of the autoinhibitory domain, leading to increased actin polymerization, disruption of mitosis, genomic instability and apoptosis of neutrophils. (Devriendt, Kim et al. 2001)

Germline G-CSFR mutations are a rare cause of K/SCN. One patient in our registry had digenic germ line mutations in *ELA2* and the extracellular domain of the G-CSFR. Others have also described digenic mutations in patients with K/SCN. (Germeshausen, Zeidler et al. 2010)

Some patients with K/SCN acquire mutations in the intracytoplasmic domain of the G-CSF receptor. The mutations are restricted to the myeloid lineage and a proliferation but not differentiation signal. Alterations are associated with the development of MDS/AML, and are not the cause of the neutropenia. (Dong, Brynes et al. 1995)

Severe other types of inherited neutropenia with more distinct phenotype are discussed in Section 2.7 "Other inherited bone marrow failure syndromes with predominantly neutroepnia"

2.5.3 Genotype phenotype correlation

ELA2 mutations are associated with severe and early onset neutropenia with differentiation arrest at the stage of promyelocyte-meylocyte. Typically the patients do not have physical malformations. The patients have a high risk of MDS/AML, but no known risk of solid tumors.

Patients with mutations in *HAX1* typically have severe and early onset neutropenia with differentiation arrest at the stage of promyelocyte-meylocyte. They also have a high risk of MDS/AML, but no know risk of solid tumors. About 30% of the patients have neurological abnormalities such as seizures, learning disabilities and developmental delay. This is usually due to nonsense mutations that affect both *HAX1* transcripts (e.g. p.Gln155ProfsX14).

Mutations in *WAS* are associated with moderate to severe neutropenia, reduced phagocyte activity; monocytopenia, lymphopenia, reduced NK cells, reduced lymphocyte proliferation and recurrent infections (Usually not as frequent as in the classical K/SCN). MDS/monosomy 7 has also been reported.

GFI mutations are associated with severe to moderate neutropenia, monocytosis, reduced B and T cells with normal lymphocytic function. There is no clear data about the bone marrow findings in this type of neutropenia and the risks of MDS/AML is unknown.

2.6 Congenital amegakaryocytic thrombocytopenia

2.6.1 Clinical feature of congenital amegakaryocytic thrombocytopenia

Congenital amegakaryocytic thrombocytopenia (CAMT) is an IBMFS, which typically presents in infancy with predominantly thrombocytopenia due to reduced or absent marrow megakaryocytes. It commonly progresses to pancytopenia and severe bone marrow failure. In untreated cases, MDS with monosomy 7 and AML can develop at a later stage. (Lau, Ha et al. 1999) Non-hematological manifestations occur in about one fifth of the patients and include cardiac defects, growth abnormalities, psychomotor retardation (King, Germeshausen et al. 2005) and brain structural malformations (Dror, Unpublished Data). The only curative treatment is HSCT and is indicated in patients who persistently manifest severe cytopenia.

2.6.2 Congenital amegakaryocytic thrombocytopenia genes

Biallelic mutations in the *MPL* (thrombopoietic receptor) gene are the cause for the disorder in 94% of the patients with CAMT,[26] particularly,(Ballmaier, Germeshausen et al. 2001) but not exclusively,(King, Germeshausen et al. 2005) (Dror, Unpublished Data) in those without physical anomalies. MPL mutations cause inactivation of the thrombopoietin receptor. The compensatory elevated levels of thrombopoietin(van den Oudenrijn, Bruin et al. 2000; Van Den Oudenrijn, Bruin et al. 2002) do not result in transmitting its signaling.(Muraoka, Ishii et al. 1997; Ballmaier, Germeshausen et al. 2003) Thrombopoietin plays a critical role in the proliferation, survival and differentiation of early and late megakaryocytes. This clearly explains the thrombocytopenia. However, *MPL* is highly expressed in hematopoietic stem cells and promotes their quiescence and survival;(Arai, Yoshihara et al. 2009) thus, insufficiency may account to depletion of hematopoietic stem cells and pancytopenia. The number of CFU-Meg progenitors might be normal initially, but declines as the disease progresses (Freedman and Estrov 1990; Guinan, Lee et al. 1993)

2.6.3 Genotype phenotype correlation

Data about genotype-phenotype correlation is scarce. Nonesense or frameshift mutations that entirely abrogate the thrombopoietin receptor signaling are associated with early development of pancytopenia and more severe bone marrow failure. Missense mutations which only partially reduce receptor signaling are associated with relatively milder initial phenotype and slow progression into pancytopenia.(King, Germeshausen et al. 2005; Ballmaier and Germeshausen 2009) However, the overall outcome might not be different.(Ballmaier and Germeshausen 2009)

2.7 Other inherited bone marrow failure syndromes with predominantly neutropenia

Cyclic neutropenia is an autosomal dominant disorder characterized by a regular, repetitive decrease in peripheral blood neutrophils for 3-4 days every 19-23 days.(Page and Good 1957) Between nadirs the patients have normal or nearly normal neutrophil counts. Patients usually present in infancy or childhood, and have a less severe infectious course compared to Kostmann/severe congenital neutropenia. However, life threatening infections have been reported.(Jonsson and Buchanan 1991; Dale, Bolyard et al. 2002) Daily treatment with G-CSF typically improves symptoms in most patients. Cyclic neutropenia is caused by heterozygous mutations in the *ELA2* gene usually at the active site of neutrophil elastase,(Horowitz, Benson et al. 1999; Ancliff, Gale et al. 2001) without disrupting the enzymatic substrate cleavage by the active site.(Ancliff, Gale et al. 2001) The mutations seem to disturb a predicted transmembrane domain, leading to excessive granular accumulation of elastase and defective membrane localization of the enzyme.(Benson, Li et al. 2003) The myeloid precursors are characterized by cyclic increase in apoptosis.(Aprikyan, Kutyavin et al. 2003) However, the precise molecular mechanism of the cycling hematopoiesis in the disease and why the same mutations in *ELA2* are associated with both cyclic and Kostmann/severe congenital neutropenia phenotype are unknown.

Myelokathexis is a rare autosomal dominant disorder with recurrent bacterial infections caused by reduced number and function of neutrophils.(Zuelzer 1964) Neutropenia is typically moderate to severe. Degenerative changes in the granulocytes are characteristic and include pyknotic nuclear lobes, fine chromatin filaments and hypersegmentation. (Zuelzer 1964) Bone marrow specimens are usually hypercellular with granulocytic hyperplasia. The pathophysiology of myelokathexis has been attributed to a defective release of marrow cells into the peripheral blood.(Zuelzer 1964) Neutrophil precursors are characterized by depressed expression of BCL-X and accelerated apoptosis.(Aprikyan, Liles et al. 2000) G-CSF ameliorate the neutropenia and lead to clinical improvement during episodes of bacterial infection. (Zuelzer 1964; Wetzler, Talpaz et al. 1992) WHIM syndrome

refers to an association of myelokatheksis with other features (warts, hypogammaglobulinemia, infections and myelokalthexis). Most cases studied are caused by mutations in the chemokine receptor gene *CXCR4.* (Hernandez, Gorlin et al. 2003) The mutations result in enhanced chemotactic response of neutrophils in response to the CXCR4 ligand CXCL12 (stroma-derived factor 1) and pathological retention of neutrophils in the bone marrow.(Gulino, Moratto et al. 2004) Patients with wild type *CXCR4* might have other genetic defects that lead to enhanced interaction between CXCR4 and CXCL12 and enhanced chemotactic response, such as reduced inhibition of CXCL12-promoted internalization and desensitization of CXCR4 by GPCR kinase-3 due to decreased transcription of the GPCR kinase-3.(Balabanian, Levoye et al. 2008)
Dursun syndrome is an autosomal recessive disorders with cardiac anomalies (particularly atrial septal defect), urogenital anomalies, vascular anomalies (prominent skin blood vessels), mild immune deficiency and intermittent mild thrombocytopenia.(Dursun, Ozgul et al. 2009) The bone marrow shows either normal maturation or promyelocyte-meylocyte arrest. The risk of MDS/AML is unknown. It is caused by mutation in *G6PC3,* the gene encodes for glucose-6-phosphatase catalytic unit 3.(Banka, Newman et al. ; Boztug, Appaswamy et al. 2009) *G6PC3* is expressed ubiquitously. It is located in the endoplasmic reticulum and hydrolyses glucose-6-phosphate to glucose and phosphate. G6PC3 function loss causes impaired glucose recycling from the endoplasmic reticulum to the cytoplasm in neutrophils.(Jun, Lee et al.) Neutrophil endoplasmic reticulum stress increases susceptibility of neutrophils and myeloid cells to apoptosis,(Boztug, Appaswamy et al. 2009) possibly due to unfolded protein response as evident by enlarged rough endoplasmic reticulum and overexpression of BiP.(Cheung, Kim et al. 2007)
Other disorders with isolated neutrophil production defects such as glycogen storage disease type Ib.(Annabi, Hiraiwa et al. 1998; Calderwood, Kilpatrick et al. 2001)and Barth syndrome (Bione, D'Adamo et al. 1996; Kuijpers, Maianski et al. 2004) are listed in Table 1.

2.8 Selected other inherited bone marrow failure syndromes with predominantly anemia

Congenital dyserythropoietic anemias (CDAs) are inherited disorders with prominent morphological dyserythropoiesis and ineffective erythropoiesis. Three main types of CDA exist: CDA I, II, and III, which differ in marrow morphology, serologic findings and inheritance patterns (Table 1). The anemia in most patients is not severe and does not mandate chronic therapy. In cases with severe anemia splenectomy, a chronic RBC transfusion program, or HSCT should be considered. Due to ineffective erythropoiesis and multiple transfusions, patients can develop iron overload necessitating iron chelation. CDAI is characterized by megaloblastic appearance of erythroid bone marrow precursors with some binucleated cells and internuclear chromatin bridges. The CDA I gene was identified as *CDA1,* which encodes for codanin-1. (Dgany, Avidan et al. 2002) The protein was shown and was entitled to be during cell cycle; it is localized to heterochromatin in interphase cells, overexpressed during the S phase and phosphorylated at mitosis. (Noy-Lotan, Dgany et al. 2009) Another group found that codanin-1 interacts with HP1α. Mutant codanin-1 results in abnormal accumulation of HP1α in the Golgi apparatus. (Renella, Roberts et al.) CDA II is characterized by larger number of binucleated cells and some multinuclear cells. Abnormally high protein, lipid dysglycosylation and endoplasmic reticulum double-membrane remnants are seen in erythroid cells. The gene for CDAII was identified as

SEC23B. The *SEC23B* protein is an essential component of protein complex II-coated vesicles that transport secretory proteins from the endoplasmic reticulum to the Golgi apparatus. Knockdown of *SEC23B* in zebrafish leads to aberrant erythrocyte development. The gene for CDA III has not been identified.

Inherited sideroblastic anemias are disorders of mitochondrial iron utilization. Iron accumulation occurs in the mitochondria of red blood cell precursors. Perl's Prussian-blue shows iron accumulation in a circular or ringed pattern around the nucleus in greater than 10% of the erythroblasts. Treatment depends on the specific syndrome. Patients with X-linked sideroblastic anemia respond to pyridoxine. Patients with thiamine responsive megaloblastic anemia respond to thiamine. In the other types of inherited sideroblastic anemia RBC transfusions are the mainstay of treatment. HSCT is curative.(Urban, Binder et al. 1992) The genes mutated in sideroblastic anemias are involved in heme biosynthesis, iron-sulfur cluster biogenesis, iron-sulfur cluster transport or mitochondrial metabolism (Table 1).

2.9 Selected other inherited bone marrow failure syndromes with predominantly thrombocytopenia

The syndrome of thrombocytopenia with absent radii (TAR) was first described in 1929,(Greenwald and Sherman 1929) and subsequently defined in 1969,(Hall, Levin et al. 1969) The two features, which are currently essential for the definition of the syndrome are hypomegakaryocytic thrombocytopenia and bilateral radial aplasia. The definition of the syndrome may change once the genetic basis is deciphered, and its inheritance mode may be clarified. Typically, parents of TAR syndrome patients are phenotypically normal, and females with TAR syndrome can conceive and give birth to hematologically and phenotypically normal offspring. Klopocki and colleagues reported deletion on chromosome 1q21.1 in TAR syndrome patients;(Klopocki, Schulze et al. 2007) however, the etiological significance of this finding is still unclear. Another group found that bone marrow adherent stromal cells from patients with TAR syndrome do not express CD105 antigen, a protein component of the transforming growth factor-β1 and β3 receptor complex which is normally expressed in mesenchymal cells.(Bonsi, Marchionni et al. 2009) They hypothesized that the clinical phenotype of TAR could derive from damage to a common osteo/chondrogenic and hematopoietic progenitors.

MYH9-assocaited familial macrothrombocytopenia comprises an array of several syndromes; Alport, Fetchner, Ebstein, Sabastian and May-Hegglin, which have traditionally been classified according to their non-hematologtical manifestations.(Drachman 2004; Geddis and Kaushansky 2004). MYH9 encodes for nonmuscle myosin-heavy chain IIA, cytoskeletal contractile protein.(Seri, Pecci et al. 2003) The common features include autosomal dominant inheritance, large platelets, mild to moderated thrombocytopenia, normal numbers of megakaryocytes in the bone marrow and variable platelet aggregation and secretion defects which may rarely cause bleeding, requiring platelet transfusions.(Peterson, Rao et al. 1985) Progression into aplastic anemia or leukemia has not been reported thus far. Myosin-heavy chain IIA normally exists as a large hexamer, comprised of two heavy chains and 4 myosin light chains. The N-terminal head interacts with actin. An intermediate neck domain binds myosin light chains. Phosphorylation of myosin light chains result in activation of myosin and interaction with actin filaments. The C-terminal tail domain is important for filament assembly and cargo binding. Mutations in the head region directly affect important functions of the motor protein and have a critical effect on function. Mutated myosin-heavy chain IIA light chains forms aggregates in neutrophils, which bind other proteins including normal myosin-heavy chain IIA from the normal allele.

Familial non-syndromic thrombocytopenia is characterized by an autosomal dominant inheritance, mild to moderate thrombocytopenia, normal platelet size and morphology and mild bleeding tendency. There is no known increased risk of progression to leukemia. Bone marrow specimens are of normal cellularity with normal to mildly reduced numbers of megakaryocytes, which can be small and have hypolobulated nuclei. Clonogenic assays show increased megakaryocytic colony growth.(Drachman, Jarvik et al. 2000) Three genes have been reported as mutated in this disease (Table 1). The most common one is *MASTL*, which encodes for a putative kinase.(Gandhi, Cummings et al. 2003) *MASTL* expression is restricted to hematopoietic and cancer cell lines and localizes to the nucleus in overexpression studies.(Johnson, Gandhi et al. 2009) A transient knockdown of *MASTL* in zebrafish reduced platelet counts.

Radioulnar synostosis with bone marrow failure is an autosomal dominant disorder with proximal radio-ulnar synostosis, clinodactyly, syndactyly, congenital hip dysplasia and sensorineural deafness.(Thompson, Woodruff et al. 2001) The thrombocytopenia can be severe and require platelet transfusions. The bone marrow shows absence of megakaryocytes. Progression into pancytopenia is common. If the thrombocytopenia is severe or progresses to aplastic anemia, allogeneic HSCT can be curative.(Thompson, Woodruff et al. 2001),(Castillo-Caro, Dhanraj et al.) Most patients are heterozygous for mutations in the *HOXA11* gene, which lead to truncation of the protein.(Thompson and Nguyen 2000) Some patients with classical presentation are negative for *HOXA11*.(Castillo-Caro, Dhanraj et al.)

Familial platelet disorder with predisposition to AML is an autosomal dominant disease and a striking predisposition for hematological malignancy.(Michaud, Wu et al. 2002) The thrombocytopenia is mild to moderate, and platelets have normal size and morphology. Treatment of the thrombocytopenia is usually not required, but periodic screening for pancytopenia and MDS/AML is advisable. HSCT is potentially curative in the leukemic phase. The disorder is caused by mutations in the *RUNX1* gene.(Song, Sullivan et al. 1999) The thrombocytopenia may result from reduced *MPL* expression possibly by decreased binding of RUNX1 to the *MPL* promotor.(Heller, Glembotsky et al. 2005) RUNX1 acts as a tumor suppressor and promotes differentiation.

Familial thrombocytopenia with dyserythropoiesis is an X-linked disease with mild to severe bleeding tendency and mild to moderate dyserythropoiesis.(Nichols, Crispino et al. 2000; Mehaffey, Newton et al. 2001) Platelets are hypogranular and of normal-to large size. Platelet counts are moderately to severely affected ($10\text{-}40 \times 10^9/L$), have variably low expression of glycoprotein Ib, and their aggregation in response to ristocitin is reduced.(Freson, Devriendt et al. 2001) The anemia is variable in severity. Bone marrow biopsy specimens are hypercellular with dysplastic megakaryocytes having peripheral location of the nucleus and lack of nuclear segmentation or fragmentation. Dysplastic erythroid precursors with mild megaloblastic changes and delayed nuclear maturation are also seen.(Mehaffey, Newton et al. 2001) There are no reports of progression to severe aplastic anemia, MDS or AML. The treatment consists of platelet transfusion in case of bleeding, trauma or preparation for surgery. Severe cases can be cured by allogeneic related or unrelated HSCT.(Nichols, Crispino et al. 2000) The disorder is caused by missense mutations in the GATA1 protein domain between 205-218 amino acids,(Nichols, Crispino et al. 2000) a transcription factor important for both magakaryopoiesis and erythropoiesis. Other IBMFSs with predominantly thrombocytopenia are listed in Table 1.

3. Conclusion

Multiple genes which function in many different pathways are associated with IBMFSs. However, about 45% of the patients do not have mutations in known genes; thus it is likely that many more genes remained to be identified. Despite accumulation of substantial knowledge about the functions of the IBMFS proteins, the mechanism of bone marrow failure in most of the conditions is still unknown.

4. Acknowledgment

The author thanks Dr. Mary Shago, the Hospital for Sick Children, Toronto, for kindly providing Figure. Elena Tsangaris and Santhosh Dhanraj for preparation of data and to Philippa McCaffrey for assistance in preparing the chapter.

5. References

Aggett, P. J., N. P. Cavanagh, et al. (1980). Shwachman's syndrome. A review of 21 cases. *Archives of Disease in Childhood* 55(5): 331-347.

Allikmets, R., W. H. Raskind, et al. (1999). Mutation of a putative mitochondrial iron transporter gene (ABC7) in X-linked sideroblastic anemia and ataxia (XLSA/A). *Hum Mol Genet* 8(5): 743-749.

Alter, B. P. (2003). Inherited bone marrow failure syndromes. Hematology of Infancy and Childhood. D. G. Nathan, Orkin S.H., Ginsberg, D., Look, A.T. Philadelphia, W.B. Saunders: 280-365.

Alter, B. P. (2007). Diagnosis, genetics, and management of inherited bone marrow failure syndromes. *Hematology Am Soc Hematol Educ Program 2007: 29-39.*

*Ancliff, P., R. Gale, et al. (2002). Paternal mosaicism proves t*he pathogenic nature of mutations in neutrophil elastase in severe congenital neutropenia. *Blood* 100(2): 707-709.

Ancliff, P. J., R. E. Gale, et al. (2001). Mutations in the ELA2 gene encoding neutrophil elastase are present in most patients with sporadic severe congenital neutropenia but only in some patients with the familial form of the disease. *Blood* 98(9): 2645-2650.

Annabi, B., H. Hiraiwa, et al. (1998). The gene for glycogen-storage disease type 1b maps to chromosome 11q23. *Am J Hum Genet* 62: 400-405.

Antonio Casado, J., E. Callen, et al. (2007). A comprehensive strategy for the subtyping of patients with Fanconi anaemia: conclusions from the Spanish Fanconi Anemia Research Network. *J Med Genet* 44(4): 241-249.

Aprikyan, A. A., T. Kutyavin, et al. (2003). Cellular and molecular abnormalities in severe congenital neutropenia predisposing to leukemia. *Exp Hematol* 31(5): 372-381.

Aprikyan, A. A., W. C. Liles, et al. (2000). Myelokathexis, a congenital disorder of severe neutropenia characterized by accelerated apoptosis and defective expression of bcl-x in neutrophil precursors. *Blood* 95(1): 320-327.

Arai, F., H. Yoshihara, et al. (2009). Niche regulation of hematopoietic stem cells in the endosteum. *Ann N Y Acad Sci* 1176: 36-46.

Arnaud, L., C. Saison, et al. A dominant mutation in the gene encoding the erythroid transcription factor KLF1 causes a congenital dyserythropoietic anemia. *Am J Hum Genet* 87(5): 721-727.

Aubert, G. and P. M. Lansdorp (2008). Telomeres and aging. *Physiol Rev* 88(2): 557-579.

Auerbach, A. D., A. Rogatko, et al. (1989). International Fanconi Anemia Registry: relation of clinical symptoms to diepoxybutane sensitivity. *Blood* 73(2): 391-396.

Austin, K. M., M. L. Gupta, et al. (2008). Mitotic spindle destabilization and genomic instability in Shwachman-Diamond syndrome. *J Clin Invest* 118(4): 1511-1518.

Austin, K. M., R. J. Leary, et al. (2005). The Shwachman-Diamond SBDS protein localizes to the nucleolus. *Blood* 106(4): 1253-1258.

Bagnara, G. P., G. Zauli, et al. (1991). In vitro growth and regulation of bone marrow enriched CD34+ hematopoietic progenitors in Diamond-Blackfan anemia. *Blood* 78(9): 2203-2210.

Balabanian, K., A. Levoye, et al. (2008). Leukocyte analysis from WHIM syndrome patients reveals a pivotal role for GRK3 in CXCR4 signaling. *J Clin Invest* 118(3): 1074-1084.

Ballmaier, M. and M. Germeshausen (2009). Advances in the understanding of congenital amegakaryocytic thrombocytopenia. *Br J Haematol* 146(1): 3-16.

Ballmaier, M., M. Germeshausen, et al. (2003). Thrombopoietin is essential for the maintenance of normal hematopoiesis in humans: development of aplastic anemia in patients with congenital amegakaryocytic thrombocytopenia. *Ann N Y Acad Sci* 996: 17-25.

Ballmaier, M., M. Germeshausen, et al. (2001). c-mpl mutations are the cause of congenital amegakaryocytic thrombocytopenia. *Blood* 97(1): 139-146.

Balmain, A., J. Gray, et al. (2003). The genetics and genomics of cancer. *Nat Genet* 33 Suppl: 238-244.

Banka, S., W. G. Newman, et al. Mutations in the G6PC3 gene cause Dursun syndrome. Am *J Med Genet A* 152A(10): 2609-2611.

Barrios, N., D. Kirkpatrick, et al. (1991). Bone marrow transplant in Shwachman Diamond syndrome. *Br J Haematol* 79(2): 337-338.

Baumann, C., R. Korner, et al. (2007). PICH, a centromere-associated SNF2 family ATPase, is regulated by Plk1 and required for the spindle checkpoint. *Cell* 128(1): 101-114.

Belaaouaj, A., R. McCarthy, et al. (1998). Mice lacking neutrophil elastase reveal impaired host defense against gram negative bacterial sepsis. *Nat Med* 4(5): 615-618.

Benson, K. F., F. Q. Li, et al. (2003). Mutations associated with neutropenia in dogs and humans disrupt intracellular transport of neutrophil elastase. *Nat Genet* 35(1): 90-96.

Bianchi, P., E. Fermo, et al. (2009). Congenital dyserythropoietic anemia type II (CDAII) is caused by mutations in the SEC23B gene. *Hum Mutat* 30(9): 1292-1298.

Bijangi-Vishehsaraei, K., M. R. Saadatzadeh, et al. (2005). Enhanced TNF-alpha-induced apoptosis in Fanconi anemia type C-deficient cells is dependent on apoptosis signal-regulating kinase 1. *Blood* 106(13): 4124-4130.

Bione, S., P. D'Adamo, et al. (1996). A novel x-linked gene, G4.5 is responsible for Barth syndrome. *Nat Genet* 12(4): 385-389.

Birney, E., S. Kumar, et al. (1993). Analysis of the RNA-recognition motif and RS and RGG domains: conservation in metazoan pre-mRNA splicing factors. *Nucleic Acids Res* 21(25): 5803-5816.

Bonsi, L., C. Marchionni, et al. (2009). Thrombocytopenia with absent radii (TAR) syndrome: from hemopoietic progenitor to mesenchymal stromal cell disease? *Exp Hematol* 37(1): 1-7.

Boocock, G. R., J. A. Morrison, et al. (2003). Mutations in SBDS are associated with Shwachman-Diamond syndrome. *Nature Genetics* 33(1): 97-101.

Boria, I., E. Garelli, et al. (2010). The ribosomal basis of Diamond-Blackfan Anemia: mutation and database update. *Hum Mutat* 31(12): 1269-1279.

Boztug, K., G. Appaswamy, et al. (2009). A syndrome with congenital neutropenia and mutations in G6PC3. *N Engl J Med* 360(1): 32-43.

Byrd, R. S., T. Zwerdling, et al. Monosomy 21q22.11-q22.13 presenting as a Fanconi anemia phenotype. *Am J Med Genet A* 155A(1): 120-125.

Calderwood, S., L. Kilpatrick, et al. (2001). Recombinant human granulocyte colony-stimulating factor therapy for patients with neutropenia and/or neutrophil dysfunction secondary to glycogen storage disease type 1b. *Blood* 97(2): 376-382.

Castella, M., R. Pujol, et al. (2011). Chromosome fragility in patients with Fanconi anaemia: diagnostic implications and clinical impact. *J Med Genet.*

Castillo-Caro, P., S. Dhanraj, et al. Proximal radio-ulnar synostosis with bone marrow failure syndrome in an infant without a HOXA11 mutation. *J Pediatr Hematol Oncol* 32(6): 479-485.

Chan, H. S., E. F. Saunders, et al. (1982). Diamond-Blackfan syndrome. I. Erythropoiesis in prednisone responsive and resistant disease. *Pediatr Res* 16(6): 474-476.

Chan, K. L., P. S. North, et al. (2007). BLM is required for faithful chromosome segregation and its localization defines a class of ultrafine anaphase bridges. *Embo J* 26(14): 3397-3409.

Chan, K. L., T. Palmai-Pallag, et al. (2009). Replication stress induces sister-chromatid bridging at fragile site loci in mitosis. *Nat Cell Biol* 11(6): 753-760.

Cheung, Y. Y., S. Y. Kim, et al. (2007). Impaired neutrophil activity and increased susceptibility to bacterial infection in mice lacking glucose-6-phosphatase-beta. *J Clin Invest* 117(3): 784-793.

Choesmel, V., D. Bacqueville, et al. (2007). Impaired ribosome biogenesis in Diamond-Blackfan anemia. *Blood* 109(3): 1275-1283.

Cmejla, R., J. Cmejlova, et al. (2009). Identification of mutations in the ribosomal protein L5 (RPL5) and ribosomal protein L11 (RPL11) genes in Czech patients with Diamond-Blackfan anemia. *Hum Mutat* 30(3): 321-327.

Cohn, M. A. and A. D. D'Andrea (2008). Chromatin recruitment of DNA repair proteins: lessons from the fanconi anemia and double-strand break repair pathways. *Mol Cell* 32(3): 306-312.

Cole, H., J. Rauschkolb, et al. (1920). Dyskeratosis congenita with pigmentation, dystrophia unguis and leukokeratosis oris. *Arch Dermatol Syphiligraph* 21: 71-95.

Cotter, P. D., M. Baumann, et al. (1992). Enzymatic defect in X-linked sideroblastic anemia: molecular evidence for erythroid delta-aminolevulinate synthase deficiency. *Proc Natl Acad Sci U S A* 89(9): 4028-4032.

Cowland, J. and N. Borregaard (1999). The individual regulation of granule protein mRNA levels during neutrophil maturation explains the heterogeneity of neutrophil granules. *J Leukoc Biol* 66(6): 989-995.

Cumming, R. C., J. Lightfoot, et al. (2001). Fanconi anemia group C protein prevents apoptosis in hematopoietic cells through redox regulation of GSTP1. *Nat Med* 7(7): 814-820.

Da Costa, L., G. Narla, et al. (2003). Ribosomal protein S19 expression during erythroid differentiation. *Blood* 101(1): 318-324.

Da Costa, L., G. Tchernia, et al. (2003). Nucleolar localization of RPS19 protein in normal cells and mislocalization due t mutations in the nucleolar localization signals in 2 Diamond-Blackfan anemia patients: potential insights into pathophysiology. *Blood* 101(12): 5039-5045.

Dale, D. C., A. A. Bolyard, et al. (2002). Cyclic neutropenia. *Seminars in Hematology* 39(2): 89-94.

Dale, D. C., R. E. Person, et al. (2000). Mutations in the gene encoding neutrophil elastase in congenital and cyclic neutropenia.[see comment]. Blood 96(7): 2317-2322.

de Oliveira, J. F., M. L. Sforca, et al. Structure, Dynamics, and RNA Interaction Analysis of the Human SBDS Protein. *J Mol Biol.*

de Winter, J. P. and H. Joenje (2008). The genetic and molecular basis of Fanconi anemia. *Mutat Res.*

de Winter, J. P., F. Leveille, et al. (2000). Isolation of a cDNA representing the Fanconi anemia complementation group E gene. *Am J Hum Genet* 67(5): 1306-1308.

de Winter, J. P., M. A. Rooimans, et al. (2000). The Fanconi anaemia gene FANCF encodes a novel protein with homology to ROM. *Nat Genet* 24(1): 15-16.

de Winter, J. P., Q. Waisfisz, et al. (1998). The Fanconi anaemia group G gene FANCG is identical with XRCC9. *Nat Genet* 20(3): 281-283.

Devriendt, K., A. S. Kim, et al. (2001). Constitutively activating mutation in WASP causes X-linked severe congenital neutropenia. *Nature Genetics* 27(3): 313-317.

Dgany, O., N. Avidan, et al. (2002). Congenital dyserythropoietic anemia type I is caused by mutations in codanin-1. *Am J Hum Genet* 71(6): 1467-1474.

Diamond, L. and K. Blackfan (1938). Hypoplastic anemia. *Am J Dis Child* 56(464-467).

Doherty, L., M. R. Sheen, et al. Ribosomal protein genes RPS10 and RPS26 are commonly mutated in Diamond-Blackfan anemia. *Am J Hum Genet* 86(2): 222-228.

Doherty, L., M. R. Sheen, et al. (2010). Ribosomal protein genes RPS10 and RPS26 are commonly mutated in Diamond-Blackfan anemia. *Am J Hum Genet* 86(2): 222-228.

Dokal, I. (2000). Dyskeratosis congenita in all its forms. *Br J Haematol* 110(4): 768-779.

Dokal, I. and T. Vulliamy (2008). Inherited aplastic anaemias/bone marrow failure syndromes. *Blood Rev* 22(3): 141-153.

Donadieu, J., T. Leblanc, et al. (2005). Analysis of risk factors for myelodysplasias, leukemias and death from infection among patients with congenital neutropenia. Experience of the French Severe Chronic Neutropenia Study Group. *Haematologica* 90(1): 45-53.

Donadieu, J., G. Michel, et al. (2005). Hematopoietic stem cell transplantation for Shwachman-Diamond syndrome: experience of the French neutropenia registry. *Bone Marrow Transplant* 36(9): 787-792.

Dong, F., R. K. Brynes, et al. (1995). Mutations in the gene for the granulocyte colony-stimulating-factor receptor in patients with acute myeloid leukemia preceded by severe congenital neutropenia. *N Engl J Med* 333(8): 487-493.

Drachman, J. G. (2004). Inherited thrombocytopenia: when a low platelet count does not mean ITP. *Blood* 103(2): 390-398.

Drachman, J. G., G. P. Jarvik, et al. (2000). Autosomal dominant thrombocytopenia: incomplete megakaryocyte differentiation and linkage to human chromosome 10. *Blood* 96(1): 118-125.

Draptchinskaia, N., P. Gustavsson, et al. (1999). The gene encoding ribosomal protein S19 is mutated in Diamond-Blackfan anaemia. *Nat Genet* 21(2): 169-175.

Dror, Y. (2006). Inherited Bone Marrow Failure Syndromes. Oxford, Blackwell Publishing.

Dror, Y. and M. H. Freedman (1999). Shwachman-Diamond syndrome: An inherited preleukemic bone marrow failure disorder with aberrant hematopoietic progenitors and faulty marrow microenvironment. *Blood* 94(9): 3048-3054.

Dror, Y. and M. H. Freedman (2001). Shwachman-Diamond syndrome marrow cells show abnormally increased apoptosis mediated through the Fas pathway. *Blood* 97(10): 3011-3016.

Dror, Y., H. Ginzberg, et al. (2001). Immune function in patients with Shwachman-Diamond syndrome. *British Journal of Haematology* 114(3): 712-717.

Duckworth-Rysiecki, G., K. Cornish, et al. (1985). Identification of two complementation groups in Fanconi anemia. *Somat Cell Mol Genet* 11(1): 35-41.

Dufour, C., A. Corcione, et al. (2003). TNF-alpha and IFN-gamma are overexpressed in the bone marrow of Fanconi anemia patients and TNF-alpha suppresses erythropoiesis in vitro. *Blood* 102(6): 2053-2059.

Dursun, A., R. K. Ozgul, et al. (2009). Familial pulmonary arterial hypertension, leucopenia, and atrial septal defect: a probable new familial syndrome with multisystem involvement. *Clin Dysmorphol* 18(1): 19-23.

Faivre, L., P. Guardiola, et al. (2000). Association of complementation group and mutation type with clinical outcome in fanconi anemia. European Fanconi Anemia Research Group. *Blood* 96(13): 4064-4070.

Fanconi, G. (1927). Familiäre infantile perniziosaartige Anämie (perniziöses Blutbild and Konstitution). *Jahrbuch Kinder* 117(257): 258.

Farrar, J. E., M. Nater, et al. (2008). Abnormalities of the large ribosomal subunit protein, Rpl35a, in Diamond-Blackfan anemia. *Blood* 112(5): 1582-1592.

Fekairi, S., S. Scaglione, et al. (2009). Human SLX4 is a Holliday junction resolvase subunit that binds multiple DNA repair/recombination endonucleases. *Cell* 138(1): 78-89.

Fleming, J. C., E. Tartaglini, et al. (1999). The gene mutated in thiamine-responsive anaemia with diabetes and deafness (TRMA) encodes a functional thiamine transporter. *Nat Genet* 22(3): 305-308.

Flygare, J., A. Aspesi, et al. (2007). Human RPS19, the gene mutated in Diamond-Blackfan anemia, encodes a ribosomal protein required for the maturation of 40S ribosomal subunits. *Blood* 109(3): 980-986.

Flygare, J., T. Kiefer, et al. (2005). Deficiency of ribosomal protein S19 in CD34+ cells generated by siRNA blocks erythroid development and mimics defects seen in Diamond-Blackfan anemia. *Blood* 105(12): 4627-4634.

Fouret, P., R. M. du Bois, et al. (1989). Expression of the neutrophil elastase gene during human bone marrow cell differentiation. *J Exp Med* 169(3): 833-845.

Freedman, M. H. and Z. Estrov (1990). Congenital amegakaryocytic thrombocytopenia: an intrinsic hematopoietic stem cell defect. *Am J Pediatr Hematol Oncol* 12(2): 225-230.

Freson, K., K. Devriendt, et al. (2001). Platelet characteristics in patients with X-linked macrothrombocytopenia because of a novel GATA1 mutation. *Blood* 98(1): 85-92.

Friedenson, B. (2007). The BRCA1/2 pathway prevents hematologic cancers in addition to breast and ovarian cancers. *BMC Cancer* 7: 152.

Futaki, M., T. Yamashita, et al. (2000). The IVS4 + 4 A to T mutation of the fanconi anemia gene FANCC is not associated with a severe phenotype in Japanese patients. *Blood* 95(4): 1493-1498.

Ganapathi, K. A., K. M. Austin, et al. (2007). The human Shwachman-Diamond syndrome protein, SBDS, associates with ribosomal RNA. *Blood* 110(5): 1458-1465.

Gandhi, M. J., C. L. Cummings, et al. (2003). FLJ14813 missense mutation: a candidate for autosomal dominant thrombocytopenia on human chromosome 10. *Hum Hered* 55(1): 66-70.

Garcia-Higuera, I., T. Taniguchi, et al. (2001). Interaction of the Fanconi anemia proteins and BRCA1 in a common pathway. *Mol Cell* 7(2): 249-262.

Gari, K., C. Decaillet, et al. (2008). Remodeling of DNA replication structures by the branch point translocase FANCM. *Proc Natl Acad Sci U S A* 105(42): 16107-16112.

Gazda, H. T., A. Grabowska, et al. (2006). Ribosomal protein S24 gene is mutated in Diamond-Blackfan anemia. *Am J Hum Genet* 79(6): 1110-1118.

Gazda, H. T., M. R. Sheen, et al. (2008). Ribosomal protein L5 and L11 mutations are associated with cleft palate and abnormal thumbs in Diamond-Blackfan anemia patients. *Am J Hum Genet* 83(6): 769-780.

Geddis, A. E. and K. Kaushansky (2004). Inherited thrombocytopenias: toward a molecular understanding of disorders of platelet production. *Curr Opin Pediatr* 16(1): 15-22.

Germeshausen, M., H. Schulze, et al. (2001). Mutations in the gene encoding neutrophil elastase (ELA2) are not sufficient to cause the phenotype of congenital neutropenia. *Br J Haematol* 115(1): 222-224.

Germeshausen, M., C. Zeidler, et al. (2010). Digenic mutations in severe congenital neutropenia. *Haematologica* 95(7): 1207-1210.

Gillio, A. P., P. C. Verlander, et al. (1997). Phenotypic consequences of mutations in the Fanconi anemia FAC gene: an International Fanconi Anemia Registry study. *Blood* 90(1): 105-110.

Giri, N., E. Kang, et al. (2000). Clinical and laboratory evidence for a trilineage haematopoietic defect in patients with refractory Diamond-Blackfan anaemia. *Br J Haematol* 108(1): 167-175.

Godthelp, B. C., F. Artwert, et al. (2002). Impaired DNA damage-induced nuclear Rad51 foci formation uniquely characterizes Fanconi anemia group D1. *Oncogene* 21(32): 5002-5005.

Greenwald, H. and I. Sherman (1929). Congenital essential thrombocytopenia. *Am J Dis Child* 38: 1245-1251.

Grenda, D. S., M. Murakami, et al. (2007). Mutations of the ELA2 gene found in patients with severe congenital neutropenia induce the unfolded protein response and cellular apoptosis. *Blood* 110(13): 4179-4187.

Guernsey, D. L., H. Jiang, et al. (2009). Mutations in mitochondrial carrier family gene SLC25A38 cause nonsyndromic autosomal recessive congenital sideroblastic anemia. *Nat Genet* 41(6): 651-653.

Guinan, E. C., Y. S. Lee, et al. (1993). Effects of interleukin-3 and granulocyte-macrophage colony-stimulating factor on thrombopoiesis in congenital amegakaryocytic thrombocytopenia. *Blood* 81(7): 1691-1698.

Gulino, A. V., D. Moratto, et al. (2004). Altered leukocyte response to CXCL12 in patients with warts hypogammaglobulinemia, infections, myelokathexis (WHIM) syndrome. *Blood* 104(2): 444-452.

Hall, J. G., J. Levin, et al. (1969). Thrombocytopenia with absent radius (TAR). *Medicine* (Baltimore) 48(6): 411-439.

Halperin, D. S. and M. H. Freedman (1989). Diamond-blackfan anemia: etiology, pathophysiology, and treatment. *Am J Pediatr Hematol Oncol* 11(4): 380-394.

Hamaguchi, I., A. Ooka, et al. (2002). Gene transfer improves erythroid development in ribosomal protein S19-deficient Diamond-Blackfan anemia. *Blood* 100(8): 2724-2731.

Hashmi, S., C. Allen, et al. (2010). Comparative analysis of Shwachman-Diamond syndrome to other inherited bone marrow failure syndromes and genotype-phenotype correlation. *Clinical Genetics.*

Heiss, N. S., S. W. Knight, et al. (1998). X-linked dyskeratosis congenita is caused by mutations in a highly conserved gene with putative nucleolar functions. *Nat Genet* 19(1): 32-38.

Heller, P. G., A. C. Glembotsky, et al. (2005). Low Mpl receptor expression in a pedigree with familial platelet disorder with predisposition to acute myelogenous leukemia and a novel AML1 mutation. *Blood* 105(12): 4664-4670.

Hernandez, P. A., R. J. Gorlin, et al. (2003). Mutations in the chemokine receptor gene CXCR4 are associated with WHIM syndrome, a combined immunodeficiency disease. *Nat Genet* 34(1): 70-74.

Horowitz, M., K. F. Benson, et al. (1999). Mutations in ELA2, encoding neutrophil elastase, define a 21-day biological clock in cyclic haematopoiesis. *Nat Genet* 23(4): 433-436.

Horwitz, M., K. Benson, et al. (2003). Role of neutrophil elastase in bone marrow failure syndromes: molecular genetic revival of the chalone hypothesis. *Curr Opin Hematol* 10(1): 49-54.

Horwitz, M., K. F. Benson, et al. (1999). Mutations in ELA2, encoding neutrophil elastase, define a 21-day biological clock in cyclic haematopoiesis. *Nat Genet* 23(4): 433-436.

Howlett, N. G., T. Taniguchi, et al. (2002). Biallelic inactivation of BRCA2 in Fanconi anemia. *Science* 297(5581): 606-609.

Huang, K. (2010). The FANCM/FAAP24 complex is required for the DNA interstrand crosslink-induced checkpoint response. *Mol Cell* 39(2): 259-268.

Hudson, E. and T. Aldor (1970). Pancreatic insufficiency and neutropenia with associated immunoglobulin deficit. *Arch Intern Med* 125(2): 314-316.

Ihara, K., E. Ishii, et al. (1999). Identification of mutations in the c-mpl gene in congenital amegakaryocytic thrombocytopenia. *Proc Natl Acad Sci U S A* 96(6): 3132-3136.

Ishiai, M., H. Katao, et al. (2008). FANCI phosphorylation functions as a molecular switch to turn on the Fanconi anemia pathway. *Mol Biol* 15(11): 1138-1146.

Johnson, H. J., M. J. Gandhi, et al. (2009). In vivo inactivation of MASTL kinase results in thrombocytopenia. *Exp Hematol* 37(8): 901-908.

Jonsson, O. G. and G. R. Buchanan (1991). Chronic neutropenia during childhood. A 13-year experience in a single institution. *Am J Dis Child* 145(2): 232-235.

Jun, H. S., Y. M. Lee, et al. Lack of glucose recycling between endoplasmic reticulum and cytoplasm underlies cellular dysfunction in glucose-6-phosphatase-beta-deficient neutrophils in a congenital neutropenia syndrome. *Blood* 116(15): 2783-2792.

Karsunky, H., H. Zeng, et al. (2002). Inflammatory reactions and severe neutropenia in mice lacking the transcriptional repressor Gfi1. *Nat Genet* 30(3): 295-300.

King, S., M. Germeshausen, et al. (2005). Congenital amegakaryocytic thrombocytopenia: a retrospective clinical analysis of 20 patients. *Br J Haematol* 131(5): 636-644.

Klein, C., M. Grudzien, et al. (2007). HAX1 deficiency causes autosomal recessive severe congenital neutropenia (Kostmann disease). *Nat Genet* 39(1): 86-92.

Klopocki, E., H. Schulze, et al. (2007). Complex inheritance pattern resembling autosomal recessive inheritance involving a microdeletion in thrombocytopenia-absent radius syndrome. *Am J Hum Genet* 80(2): 232-240.

Kostmann, R. (1956). Infantile genetic agranulocytosis: A new recessive lethal disease in man. . *Acta Paediatr Scand* 45((suppl 105)): 361-368.

Kuijpers, T. W., N. A. Maianski, et al. (2004). Neutrophils in Barth syndrome (BTHS) avidly bind annexin-V in the absence of apoptosis. *Blood* 103(10): 3915-3923.

Kutler, D. I., B. Singh, et al. (2003). A 20-year perspective on the International Fanconi Anemia Registry (IFAR). *Blood* 101(4): 1249-1256.

Lagresle-Peyrou, C., E. M. Six, et al. (2009). Human adenylate kinase 2 deficiency causes a profound hematopoietic defect associated with sensorineural deafness. *Nat Genet* 41(1): 106-111.

Lai, C. H., C. Y. Chou, et al. (2000). Identification of novel human genes evolutionarily conserved in Caenorhabditis elegans by comparative proteomics. *Genome Research* 10(5): 703-713.

Lau, Y. L., S. Y. Ha, et al. (1999). Bone marrow transplant for dyskeratosis congenita. *Br J Haematol* 105(2): 571.

Levitus, M., M. A. Rooimans, et al. (2004). Heterogeneity in Fanconi anemia: evidence for 2 new genetic subtypes. *Blood* 103(7): 2498-2503.

Lipton, J. M., E. Atsidaftos, et al. (2006). Improving clinical care and elucidating the pathophysiology of Diamond Blackfan anemia: an update from the Diamond Blackfan Anemia Registry. *Pediatr Blood Cancer* 46(5): 558-564.

Lipton, J. M. and S. R. Ellis (2009). Diamond-Blackfan anemia: diagnosis, treatment, and molecular pathogenesis. *Hematol Oncol Clin North Am* 23(2): 261-282.

Lo Ten Foe, J. R., M. A. Rooimans, et al. (1996). Expression cloning of a cDNA for the major Fanconi anaemia gene, FAA. *Nat Genet* 14(3): 320-323.

Londono-Vallejo, J. A. (2008). Telomere instability and cancer. *Biochimie* 90(1): 73-82.

Luke-Glaser, S., B. Luke, et al. (2010). FANCM regulates DNA chain elongation and is stabilized by S-phase checkpoint signalling. *Embo J* 29(4): 795-805.

Luscombe, N. M., S. E. Austin, et al. (2000). An overview of the structures of protein-DNA complexes. *Genome Biol* 1(1): 1-37.

Majeed, F., S. Jadko, et al. (2005). Mutation analysis of SBDS in pediatric acute myeloblastic leukemia. *Pediatr Blood Cancer* 45(7): 920-924.

Makitie, O., L. Ellis, et al. (2004). Skeletal phenotype in patients with Shwachman-Diamond syndrome and mutations in SBDS. *Clinical Genetics* 65(2): 101-112.

Marrone, A., A. Walne, et al. (2007). Telomerase reverse-transcriptase homozygous mutations in autosomal recessive dyskeratosis congenita and Hoyeraal-Hreidarsson syndrome. *Blood* 110(13): 4198-4205.

Marsh, J. C., A. J. Will, et al. (1992). Stem cell origin of the hematopoietic defect in dyskeratosis congenita. *Blood* 79(12): 3138-3144.

Massullo, P., L. J. Druhan, et al. (2005). Aberrant subcellular targeting of the G185R neutrophil elastase mutant associated with severe congenital neutropenia induces premature apoptosis of differentiating promyelocytes. *Blood* 105(9): 3397-3404.

Mavaddat, N., P. D. Pharoah, et al. (2010). Familial relative risks for breast cancer by pathological subtype: a population-based cohort study. *Breast Cancer Res* 12(1): R10.

McGowan, K. A., J. Z. Li, et al. (2008). Ribosomal mutations cause p53-mediated dark skin and pleiotropic effects. *Nat Genet* 40(8): 963-970.

Meetei, A. R., J. P. de Winter, et al. (2003). A novel ubiquitin ligase is deficient in Fanconi anemia. *Nat Genet* 35(2): 165-170.

Meetei, A. R., M. Levitus, et al. (2004). X-linked inheritance of Fanconi anemia complementation group B. *Nat Genet* 36(11): 1219-1224.

Meetei, A. R., A. L. Medhurst, et al. (2005). A human ortholog of archaeal DNA repair protein Hef is defective in Fanconi anemia complementation group M. *Nat Genet* 37(9): 958-963.

Mehaffey, M. G., A. L. Newton, et al. (2001). X-linked thrombocytopenia caused by a novel mutation of GATA-1. *Blood* 98(9): 2681-2688.

Menne, T. F., B. Goyenechea, et al. (2007). The Shwachman-Bodian-Diamond syndrome protein mediates translational activation of ribosomes in yeast. *Nat Genet* 39(4): 486-495.

Michaud, J., F. Wu, et al. (2002). In vitro analyses of known and novel RUNX1/AML1 mutations in dominant familial platelet disorder with predisposition to acute myelogenous leukemia: implications for mechanisms of pathogenesis. *Blood* 99(4): 1364-1372.

Miyake, K., J. Flygare, et al. (2005). Development of cellular models for ribosomal protein S19 (RPS19)-deficient diamond-blackfan anemia using inducible expression of siRNA against RPS19. *Molecular Therapy: the Journal of the American Society of Gene Therapy* 11(4): 627-637.

Miyake, K., T. Utsugisawa, et al. (2008). Ribosomal protein S19 deficiency leads to reduced proliferation and increased apoptosis but does not affect terminal erythroid differentiation in a cell line model of Diamond-Blackfan anemia. *Stem Cells* 26(2): 323-329.

Muraoka, K., E. Ishii, et al. (1997). Defective response to thrombopoietin and impaired expression of c-mpl mRNA of bone marrow cells in congenital amegakaryocytic thrombocytopenia. *Br J Haematol* 96(2): 287-292.

Naim, V. and F. Rosselli (2009). The FANC pathway and BLM collaborate during mitosis to prevent micro-nucleation and chromosome abnormalities. *Nat Cell Biol* 11(6): 761-768.

Nichols, K. E., J. D. Crispino, et al. (2000). Familial dyserythropoietic anaemia and thrombocytopenia due to an inherited mutation in GATA1. *Nat Genet* 24(3): 266-270.

Noy-Lotan, S., O. Dgany, et al. (2009). Codanin-1, the protein encoded by the gene mutated in congenital dyserythropoietic anemia type I (CDAN1), is cell cycle-regulated. *Haematologica* 94(5): 629-637.

O'Driscoll, M., K. M. Cerosaletti, et al. (2001). DNA ligase IV mutations identified in patients exhibiting developmental delay and immunodeficiency. *Mol Cell* 8(6): 1175-1185.

Olivieri, N. F., T. Grunberger, et al. (1991). Diamond-Blackfan anemia: heterogenous response of hematopoietic progenitor cells in vitro to the protein product of the steel locus. *Blood* 78(9): 2211-2215.

Page, A. and R. Good (1957). Studies on cyclic neutropenia. *Am J Dis Child* 94: 623.

Pai, G. S., Y. Yan, et al. (1989). Bleomycin hypersensitivity in dyskeratosis congenita fibroblasts, lymphocytes, and transformed lymphoblasts. *Cytogenet Cell Genet* 52(3-4): 186-189.

Pang, Q., W. Keeble, et al. (2001). FANCC interacts with Hsp70 to protect hematopoietic cells from IFN-gamma/TNF-alpha-mediated cytotoxicity. *Embo J* 20(16): 4478-4489.

Pannicke, U., M. Honig, et al. (2009). Reticular dysgenesis (aleukocytosis) is caused by mutations in the gene encoding mitochondrial adenylate kinase 2. *Nat Genet* 41(1): 101-105.

Perdahl, E. B., B. L. Naprstek, et al. (1994). Erythroid failure in Diamond-Blackfan anemia is characterized by apoptosis. *Blood* 83(3): 645-650.

Person, R. E., F. Q. Li, et al. (2003). Mutations in proto-oncogene GFI1 cause human neutropenia and target ELA2. *Nature Genetics* 34(3): 308-312.

Peterson, L. C., K. V. Rao, et al. (1985). Fechtner syndrome--a variant of Alport's syndrome with leukocyte inclusions and macrothrombocytopenia. *Blood* 65(2): 397-406.

Pippucci, T., A. Savoia, et al. Mutations in the 5' UTR of ANKRD26, the ankirin repeat domain 26 gene, cause an autosomal-dominant form of inherited thrombocytopenia, THC2. *Am J Hum Genet* 88(1): 115-120.

Punzo, F., E. J. Mientjes, et al. (2010). A mutation in the acyl-coenzyme A binding domain-containing protein 5 gene (ACBD5) identified in autosomal dominant thrombocytopenia. *J Thromb Haemost* 8(9): 2085-2087.

Reid, S., D. Schindler, et al. (2007). Biallelic mutations in PALB2 cause Fanconi anemia subtype FA-N and predispose to childhood cancer. *Nat Genet* 39(2): 162-164.

Renella, R., N. A. Roberts, et al. Codanin-1 mutations in congenital dyserythropoietic anemia type 1 affect HP1α localization in erythroblasts. *Blood*.

Rotig, A., V. Cormier, et al. (1990). Pearson's marrow-pancreas syndrome. A multisystem mitochondrial disorder in infancy. *J Clin Invest* 86(5): 1601-1608.

Rujkijyanont, P., K. Watanabe, et al. (2008). SBDS-deficient cells undergo accelerated apoptosis through the Fas-pathway. *Haematologica* 93(3): 363-371.

Saadatzadeh, M. R., K. Bijangi-Vishehsaraei, et al. (2009). Distinct roles of stress-activated protein kinases in Fanconi anemia-type C-deficient hematopoiesis. *Blood* 113(12): 2655-2660.

Sabatier, L. and B. Dutrillaux (1988). Effect of caffeine in Fanconi anemia. I. Restoration of a normal duration of G2 phase. *Hum Genet* 79(3): 242-244.

Santucci, M. A., G. P. Bagnara, et al. (1999). Long-term bone marrow cultures in Diamond-Blackfan anemia reveal a defect of both granulomacrophage and erythroid progenitors. *Exp Hematol* 27(1): 9-18.

Saunders, E. F. and M. H. Freedman (1978). Constitutional aplastic anaemia: defective haematopoietic stem cell growth in vitro. *Br J Haematology* 40(2): 277-287.

Savage, S. A., N. Giri, et al. (2008). TINF2, a component of the shelterin telomere protection complex, is mutated in dyskeratosis congenita. *Am J Hum Genet* 82(2): 501-509.

Savchenko, A., N. Krogan, et al. (2005). The Shwachman-Bodian-Diamond syndrome protein family is involved in RNA metabolism. *Journal of Biological Chemistry* 280(19): 19213-19220.

Savoia, A., C. Balduini, et al. (2001). Autosomal dominant macrothrombocytopenia in Italy is most frequently a type of heterozygous Bernard-Soulier syndrome. *Blood* 97(5): 1330-1335.

Schofield, K. P. and D. I. Evans (1991). Diamond-Blackfan syndrome and neutropenia. *J Clin Pathol* 44(9): 742-744.

Schwarz, K., A. Iolascon, et al. (2009). Mutations affecting the secretory COPII coat component SEC23B cause congenital dyserythropoietic anemia type II. *Nat Genet* 41(8): 936-940.

Sejas, D. P., R. Rani, et al. (2007). Inflammatory reactive oxygen species-mediated hemopoietic suppression in Fancc-deficient mice. *J Immunol* 178(8): 5277-5287.

Seri, M., A. Pecci, et al. (2003). MYH9-related disease: May-Hegglin anomaly, Sebastian syndrome, Fechtner syndrome, and Epstein syndrome are not distinct entities but represent a variable expression of a single illness. *Medicine* 82(3): 203-215.

Shammas, C., T. F. Menne, et al. (2005). Structural and mutational analysis of the SBDS protein family. Insight into the leukemia-associated Shwachman-Diamond Syndrome. *J Biol Chem* 280(19): 19221-19229.

Shimamura, A. (2006). Inherited bone marrow failure syndromes: molecular features. *Hematology Am Soc Hematol Educ Program*: 63-71.

Shwachman, H. (1964). The syndrome of pancreatic insufficiency and bone marrow dysfunction. *J Pediatr* 65: 645-663.

Smeenk, G., A. J. de Groot, et al. (2010). Rad51C is essential for embryonic development and haploinsufficiency causes increased DNA damage sensitivity and genomic instability. *Mutat Res* 689(1-2): 50-58.

Song, W. J., M. G. Sullivan, et al. (1999). Haploinsufficiency of CBFA2 causes familial thrombocytopenia with propensity to develop acute myelogenous leukaemia. *Nat Genet* 23(2): 166-175.

Stepanovic, V., D. Wessels, et al. (2004). The chemotaxis defect of Shwachman-Diamond Syndrome leukocytes. *Cell Motil Cytoskeleton* 57(3): 158-174.

Stoepker, C., K. Hain, et al. SLX4, a coordinator of structure-specific endonucleases, is mutated in a new Fanconi anemia subtype. *Nat Genet* 43(2): 138-141.

Strathdee, C., H. Gavish, et al. (1992). Cloning of cDNAs for Fanconi's anaemia by functional complementation. *Nature* 356: 763-767.

Teo, J. T., R. Klaassen, et al. (2008). Clinical and genetic analysis of unclassifiable inherited bone marrow failure syndromes. *Pediatrics* 122(1): 139-148.

Thompson, A. A. and L. T. Nguyen (2000). Amegakaryocytic thrombocytopenia and radio-ulnar synostosis are associated with HOXA11 mutation. *Nat Genet* 26(4): 397-398.

Thompson, A. A., K. Woodruff, et al. (2001). Congenital thrombocytopenia and radio-ulnar synostosis: a new familial syndrome. *Br J Haematol* 113(4): 866-870.

Timmers, C., T. Taniguchi, et al. (2001). Positioning cloning of a novel Fanconi anemia gene, FANCD2. *Mol Cell* 7(2): 241-248.

Trahan, C. and F. Dragon (2009). Dyskeratosis congenita mutations in the H/ACA domain of human telomerase RNA affect its assembly into a pre-RNP. *RNA* 15(2): 235-243.

Trahan, C., C. Martel, et al. (2010). Effects of dyskeratosis congenita mutations in dyskerin, NHP2 and NOP10 on assembly of H/ACA pre-RNPs. *Hum Mol Genet* 19(5): 825-836.

Tsai, P. H., S. Arkin, et al. (1989). An intrinsic progenitor defect in Diamond-Blackfan anaemia. *Br J Haematol* 73(1): 112-120.

Tsai, P. H., I. Sahdev, et al. (1990). Fatal cyclophosphamide-induced congestive heart failure in a 10-year-old boy with Shwachman-Diamond syndrome and severe bone marrow failure treated with allogeneic bone marrow transplantation. *Am J Pediatr Hematol Oncol* 12(4): 472-476.

Tsangaris, E., R. Klaassen, et al. (2011). Genetic analysis of inherited bone marrow failure syndromes from one prospective, comprehensive and population-based cohort and identification of novel mutations. *Journal of Medical Genetics*.

Urban, C., B. Binder, et al. (1992). Congenital sideroblastic anemia successfully treated by allogeneic bone marrow transplantation. *Bone Marrow Transplant* 10(4): 373-375.

Van Den Oudenrijn, S., M. Bruin, et al. (2002). Three parameters, plasma thrombopoietin levels, plasma glycocalicin levels and megakaryocyte culture, distinguish between different causes of congenital thrombocytopenia. *Br J Haematol* 117(2): 390-398.

van den Oudenrijn, S., M. Bruin, et al. (2000). Mutations in the thrombopoietin receptor, Mpl, in children with congenital amegakaryocytic thrombocytopenia. *Br J Haematol* 110(2): 441-448.

Vaz, F., H. Hanenberg, et al. Mutation of the RAD51C gene in a Fanconi anemia-like disorder. *Nat Genet* 42(5): 406-409.

Vinciguerra, P., S. A. Godinho, et al. (2010). Cytokinesis failure occurs in Fanconi anemia pathway-deficient murine and human bone marrow hematopoietic cells. *J Clin Invest* 120(11): 3834-3842.

Vlachos, A., S. Ball, et al. (2008). Diagnosing and treating Diamond Blackfan anaemia: results of an international clinical consensus conference. *Br J Haematol* 142(6): 859-876.

Volpi, L., G. Roversi, et al. Targeted next-generation sequencing appoints c16orf57 as clericuzio-type poikiloderma with neutropenia gene. *Am J Hum Genet* 86(1): 72-76.

Vulliamy, T., R. Beswick, et al. (2008). Mutations in the telomerase component NHP2 cause the premature ageing syndrome dyskeratosis congenita. *Proc Natl Acad Sci* U S A 105(23): 8073-8078.

Vulliamy, T., A. Marrone, et al. (2002). Association between aplastic anaemia and mutations in telomerase RNA. *Lancet* 359(9324): 2168-2170.

Vulliamy, T., A. Marrone, et al. (2001). The RNA component of telomerase is mutated in autosomal dominant dyskeratosis congenita. *Nature* 413(6854): 432-435.

Vulliamy, T. J. and I. Dokal (2008). Dyskeratosis congenita: the diverse clinical presentation of mutations in the telomerase complex. *Biochimie* 90(1): 122-130.

Vulliamy, T. J., S. W. Knight, et al. (2001). Very short telomeres in the peripheral blood of patients with X-linked and autosomal dyskeratosis congenita. *Blood Cells Mol Dis* 27(2): 353-357.

Vulliamy, T. J., A. Walne, et al. (2005). Mutations in the reverse transcriptase component of telomerase (TERT) in patients with bone marrow failure. *Blood Cells Mol Dis* 34(3): 257-263.

Walne, A. J., T. Vulliamy, et al. (2008). TINF2 mutations result in very short telomeres: analysis of a large cohort of patients with dyskeratosis congenita and related bone marrow failure syndromes. *Blood* 112(9): 3594-3600.

Walne, A. J., T. Vulliamy, et al. (2007). Genetic heterogeneity in autosomal recessive dyskeratosis congenita with one subtype due to mutations in the telomerase-associated protein NOP10. *Hum Mol Genet* 16(13): 1619-1629.

Watanabe, K., C. Ambekar, et al. (2009). SBDS-deficiency results in specific hypersensitivity to Fas stimulation and accumulation of Fas at the plasma membrane. *Apoptosis* 14(1): 77-89.

Wessels, D., T. Srikantha, et al. (2006). The Shwachman-Bodian-Diamond syndrome gene encodes an RNA-binding protein that localizes to the pseudopod of Dictyostelium amoebae during chemotaxis. *J Cell Sci* 119(Pt 2): 370-379.

Wetzler, M., M. Talpaz, et al. (1992). Myelokathexis: normalization of neutrophil counts and morphology by GM-CSF. *Jama* 267(16): 2179-2180.

Woloszynek, J. R., R. J. Rothbaum, et al. (2004). Mutations of the SBDS gene are present in most patients with Shwachman-Diamond syndrome. *Blood* 104(12): 3588-3590.

Xia, J., A. A. Bolyard, et al. (2009). Prevalence of mutations in ELANE, GFI1, HAX1, SBDS, WAS and G6PC3 in patients with severe congenital neutropenia. *Br J Haematol* 147(4): 535-542.

Yoshida, M. C. (1980). Suppression of spontaneous and mitomycin C-induced chromosome aberrations in Fanconi's anemia by cell fusion with normal human fibroblasts. *Hum Genet* 55(2): 223-226.

Zeharia, A., N. Fischel-Ghodsian, et al. (2005). Mitochondrial myopathy, sideroblastic anemia, and lactic acidosis: an autosomal recessive syndrome in Persian Jews caused by a mutation in the PUS1 gene. *J Child Neurol* 20(5): 449-452.

Zhang, S., M. Shi, et al. (2006). Loss of the mouse ortholog of the shwachman-diamond syndrome gene (Sbds) results in early embryonic lethality. *Molecular & Cellular Biology* 26(17): 6656-6663.

Zhang, X., J. Li, et al. (2004). The Fanconi anemia proteins functionally interact with the protein kinase regulated by RNA (PKR). *J Biol Chem* 279(42): 43910-43919.

Zhong, F., S. A. Savage, et al. (2011). Disruption of telomerase trafficking by TCAB1 mutation causes dyskeratosis congenita. *Genes Dev* 25(1): 11-16.

Zinnsser, F. (1906). Atrophia cutis reticularis cum pigmentatione, dystrophia unguium et leukoplakia oris. *Ikonogr Dermatol* (Hyoto) 5: 219-223.

Zuelzer, W. W. (1964). Myelokathexis--a New Form of Chronic Granulocytopenia. Report of a Case. *N Engl J Med* 270: 699-704.

19

Bernard Soulier Syndrome: A Genetic Bleeding Disorder

Basma Hadjkacem[1], Jalel Gargouri[2] and Ali Gargouri[1]
[1]*Laboratoire de Valorisation de la Biomasse et Production de Protéines chez les Eucaryotes, Centre de Biotechnologie de Sfax, université de Sfax, Sfax*
[2]*Laboratoire d'Hématologie (99/UR/08-33), Faculté de Médecine de Sfax, Université de Sfax, Centre régionale de transfusion sanguine de Sfax*
Tunisie

1. Introduction

Platelets and other coagulation factors play an important role in the primary haemostasis mechanism, a multistep process of platelets interaction with elements of the damaged vessel wall, leading to the initial formation of a platelet plug (Ahmad et al., 2008). This mechanism requires the synergistic action of several different platelet receptors which play an essential role in each step of aggregation. Platelet adhesion, activation and aggregation are in fact regulated by specific glycoprotein on the platelet cell surface. Genetic defects in one of these glycoprotein led to bleeding symptoms due to inability of blood platelets to provide their hemostatic function in the vessel injury.

Inherited platelet defects cause bleeding symptoms of varying severity. Typically, easy bruising, epistaxis, gingival and mucocutaneous bleeding are observed in affected patients.

Different diagnostic parameters have been used to classify inherited thrombocytopenia including the degree of bleeding, inheritance trait, platelet function and kinetics, and clinical abnormalities (see table 1).

The platelet defects are classified into disorders affecting either intracellular organelle of platelets, signalling pathway or surface receptors.

Currently, much effort is being put into methods to more rapidly and accurately diagnose patients with platelet disorders and to initiate appropriate therapy and prevent life threatening bleeding (Simon et al., 2008).

In this chapter, we describe many platelets disease caused by secretion defects like in Grey Platelet Syndrome (GPS), Quebec platelet disorder (QPD) or Wiscott-Aldrich syndrome (WAS), other diseases due to signal transduction shortcoming. Finally, we detail some diseases caused by deficiency of platelet complex expression in the cell surface and we develop especially Bernard Soulier syndrome (BSS).

2. Defects of secretion

Many disorders are classified in this category and are known as "storage pool disease". This group contain several congenital diseases characterized by defects in intracellular organelle

especially α-granule and dense granule (Simon et al., 2008)..The absence of platelet granules results in a defective secretion from activated platelets as well as abnormal secretion-dependent platelet aggregation (Sandrock & Zieger, 2010).
Deficiencies can alter the contents of α-granules, dense granules or both. In many patients the storage pool defect is the only abnormality detected. Nevertheless, the association with other congenital abnormalities was also shown like in Hermansky-Pudlak syndrome (HPS), Chediak-Higashi syndrome (CHS) and Wiskott-Aldrich syndrome (David et al., 2001).

Syndrome	Bleeding symptoms	Platelet count (10^9/l)	Platelet aggregation	Inheritance	Gene
GPS	Mild to moderate	30-100	normal or ↓ aggregation with thrombin, collagen	autosomal recessive (most) or dominant	unknown
QPD	Mild to moderate	Normal or less	↓ aggregation with epinephrine	Autosomal dominant	uPA gene (PLAU)
HPS	Moderate to severe	normal	↓ second wave of aggregation	Autosomal recessive	HPS1-HPS8
CHS	Moderate to severe	normal	↓ second wave of aggregation	Autosomal recessive	LYST
WAS	Moderate to severe	10-100	↓ aggregation	X-linked recessive	WAS
XLT	moderate	decreased	↓ aggregation	X-linked	WAS
GT	Moderate to severe	Normal	Reduced or absence of aggregation	Autosomal recessive	GPIIb and GPIIIa
BSS	Moderate to severe	10-100	Absence of Aggregation with ristocetin	Autosomal recessive (most) or dominant	GPIbα, GPIbβ and GPIX

Table 1. Clinical symptoms and candidate genes of several inherited platelet diseases

2.1 Abnormalities of α-granule

2.1.1 Grey Platelet Syndrome

The first case has been reported by Raccuglia in 1971 as a qualitative defect in platelets (Raccuglia, 1971). This rare hereditary disease is characterized by a bleeding tendency, moderate thrombocytopenia and decrease or absence of platelet α-granules and their contents probably due to the failure of maturation during megakaryocyte differentiation (White, 1979). GPS platelets are unsuitable to get and store endogenously synthesized proteins such as platelet factor-4, β-thromboglobulin, Von Willebrand Factor (vWF) as well as exogenous proteins such as fibrinogen, albumin, or factor V (Sandrock & Zieger, 2010).

Microscopic observations of patients blood smear revealed mild to moderate thrombocytopenia and enlarged (but not giant) platelets that have a gray appearance. Platelet aggregation studies are variable with no classical response pattern to ADP, epinephrine, thrombin, or collagen (Nurden, 2007).
Both autosomal recessive and autosomal dominant inheritance have been reported suggesting that this syndrome is genetically heterogeneous (Mori et al, 1984) (Nurden et al., 2004). The molecular basis of GPS is unknown but could involve a "sorting" receptor for vesicles leaving the Golgi apparatus (Nurden, 2005).

2.1.2 Quebec platelet disorder

Quebec platelet disorder (QPD) is a defect in α-granule proteolysis of proteins and a deficiency of α- granule multimerin, a protein that binds factor V within the granule, thus leading to a decreased content of platelet factor V along with several other proteins like fibrinogen and vWF (Shapiro, 1999).
In addition to α-granule protein degradation, this inherited bleeding disorder is associated with increased expression and storage of the fibrinolytic enzyme urokinase plasminogen activator (uPA) in platelets and intra-platelet plasmin generation (Diamandis et al., 2009). Patients showed mild thrombocytopenia, absence of aggregation with epinephrine and moderate to severe delayed bleeding following trauma or surgery that responds only to fibrinolytic inhibitor therapy (Veljkovic et al., 2009).
This syndrome is inherited as an autosomal dominant manner. The genetic cause of QPD has recently been linked to inheritance of a region on chromosome 10 that contains the uPA gene (PLAU) (Diamandis et al., 2009).

2.2 Abnormalties of dense granule

Dense granule deficiency is often, but not always, associated with impaired secondary aggregation responses to some agonists (Ahmad et al., 2008).

2.2.1 Hermansky-Pudlak syndrome

Hermansky–Pudlak syndrome (HPS) is a rare autosomal recessive disorder. First HPS cases were reported on 1959 by Hermansky and Pudlak: Two unrelated patients suffered from oculocutaneous albinism, a history of frequent bruising following minimal trauma, lifelong bleeding tendency and unusual pigmented macrophages in bone marrow (Hermansky & Pudlak, 1959).
This syndrome results from abnormal formation or trafficking of intracellular vesicles. The specific organelles affected in HPS are the lysosomes and lysosome-related organelles such as the melanosomes and the platelet dense granule (Cutler, 2002).
Clinical manifestations showed hypopigmentation, platelet dense granule deficiency and accumulation of ceroid pigment in lysosomal organelles (Ramasamy, 2004).
HPS patients have been described in different ethnic groups. However, this syndrome is frequent in Puerto Rico and in an isolated mountain village in the Swiss Alps (Schallreuter et al., 1993; Witkop et al., 1990).
Eight human HPS genes (HPS1–HPS8) have been found causing hypopigmentation and platelet storage pool deficiency. All HPS proteins are associated in multi-protein complexes essential for biogenesis and intracellular trafficking of intracellular vesicles of lysosomal lineage (Li et al., 2004). Mutations within particular HPS genes can lead to dysfunction of

the corresponding protein complex and thus to defective maturation of melanosomes and platelet dense bodies (Sandrock & Zieger, 2010).

2.2.2 Chediak-Higashi syndrome

Chediak-Higashi syndrome (CHS) is a rare autosomal recessive disease described since 1955 by Sato (Sato, 1955). Like HPS, CHS is also characterized by oculocutaneous albinism and dense granule deficiency leading to platelet disorder and prolonged bleeding tendency. In addition, CHS patients showed severe immunologic defects and progressive neurological dysfunction making this disease lethal. If patients survive until adulthood, they develop neurological defects including neuropathies, autonomic dysfunction, atrophy, sensory deficits, seizures, and cognitive defects (Sandrock & Zieger, 2010). Only hematopoietic stem cell transplantation can improve the health status of patients (Eapen et al., 2007).

The canditate gene for this syndrome is named LYST (lysosomal trafficking regulator) (Barbosa et al., 1996; Nagle et al., 1996). The gene product is a protein which regulates the size and movement of lysosome-related organelles. LYST is predicted to be a cytosolic protein that mediates membrane interactions. Genetic defects are usually frameshift and nonsense mutations in LYST gene giving rise to truncated protein and a severe phenotype (Certain et al., 2000; Moore et al., 2002). Rarely, missense mutations are associated with a milder form of the disease.

2.3 Abnormalities of both granules

2.3.1 Wiskott-Aldrich syndrome

Wiskott–Aldrich syndrome (WAS) is a rare X-linked recessive disease. The inheritance of this syndrome explains why symptomatic individuals were all male (Aldrich et al., 1954). This syndrome has been observed first in 1939 by Alfred Wiskott. This paediatrician described three brothers who suffer from thrombocytopenia, bloody diarrhea, eczema, and recurrent ear infections; all three died early in life from intestinal bleeding and sepsis (Wiskott et al., 1939). The WAS phenotype consists of immunodeficiency, eczema, thrombocytopenia and is associated with extensive clinical heterogeneity. The immune deficiency is caused by decreased antibody production, although T cells are also affected (Vera Binder et al., 2006).

WAS is caused by mutations in WAS gene located at Xp11.22–p11.23, encoding Wiskott-Aldrich syndrome protein (WASP). This protein seems to be involved in signal transduction pathways in which tyrosine phosphorylation and adapter protein function have been suggested. Deficiency of WASP induces premature proplatelet formation in the bone marrow and cancels megakaryocytes migration (Sabri et al., 2006).

WASP is involved in innate immunity, cell motility and protection against autoimmune disease. The success of hematopoietic stem cell transplantation is related to the patient's age, donor selection, the conditioning regimen and the extent of reconstitution. Gene therapy is expected to cure the disease because WASP is expressed exclusively in hematopoietic stem cells and it exerts a robust selective pressure (Notarangelo et al., 2008).

2.4 X-linked thrombocytopenia

X-linked thrombocytopenia (XLT) was recognized in 1960 and was suspected to be a variant of WAS. This was confirmed when XLT patients showed mutations in the WAS protein gene.

XLT patients have moderate symptoms when compared with WAS. They showed mild eczema and/or infections and they have a lower risk of cancer or autoimmunity than patients with WAS. XLT phenotype is often resulting from missense mutations given rise to defective expression of WASP (Albert et al., 2010).

3. Defects of intracellular signalling pathway

For many patients with platelet aggregation defects, the abnormalities lie in early signal transduction events. Those patients have a prolonged bleeding time on most occasions, they have an impaired dense granule secretion although their platelets have normal granule storage and generally synthesise substantial amounts of thromboxane A2 (Ramasamy, 2004). Platelet pathologies involving the signal transduction pathways mostly concern patients with mild bleeding disorders and defects of platelet aggregation which affect some stimuli more than others.

Concerned patients showed:

Impaired Ca2+ mobilisation.

Defective inositol-triphosphate production and a reduced phosphorylation of the protein, plekstrin, by protein kinase C.

Deficiency of the phospholipase C-γ2 isoform,

Specific decrease in platelet membrane Gαq and decrease in platelets response to several agonists including a decreased activation of αIIbβ3.

A major effort is underway to uncover the genetic defects responsible of these phenotypes. (Nurden & Nurden, 2008)

4. Disorders of the surface membrane

Most studied disease affecting membrane receptors are Bernard Soulier syndrome which concern GPIb-IX-V complex and Glanzmann thrombasthenia with deficiency in GPIIb-IIIa complex.

4.1 Glanzmann thrombasthenia

Glanzmann thrombasthenia (GT) is the most common of the platelets diseases. It is characterized by the absence or deficiency of GPIIb-IIIa platelet complex. This complex play an essential role in platelets aggregation by fixing several ligand, like von Willebrand Factor and fibrinogen (Bellucci et al., 1983; Giltay et al., 1987). GP IIb–IIIa is one of the most abundant platelet surface receptors (about 80 000 per platelet) (Wagner et al., 1996).

The patients present normal platelet morphology, prolonged bleeding time, severe mucocutaneous diasthesis and series of epistaxis, purpura or menorrhagia (Sherer & Lerner, 1999). The hallmark of this disease is a severely reduced or absent platelet aggregation in response to multiple physiological agonists such as ADP, epinephrine, thrombin and collagen. (Ahmad et al., 2008).

This disease is inherited as an autosomal recessive manner (Sherer & Lerner, 1999). Genetic defects are distributed in GPIIb or GPIIIa genes resulting in qualitative or quantitative abnormalities of the proteins. Both genes are present in our genome as single copies and are localized on chromosome 17 (table 2) (Rosenberg *et al.*, 1997). More than 70 mutations have been described. Large deletions are very rare. Most of them are missense or nonsense mutation, insertion, small deletion and splicing defects; some of the punctual mutations affected the mRNA production or stability (Nurden, 2005). This large number of identified mutations offers an opportunity to investigate phenotype/genotype correlations (Ramasamy, 2004).

	GPIIb	GPIIIa
Size (Kb)	17	65
Number of exons	30	15
Chromosome Localisation	17q21-23	17q21-23

Table 2. Characteristics of GPIIb and GPIIIa genes

4.2 Bernard Soulier syndrome
4.2.1 History
BSS was described more than 60 years ago as a severe and potentially fatal, congenital bleeding disorder. The first case was reported in 1948 by two French hematologists (Jean Bernard and Jean-Pierre Soulier) in a young male patient from a consanguineous family with severe bleeding episodes, a prolonged bleeding time, low platelet counts and very large platelets. They termed the disorder ''congenital hemorrhagiparous thrombocytic dystrophy'' (Bernard & Soulier, 1948). Since then, several individuals have been described with a similar disorder.

4.2.2 Clinical manifestations
BSS patients present early many bleeding symptoms, most commonly epistaxis, ecchymosis, cutaneous and gingival bleeding. Some patients can show gastrointestinal haemorrhage. Severe bleeding occurred in the case of trauma, surgical intervention and in menses (Lanza, 2006). Chronic easy bruising and frequent hematomas are rarely reported (Kenny et al., 1999). Pregnancy in BSS patients may present complications of varying gravity.

The severity of these bleeding symptoms is variable among patients and may range from mild to life-threatening and may become more or less severe during puberty and adulthood. Some rare BSS patients suffered fatal haemorrhage (Hadjkacem et al., 2010a). Heterozygous patients may have mild to moderate bleeding tendencies (Pham & Wang, 2007).

4.2.3 Etiology
The molecular defect alters platelet complex named GPIb-IX-V. It is the surface receptor for von Willebrand factor that mediates both platelet agglutination in response to ristocetin and platelet adhesion under conditions of rapid blood flow. This complex plays an essential role in primary haemostasis ensuring platelets adhesion by its binding to von Willebrand factor, itself captured from plasma by sub-endothelial collagen (Berndt et al., 1989).

GPIb-IX-V complex is composed by four glycoproteins designated GPIbα, GPIbβ, GPIX and GPV. They are expressed on the platelets surface in an apparent molar ratio of 2:2:2:1 respectively (figure 1). Approximately, 24000 copies of this complex are presents on the membrane of activated platelets (Strassel et al., 2009).

GPIbα, consists of 610 amino acids (MW 145 kDa), GPIbβ of 181 (22 kDa), GPIX of 160 (20 kDa), and GPV of 544 amino acids (82 kDa). GPIbα is disulfide linked to GPIbβ constituting GPIb dimer while GPIX and GPV bind to GPIb non-covalently (Lopez et al., 1998).

The vWF binding domain is located at the N-terminus of GPIbα. The GPIbα chain also binds a number of other ligands, including thrombin. The GPIbβ protein has N-terminal extra cellular domain that contains a cysteine knot region, which is essential for interaction with GPIX. The letter is essential for the correct assembly of the GPIb-IX-V complex on the platelet membrane. GPV is required for thrombin binding, possibly through an interaction with GPIbα. In addition, GPV binds to collagen and appears to be required for normal platelet responses to this agonist (Dong et al., 1998; Lopez et al., 1998).

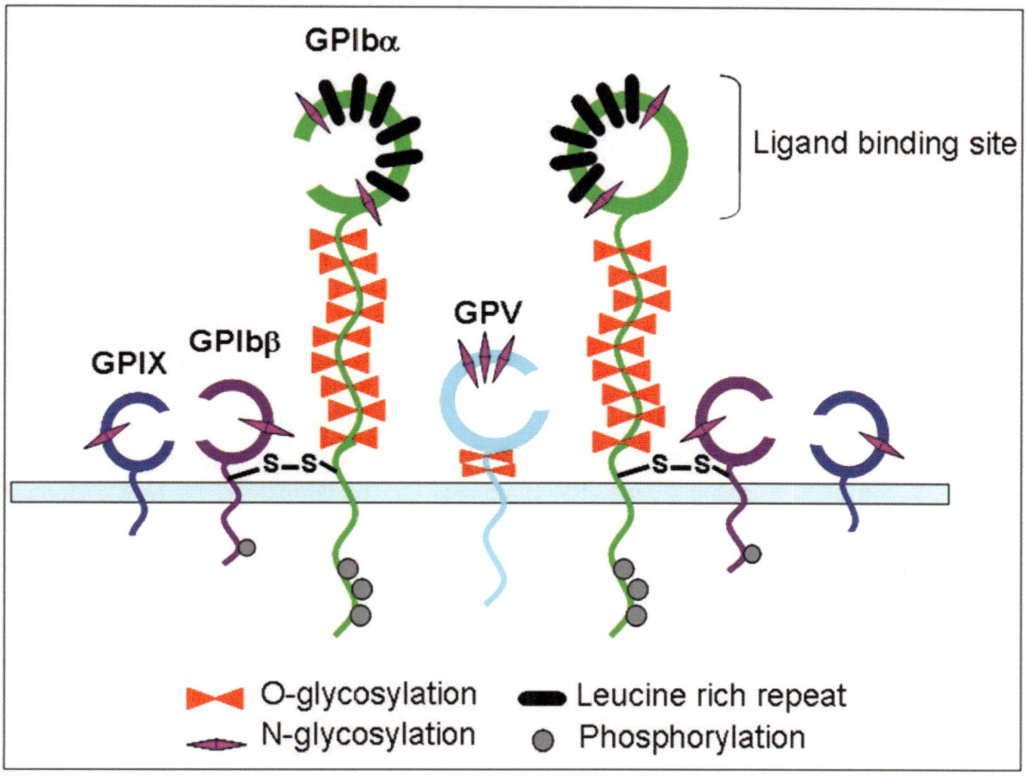

Fig. 1. GPIb-IX-V complex

The GPIb-IX-V complex is formed within minutes in the endoplasmic reticulum before being transported into the Golgi cisternae to undergo post-translational modifications. Only complete complexes were expressed on the platelets membrane. The absence of one component of the complex increases the rate of degradation (Dong et al., 1998)

4.2.4 Diagnosis

The diagnosis is based on the presence of a prolonged skin bleeding time (more then 15 min), giant circulating platelets observed on a peripheral blood smear (larger than 4 µm and being able to reach 10 mm, while normal platelets are 2-3 µm) (figure 2) and thrombocytopenia (between 10^{10} to 10^{11} platelets/l compared to 1.5×10^{11} to 4×10^{11} platelets/l in healthy persons) (Hadjkacem et al., 2010a; Lanza, 2006)

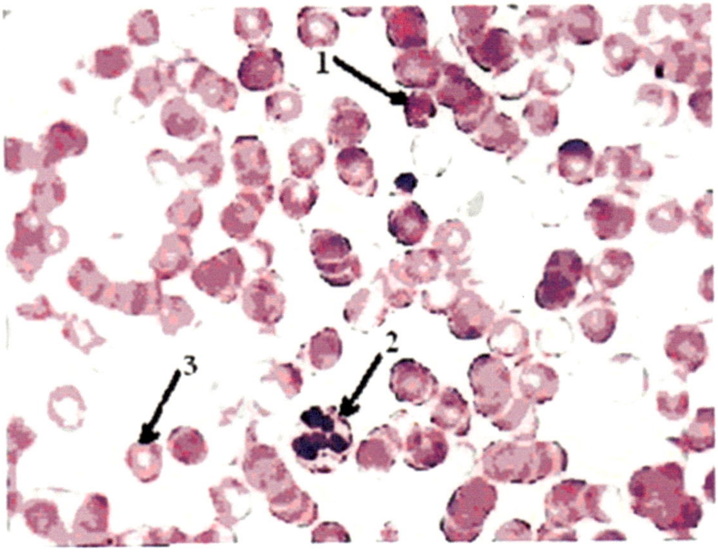

Fig. 2. Blood smear of a BSS patient demonstrating giant platelet (1), white blood cell (2) and red cell (3)

BSS diagnosis is based mainly on aggregation test using an aggregometer since the platelets of patients aggregate normally in response to agonists such as adenosine diphosphate (ADP), collagen, epinephrine, arachidonic acid but they failed to aggregate in presence of ristocetin (figure 3). In addition, all BSS patients have decreased or absent expression of the GPIb-IX-V complex. For this reason, the diagnosis can be confirmed by flow cytometry using specific antibodies recognizing one or more proteins of the complex (figure 4) (Hadjkacem et al., 2010a; Ware et al., 1998).

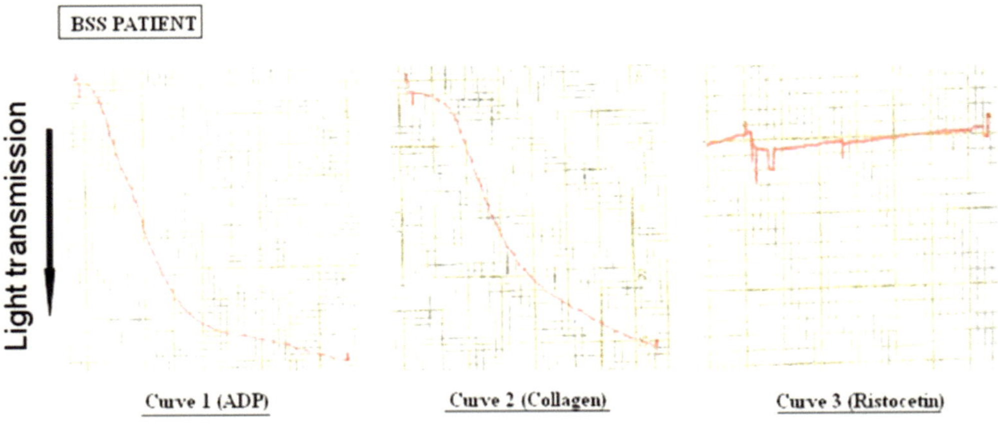

Fig. 3. BSS platelets aggregation

The curve 1 and 2 showed an increasing of light transmission that indicates positive wave aggregation, so BSS platelets aggregate normally with ADP and collagen but failed to aggregate in presence of ristocetin (curve 3).

The GPIIb-IIIa complex, normally expressed on the platelets surface of healthy persons and BSS patients, serves as a positive control. Those specialized laboratory tests are essential to avoid confusion between BSS and other similar platelet disorders (Hadjkacem et al., 2010a). Based only on clinical manifestations, many patients had been erroneously diagnosed with immune thrombocytopenia and were treated with steroids without response (Sachs et al., 2003).

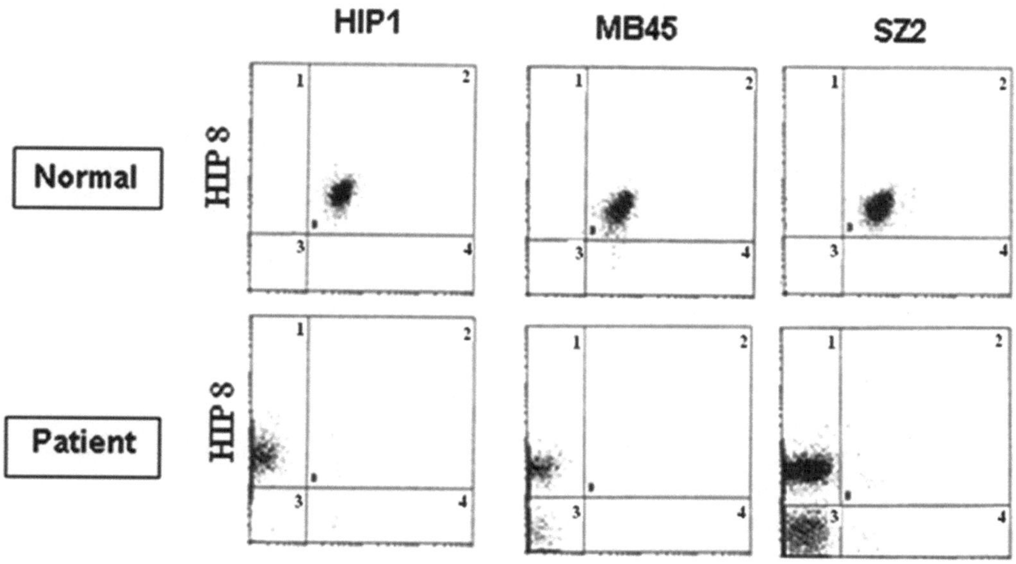

Fig. 4. Flow cytometric analysis of normal and BSS platelets. (Hadjkacem et al., 2010b)

HIP8 is an antibody recognizing GPIIb-IIIa complex and serves as positive control. HIP1, MB45 and SZ2 are antibodies directed against different epitope on GPIbα. We have used simultaneously two antibodies for each platelets marking: the HIP8 and one of the GPIbα antibodies. The result is considered as double positive when the fluorescence is observed in the square 2 and it is considered as only HIP8 positive when fluorescence exist in square 1. If the fluorescence is localized in the square 3, we concluded that the GPIbα antibody failed to bind to the specific protein.

For healthy person, response is positive with all antibodies but in BSS patient, anti-GPIbα failed to bind on platelets surface because the absence of this protein.

4.2.5 Transmission mode

The BSS is an inherited disorder usually transmitted in an autosomal recessive manner and occurring in persons whose parents are close relatives. Both male and females are concerned by this disease; the male/female ratio is 1:1. An autosomal dominant with heterozygous state has also been found but rarely reported. This form was characterized by mild or no clinical symptoms and normal in vitro platelet function (Miller et al., 1992; Savoia et al., 2001).

Genetic counselling is done according to established standards for all autosomal recessive diseases.

4.2.6 Frequency

BSS is a rare disease, the frequency of homozygous has been estimated to be approximately one in one million (Lopez et al., 1998) and, according to the Hardy-Weinberg Law, the frequency of heterozygotes is 1 in 500 (Savoia et al., 2001).

4.2.7 Canditates genes

Molecular investigations of numerous BSS patients showed that only three genes are responsible of the disease: GPIbα, GPIbβ, and GPIX. No mutations have been reported in the GPV gene (Moran et al., 2000). These genes belong to the leucine-rich family of proteins and are exclusively expressed in megakaryocytes and platelets lineage. They showed common structural features except for their different chromosomal locations (Table 3). All candidate genes are present in monocopie. They are relatively poor in intron and contain their open reading frame (ORF) and the 3'UTR in a single exon except the GPIbβ where the ORF is contained in two exons (Antonucci et al., 2000; Lopez et al., 1998). GPIbα and GPIX genes shared promoter consensus sequences especially GATA and ETS sites (Mayumi et al., 1994).

	GPIbα	GPIbβ	GPIX
Size of mRNA (kb)	2.5	1	1
Number of exons	2	2	3
Number of coding exons	1	2	1
Chromosome localization	17-p12	22-q11.2	3q-21

Table 3. Characteristics of BSS candidates genes

4.2.8 BSS mutations

Until now, more then fifty mutations responsible for BSS have been described: 25 mutations in the gene GPIbα, 18 mutations in GPIbβ and 11 in GPIX. These defects can be classified into three groups (table 4):

- missense mutations or short deletions, often resulting in abnormal and/or unsuitable complex with a significant reduction of protein expression on the platelets surface.
- nonsense mutations giving truncated subunits, often without the transmembrane domain.
- frameshift insertions or deletions leading to a new polypeptide with premature stop codon (Hadjkacem et al., 2010a; Lanza, 2006).

Gene	Missense mutation	Nonsense mutations	Frameshift or short deletions	Others
GPIbα	10	3	11	1
GPIbβ	9	4	3	2
GPIX	9	1	1	0

Table 4. Different type of mutations described in literature in each BSS candidate gene

Compound heterozygote has been also described in BSS patients. It was relatively frequent as approximately 1/5 of described BSS mutations are of this form (Hadjkacem et al., 2010a). The genetic defects observed in BSS patients affect the von Willebrand binding site on GPIbα, inhibit the association between GPIbβ and GPIX after protein synthesis, or affect post-translational modifications that may influence the function of the complex. In very few cases, a point mutation predominantly affects receptor function as some described mutations in GPIbα and GPIX (Antonucci et al., 2000).

4.2.9 BSS founder mutations

Most mutations affect only one patient or one family but few exceptions do exist, such as the Asn45Ser identified in GPIX in several families from different nations (Koskela et al., 1999), Ala156Val in GPIbα frequently observed in Italian families (Budarf et al., 1995) and a recently identified Tunisian mutation (Hadjkacem et al., 2009, 2010).

Bernard Soulier syndrome was the focus of several studies in European, Japanese and North American populations. African and Arab populations have not been studied, with few exceptions. Our laboratory studied this syndrome for the first time in Tunisia.

Initially, our study concerned only one family consisting of five members: parents and three children including a boy suffering from BSS. Intermarriage increased the risk of developing the disease. We have identified a novel mutation in GPIbβ gene responsible for BSS in this family. The Ser23Stop so identified can be followed by MnlI restriction analysis of PCR amplified fragment. It is inherited as an autosomal recessive manner. Studies of protein expression of GPIb-IX-V complex showed the absence of GPIbα on the platelets surface of the patient (Hadjkacem et al., 2009).

Subsequently, our study included two other unrelated Tunisian families with BSS cases. In one of these families, we have revealed the same Ser23Stop mutation while in the second we observed compound heterozygosity including Ser23Stop in addition to two others missense mutations located in GPIbβ gene: Asp51Gly and Ala55Pro (Hadjkacem et al., 2010b).

Given that most of described BSS mutations are unique and the same Ser23Stop mutation being found in three unrelated Tunisian families, we suggested that it is an ancient mutation having a founder effect and can be used in genotyping for BSS diagnosis in further exploration of other Tunisian families. Indeed, the identification of a founder mutation can help physicians to avoid misdiagnosis.

4.2.10 Treatment

The severity of bleeding is unpredictable in the BSS, however most patients require transfusion in case of excessive bleeding (Nurden, 2005). The benefits of receiving the transfusions must be evaluated against the risks of exposure. Repeated exposure to blood products raises concern for alloimmunization and platelet refractoriness. Although some authors have suggested that patients should receive platelets from human leukocyte antigen-matched donors in order to avoid alloimmunization (Balduini et al., 2002),

Some patients should be warned to avoid trauma and antiplatelet drugs such as aspirin, to maintain dental hygiene and use of contraceptive devices to puberty (Lanza, 2006).

The administration of rFVIIa and Desmopressin is used to shorten the bleeding time in some patients. In rare cases of patients with serious and repetitive bleeding, bone marrow transplantation is used (Lanza, 2006).

5. Conclusion

The inherited platelet disorders are functional abnormalities of platelets due to genetic defects and lead to bleeding symptoms of varying severity. They constitute a large group of rare diseases caused by one or more mutations affecting one or more genes. These genetic defects may affect platelet granules or proteins involved in signaling pathways. Nevertheless, diseases caused by abnormalities of platelet membrane receptors are the best known platelets diseases especially the Glanzmann thrombasthenia and the Bernard Soulier syndrome. Their diagnosis is relatively easy to perform but they are manifested by severe bleeding.

Despite advances in the understanding of the etiology of these deseases, usually the underlying mechanisms remain unknown and treatment is relatively rudimentary.

6. References

Ahmad, F.; Kannan, M.; Ranjan, R.; Bajaj, J.; Choudhary, VP. & Saxena, R. (2008). Inherited platelet function disorders versus other inherited bleeding disorders: An Indian overview. *Thrombosis Research.*, Vol. 121, pp. 835–841,

Albert, MH.; Bittner, TC.; Nonoyama, S.; Notarangelo, LD.; Burns, S.; Imai, K.; Espanol, T.; Fasth, A.; Pellier, I.; Strauss, G.; Morio, T.; Gathmann, B.; Noordzij, JG.; Fillat, C.; Hoenig, M.; Nathrath, M.; Meindl, A.; Pagel, P.; Wintergerst, U.; Fischer, A.; Thrasher, AJ.; Belohradsky, BH. & Ochs, HD. (2010). X-linked thrombocytopenia (XLT) due to*WAS* mutations: clinical characteristics, long-term outcome, and treatment options. *Blood.*, vol. 115, No. 16, pp. 3231-3238,

Aldrich, RA.; Steinberg, AG. & Campbell, DC. (1954). Pedigree demonstrating a sex-linked recessive condition characterized by draining ears, eczematoid dermatitis and bloody diarrhea. *Pediatrics*, vol. 13, pp. 133-139,

Antonucci, JV.; Martin, ES.; Hulick, PJ.; Joseph, A. & Martin, ES. (2000). Bernard-Soulier Syndrome: Common Ancestry in Two African American Families with the GPIbα Leu129Pro Mutation. *Am J Hematol*, vol. 65, pp. 141-148,

Balduini, CL., Iolascon, A. & Savoia, A. (2002). Inherited thrombocytopenias: from genes to therapy. *Hematologica*, vol. 87, pp. 860–880,

Barbosa, MD.; Nguyen, QA.; Tchernev, VT.; Ashley, JA.; Detter, JC.; Blaydes, SM.; Brandt, SJ.; Chotai, D.; Hodgman, C.; Solari, RC.; Lovett, M. & Kingsmore, SF. (1996). Identification of the homologous beige and Chediak-Higashi syndrome genes. *Nature*, vol. 382, pp.262–265,

Bellucci, S.; Tobelem, G. & Caen, J. (1983). Inherited platelet disorders. *Prog Hematol*, vol. 13, pp. 223-263.

Bernard, J. & Soulier, JP. (1948). Sur une nouvelle variété de dystrophie thrombocytaire-hémorragipare congénitale. *Sem Hop Paris*, vol. 24, pp. 3217-3222,

Berndt, MC.; Fournier, DJ. & Castaldi, PA. (1989). Bernard-Soulier syndrome. *Clin Haematol*, vol. 2, pp. 585,

Biddle, DA.; Neto, TG. & Nguyen, AND. (2001). Platelet Storage Pool Deficiency of α and δ Granules. *Archives of Pathology & Laboratory Medicine*, vol. 125, No. 8, pp. 1125-1126,

Binder, V.; Albert, MH.; Kabus, M.; Bertone, M.; Meindl, A. & Belohradsky, BH. (2006). The Genotype of the Original Wiskott Phenotype. *N Engl J Med,* vol. 355. pp. 1790-1793,

Budarf, ML.; Konkle, BA. ; Ludlow, LB. ; Michaud, D. ; Li, M.; Yamashiro, DJ.; McDonald-McGinn, D.; Zackai, EH. & Driscoll, DA. (1995). Identification of a patient with Bernard-Soulier syndrome and a deletion in the DiGeorge/velo-cardio-facial chromosomal region in 22q11.2. *Hum Mol Genet,* vol. 4, pp. 763-766,

Certain, S., Barrat, F.; Pastural, E.; Le, DF.; Goyo-Rivas, J.; Jabado, N.; Benkerrou, M.; Seger, R.; Vilmer, E.; Beullier, G.; Schwarz, K.; Fischer, A. & de Saint, BG. (2000). Protein truncation test of LYST reveals heterogenous mutations in patients with Chediak-Higashi syndrome. *Blood,* vol. 95, pp. 979–983,

Cutler, DF. (2002). Introduction: lysosome-related organelles. *Semin Cell Dev Biol,* vol. 13. pp. 261–262.

Diamandis, M.; Paterson, AD.; Rommens, JM.; Veljkovic, DK.; Blavignac, J.; Bulman, DE.; Waye, JS.; Derome, F.; Rivard, GE & Hayward, CP. (2009). Quebec platelet disorder is linked to the urokinase plasminogen activator gene (PLAU) and increases expression of the linked allele in megakaryocytes. *Blood,* vol. 113. pp. 1543-1546.

Dong, JF.; Gao, S. & Lopez, JA. (1998). Synthesis, assembly, and intracellular transport of the platelet glycoprotein Ib-IX-V complex. *J Biol Chem,* vol. 273, No. 47, pp. 31449-31454.

Eapen, M.; DeLaat, CA.; Baker, KS.; Cairo, MS.; Cowan, MJ.; Kurtzberg, J.; Steward, CG.; Veys, PA. & Filipovich, AH. (2007). Hematopoietic cell transplantation for Chediak-Higashi syndrome. *Bone Marrow Transplant,* vol. 39, pp. 411–415.

Giltay, JC.; Leeksma, OC.; Breederveld, C. & van Mourik, JA. (1987). Normal synthesis and expression of endothelial IIb/IIIa in Glanzmann's thrombasthenia. *Blood,* vol. 69, No. 3. pp. 806-812.

Hadjkacem, B.; Elleuch, H.; Gargouri, J. & Gargouri, A. (2009). Bernard Soulier syndrome: novel nonsense mutation in GPIbbeta gene affecting GPIb-IX complex expression. *Ann Hematol,* vol. 88, No. (5), pp. 465-472.

Hadjkacem, B.; Ben Amor, I.; Smaoui, M.; Maalej, L.; Gargouri, J. & Gargouri, A. (2010a). Bernard Soulier Syndrome: a rare bleeding disorder with a wide range of genetic defects. *Journal of coagulation disorders,* vol. 2, No. 3.

Hadjkacem, B.; Elleuch, H.; Trigui, R.; Gargouri, J. & Gargouri, A. (2010b). The same genetic defect in three Tunisian families with Bernard Soulier syndrome: a probable founder stop mutation in GPIbbeta. *Ann Hematol,* vol. 89, pp. 75-81.

Hermansky, F. & Pudlak, P. (1959). Albinism associated with hemorrhagic diathesis and unusual pigmented reticular cells in the bone marrow: report of two cases with histochemical studies. *Blood,* vol. 14, pp. 162-169.

Kenny, D.; Morateck, PA.; Gill, JC. & Montgomery, RR. (1999). The critical interaction of glycoprotein (GP)Ib beta with GPIX- a genetic cause of Bernard Soulier syndrome. *Blood,* vol. 93, pp. 2968-2975.

Koskela, S.; Javela, K.; Jouppila, J.; Juvonen, E.; Nyblom, O.;, Partanen, J. & Kekomäki, R. (1999). Variant Bernard-Soulier syndrome due to homozygous Asn45Ser mutation in the platelet glycoprotein (GP)IX in eleven patients of five unrelated Finnish families. *Eur J Haematol,* vol. 62, pp. 256-264.

Lanza, F. (2006). Bernard-Soulier syndrome (Hemorrhagiparous thrombocytic dystrophy). *Orphanet Journal of Rare Diseases*, vol. 1, pp. 46-51.

Li, W.; Rusiniak, ME.; Chintala, S.; Gautam, R.; Novak, EK. & Swank, RT. (2004). Murine Hermansky-Pudlak syndrome genes: regulators of lysosome-related organelles. *Bioessays*, vol. 26, No. 6, pp. 616-28.

Lopez JA, Andrews RK, Afshar-Kharghan V & Berndt MC. (1998). Bernard-Soulier Syndrome. *Blood*, vol. 91, pp. 4397-4418.

Mayumi, Y. ; Edelhoff, S. ; Disteche, CM. & Roth, GJ. (1994). Structural Characterization and Chromosomal Location of the Gene Encoding Human Platelet Glycoprotein Ibβ. *The Journal of Biological Chemistry*, vol. 269, No. 26, pp. 17424-17427.

Miller, JL.; Lyle, VA. & Cunningham, D. (1992). Mutation of Leucine 57 to phenylalanine in a platelet glycoprotein Iba leucine tandem repeat occurring patients with an autosomal dominant variant of Bernard-Soulier disease. *Blood*, vol. 79, pp. 439-446.

Moore, KJ.; Barbosa, E.; Falik-Borenstein, T.; Filipovich, A.; Ishida, Y.; Kivrikko, S.; Klein, C.; Kreuz, F.; Levin, A.; Miyajima, H.; Regueiro, J.; Russo, C.; Uyama, E.; Vierimaa, O. & Spritz, RA. (2002). Apparent genotype-phenotype correlation in childhood, adolescent, and adult Chediak-Higashi syndrome. *Am J Med Genet*, vol. 108, pp. 16–22.

Moran, N.; Morateck, PA.; Deering, A.; Ryan, M.; Montgomery, RR.; Fitzgerald, DJ. & Kenny, D. (2000). Surface expression of GPIb alpha is dependent on GPIb beta: evidence from a novel mutation causing Bernard-Soulier syndrome. *Blood*, vol. 96, pp. 532-539.

Mori, K.; Suzuki, S. & Sugai, K. (1984). Electron microscopic and functional studies on platelets in gray platelet syndrome. *Tohoku J Exp Med*, vol. 143, No. 3, pp.261-87.

Nagle, DL. ; Karim, MA.; Woolf, EA. ; Holmgren, L.; Bork, P.; Misumi, DJ.; McGrail, SH.; Dussault, BJ.; Perou, CM.; Boissy, RE.; Duyk, GM.; Spritz, RA. & Moore, KJ. (1996). Identification and mutation analysis of the complete gene for Chediak-Higashi syndrome. *Nat Genet*, vol. 14, pp. 307–311.

Notarangelo, LD.; Miao, CH. & Ochs, HD. (2008). Wiskott-Aldrich syndrome. *Curr Opin Hematol*, vol. 15, No. 1, pp. 30-6.

Nurden, P.; Jandrot-Perrus, M.; Combrié, R.; Winckler, J.; Arocas, V.; Lecut, C.; Pasquet, JM.; Kunicki, TJ. & Nurden, AT. (2004). Severe deficiency of glycoprotein VI in a patient with gray platelet syndrome. *Blood*, vol. 104, No. 1, pp. 107-14.

Nurden, AT. (2005). Qualitative disorders of platelets and megakaryocytes. *J Throm Haemost*, vol. 3, pp. 1773-82.

Nurden, AT. & Nurden, P. (2007). The gray platelet syndrome: clinical spectrum of the disease. *Blood Rev*, vol. 21, No. 1, pp. 21-36.

Nurden, P. & Nurden, AT. (2008). Congenital disorders associated with platelet dysfunctions. *Thromb Haemost*, vol. 99, pp. 253–263

Raccuglia, G. (1971). Gray platelet syndrome. A variety of qualitative platelet disorder. *Am J Med*, vol. 51, No. 6, pp. 818-28.

Pham, A. & Wang, J. (2007). Bernard-Soulier Syndrome: An Inherited Platelet Disorder. *Arch Pathol Lab Med*, vol. 131, pp. 1834–1836.

Ramasamy, I. (2004). Inherited bleeding disorders: disorders of platelet adhesion and aggregation. *Critical Reviews in Oncology/Hematology*, vol. 49, pp. 1–35.

Rosenberg, N.; Yatuv, R.; Orion, Y.; Zivelin, A.; Dardik, R.; Peretz, H. & Seligsohn, U. (1997). Glanzmann thrombasthenia caused by an 11.2-kb deletion in the glycoprotein IIIa (beta-3) is a second mutation in Iraqi Jews that stemmed from a distinct founder. *Blood*, vol. 89, pp. 3654-3662.

Sabri, S.; Foudi, A.; Boukour, S.; Franc, B.; Charrier, S.; Jandrot-Perrus, M.; Farndale, RW.; Jalil, A.; Blundell, MP.; Cramer, EM.; Louache, F.; Debili, N.; Thrasher, AJ. & Vainchenker, W. (2006). Deficiency in the Wiskott-Aldrich protein induces premature proplatelet formation and platelet production in the bone marrow compartment. *Blood*, vol. 108, No. 1, pp. 134-40.

Sachs, UJ.; Kroll, H.; Matzdorff, AC.; Berghofer, H.; Lopez, JA. & Santoso, S. (2003). Bernard-Soulier syndrome due to the homozygous Asn-45Ser mutation in GPIX: an unexpected, frequent finding in Germany. *Br J Haematol,* vol. 123, No. 1, pp. 127-131.

Sandrock, K. & Zieger, B. (2010). Current Strategies in Diagnosis of Inherited Storage Pool Defects. *Transfus Med Hemother,* vol. 37, No. 5, pp. 248–258.

Sato, A. (1955). Chédiak and Higashi's disease: probable identity of a new leucocytal anomaly (Chédiak) and congenital gigantism of peroxidase granules (Higashi). *Tohoku J Exp Med,* vol. 61, pp. 201-10.

Savoia, A.; Balduini, CL.; Savino, M.; Noris, P.; Del Vecchio, M.; Perrotta, S.; Belletti, S & Poggi Iolascon, A. (2001). Autosomal dominant macrothrombocytopenia in Italy is most frequently a type of heterozygous Bernard-Soulier syndrome. *Blood*, vol. 97, No. 5, pp. 1330-1335.

Schallreuter, KU.; Frenk, E.; Wolfe, LS.; Witkop, CJ. & Wood, JM. (1993). Hermansky-Pudlak syndrome in a Swiss population. *Dermatology*, vol. 187, pp. 248–256.

Shapiro, AD. (1999). Platelet function disorders, in *Treatment of hemophilia,* Sam Schulman, pp. 1-11, World Federation of Hemophilia, Canada

Sherer, DM. & Lerner, R. (1999). Glanzmann's thrombasthenia in pregnancy: a case and review of the literature. *Am J Perinatol*, vol. 16, No. 6, pp. 297-301.

Simon, D;, Kunicki, T. & Nugent, D. (2008). Platelet function defects. *Haemophilia,* vol. 14, No. 6, pp. 1240-9.

Strassel, C.; Eckly, A.; Léon, C.; Petitjean, C.; Freund, M.; Cazenave, JP.; Gachet, C & Lanza, F. (2009). Intrinsic impaired proplatelet formation and microtubule coil assembly of megakaryocytes in a mouse model of Bernard-Soulier syndrome. *Haematologica.* vol. 94, No. 6, pp. 800-810.

Veljkovic, DK.; Rivard, GE.; Diamandis, M.; Blavignac, J.; Cramer-Borde, EM. & Hayward, CPM. (2009). Increased expression of urokinase plasminogen activator in Quebec platelet disorder is linked to megakaryocyte differentiation. *Blood*, vol. 113, pp. 1535-1542

Wagner, CL.; Mascelli, MA.; Neblock, DS.; Weisman, HF.; Colle, BS. & Jordan, RE. (1996). Analysis of GP IIb–IIIa receptor number by quantitation of 7E3 binding to human platelets. *Blood*, vol. 88, pp. 907–914.

Ware, J. (1998). Molecular analysis of the platelet glycoprotein Ib-IX-V receptor. *Thromb Haemost*, vol. 79, pp. 466-478.

White, JG. (1979). Ultrastructural studies of the gray platelet syndrome. Am J Pathol, vol. 95, No. 2, pp. 445-62.

Wiskott, A. (1937). Familiärer, angeborener Morbus Werlhofii? *Monatsschr Kinderheilkd,* vol. 68, pp. 212-216.

Witkop, CJ.; Nunez, BM.; Rao, GH.; Gaudier, F.; Summers, CG.; Shanahan, F.; Harmon, KR.; Townsend, D.; Sedano, HO.; King, RA.; et al: Albinism and Hermansky-Pudlak syndrome in Puerto Rico. *Bol Asoc Med P R,* vol. 82, pp. 333–339.

20

Prader–Willi Syndrome, from Molecular Testing and Clinical Study to Diagnostic Protocols

Maria Puiu[1] and Natalia Cucu[2]
[1]"Victor Babes" University of Medicine and Pharmacy Timisoara,
Department of Medical Genetics,
[2]University of Bucharest, Faculty of Biology,
Department of Genetics/Epigenetic Research Center
Romania

1. Introduction

Prader-Willi syndrome (PWS) is a complex and fascinating human disease, whose patophisiological characteristics are still the targets of research in teams that can afford multidisciplinary approaches for seeking the link between the genetic, epigenetic and phenotypic aspects. The genetic complexity of the PWS chromosomal region, 15q11-q13, relies on the multiple clustered imprinted genes, alternative splice variants, gene duplications and variant copies, that control the epigenetic phenomenon of the imprinting itself. These DNA and transcriptome levels are matched by the wide variety of phenotypes that involve multiple organ systems and the complexity of brain functions influenced by the expression of the PWS critical genes.

In this review a general description of the clinical diagnostic criteria will be linked with the most recent knowledge described for the structure of the 15 critical chromosomal region and candidate genes, as well as the model mechanisms explaining the interaction of the cis- and trans- genetic factors and the epigenetic ones during the establishment and maintenance of the imprinting marks that define the parental characteristic contribution to the critical genes expression. This review aims at explaining the criteria of molecular diagnosis and genetic counceling based on the techniques that are currently used and that will be used in the future approaches for the improvement of the diagnosis and treatment schemes.

PWS has been initially linked with its main characteristic phenotype, the obesity, and therefore was the first described genetic human obesity syndrome. The main etiology of this disease included: gross hyperphagia, hypogonadism and growth hormone deficiency, indicating hypothalamic dysfunction. A neurodegenerative aspect was also appreciated as a major contributor to the complex PWS phenotype. Recent epidemiological study proved that PWS is a rare disease with an estimated incidence of about 1 in 25 000 births, and a population prevalence of about 1 in 50 000 (Buiting, 2010). An interesting feature linked with the diagnosis and the treatment impact is that this syndrome develops during late development of neonate. Initially, the signs like hypotonia had not suggested a suspicion for PWS, nor the consideration of further clinical and molecular cytogenetic investigations, until the moment when the feeding habits started to restore but meantime to initiate an uncontrolled rate of weight gaining leading to the obesity state and the linked illness conditions. The wrong concept according to which the genetic disorder involves solely genetic modifications that may be monitored at the chromosomal level has not been proved by the classical cytogenetic approaches : the affected child commonly presents a normal karyotype and rarely a translocation or a gross deletion; this fact was misleading the medical geneticians towards wrong conclusions and hence incorrect strategy for treatment and social integration.

The initial genetic investigations on PWS and its sister syndrome, the Angelmann syndrome (AS), have driven the research towards the first proof of the epigenetic regulation of the gene function: AS was detected by the same genetic defect, a deletion on the same critical 15q11.q13 region, however it was defined by quite different phenotypes. This fact lead to the conclusion that beyond the identical affected chromosomal region there were involved certain other factors, such as the parental allele contribution to the candidate genes expression. Once the specific epigenetic marking of the allele for their expression was discovered in terms of the DNA methylation, the corresponding histone modifications and RNA processing, the research in this domain has been oriented towards new clues that could link the two types of hereditary information: genetic information, defined by either deletions as cis-acting factors and those coded by the single nucleotide polymorphisms (SNPs) as trans-acting factors, and the epigenetic information used in the process of imprinting. Both genetic and epigenetic approaches resulted finally in a more correct estimation of the types of defect frequencies and focused also on the right moment for diagnosis, and the right tissue type for the imprinted gene expression. Once the molecular mechanism of the defect establishment and maintenance is designed based on aberrant germ cells reprogramming during the parental meiosis, then after fertilization, during embryogenesis and fetal development, an improvement of the genetic counceling activities may be envisaged in the future for the patient and genitors' benefit.

Based on the newly established relationship between genotype-epigenotype and phenotye, new approach of the clinical diagnosis was initiated, that considers actually the dynamics of the epigenome reprogramming and hence the spatio-temporal variation in gene expression, that is imposed by the epigenetic control of cytodifferentiation processes. It became commonly apparent that clinical features of PWS appear during different developmental moments: severe hypotonia and consequently feeding difficulties concomitant with low birth weight- in early infancy, followed by hyperphagia and obesity - starting in early childhood. These general characteristics are accompanied by certain common features that determined the establishment of consensus diagnostic clinical criteria for PWS (Holm et al., 1993; Cassidy and Driscoll, 2009). They include both physical features such as facial appearance (like almond-shaped eyes, triangular mouth and narrow bifrontal diameter), short stature and small hands and feet, and distinctive behavioral traits due to mild and moderate mental retardation (such as temper tantrums, obsessive-compulsive characteristics and psychiatric disturbance as well as motor milestones and language development delay). The score includes also features that appear later during the child development; these are defects in sexual development (genital hypoplasia that may result in hypogonadism in both sexes and incomplete pubertal development and frequent infertility) and the obesity linked

features, among which the most frequent one is the non-insulin-dependent diabetes mellitus (Buiting, 2010).
Structural characteristics of the critical chromosomal 15q11.q13 region explain its genomic instability and its special behavior during the primary imprinting process, during the genitor's meiosis and germ line establishment, followed by the secondary imprinting process, that occurs during the affected offspring PCG (primordial germ cells) determination and germ cells specialization.
The major determinant feature of the critical chromosomal region is the abundant imprinted genes arranged in clusters together with numerous variable sequences (CNVs) (such as interstitial microdeletions, duplications, triplications) that are flanking the critical breakpoints (BPs) defining the around 5 Mb deletions. Due to the presence of these critical instability regions on chromosome 15, another critical region, named IC for imprinting control region, apparently contributed to defects that determines wrong marking of parental alleles and hence their gene expression in all somatic cells of the offspring. The structure and control of functions in this region will be discussed below.

2. PWS genetics

A genetic approach of the PWS includes the description of the candidate genes and their expression which is epigenetically controlled based on the parental contribution. PWS arises when the lack of contribution from the paternally derived chromosome 15q11-q13 occurs (Goldstone, 2003). Normally, candidate genes for PWS in this region are imprinted and silenced on the maternally inherited chromosome. The causes of the lack of contribution are multiple in PWS: either paternal alleles are sequence defective (mutant or missing) or silenced by wrong, repressive epigenetic marking. The imprinting marking determines in normal, healthy individuals, the expression of critical genes only from the paternal allele. Paternally expressed genes are particularly important in hypothalamic development, this fact explaining the spectrum of neuroendocrine disturbances in PWS. These genes are located in the centromeric part of the 15q11q13 region and are as follows: MKRN3, MAGEL2, NDN, C15orf2, SNURF-SNRPN and the C/D box small nucleolar (sno)-RNA genes. The latter genes are represented by numerous, so-called SNORD genes, previously named HB (human brain) II genes (SNORD107, previously named HBII-436; SNORD64, previously named HBII-13; SNORD108, previously named HBII-437; SNORD109A, previously named HBII- 438A; SNORD116, previously named HBII- 85; SNORD115, previously named HBII- 52 and SNORD109B, previously named HBII- 438B) (Buiting, 2010). These genes are differentiated based on their repetitive state: SNORD 115 and SNORD116 genes are present as multiple copy clusters, whereas the other SNORD genes are single copy genes. The snoRNA genes in the critical chromosomal 15 region might have a role in modulating alternative splicing and thus be involved in the modification of mRNA (Cavaille et al., 2000; Bazeley et al., 2008). Recent investigations revealed that SNORD116 gene is the minimal region linked with the PWS phenotypes (Buiting, 2010).
The most frequent genetic causes linked with the paternal contribution are large (a typical 5-7 Mb) chromosomal de novo interstitial deletions (either type I or type II deletions detected in around 70%, of PWS cases) and the double maternal chromosomal contribution by uniparental maternal disomy (UPD), with 22% frequency (Fig.1). With much lower

frequency were detected paternal chromosomal translocations (less that 1% of cases). Other explanations of the lack of paternal contribution are grouped in the class of epigenetic defects that impaired the imprinting process (around 3% of cases).

In Fig. 1 a schematic view of the human chromosomal region 15q11q13 the genes expressed from different alleles are differently colored; there is evidenced also the localization of two common deletions [del (15)(q11-q13)] (class or type I and class II deletions) and their localization. Such deletions include the entire imprinted domain plus certain non-imprinted (green boxes) genes.

Different allelic localizations of such large deletions demonstrated the involvement of the parent of origin marking by epigenetic factors. In PWS, they are always on the paternal allele, whereas in AS, they occur on the maternal chromosome. The deletion regions are flanked by the three break-points (BP1, BP2 and BP3) (Fig.1). In certain rare cases even larger deletions were detected extending telomeric region including the more distal break-points, named BP4 and BP5 (Sahoo et al., 2007).

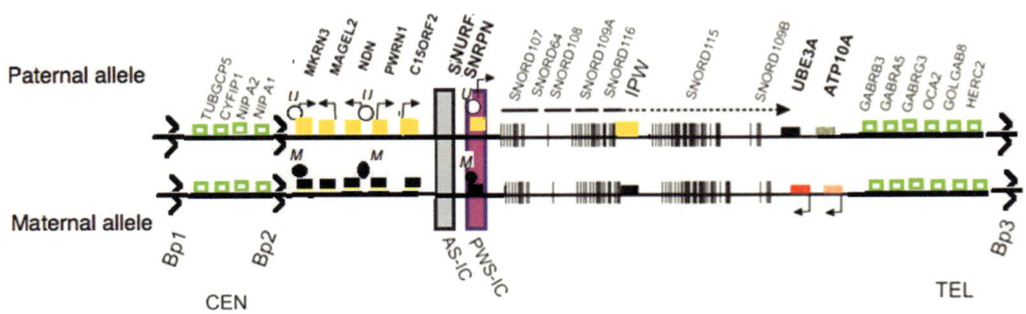

Fig. 1. A map of the 15q11–q13 critical region. Imprinted, paternally-expressed genes are represented by yellow boxes, while imprinted, maternally-expressed genes are represented by red boxes. Black boxes represent imprinted (silenced) genes and green boxes respresent genes expressed biallelically. Dashed and dotted lines demarcate the snoRNA clusters. The PWS- and AS-ICs are represented by two differently colored domains. Black circles indicate methylated (M) CpG islands and the white circles the unmethylated (U) CpG islands. BP1, BP2, and BP3 are the common deletion breakpoints and are represented by zigzag lines. (Chamberlain and Lalande 2010)

The structure of these BPs consists of repetitive blocks of 250-400 kb, that explains their instability and hence their role in non-homologous recombination events during parental meiosis (Christian et al., 1998, Amos-Landgraf et al., 1999). It was demonstrated that the deletions can occur via cross-over interchromosomal (between the two homologous chromosomes) or intrachromosomal (between different regions of one chromosome 15) events (Carrozzo et al., 1997; Robinson et al., 1998).

The causes of maternal uniparental disomy [upd(15)mat] occurrence was ascribed to maternal meiotic non-disjunction followed by mitotic loss of the paternal chromosome 15, during fertilization (Buiting, 2010).

PWS epigenetics investigates the causes of the imprinting defects and hence the occurrence of the lack of expression of the paternally inherited genes. In patients with PWS and an imprinting defect, the paternal chromosome carries a wrong (maternal) imprint in terms of the epigenetic marks on DNA and histones or noncoding RNA (wrong distribution of DNA methylated cytidine residues in the paternal and maternal genes concomitant with wrong histone modifcation and ncRNA expression). In PWS, these epigenetic modifications are repressive not only for the maternal allele, but also, in a wrong way for the paternally expressed genes in the 15q11q13 region.

Much of research has been performed in order to find the causes of such non-genetic defect. This epigenetic factor in PWS may be or may be not accompanied by deletions. The first situation was rarely observed (8-15%), but the second one is more frequent (85% in PWS cases).

The discovery of cases of critical DNA regions containing both small deletions and the imprinting defect led to the definition of a bipartite imprinting controlling (IC) region: its role is regulation in cis- the process of imprint resetting and imprint maintenance in the whole critical chromosomal region 15q11q13 (Sutcliffe et al., 1994; Buiting et al., 1995). Thus the paternal-only expression of MKRN3, NDN, and SNURF-SNRPN genes is regulated by the parent-of-origin epigenetic modification of the promoter regions of these genes. Another parental expressed gene, C15orf2 has a special feature of expression: it has been reported to be biallelically expressed in testis, however, in brain its expression is restricted to the paternal allele (Wawrzik et al., 2010). A recent review of the genetics and epigenetics in PWS revealed about 21 IC-deletions in patients with PWS (Buiting, 2010).

The most complex gene in the critical chromosome 15 region is linked with the IC region and is considered SNURF- SNRPN gene. IC contains the major transcriptional start site of SNURF- SNRPN gene. It consists of 10 exons which encodes in fact two different proteins: exons 1-3 encode SNURF (SNRPN upstream reading frame), a small polypeptide of unknown function (Gray et al., 1999), while exons 4-10 encodes a small nuclear (SmN) ribonucleoprotein named SNRPN, a spliceosomal protein involved in mRNA splicing in the brain (Ozcelik et al., 1992). SNURF gene, along with upstream noncoding exons, has been considerred the major site of imprinting defects, because disruption of this gene leads to altered imprinting of SNRPN and many other 15q11-q13 imprinted genes. However, numerous 5′ and 3′ exons of SNURF- SNRPN gene identified up to now do not encode proteins and they occur in many splice forms of the primary transcript (Dittrich et al., 1996; Farber et al., 1999). Exon 1 and the promoter region of this complex genetic locus overlap with the IC. Also, as it has been mentioned earlier, the SNURF-SNRPN region also serves as a host for all snoRNA genes encoded within its introns. These genes lack a direct methylation imprint, but their imprinted expression is indirectly regulated by the same SNURF-SNRPN methylation (Horsthemke and Buiting, 2008; Buiting, 2010).

The IC region investigations resulted in its definition by two critical elements that are named the smallest regions of overlap (SRO) that control the imprinting process in PWS and AS: the AS-SRO and the PWS-SRO (Buiting et al., 1995; Buiting, 2010). The 4.3 kb long PWS-SRO overlaps with the SNURF-SNRPN exon 1/promoter region (Ohta et al., 1996b). This IC element is required for the maintenance of paternal imprint during early embryonic developments (El-Maarri et al., 2001).

The cases of imprinting defects with no IC deletion are classified in a subgroup of cases defined by primary epimutations or epigenetic modification (Buiting et al., 2003; Horsthemke and Buiting, 2008).

3. Clinically PWS diagnosed cases in Romanian population

Diagnostic testing: approaching classical genetic and epigenetic methods, as well as advanced combined sequencing and epigenetic methods, in a study of a cohort of 17 clinically PWS diagnosed cases in Romanian population (Table 1).

Nr crt	Clinical diagnosis	Molecular tests confirmation			Classical cytogenetic confirmation
		MSPCR	FISH	MLPA	Karyotype
1	PWS	-	-	-	-
2	PWS	-	-	-	-
3	PWS	-	-	-	-
4	PWS	-	-	-	-
5	PWS	-	-	-	-
6	PWS	-	-	-	-
7	PWS	-	-	-	-
8	PWS	+	+	del NDN, SNRPN, UBE3A	-
9	PWS	-	-	-	-
10	PWS	+	+	-	-
11	PWS	-	-	-	-
12	PWS	+	+	-	-
13	PWS	-	-	-	-
14	PWS	+	-	Nondeleted NDN, SNRPN, UBE3A	-
15	PWS	+	+	-	-
16	PWS	+	-	Nondeleted NDN, SNRPN, UBE3A	-
17	PWS	-	-	-	-
18	PWS	-	-	-	-
19	PWS	-	-	-	-

Nr crt	Clinical diagnosis	Molecular tests confirmation			Classical cytogenetic confirmation
		MSPCR	FISH	MLPA	Karyotype
20	PWS	-	-	-	-
21	PWS	+	+	-	-
22	PWS	+	+	-	-
23	PWS	-	-	-	-
24	PWS	+	+	-	-
25	PWS	-	-	-	-
26	PWS	-	-	-	-
27	PWS	+	+	del NDN, SNRPN, UBE3A, TUBGCP5, MKRN3, APBA2	-
28	PWS	+	-	-	-
29	PWS	+	+	-	-
30	PWS	-	-	-	-

Table 1. Patient Sample characterstics: clinical, karyotipical and molecular aspects

3.1 Clinical methods

The most obvious features observed were obesity and mental retardation and the rest of criteria being variable. Our survey in Romanian population resulted in a DNA bank designed to characterize the PWS features. Initial surveys contributed to gathering 13 females and 7 males, between 6 month and 28 years old. Positive clinical diagnosis of PWS was based on major and minor criteria, the minimum diagnostic score being 3 - up to age 3 and 5 – for patients older than 3 (up to the adult age) (Gunay-Aygun M et al., 2001, Holm VA et al., 1993, P. Goldstone et al., 2008, Suzanne B Cassidy and Daniel J Driscoll, 2008). Consequently, clinical diagnosis of PWS has been established based on characteristic clinical features that differ with age (Ledbetter DH and Engel E, 1995, Ohta T et al., 1999). In the newborn infant, the suggestive feature remained hypotonia; it resulted from the history in our study (patients aged 6 month to 7 years – 6 cases and more than 14 years – 11 cases) (Table 2 in Annexes).

Obesity, moderate mental retardation, behavioral disturbances related to food and learning difficulties are present in all studied cases. Facial features of PWS (periorbital fullness, almond-shaped and down-slanting palpebral fissures, malar hypoplasia, down-turned mouth corners and thin upper lip) are also present (Figs.2, 3, 4).

3.2 Classical genetic approach

Karyotyping- for the monitoring of the variations in chromosomal morphology as a result of DNA sequence modifications (deletions, translocations) is the classical genetic approach. Initially, the gold standard was thought to be the karyotype. But this classical chromosome investigation commonly did not reveal any of the complex genetic and epigenetic defects lately described for PWS patients (Fig. 3). Also, only very rare paternal translocations and even more rare deletions have been detected in the restricted HBII-85 region, more recently.

A

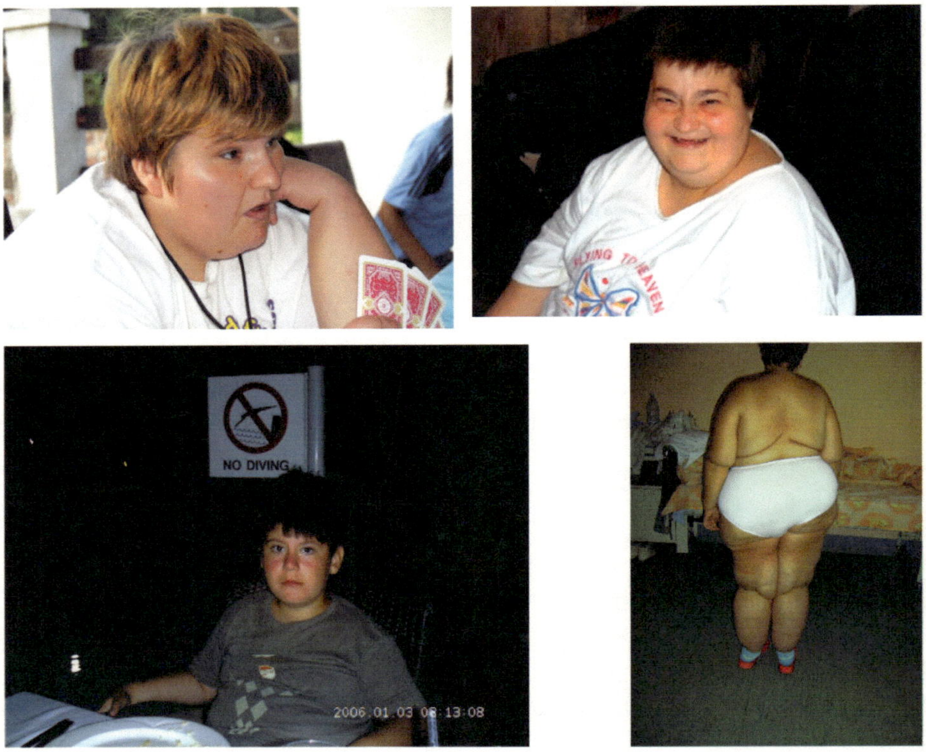

B

Fig. 2. A,B. Typical features with PWS cases. A. Facial features of the Prader Willi syndrome (periorbital fullness, almond-shaped palpebral fissures, malar hypoplasia, down-turned mouth corners and thin upper lip). FISH test identified 15q deletion in these patients with typical clinical features. B. Short stature and typical feet and hands dimensions. Obesity is another typical feature with all represented cases

3.3 Molecular tests

Confirmation of the clinical phenotypes has been realized by approaching molecular methods. Molecular cytogenetic approach (FISH fluorescence in situ hybridization technique) brought numerous PWS cases that presented deletions as detected by fluorescent probes in FISH. Further investigations by this method revealed an interesting, non-mendelian transmittance aspect with PWS, that required another molecular approach ,based on the epigenetic, methylation method. The need for discussing the recurrence risk with any of these situations determined a new, more precise approach, by sequencing methods (MLPA or even MS-MLPA) for the detection of the microdeletions as causes of the impaired IC role in imprinting control concomitant with the estimation of the methylation status on paternal allele.

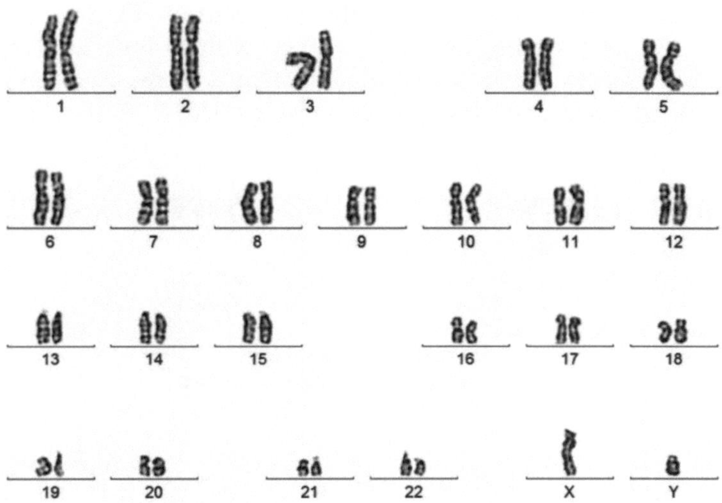

Fig. 3. A normal karyotype frequently obtained for the PWS patients

A more efficient and correct scheme of molecular testing have been suggested in the recent literature that included the following sequence of techniques in order to reveal not only the causes of genetic and epigenetic defects, but meantime to decipher the molecular mechanism involved in the establishment of the birth defect:

- Methylation analysis for the general diagnosis (about 99% cases confirmed);
- FISH detection of deletions for the establishment of the disease mechanism
- Sequencing methods that were imposed in the cases when FISH was negative and suspicion for UPD had to be solved- MLPA and MS-MLPA.

3.3.1 Methylation analysis

The detection of methylation status solely at the SNRPN locus may be performed by using methylation specific PCR (MS-PCR) . This approach confirms a diagnosis but provides no further information regarding the disease mechanism requiring follow up studies (FISH and/or microsatellite analysis).

The(PCR)-based assay MS-PCR allows rapid diagnosis of PWS and AS. Methylated cytosines in the CpG dinucleotide are resistant to chemical modification by sodium bisulfite. In contrast, bisulfite treatment converts all unmethylated cytosines to uracil. Based on this differential effect, the bisulfite modified DNA sequence of a methylated allele was successfully distinguished from that of an unmethylated allele using 2 sets of allele-specific primer pairs: a methylated allele-specific primer pair (M) and an unmethylated allele-specific primer pair (U). Bisulfite-modified DNA from patients with PWS amplified only with the M pair while modified DNA from patients with AS amplified only with the U pair (Jones et al. 1997) (Fig. 4). The results of MSPCR tests performed on clinically diagnosed individuals are represented in Figures 5 a,b.

This method has the following significant advantages over conventional analysis using methylation-sensitive enzymes and Southern blotting: (1) MSPCR can be completed in 2 days. Rapid turnaround of the test result may be especially useful when evaluating hypotonic newborn infants among whom the incidence of PWS is high [Gillessen-Kaesbach et al., 1995]; (2) Testing can be performed with as little as 50 ng of genomic DNA. Thus, in addition to whole blood, other potential sources of genomic DNA for analysis include dried blood spots and oral cell smears; (3) MSPCR does not require use of radioactivity.

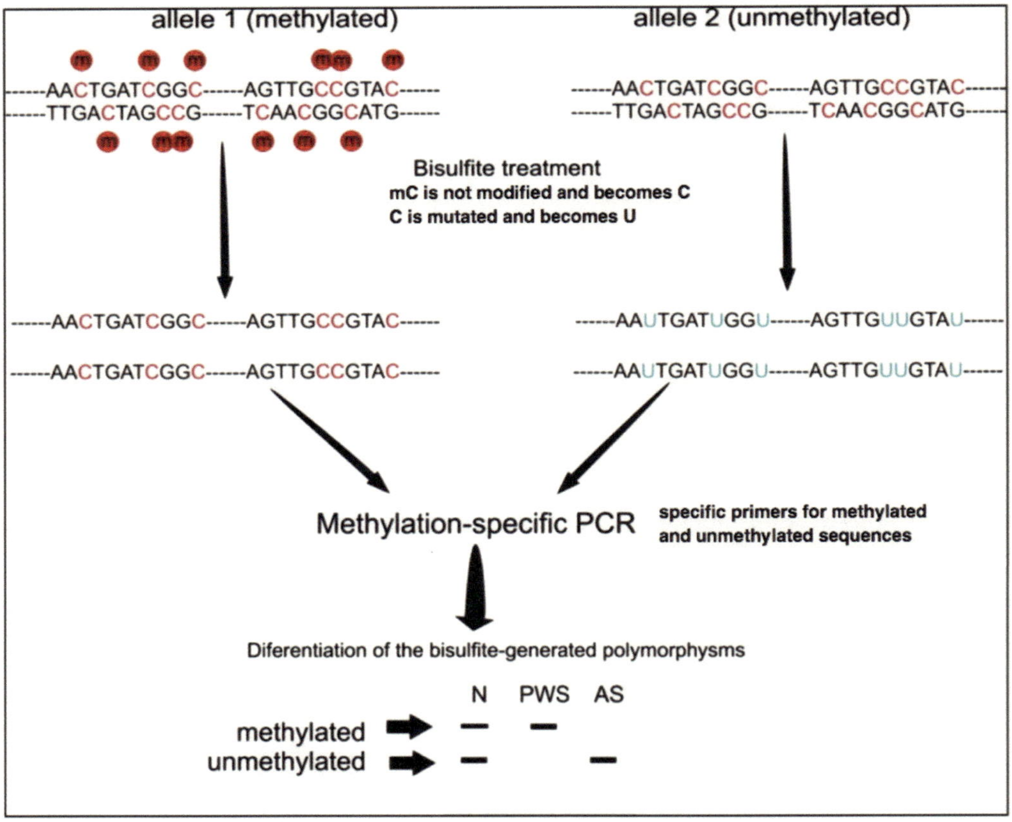

Fig. 4. The scheme of the steps in the methylation specific PCR protocol. It includes the mutagenesis by bisulfite conversion treatment, followed by the converted DNA purification and the PCR amplification of the methylated/unmethylated DNA fragment. The amplicon resulted from the amplification of the fragment flanked by the U primers stands for the fragment that was unmethylated. It is detected after its electrophoresis and its visualization in agarose gels by ethidium bromide in uv light

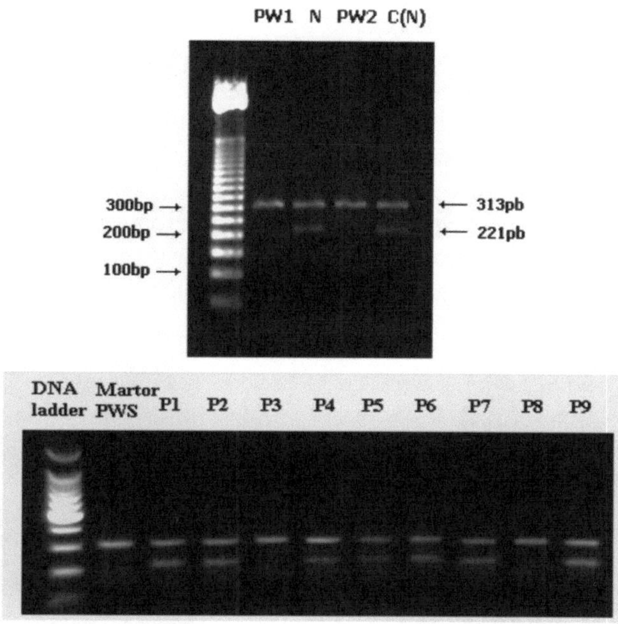

Fig. 5. a,b MSPCR analysis based on the distribution of the two MSPCR products (amplicons) of 313 and 221bp corresponding to the methylated (imprinted) maternal allele and, respectively, the unmethylated paternal allele. "PW" - individuals have an electrophoresis pattern specific for PWS - maternal only 313bp MSPCR product; "N" - individuals suspected of PWS based on clinical diagnosis,but not confirmed by methylation test- both MSPCR products are present - "C(N)"- normal individuals used as control, both MSPCR products are present

In Table 1 there are represented the results of our methylation analysis for the confirmation of the clinically diagnosed cases. From 3o clinically diagnosed cases, only 12 have been confirmed by methylation analysis. And among these latter ones, only 9 presented deletions, as confirmed by FISH method.

3.3.2 FISH method

Fluorescence in situ hybridization technique offers the possibility to use fluorochromes in order to specifically mark individual chromosomes over their entire length or defined chromosome regions in meta- and interphase preparations (Chevret et al. 2000); their presence is proved by using fluorescence microscopy. The first step in FISH procedures is the procurement of cells. Unlike many other chromosomal visualization techniques, FISH can be conducted on currently dividing or terminally differentiated cells. Cells are grown to a specific culture density and fixed with formaldehyde and placed on a functionalized glass slide. This slide is then allowed to dry, dehydrated with ethanol, and then treated with the hybridization buffer. DNA probes are then added and the slide is allowed to incubate. This gives the DNA probes enough time to hybridize with their complementary sequences.

Following hybridization, the slides are allowed to air dry and then are examined under microscope (Langedijk et al. 1995).
Many PWS/AS deletions are not detectable by G-banding. Even at higher band levels, variable G-banding quality, differences in homologue condensation/splitting of band 15q12, and possible presence of extra clinically benign G-bands in this region made interpretation difficult [Hoo et al., 1990; Ludowese et al., 1991). Unreliability of G-banding for deletion detection in the region 15q11-q13 in comparison with FISH has been well documented[Delach et al., 1994; Butler, 1995; Bettio et al., 1995; Smith et al., 1995). The development of molecular probes for the Prader-Willi syndrome and Angelman's syndrome region of 15(ql1-13) enabled alternate or complementary means for the detection of deletions in patients (Chan et al., 1993; Butler, 1990; Knoll et al., 1989).

A. Deletion in PWS/AS critical region B. Normal PWS/AS critical region

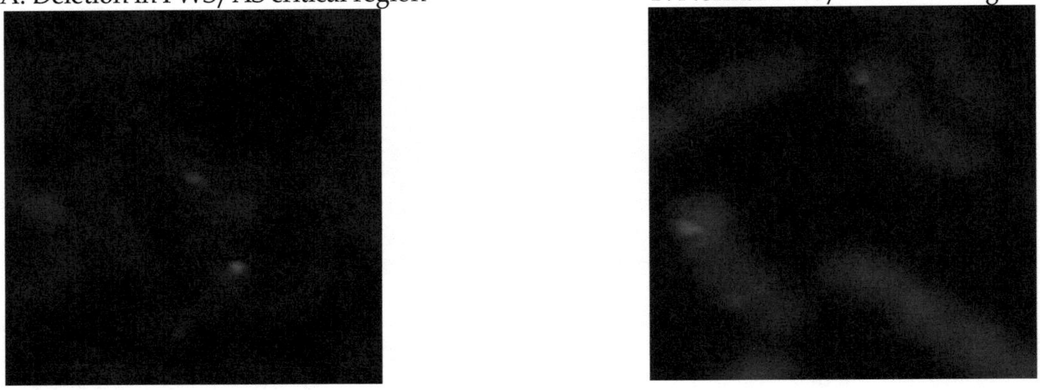

Fig. 6. FISH (fluorescent in situ hybridization for the region 15q11-q13) results for A-PWS case and B- normal case. The probes used: LSI for the common deletion D15S10 (spectrum orange/PML) and spectrum orange/CEP15 spectrum green for the common chromosome 15 mark (centromere) (Vysis, Abbott inc.)

For FISH analysis, probes for loci D15Sl1, SNRPN, D15S10, and GABRB3 within 15qll-13, and for identification of the chromosome 15 homologues an internal control probe for locus PML at 15q22, were co-hybridized to chromosomes following protocols provided by the manufacturer (Oncor, Gaithersburg, MD). Although it's an expensive and time-consuming, this method confirms the diagnosis of ~ 70% PWS and AS , and reveals the mosaic and translocation cases.
Patients with clinical features suggestive of Prader-Willi Syndrome and confirmed by MSPCR were tested for deletions of 15q11-q13 region and the results are illustrated in Figures 6 A and B.

3.3.3 Sequencing methods

The detection of microdeletions or duplications (CNVs) in critical 15 chromosomal region may be performed by classical MLPA method. MLPA is a technique based on semiquantitative genetic molecular method, initially developed by Schouten group (Shouten et al., 2002) while attempting to target 40 genomic loci containing variable copy numbers (deletions, duplications, triplications) by using a pair of probes for each target. Each probe contains a universal primer sequence and a sequence that is complementary to the target

DNA, named hybridization sequence. Both probes are hybridized adjacent one for the other avoiding the gap formation. When the probes are correctly hybridized to the target sequence, they are ligated by a thermostable enzyme (named ligase). Later the PCR primers contribute to the amplification of the linked probes during the exponential process that leads to a unique molecule. One of the primers is fluorescent labeled releasing a specific color, and therefore its amplification products to be visualized and thus detected and registered. Capillary electrophoresis enable after this the analysis of the PCR products and their comparison based on their dimensions.

In our first approach the MRC-Holland kit SALSA MLPA P245-A2 was used on the Applied Biosystem sequencer. It contained probes for the genes coding for: UBE3A, Necdin (NDN) and (2 probes) SNRPN (for two different regions a,b). The reactions were performed according to the producer's instructions and the DNA quantity was 150µg genomic DNA in sufficient concentration, optimum 75-100ng/ml) in a volume of 5µl water. The identification of the altered peak height is basically the principle for the estimation of deletions. This is done by comparing the MLPA profiles obtained from the patients and the controls (parents). Softgenetics, LLC, State College, PA USA software was used in order to realize this comparisons.

In Figures 7 and 8 there are represented the normalized profiles of two individuals. Each peak represents the amplicon signal obtained from the corresponding exon, that is designed on X axis. The Y axis indicates the fluorescent intensity and the arrows indicate the positions of the four genomic targets on chromosome 15, analyzed by the kit.

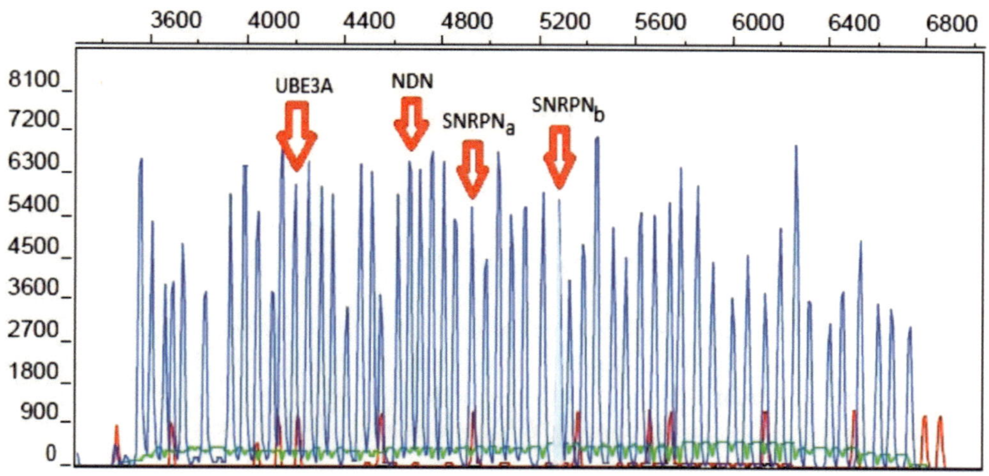

Fig. 7. The MLPA diagram obtained for a PWS patient, clinically diagnosed and confirmed by the molecular methylation test – the normal peak height does not suggest a deletion: UBE3A(15q12) – 6103, NDN (15q11.2) - 6593, SNRPN a (15q12) - 5653, SNRPN b (15q12) – 5802

The MLPA test is essentially a PCR technique. The characteristics that make it distinct from the other common techniques are as follows: 1. The amplification is dependent on the ligation process, as the unligated oligomers are not amplified; 2. High ligation temperatures assure the specificity; 3. Amplification is performed in multiplex systems, thus enabling the analysis of up to 50 genomic targets, by a single test. This results in an effective low cost of the test, similarly to a mean high-throughput (HT) test. This type of analysis differs from the RT-PCR as the primers are in excess to the template, and the amplification is performed on a linear domain; therefore the number of generated amplicons is proportional with the template (the ligation products).

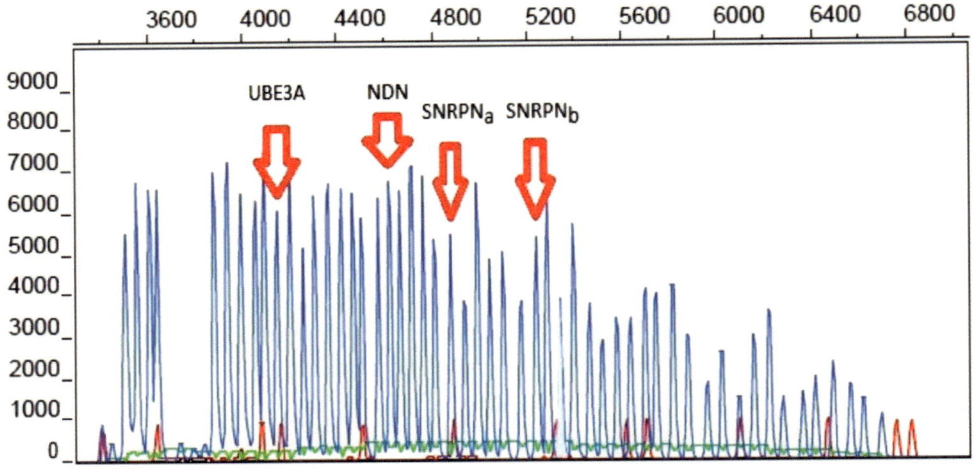

Fig. 8. The MLPA diagram obtained for a parent (normal control-mother); the normal height of the peak does not suggest a deletion: UBE3A(15q12) – 7530, NDN (15q11.2) - 6790, SNRPN a (15q12) - 5464, SNRPN b (15q12) - 5455

Due to its low cost and excellent sensibility and to the easy steps, the MLPA test is actually becoming a frequent tool approached in research and routine diagnosis. One negative aspect is however linked with the fact that it is not enough informative regarding the localization of the duplicated sequences as compared with the original copy, nor regarding their orientation.

The analysis of the genomic instability on chromosome 15 by this method resulted in the following conclusions: the chosen samples corresponded to a patient that was confirmed clinically and by molecular MSPCR and to his mother (control). The lack of the deletion in SNRPN region suggested an imprinting defect with no deletion, thus it is suggested a primary imprinting defect.

A more complete molecular approach is presently running in our investigations and would further involve the following test for a correct conclusion regarding the mechanism that led to the imprinting defect, a conclusion valuable for the genetic councelling: the confirmation or exclusion of UPD by microsatellite detection testing and the use of other, more informative MS-MLPA kits, in order to target the unique HBII-85 sequence, presently considered as characteristic for the PWS phenotypes. The simultaneous assessment of methylation status and genomic dosage at numerous sites across the 15q11-q13 region may be performed by the use of methylation sensitive multiplex ligation-dependent probe amplification (MS-MLPA). This approach will confirm the diagnosis and further identify the presence of a causative deletion. However, in the absence of a deletion follow up studies (microsatellite analysis) are required to distinguish between UPD and an imprinting defect (Ramsden et al. 2010).

Trans factors influencing the imprinting process through the maintenance of proper cell methylome, such as the polymorphism in the critical gene *mthfr* (a gene encoding methylenetetrahydrofolate reductase) are also reported in numerous literature. Our analysis on three families with one PWS proband reveals only one affected family, where the mother was a carrier of a homozigous C677T mutation; the other two families had a polymorphic profile with only one father being heterozygous for the same mutation. Hence this approach need a larger individual group for the *mthfr* SNP test and perhaps the inclusion of other SNPs that may be relevant for the genome instability during gestational period or for the genome instability during the perinatal periods. The more cases will be accessible for providing the parental state of this gene, the more informative will be this algorithm for the detection of trans-factors influencing the mechanism of the imprinting process.

3.3.4 Interpretation of the analysis and further molecular approaches

For the laboratory diagnostic of the PWS one should start with the methylation analysis because it is the most sensitive method, confirming over 99% of the cases. If we start the diagnostic test with the MS-PCR (which will confirm a diagnosis but will provide no further information regarding the disease mechanism - i.e. about deletion, UPD, ID) and the result is positive, for genetic counseling, the next step is to perform a FISH or MLPA analysis (asking for deletion) and microsatellites analysis (asking for UPD) to determine the genetic mechanism and recurrence risk.

In the case the methylation test is negative, this result excludes paternal deletion, uniparental disomy and an imprinting defect result makes a diagnosis of PWS highly unlikely.

The other approach for the diagnosis of PWS is to start with the MS-MLPA assay. This test shows the methylation status and the dosage at 15q11-q13; it is more precise then MS-PCR as it investigates methylation status at several loci, thereby reducing the risk of a false positive or false negative result due to SNPs, and can also identify micro deletions in the IC as it uses many probes in the same reaction (up to 40). A positive result may indicate either a) the molecular cause of PWS is due to 15q11-q13 deletion, or b) the molecular cause of PWS may be due the molecular cause of PWS may be due to maternal UPD or an imprinting defect. Laboratories should recommend in the later case microsatellite studies to confirm or exclude UPD.

In the case the methylation test is negative (in either MS-PCR and MS-MLPA), the result will exclude paternal deletion, uniparental disomy and an imprinting defect, but to be more accurate, FISH analysis is still recommended in order to confirm a translocation or a mosaic form of the syndrome.

Our work presents the simple MLPA method that used only few kits for the detection of deletions in critical 15 chromosome region. MS-MLPA assay may confer further both information about the methylation status and the dosage at 15q11-q13, and as described earlier it has some characteristics which makes it more reliable than MS-PCR. A deletion and methylation positive result suggests the following mechanisms: a) deletion confirms a

genetic cause; b) aberrant methylation suggests either maternal UPD or an imprinting defect.
PWS deletion patients present the classical clinical picture of the disorder (fig. 2), whereas negative FISH patients are characterized by absence of the particular facies, higher IQ and moderate behavioral problems.
Because the genetics of PWS is complicated it usually takes more than one test to ascertain the diagnosis and the form of disease (Roberts SE and Thomas NS. , 2003, Roof E et al., 2000). The genetic tests used and the order depend on a number of considerations for each individual case. Genetic testing usually requires a blood sample from the child and possibly from the parents as well (Simon C Ramsden et al., 2010, Gillessen-Kaesbach G et al., 1995).
The diagnostic methods used in our study allowed PWS diagnosis confirmation in 14 out of the 17 cases. The 3 cases left will be analyzed with specific molecular tests to identify possible mutations of the imprinting center.

4. Differential diagnosis

For PWS, there were described several disorders with a phenotype that can strongly resemble PWS consisting in neonatal hypotonia and later onset obesity. Their associated mechanisms implied: (i) upd(14)mat, which can be caused by uniparental disomy 14 and imprinting defects or deletions affecting the DLK1/GTL2 locus in the chromosomal region 14q32 (Temple et al., 2007; Buiting et al. 2008); (ii) a number of other conditions associated with obesity and developmental disability including Cohen syndrome, Bardet- Biedl syndrome, Alstrom syndrome, and (iii) the 1p36 microdeletion which characterize a specific syndrome (Goldstone and Beales, 2008).

5. Conclusions

The establishment of a practical set of molecular genetic testing guidelines for PWS and AS has been succeeded through numerous experiences linked with the technical performance, the complexity of the imprinting diseases and the basic concepts linked with the hereditary transmittance.
This study is part of a research programme for PWS and Angelman Syndrome (AS) patients. The diagnostic protocol applied with this group included: physical examination, cytogenetic investigations (karyotype and FISH) and methylation analysis (after a model of Glenn CC et al., 1996, Kubota T et al., 1997).
Multidisciplinary physical examination (geneticist, pediatrician, endocrinologist, orthopedist, neuropsychiatrist, pneumologist etc) allows for the correct establishing of the clinical score (Gunay-Aygun M et al., 2001, Holm VA et al., 1993, P. Goldstone et al., 2008).
The strategy we propose for the confirmation of the clinical PWS diagnosis includes initially a methylation analysis (MSPCR). This test is used as a diagnostic instrument for PWS, because the methylation pattern is parental specific in this region (Butler MG, 19990, Carrel AL et al., 2002) and detects patients with deletions, UPD and imprinting defects that represent 99% of PWS cases.
Thus, an efficient strategy for the routine diagnosis of PWS patients includes: a) methylation analysis which allows diagnosis for 99% of PWS patients and doesn't need parental samples; b) analysis of the microsatellite genotype of the family (child, mother and father), in order to identify deletions, UPD and mutations of the imprinting center; c) in noninformative cases

or if the parental samples are not available FISH technique is indicated because it can identify deletions (~ 75% of PWS patients). Cytogenetic studies using G banding should be routinely used in all patients in whom the clinical score highly suggests the PWS diagnosis, as approximately 5% of the PWS patients reported in the literature have a chromosomal rearrangement (Cassidy SB, et al., 1994).
Even if this study group size does not allow important statistic conclusions, the results obtained differ from those reported in the specialized literature both in the proportion of PWS cases confirmed by methylation analysis (82.35% compared to 99% in the literature) (Suzanne B Cassidy, 2008, Mellissa R. W. Mann, 1999), and in the number of cases confirmed by FISH analysis (41,1% compared to 70% in the literature) (Mellissa R. W. Mann , 1999).
The explanations could be related to a particular molecular profile of PWS patients in Romania. Such studies do not exist for the moment in our country and the confirmation will be possible by investigating a larger number of patients. In patients with a normal methylation pattern and without chromosomal abnormalities, we propose a clinical reevaluation in order to establish if further molecular investigations are indicated.
Due to the variability of expression and the importance of early diagnosis awareness is growing, and looking for evocative signs increases detection rate of patients with PWS (Gunay-Aygun M, et al., 2001, Holm VA, et al., 1993).
The study showed the relative correlation between clinical score and cytogenetic and molecular confirmation of PWS. The presence of short fingers seems likely to confirm the diagnosis. The triad brachydactyly - obesity - mental retardation is easy to follow by your practitioner, for the correct guidance of suspected cases to the specialist. The differential diagnosis of PWS, Fragile X and Prader-Willi-like syndrome has to be considered, especially when laboratory workup for PWS is negative.
Clinical behavioral pattern can be of assistance in guiding the investigations and final diagnosis. Further study and experience gathered by the project team will allow a refinement of techniques and an accurate diagnosis. Knowledge of the so called "open windows" of vulnerability of the genome during the crucial stages of development and their interaction with the environment would be beneficial for the activities of deciphering the cis and trans-acting factors in the altered imprinting mechanism that may lead to establishment of optimal diagnosis and therapeutic or preventive schemes.

6. Acknowledgements

The authors are grateful for the support with funding on CNMP Grant 42-113. We regret the omission of many deserving reference citations because of the limitation on the number of references. The authors declare no competing financial interests. The graphic and testing work of molecular techniques of drd. Cosmin Arsene and Anca-Loredana Alungulese is also acknowledged.

7. References

Amos-Landgraf JM, Ji Y, Gottlieb W, Depinet T, Wandstrat AE, Cassidy SB, Driscoll DJ, Rogan PK, Schwartz S, Nicholls RD. 1999. Chromosome breakage in the Prader-Willi and Angelman syndromes involves recombination between large, transcribed repeats at proximal and distal breakpoints. Am J Hum Genet 65:370–386.

Anders O. H. Nygren, Najim Ameziane, Helena M. B. Duarte, Raymon N. C. P. Vijzelaar, Quinten Waisfisz, Corine J. Hess, Jan P. Schouten and Abdellatif Errami (2005) : Methylation-Specific MLPA (MS-MLPA): simultaneous detection of CpG methylation and copy number changes of up to 40 sequences. Nucleic Acids Research, Vol. 33, No. 14, e128

Arn PH, Williams CA, Zori RT, Driscoll DJ, Rosenblatt DS: Methylenetetrahydrofolate reductase deficiency in a patient with phenotypic findings of Angelman syndrome. Am J Med Gen 1998, 77:198-200.

Bettio D, Rizzi N, Giardino D, Grugni G, Briscioli V, Selicorni A, Carnevale F, Larizza L (1995): FISH analysis in Prader-Willi and Angelman syndrome patients. Am J Med Genet 56:224-228.

Buiting K, Gross S, Lich C, Gillessen-Kaesbach G, El-Maarri O, Horsthemke B. 2003. Epimutations in Prader-Willi and Angelman syndromes: A molecular study of 136 patients with an imprinting defect. Am J Hum Genet 72: 571–577

Buiting K, Kanber D, Martín-Subero JI, Lieb W, Terhal P, Albrecht B, Purmann S, Gross S, Lich C, Siebert R, Horsthemke B, Gillessen-Kaesbach G: Clinical features of maternal uniparental disomy 14 in patients with an epimutation and a deletion of the imprinted DLK1/GTL2 gene cluster. Hum Mutat 2008, 29:1141-6.

Buiting K. 2010. Prader–Willi syndrome and Angelman syndrome. Am J Med Genet Part C Semin Med Genet 154C:365–376.

Butler JV, Whittington JE, Holland AJ, Boer H, Clarke D, Webb T. Prevalence of, and risk factors for, physical ill-health in people with Prader-Willi syndrome: a population-based study. Dev Med Child Neurol 2002, 44:248-55

Butler MG (1995): High resolution chromosome analysis and fluorescence in situ hybridization in patients referred for Prader-Willi or Angelman syndrome. Am J Med Genet 56:420422.

Butler MG Prader-Willi syndrome: Current understanding of cause and diagnosis. Am J Med Genet, 1990, 35:319–332

Butler MG. Prader-Willi syndrome: current understanding of cause and diagnosis. Am J Med Genet 1990; 35: 319-32. Knoll JH, Nicholls RD, Magenis RE, Graham JM, Lalande M, Latt SA. Angelman and Prader-Willi syndromes share a common chromosome 15 deletion but differ in parental origin of the deletion. AmJMed Genet 1989; 32: 285-90.

Carrel AL, Myers SE, Whitman BY, Allen DB. Benefits of long-term GH therapy in Prader-Willi syndrome: a 4-year study. J Clin Endocrinol Metab 2002, 87:1581-5

Cassidy SB, Devi A, Mukaida C. Aging in Prader-Willi syndrome: 22 patients over age 30 years. Proc Greenwood Genet Center 1994, 13:102-3

Cassidy SB, Forsythe M, Heeger S, Nicholls RD, Schork N, Benn P, Schwartz S (1997): Comparison of phenotype between patients with Prader-Willi syndrome due to deletion 15q and uniparental disomy 15. Am J Med Genet 68:433–440.

Cassidy SB, Schwartz S. Prader–Willi syndrome. GeneReviews at GeneTests: Medical Genetics Information Resource (database online). Seattle: University of Washington, 2006.

Cassidy Suzanne B , Driscoll Daniel J , Prader–Willi syndrome, European Journal of Human Genetics, 2009, 17, 3–13; published online 10 September 2008

Chamberlain, S.J., Lalande, M., (2010):Neurodevelopmental disorders involving genomic imprinting at human chromosome 15q11–q13, Neurobiol. Dis. doi:10.1016/j.nbd.

Chan C-TJ, Clayton-Smith J, Cheng X-J, et al. Molecular mechanisms in Angelman syndrome: a survey of 93 patients. J Med Genet 1993; 30: 895-902.

Chevret E, Volpi EV, Sheer D 2000. Mini review: formand function in the human interphase chromosome. Cytogenet Cell Genet, 90: 13-21.

Christian SL, Bhatt NK, Martin SA, Sutcliffe JS, Kubota T, Huang B, Mutirangura A, Chinault AC, Beaudet AL, Ledbetter DH. 1998. Integrated YAC contig map of the Prader-Willi/Angelman region on chromosome 15q11-q13 with average STS spacing of 35 kb. Genome Res 8:146–157.

Christian SL, Fantes JA, Mewborn SK, Huang B, Ledbetter DH. 1999. Large genomic duplicons map to sites of instability in the Prader- Willi/Angelman syndrome chromosome region (15q11-q13). Hum Mol Genet 8:1025–1037.

Delach JA, Rosengren SS, Kaplan L, Greenstein RM, Cassidy SB, Benn PA (1994): Comparison of high resolution chromosome banding and fluorescence in situ hybridization (FISH) for the laboratory evaluation of Prader-Willi syndrome and Angelman syndrome. Am J Med Genet 52:85-91.

Donlon TA. 1988. Similar molecular deletions on chromosome 15q11.2 are encountered in both the Prader-Willi and Angelman syndromes. Hum Genet 80:322–328.

Francke U (1994): Digitized and differentially shaded human chromosome ideograms for genomic applications. Cytogenet Cell Genet 65:206-219.

Gilfillan GD, Selmer KK, Roxrud I, Smith R, Kyllerman M, Eiklid K, Kroken M, Mattingsdal M, Egeland T, Stenmark H, Sjøholm H, Server A, Samuelsson L, Christianson A, Tarpey P, Whibley A, Stratton MR, Futreal PA, Teague J, Edkins S, Gecz J, Turner G, Raymond FL, Schwartz C, Stevenson RE, Undlien DE, Strømme P: SLC9A6 mutations cause X-linked mental retardation, microcephaly, epilepsy, and ataxia, a phenotype mimicking Angelman syndrome. Am J Hum Genet 2008, 82:1003-1010.

Gillessen-Kaesbach G, Gross S, Kaya-Westerloh S, Passarge E, Horsthemke B. DNA methylation based testing of 450 patients suspected of having Prader-Willi syndrome. J Med Genet 1995, 32:88-92

Gillessen-Kaesbach G, Gross S, Kaya-Westerloh S, Passarge E, Horsthemke B 1995): DNA methylation based testing of 450 patients suspected of having Prader-Willi syndrome. J Med Genet 32:88–92.

Gillessen-Kaesbach G, Robinson W, Lohmann D, Kaya-Westerloh S, Passarge E, Horsthemke B (1995): Genotype-phenotype correlation in a series of 167 deletion and non-deletion patients with Prader-Willi syndrome. Hum Genet 96:638–643.

Glatt KA, Sinnett D, Lalande M: Dinucleotide repeat polymorphism at the GABAA receptor alpha 5 (GABRA5) locus at chromosome 15q11- q13. Hum Mol Genet 1992, 1:348.

Glenn CC, Porter KA, Jong MT, Nicholls RD, Driscoll DJ . Functional imprinting and epigenetic modification of the human SNRPN gene. Hum Mol Genet 1993, 2:2001-5

Glenn CC, Saitoh S, Jong MT, Filbrandt MM, Surti U, Driscoll DJ, Nicholls RD Gene structure, DNA methylation and imprinted expression of the human SNRPN gene. Am J Hum Genet, 1996, 58:335–346

Goldstone AP, Beales PL: Genetic Obesity Syndromes. Front Horm Res 2008, 36:37-60.

Goldstone P., A. J. Holland, B. P. Hauffa, A. C. Hokken-Koelega, M. Tauber, on behalf of speakers contributors at the Second E, (2008). Recommendations for the Diagnosis and Management of Prader-Willi Syndrome, The Journal of Clinical Endocrinology & Metabolism, 2008, Vol. 93, No. 11 4183-4197

Guerrini R, Carozzo R, Rinaldi R, Bonanni P.(2003) Angelman syndrome: etiology, clinical features, diagnosis, and management of symptoms. Pediatr Drugs. 5(10):647-61.

Gunay-Aygun M, Schwartz S, Heeger S, O'Riordan MA, Cassidy SB, The changing purpose of Prader-Willi syndrome clinical diagnostic criteria and proposed revised criteria, Pediatrics. 2001 Nov; 108(5): E92

Holm VA, Cassidy SB, Butler MG, Hanchett JM, Greenswag LR, Whitman BY, Greenberg F., Prader-Willi syndrome: consensus diagnostic criteria, Pediatrics, 1993 Feb; 91(2): 398-402

Hoo J-J, Chao MC, Samuel IP, Morgan AM (1990): Proximal 15q variant as possible pitfall in the cytogenetic diagnosis of Prader-Willi syndrome. Clin Genet 37:161-166.

Horsthemke B, Buiting K. 2006. Imprinting defects on human chromosome 15. Cytogenet Genome Res 113: 292–299.

Horsthemke B, Buiting K. 2008. Genomic imprinting and imprinting defects in humans. Adv Genet 61: 225–246.

Horsthemke B, Wagstaff J. 2008. Mechanisms of imprinting of the Prader–Willi/Angelman region. Am J Med Genet Part A 146A:2041–2052.

Kaplan LC, Wharton R, Elias E, Mandell F, Donlon T, Latt SA. 1987. Clinical heterogeneity associated with deletions in the long arm of chromosome 15: Report of 3 new cases and their possible genetic significance. Am J Med Genet 28:45–53.

Knoll JH, Nicholls RD, Magenis RE, Graham JM Jr, Lalande M, Latt SA. 1989. Angelman and Prader-Willi syndromes share a common chromosome 15 deletion but differ in parental origin of the deletion. Am J Med Genet 32:285–290.

Kosaki Kenjiro, Matthew J. McGinniss, Alexey N. Veraksa, William J. McGinnis, and Kenneth Lyons Jones (1997) : Prader-Willi and Angelman Syndromes: Diagnosis With a Bisulfite-Treated Methylation-Specific PCR Method. American Journal of Medical Genetics 73:308–313

Kozlowski Piotr, Anna J. Jasinska, and David J. Kwiatkowski (2008) : New applications and developments in the use of multiplex ligation-dependent probe amplification. Electrophoresis 29, 4627–4636

Kubota T, Das S, Christian SL, Baylin SB, Herman JG, Ledbetter DH Methylation-specific PCR simplifies imprinting analysis. Nat Genet, 1997, 16:16–17

Kubota, T., Das, S., Christian, S.L. et al, Methylation-specific PCR simplifies imprinting analysis. Nature Genet., 1997, 16, 16–17

Langedijk, P.S.; Schut, F.; Jansen, G. J.; Raangs, G. C.; Kamphuis, G. R.; Wilkinson, M. H. F.; Welling, G. W.; Applied and Environmental Microbiology 1995, 61, 3069-3075.

Ledbetter DH and Engel E. Uniparental disomy in humans: development of an imprinting map and its implications for prenatal diagnosis. Hum Mol Genet 4 1995, Spec No:1757-64

Ledbetter DH, Riccardi VM, Airhart SD, Strobel RJ, Keenan BS, Crawford JD. 1981. Deletions of chromosome 15 as a cause of the Prader-Willi syndrome. N Engl J Med 304:325–329.

Lossie, A.C., Whitney, M.M., Amidon, D., Dong, H.J., Chen, P., Theriaque, D., Hutson, A., Nicholls, R.D., Zori, R.T., Williams, C.A., Driscoll, D.J., 2001. Distinct phenotypes distinguish the molecular classes of Angelman syndrome. J. Med. Genet. 38, 834–845.

Ludowese CJ, Thompson KJ, Sekhon GS, Pauli RM (1991): Absence of predictable phenotypic expression in proximal 15q duplications. Clin Genet 40:194-201.

Magenis RE, Brown MG, Lacy DA, Budden S, LaFranchi S. 1987. Is Angelman syndrome an alternate result of del(15)(q11q13)? Am J Med Genet 28:829–838.

Mellissa R. W. Mann, Marisa S. Bartolomei, Towards a molecular understanding of Prader-Willi and Angelman syndromes, Human Molecular Genetics, 1999, 8: 1867-1873

Mitchell J, Schinzel A, Langlois S, Gillessen-Kaesbach G, Michaelis RC, Abeliovich D, Lerer I, Schuffenhauer S, Christian S, Guitart M, Mc- Fadden DE, Robinson WP (1996): Comparison of phenotype in uniparental disomy and deletion Prader-Willi syndrome: Sex specific differences. Am J Med Genet 65:133–136.

Mutirangura A, Greenberg F, Butler MG, Malcolm S, Nicholls RD, Chakravarti A, Ledbetter DH: Multiplex PCR of three dinucleotide repeats in the Prader-Willi/Angelman critical region (15q11-q13): molecular diagnosis and mechanism of uniparental disomy. Hum Mol Genet 1993, 2:143-151.

Nicholls RD, Knoll JH, Glatt K, Hersh JH, Brewster TD, Graham JM Jr, Wurster-Hill D, Wharton R, Latt SA. 1989a. Restriction fragment length polymorphisms within proximal 15q and their use in molecular cytogenetics and the Prader-Willi syndrome. Am J Med Genet 33:66–77.

Ohta T, Gray TA, Rogan PK, Buiting K, Gabriel JM, Saitoh S, Muralidhar B, Bilienska B, Krajewska-Walasek M, Driscoll DJ, Horsthemke B, Butler MG, Nicholls RD. Imprinting-mutation mechanisms in Prader-Willi syndrome. Am J Hum Genet 1999, 64:397-413

Roberts SE and Thomas NS. A quantitative polymerase chain reaction method for determining copy number within the Prader-Willi/Angelman syndrome critical region. Clin Genet 2003, 64:76-8

Roof E, Stone W, MacLean W, Feurer ID, Thompson T, Butler MG. Intellectual characteristics of Prader-Willi syndrome: comparison of genetic subtypes. J Intellect Disabil Res 2000, 44 (Pt 1):25-30

Sahoo T, del Gaudio D, German JR, Shinawi M, Peters SU, Person RE, Garnica A, Cheung SW, Beaudet AL. Prader–Willi phenotype caused by paternal deficiency for the HBII-85 C/D box small nucleolar RNA cluster. Nat Genet 2008;40:719–721.

Saitoh S, Buiting K, Cassidy SB, Conroy JM, Driscoll DJ, Gabriel JM, Gillessen-Kaesbach G, Glenn CC, Greenswag LR, Horsthemke B, Kondo I, Kuwajima K, Niikawa N, Rogan PK, Schwartz S, Seip J, Williams CA and Nicholls RD Clinical spectrum and molecular diagnosis of Angelman and Prader-Willi syndrome imprinting mutation patients. Am J Med Genet, 1997, 68:195-206

Schouten, J.P., McElgunn,C.J., Waaijer,R., Zwijnenburg,D., Diepvens,F. and Pals,G. (2002) Relative quantification of 40 nucleic acid sequences by multiplex ligation-dependent probe amplification. Nucleic Acids Res., 30, e57.

Simon C Ramsden, Jill Clayton-Smith, Rachael Birch and Karin Buiting: CPracticenc guidelines for the molecular analysis of Prader-Willi and Angelman syndromes. BMC Medical Genetics 2010, 11:70

Smith A, Prasad M, Deng ZM, Robson L, Woodage T, Trent RJ (1995): Comparison of high resolution cytogenetics, fluorescence in situ hybridisation, and DNA studies to validate the diagnosis of Prader-Willi and Angelman's syndromes. Arch Dis Child 72:397402.

Tantravahi U, Nicholls RD, Stroh H, Ringer S, Neve RL, Kaplan L, Wharton R, Wurster- Hill D, Graham JM Jr, Cantu ES, Frias JL, Kousseff BG, Latt SA. 1989. Quantitative calibration and use of DNA probes for investigating chromosome abnormalities in the Prader-Willi syndrome. Am J Med Genet 33:78–87.

Temple IK, Shrubb V, Lever M, Bullman H, Mackay DJ: Isolated imprinting mutation of the DLK1/GTL2 locus associated with a clinical presentation of maternal uniparental disomy of chromosome 14. J Med Genet 2007, 44:637-640.

Williams CA, Lossie A, Driscoll D, R.C. Phillips Unit. 2001. Angelman syndrome: mimicking conditions and phenotypes. Am J Med Genet 101:59–64.

21

Turner Syndrome and Sex Chromosomal Mosaicism

Eduardo Pásaro Méndez and Rosa Mª Fernández García
University of A Coruña, Department of Psichobiology
Spain

1. Introduction

Turner syndrome (TS) is defined as the total or partial absence of the second sex chromosome in women (Ford et al., 1959). Its incidence is 1 in every 1,850 newborn girls (7th International Conference on Turner Syndrome, 2009) although it is higher at the moment of fertilization, since it is estimated that 3% of all human fertilizations are 45,X (Urbach and Benvenisty, 2009) but only 1% survive beyond 24 weeks gestation (Hook and Warburton, 1983).

The Turner phenotype is quite variable, even among women with the same karyotype, however, there are some cardinal features: low stature (>99%), gonadal dysgenesis (>90%) and anatomic malformations such as *Pterigium colli* or *cubitus valgus* (>80%). In addition, the Turner phenotype can be associated to other less frequent characteristics such us: cardiovascular congenital defects, renal alterations, aorta anomalies, etc, besides a specific neuropsicologic profile which can include selective non-verbal deficiencies: alterations of the sight-space capacity and low capacity of abstraction (Bondy et al., 2007; Ross et al., 2000a; Ross et al., 2000b; Ross et al., 2006; Zinn et al., 2007). Mental deficiency is not a characteristic of TS.

Both the embrionary lethality and the Turner phenotype are considered the result of a haploinsufficiency of genes found on both sex chromosomes (X and Y) and that escape X-inactivation (it is assumed that these genes are expressed in both active and inactive X chromosomes as a means of ensuring the right quantity of genetic product). The sex chromosomal regions causing these two conditions are referred to as pseudoautosomal regions 1 and 2 (PAR1 and PAR2) and are found at the ends of both sex chromosomes.

The high percentage of fetal and embryonic lethality for karyotype 45,X also suggests the need of mosaicism for survival (Held et al., 1992). Natural selection is not as prevalent when mosaicism is operative (Hassold et al., 1988; Hook and Warburton, 1983) although, paradoxically, the resulting phenotype after birth is similar with or without mosaicism.

Some hypotheses argue for the existence of a feto-protective effect of one or more genes of the sex chromosomes (X or Y). According to this concept, all Turner women are mosaics since the presence of two copies of these gene(s) should be present, either in the fetus or in extra-embryonic tissues (Kalousek et al., 1987). But the detection of mosaicism is not always possible. It is mainly determined by four factors: the type and number of tissues analyzed (Held et al., 1992); the number of cells studied (Hook, 1977); the sensitivity of the techniques applied, and the possible selection which may result in the disappearance of cell lines (Procter et al., 1984). Thus, a small percentage of mosaicism cannot be detected by conventional cytogenetic techniques unless we sit down case by case in front of the microscope with much patience, analyzing at great number of metaphases. This way, the application of molecular techniques substantially improves the detection of low-frequency cell lines.

Here we present the results of hidden mosaicism on 192 women diagnosed as TS and we focus on the molecular study of the Y chromosome, since numerous studies have shown that 4-20% of Turner women present a Y-chromosome (Kocova et al., 1995), increasing the risk of developing gonadoblastoma (Coto et al., 1995). Although the identity of the gene (or genes) linked to gonadoblastoma has not been established yet, there is evidence indicating that these genes are located near the centromere of the Y chromosome (Salo et al., 1995; Tsuchiya et al., 1995).

2. Patients and methods

The selection of the 192 Turner patients was carried out with the aid of the Genetics Division of the "Materno Infantil" Hospital of A Coruña, the Endocrinology Section of the General Hospital of Galicia, the Endocrinology Section of the Hospital of Málaga, and the Turner association from Spain. The age of the analyzed population ranged between 1 month and 43 years and the average age was 13.2 years.

Blood samples were extracted using heparinized test tubes for further cytologic study, and tubes with EDTA anticoagulant for molecular analysis. Standard techniques for the cultivation of lymphocytes from peripheral blood were used (Moorhead et al., 1960), and the preparations were treated with trypsin to obtain G-banding (Seabright, 1971).

2.1 Fluorescence *in situ* hybridization

The X chromosome was studied using the probes specified in Table 1: DXZ1, Xq13.2 (XIST), DXZ4, painting for Xp and *SHOX* (short stature homeobox-containing gene) and cosmid LLNOYCO3'M'34F5 kindly provided by Dr. Andrew Zinn.

The DXZ1 probe specifically hybridizes with the centromeric region of the X chromosome. The nature of the material involved in the restructuring was determined by the Xq13.2 inactivation site probe, and the DXZ4 probe specific to the macrosatellite repeat located at Xq23-24. The absence or presence of the Y chromosome was determined with the DYZ1-DYZ3 probe (Oncor), which specifically hybridizes with the centromere and the long arm of the Y chromosome, and the chromosomal material was determinated by the painting probe from Vysis.

Independently of the karyotypes, all Turner patients where checked for the presence of the Y chromosome by PCR and FISH. Metaphases from a control male were simultaneously and identically processed, as a positive control. In the case of the DXZ1 probe, the fluorescent signal of the intact X chromosome served as an internal control. The minimum number of analyzed metaphases for each probe was 100, distributed in at least two slides.

The hybridization procedure originally described by Pinkel (Pinkel et al., 1986) was used according to commercial protocols (Oncor and Vysis). The chromosome preparations were counter-stained with propidium iodide (PI) or DAPI, and were observed and photographed by a Zeiss fluorescence photomicroscope.

To achieve simultaneous hybridization of DXZ1 and Xq13.2 probes, the Oncor sequential hybridization protocol was used. For hybridization with the SHOX probe, the cosmid was labelled by nick translation using biotin (Roche). The post-hybridization washes spent 15 min at 43°C in 50% formamide/2x SSC and then 15 min at 43°C in 2XSSC.

Probes	Characteristics of the probes	Provider
X-chromosome		
DXZ1	Specific to the centromeric region of the X chromosome	ONCOR
DXZ4	Specific to the repetitive region on Xq24	ONCOR
ToTelVysion	Specific to the telomeric regions from all chromosomes	Vysis
SHOX	Short stature homeobox. Cosmid LLNOYCO3'M'34F5	Dr. Andrew Zinn
XIST	Specific to the inactivation center at Xq13.2	ONCOR
WCP-X	Whole X chromosome painting probe	Vysis
SCPL116	Partial Xp painting probe	Dr. Rocchi
SCPL102	Partial Xq painting probe	Dr. Rocchi
Y-chromosome		
DYZ1	Specific to the heterochromatic region Yq12	ONCOR
DYZ3	Specific to the centromeric region of the Y chromosome	ONCOR
PCYq	Partial Yq painting probe	Vysis
WCP-Y	Whole Y chromosome painting probe	Vysis

Table 1. FISH Hybridization probes and characteristics

2.2 PCR analyses

DNA extraction from peripheral blood was carried out using standard procedures. For PCR analysis, different sets of oligonucleotide primers were used to amplify X and Y-specific sequences:

1. XC1-XC2, located at the centromeric region of the X chromosome, to amplify a 130-bp fragment (Witt and Erickson, 1989; Witt and Erickson, 1991)
2. YC1-YC2, located at the centromeric region of the Y chromosome, to amplify a fragment of 170-bp (Witt and Erickson, 1989; Witt and Erickson, 1991)
3. XES7-XES2, located within the *SRY* open reading frame, to amplify a 609-bp fragment (Berta et al., 1990).
4. DYZ1A-DYZ1B to amplify a 1024-bp fragment from the DYZ1 region contained within the Yq12 (Cooke, 1976; Nakagome et al., 1991)

The PCR amplification was carried out according to standard protocols. The PCR products were detected in 1,5% agarose gels.

2.3 Cloning and DNA sequencing of the XES-PCR products

In those patients in which the amplification of the *SRY* gene was positive, we cloned and sequenced the fragment in the following way: the products from three independent PCR reactions were joined to the plasmid pGEM-T (Promega) and subsequently transformed into the E. coli JM109 under the conditions recommended by the manufacturer. Six positive clones were sequenced in both directions by using the Thermosequenase fluorescent cycle sequencing kit from Amersham. The sequence reactions were analyzed on a 6.5% polyacrylamide gel in a LICOR-400L automated sequencer.

3. Results and discussion

In 1992 Held and others (Held et al., 1992) sent an innovative idea about TS: karyotype 45,X really does not exist, all Turner patients who survive and get to be born are really mosaic.

The karyotype 45,X is really deletereous and the natural selection does not allow it, causing a spontaneous abortion in the first weeks of gestation. The presence of a second celullar line, either 46,XX or 46,XY, in embryonic or extraembryonic tissues, provides a feto-protective effect which allows the development of a Turner girl.

When only one cellular tissue (blood generally) is analyzed, the resulting karyotype might lead to error, because the second cellular line could be located in any other place, or in extraembryonic cellular tissues, which allow the fetus to develop to maturity. In addition, in order to make a diagnosis, it is necessary to analyze a high quantity of metaphases, specially if the 45,X cells immediately become very apparent through the microscope. Time is very limited and usually not enough time is spent in the detailed observation of over 1000 cells. In our opinion, and according to the words of Santiago Ramon and Cajal "*It is not enough to examine, is necessary to contemplate...*" (In the fourth edition of his book of Rules and Advice (page 166)

Even so, after applying molecular techniques and studying several cellular lines, some patients are still seemngly 45,X (see Table 2). But we do not discard hypothesis of Held since sensible techniques which discard 100% mosaicism do not exist and it is not possible to analyze all the cellular tissues from one patient because she is alive (obviously).

In the following Table we present the results obtained in our laboratory, after almost twenty years analyzing blood samples of women and children with this syndrome, within the Spanish population. The average number of analyzed metaphases (not including nucleous, which were also analyzed) for each patient was 507,73.

KARYOTYPE	Nº Patients	Percentage
No mosaicism		
45,X	20	10,42
45,X, +*SRY*	1	0,52
46,X,i(Xq)	10	5,21
46,X,del(Xp)	12	6,25
X-Mosaicism	**135**	**70,31**
45,X/46,XX	83	43,23
45,X/47,XXX	7	3,65
45,X/46,X,i(Xq)	11	5,73
45,X/46,X,+der(X)	16	8,33
45,X/46,X+r(X)	4	2,08
45,X/46,XX/47,XXX	1	0,52
Others	**11**	**5,73**
Complex mosaics (+3 cell lines)	**2**	**1,04**
Y-Mosaicism	**14**	**7,29**
45,X/46,X,+der(Y)	1	0,52
45,X/46,XY	9	4,69
46,X,der(X)t(X;Y)(qter→p22.3::q11.21→qter)	1	0,52
45,X/46,X,+i(Yq)/46,X,+der(Y)	1	0,52
idic(Y)(qter→p11.32::p11.32→qter)	2	1,04
Total	**192**	**100%**

Table 2. Distribution of the karyotypes in a Spanish population of 192 Turner women

3.1 Non-mosaic patients: The karyotype 45,X

As we can observe in table 2, of the 192 Turner patients analyzed throughout these years, only 21 (aprox. 11%) showed karyotype 45,X. Or rather we could say that there were 21 patients in whom we were not able to locate a cellular line other than the 45,X, in spite of our efforts. In addition, for those same patients, we analyzed the *AR* gene (androgen receptor gene), in particular a variable region within exon 1, located in Xq11-12 which shows tandem GCA repetitions to let us know if one or two copies of that gene exists (in blood) (Table 3). The results indicated the same outcome. There continues to be 21 patients without an apparent second cellular line (46,XX or 46,XY).

Gene	Lozalization	Position	characteristics	Primers	T° annealing
Androgen receptor (*AR*)	Xq11-12	exon 1	Tamden repetition GCA	5′-GTTCCTCATCCAGGACCAGGTA-3′ 5′-GTGCGCGAAGTGATCCAGA-3′ HEX	56° C

Table 3. PCR Primers for Androgen receptor (*AR*)

The choice of this variable region and not another one, was due to its proximity to the center of inactivation of the X cromosome, and therefore, its proximity to the centromere. It is known that a fragment without centromere is generally considered an unstable element since it cannot join the metaphase spindle and therefore, it tends to dissapear in successive mitoses. Consequently, we are able to say that a stable chromosome, capable of forming a cellular line, must have a centromere. Otherwise, we know that the loss of the inactivation center (XIC) in a small fragment from the X chromosome produces mental deficiency. Not at all a normal characteristic of this syndrome.

We can emphasize one case in this group which is striking due to its exceptional nature.

3.1.1 The tall and mathematical 45,X non mosaic woman

One of the patients showed a nonmosaic 45,X karyotype in different weaves and by means of cytogenetic and molecular techniques. Her phenotype cannot then be classified as "characteristic" because her height is 170 cm without growth hormone (GH) treatment, and whose only apparent Turner feature is gonadal dysgenesis. The only possible explanation for the absence of a Turner phenotype is the hidden mosaicism combined with an untreated gonadal dysgenesis (Fernandez and Pasaro, 2010). Another characteristic of this patient is that she has completed her studies in mathematics obtaining excellent grades. Taking into account that TS women were defined as *blind to form and space* by Money (Money, 1993) , we have to consider this woman is exceptional, since she is a 45,X non-mosaic and breaks away from all the pre-stablished standards for this syndrome.

The G-banding analysis (blood and skin fibroblast) and the FISH method using all the X probes, showed the same karyotype (45,X) whereas the DYZ1 and DYZ3 probes showed that the Y chromosome was not involved in the karyotype. The parents' karyotype was normal.

The cytogenetic and molecular analysis of the X chromosome always showed that the X present in the karyotype was a normal chromosome without duplication in the PAR1 region.

The absence of the Y chromosome was confirmed by PCR. The study of polymorphism also showed that the X present was inherited from the mother, and that this patient has only one copy of the *SHOX* gene. The analysis of the *AR* showed only one copy of the gene.
The discrepancies between the karyotype and the phenotype found in our patient suggest that previous cases of TS have been undiagnosed or misdiagnosed. Our results support the theory that significant ascertainment bias exists in our understanding of TS, with important implications for prenatal counseling. We think that the real frequency of TS can be greater than 1/1,850 due to females with a normal phenotype.
At first sight we could think that this patient discards the hypothesis of Held, because, in spite of our efforts, we have not been able to find a second cellular line. But we think that it is indeed an optimal test that the TS "always" goes accompanied by one second cellular line which protects it against natural selection and allows it to continue with its fetal development.
We cannot deny the existence of this hypothetical second cellular line which protects the embryo and the fetus, after analyzing a few cells to the microscope. Not even after carrying out a molecular study of the sex chromosomes, since we cannot exclude the different distribution possibilities of the different cellular lines in the many weaves of the organism throughout the embryonic development, which allowed, in this case, the development of a 45,X woman with an absence of a Turner phenotype.

3.2 Mosaicism in the Turner syndrome

The presence of mosaicism (small chromosomic fragments, rings, or isodiscentric chromosomes, derived from X or Y) characterized the second cellular line for the remainder of the analyzed women (70,31%). The ones who had been previously diagnosed as mosaic using G-bands, presented a more complex karyotype after the molecular study due to the presence of new cellular lines. The complex mosaics were always asociated to isodicentric chromosomes in both X and Y. The presence of two centromere leads to instability and loss of chromosomes which tend to break and to distribute themselves randomly through the succesive mitotic divisions (Fernandez-Garcia et al., 2000; Fernandez et al., 1996).

3.2.1 Implication of the Y chromosome on the chromosomic mosaicism in Turner syndrome

When the chromosome involved in the second cellular line was Y, we were able to observe isodicentric chromosomes for the short as well as the long arms. These chromosomes had been defined as monocentric fragments of unknown origin using the G-Band technique, and the existence of both centromeres was evident only using FISH. The presence of two centromeric regions unleashes great instability during mitosis, which produces a buil-up of chromosomal derivatives which are randomly distributed and which cause a high number of cellular lines due to the formation of different sized rings. An example of this type of mosaicism associated with isodiscentric chromosomes are shown below. They represent the most striking cases within the analyzed group in our laboratory.

3.2.1.1 Molecular analysis of an idic(Y)(qter→p11.32::p11.32→qter) chromosome from a female patient with a complex karyotype

Here we present a 4-year-old girl with a low to moderate height and a gonadal dysgenesis as the only features associated to TS (Fernandez and Pasaro, 2006). She exhibited a chromosome similar in size to a member of group D, which suggests two Y chromosomes united by the pter ends (Figure 1). The analysis of 506 metaphases by FISH revealed at least eight cell lines and two different derivatives from the Y chromosome. In 58% of the cells, a double-hybridization signal was observed in the derivative chromosome for probes DYZ1 and DYZ3, corresponding to double heterochromatic and centromeric regions, respectively. The cell line 45,X was found in 19% of the cells, whereas the cell line 46,X,del(Y)(p11.32) was present in 16.5%. Furthermore, five other cell lines were observed in smaller percentages, resulting from the breakage of the idic(Y) (qter→p11.32::p11.32→qter) at p11.32 and a later mitotic random distribution of the two del(Y)(p11.32) and the X chromosome:

- 3% corresponding to a cell line with an X chromosome, a Y chromosome with terminal deletion and an isodicentric Y: 47,X,del(Y)(p11.32), idic(Y) (qter→p11.32::p11.32→qter)
- 1.5% corresponding to a cell line containing two X chromosomes and one isodicentric Y chromosome 47,XX, idic(Y)(qter→p11.32::p11.32→qter).
- 1% of the cells showed a combination of one X chromosome and two isodicentric Y chromosomes 47,X, 2idic(Y)(qter→p11.32::p11.32→qter)
- 0.5% showed one X chromosome and two Y chromosomes with terminal deletion 47,X, 2del(Y)(p11.32)
- 0.5% of the cells showed two X chromosomes and one deleted Y chromosome 47,XX,del(Y)(p11.32).

The fact that an intact 46,XY line was not found and that all the der(Y) had lost the PAR1 region suggests a meiotic origin for the dicentric Y. Perhaps the isodicentric Y chromosome was present in the sperm before fertilization as a result of an error during gametogenesis. Errors occurring after the first zygotic division would result in mosaicism including a normal cell line. We think that the dic(Y) was a result of a meiosis I exchange between sister chromatids at a side between *SRY* and the *SHOX*, followed by centromere misdivision in meiosis II (Battin, 2003; Hsu, 1994; Robinson et al., 1999).

The patient showed a total of eight cell lines and at least two morphologically distinct abnormal Y derivatives, all presumably descendants of a progenitor and unstable idic(Y) chromosome. The heterogeneous cell content observed suggests a great mitotic instability of sex chromosome Y and mitotic non-disjunction.

Usually, isodicentric Y chromosomes occur in mosaic form and are generally considered unstable elements since improper alignment of two centromeres on the metaphase spindle may lead to the formation of a bridge during anaphase (Cohen et al., 1973). In the patient studied here, the isodicentric Y chromosome showed two noticeable centromeres. If both centromeres were active, it could be assumed that the Y derivatives observed in the different cell lines would be the result of the breakage of the isodicentric at Yp11:32 due to improper alignment of the two centromeres on the metaphase spindle.

As in all the cases studied in our laboratory and in most of the reports published to date (Robinson et al., 1999), the patient examined here had a 45,X cell line (19%). Such mosaic patients exhibit a phenotype ranging from female to male, depending on the presence or absence of the testis-determining gene *SRY* and, perhaps more importantly, on the degree of mosaicism and the tissue distribution of 45,X cells. It has been proposed that the predominance of XO or XY cells determines gonadal differentiation into a testis or a streak gonad (Bergada et al., 1986).

On the other hand, TS is the result of a haploinsufficiency of a specific gene(s) that must escape from X-inactivation, and also, these individuals must have a functional Y peer. The discovery of the pseudoautosomal region at the termini of Xp and Yp fits well with these two requirements: the meiotic combination maintains nucleotide sequence identity between X- and Y-linked pseudoautosomal genes, and all such genes tested to date escape X inactivation (Zinn and Ross, 1998). Nevertheless, the only TS features present in this patient were short stature and gonadal dysgenesis. The absence of the PAR1 region in all cells examined in this patient suggests that loci responsible for other Turner features lie outside the pseudoautosomal region (Haddad et al., 2003; Joseph et al., 1996; Spranger et al., 1997). Our data is in agreement with the fact that the only PAR1 gene consistently related to TS is the short stature gene or *SHOX/PHOG*. This gene is a strong candidate for a TS growth gene on the basis of its chromosomal location, its pattern of expression and a mutational analysis (Alves et al., 2003; Rao et al., 1997).

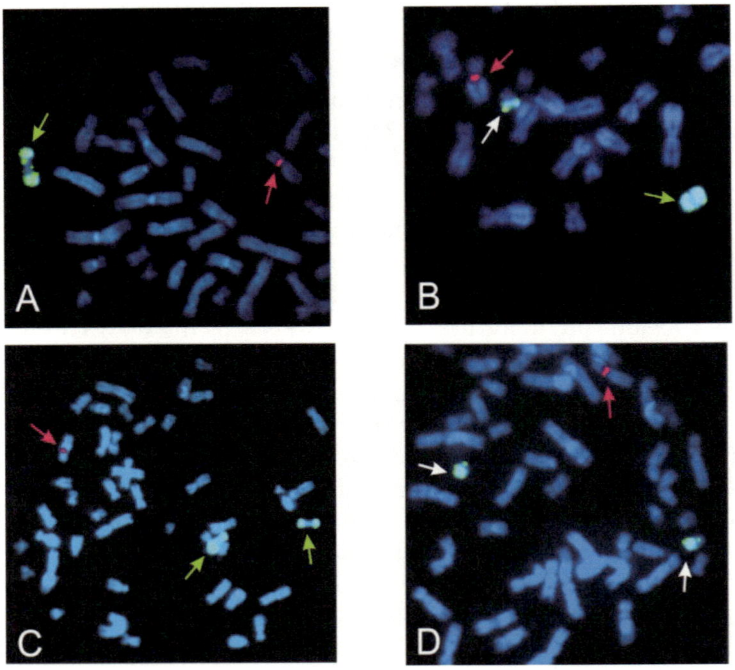

Fig. 1. FISH analysis using DXZ1 (magenta signal) and DYZ1 (green signal). A: 46,X,idic(Y)(qter→p11.32::p11.32 →qter) metaphase; the magenta arrow indicates the X chromosome and the green one indicates the idic(Y)(qter→p11.32::p11.32 →qter). B: 47,X,del(Y)(p11.32),idic(Y)(qter→p11.32::p11.32→qter) metaphase; the magenta arrow indicates the X chromosome, the white arrow indicates the del(Y)(p11.32) and the green one indicates the idic(Y)(qter→p11.32::p11.32 →qter). C: 47,X,2idic(Y)(qter→p11.32::p11.32→qter) metaphase; once again the magenta arrow indicates the X chromosome, and the green arrows indicate the two idic(Y)(qter→p11.32::p11.32→qter). D: 47,X, 2del(Y)(p11.32) metaphase; the magenta arrow indicates the X chromosome, and the white arrows indicate the two del(Y)(p11.32)

In conclusion, it appears that the most common abnormal Y chromosome present in TS patients is an isodicentric Y chromosome occurring as part of a mosaic karyotype including a 45,X cell line. It is probable that isodicentric Y chromosomes are usually generated during gametogenesis before spermatid formation, or during the first division after fertilization, and that almost all are present as part of a mosaic karyotype. The TS patients with a Y chromosome studied in our laboratory carried the testis-determining factor gene *SRY*, but the mosaic nature of their karyotypes rendered this insufficient to induce a male phenotype.

In all our patients, the degree and distribution of the 45,X cell line seem to be decisive factors in phenotype determination.

3.2.1.2 A mutation point, R59G, within the HMG-*SRY* box in a 45,X/46,X,psu dic(Y)(pter→q11::q11→pter) female

The key step in mammalian sex determination is the development of the undifferentiated embryonic gonads into either testes or ovaries. We have known since 1990 that the *SRY* gene (sex determining region Y), located at the tip of the Y short arm (Yp11.3) and proximal to the pseudoautosomal boundary, is the critical switch leading to testis development (Berta et al., 1990). Mutations in *SRY* result in XY individuals developing as females, and patients with 45,X karyotype who have insertion of *SRY* into an autosome have a male phenotype (Yenamandra et al., 1997).

Mutations in this gene can cause failure of testicular development that may result in complete or partial male to female sex reversal (Cameron and Sinclair, 1997). This means that among all the Y-chromosome-derived sequences, *SRY* is the only one that is both required and sufficient to initiate male sex determination (Gubbay et al., 1990; Koopman et al., 1990; Koopman et al., 1991)

The first evidence for the identification of *SRY* as the testis determining factor (TDF) in humans came from the study of XY females with gonadal dysgenesis harboring de novo mutations or deletions in the *SRY* open reading frame. Since 1990, analysis of a number of the XY females with gonadal dysgenesis has led to the description of 36 mutations (31 nucleotide substitutions, three small deletions, one small insertion and one complex rearrangement) in the *SRY* gene. Most of them were located in a critical portion of *SRY*, namely the HMG-box (high-mobility group). The HMG-box is essential for SRY to bind and bend DNA, as well as for transporting the protein into the nucleus (Sinclair, 2001).

On the other hand, the most common abnormal Y chromosome is a dicentric Y chromosome present as part of a mosaic karyotype including a 45,X cell line (Robinson et al., 1999). They are usually generated during gametogenesis before spermatid formation, or during the first division after fertilization, and most are present as part of a mosaic karyotype. There appears to be a region between Yq11 and Yq12 prone to breakage where sister chromatid breakage and inappropriate fusion of broken ends could occur to form isodicentric chromosomes (Kirsch et al., 1996; Robinson et al., 1999; Schwinger et al., 1996). A wide spectrum of phenotypes of patients with a 45,X/46,X,der(Y) karyotype ranges from almost normal males through mixed gonadal dysgenesis to females with TS phenotype. Factors that most influence this variability of sex differentiation are, at least: (1) the presence of certain loci, fundamentally the *SRY* gene, in the developing gonad; (2) the proportion and distribution of 45,X cell line in various tissues, specially in gonads; (3) the moment at which testes degenerate during intrauterine development (Alfaro et al., 1976).

A small marker chromosome was found in 28 of 40 G-banded metaphases from peripheral blood lymphocytes in mosaic karyotype with a 45,X cell line. The G-banding pattern exhibited a marker chromosome similar in size to a member of group F (chromosomes 19 and 20) but did not unequivocally suggest its genetic content (Figure 2) (Fernandez et al., 2002).

When 559 metaphases were analyzed by FISH, the DYZ3 probe revealed, in 60% of the cells, a double hybridization signal in the marker chromosome (Figure 2). However, when the DYZ1 probe was used, no specific hybridization signal was obtained, indicating that the marker had lost the heterochromatic region of the Y chromosome. Application of the WCP-Y probe completely tinted the marker. The study of ovarian tissue using FISH also showed the same result: double hybridization signal when the DYZ3 probe was used, and absence of specific signal with the DYZ1 probe. Therefore, the results obtained by FISH allowed the marker to be redefined as a pseudodicentric nonfluorescent Y chromosome psu dic(Y)(pter→q11::q11→pter) characterized by the presence of two copies of the short arm, two centromeres and two copies of proximal long arm. The heterochromatin region was not present. PCR analysis confirmed the deletion of the Y-heterochromatic region and also the presence of the Y-centromere and the *SRY* gene in blood.

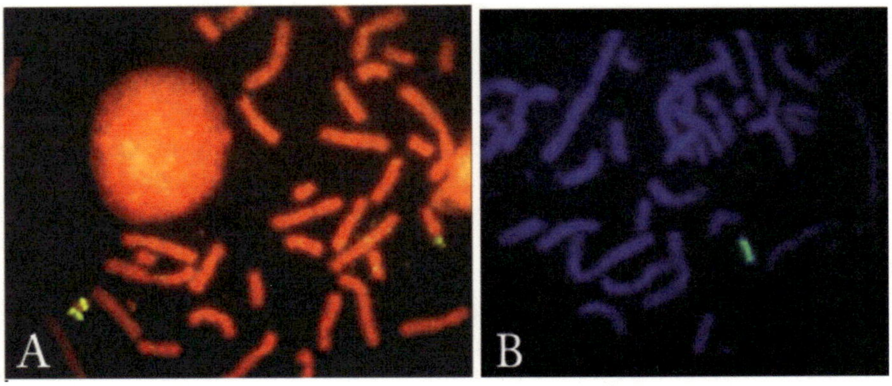

Fig. 2. A. Characterization of the psu dic(Y) in blood by FISH and DYZ3 probe. B. Characterization of the psu dic(Y) by FISH and whole painting WCP-Y probe

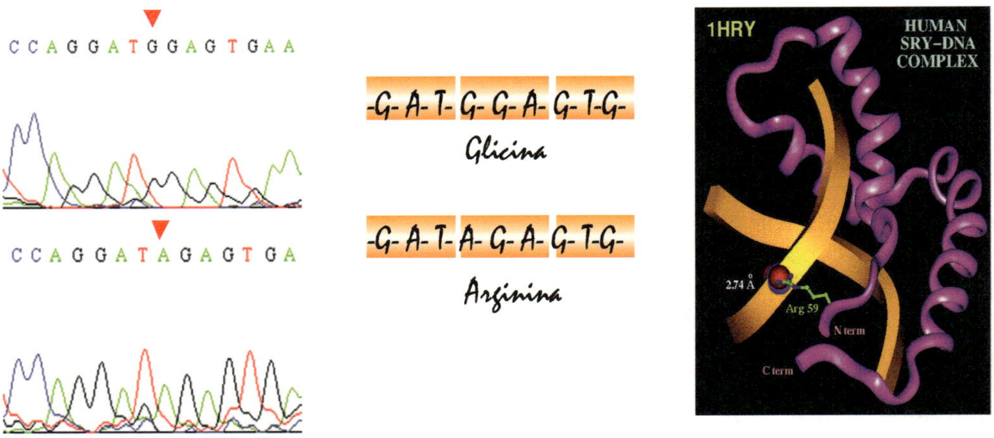

Fig. 3. Sequence of the *SRY* gene, the *top part* showing the A-G mutation produced at codon 59 of the gene and that causes a change from Arg (AGA) to Gly (GGA) within the HMG box. The *bottom* shows the other sequence, also present in the same patient, which is identical to the *SRY* sequence already published. Both copies appear in blood at a frequency of 50%

Due to the possibility of a mutation, a fragment of 609 bp of the *SRY* gene was cloned and sequenced from independent PCR products. Analysis of the sequence revealed, in blood, two copies of the gene. In three of the six clones analyzed, a sequence identical to that of the *SRY* sequence of a male was obtained, whereas the other three clones displayed a non-conservative point mutation, A>G at nucleotide 2,250, codon 59 (Su and Lau, 1993), which causes a change from arginine (AGA) to glycine (GGA) in the second codon within the DNA-binding HMG box domain (Figure 3). This Arg59 is strictly conserved among the *SRY* genes of all species studied to date, suggesting that it is essential for the function of the protein. Here, we describe a female, with gonadal dysgenesis and mosaic karyotype 45,X/46,X,dic(Y)(pter→q11::q11→pter) in blood and gonads, who displays in her dic(Y) an R59G mutation in one of the two copies of the *SRY* gene. This Arg59 is in electrostatic interaction with a phosphate of the DNA; this type of interaction plays an important role in determining the orientation of the protein in specific binding, usually to DNA bases in the major groove (Werner et al., 1995). The Arg59 is strictly conserved among the *SRY* genes of all species studied to date, suggesting that it is essential for proper protein function. We think that all these data indicate that an R59G mutation would totally, or at least partially, inhibit the capacity of SRY to interact with DNA.

On the other hand, dicentric chromosomes are among the most common structural rearrangements of the Y chromosome (Hsu, 1994). Usually these chromosomal alterations occur in mosaic form, and are generally considered unstable elements since improper alignment of two centromeres on the metaphase spindle might lead to the formation of a bridge during anaphase (Cohen et al., 1973). Nonetheless, some dicentrics do persist and replicate normally, since one of the two centromeres becomes inactive and the chromosome may behave as a monocentric marker, as in the present case. Thus, although the dicentric chromosomes showed two noticeable centromeres, one of them is not constricted and it is therefore inactive.

Dicentric Y chromosome formation may occur in different ways: (1) in meiosis, from a break in the long arm of the Y followed by a U type exchange in meiosis I, resulting in a dicentric following meiosis II; (2) a post-zygotic origin of the dicentric Y. The fact that these chromosomal rearrangements usually occur in a 45,X mosaic form would suggest a post-zygotic origin for the dicentric Y. However, a normal 46,XY cell line was absent.

In a review of Y-chromosome aneuploidy by Hsu (Hsu, 1994) no normal cell line (46,XY) was found in 99 of the 102 isodicentric Y chromosomes described. Hsu suggested that the abnormal Y chromosome was either (1) present in the sperm before fertilization and resulted from an error during gametogenesis, or (2) arose from an error in the first zygotic division. Errors occurring after the first zygotic division would result in mosaicism including a normal cell line. The absence of a detectable 46,XY cell line in all 13 isochromosome cases described by Robinson et al. (1999) and in 99 of the 102 described by Hsu et al. (1994) strongly suggests that such errors are more likely to occur during gametogenesis before the spermatid stage, or during the first division after fertilization, rather than during subsequent cell divisions.

In our case, the presence of a dicentric Y and the absence of the 46,XY cell line indicates that the chromosomic rearrangement took place previously or during early embryonic development. Also, the existence of different sequences of the *SRY* gene in the dicentric Y indicates that the formation of the dicentric took place prior to the mutation of the *SRY* gene. The data suggest that the patient suffered a postzygotic mutation early in development. She retained a remnant of functional SRY protein in an amount not sufficient to allow normal male differentiation.

The presence of a Y chromosome in gonads is in discordance with the absence of virilization features in the patient. Hence, one of the possible causes of this discordance can be the presence of the mutation R59G in one of two copies of the *SRY* gene. Furthermore, the presence of the 45,X cell line in gonads prevents the development of testicular tissue.

In conclusion, to our knowledge this is the first time that a mutation is described in codon 59 within the HMG-*SRY* box, and also the first case of a psu dic(Yp) chromosome that displays two different sequences of the *SRY* gene. We think that presence of the 45,X cell line in gonads prevents the development of testicular tissue. The magnitude in which the 45,X cell line or the *SRY* mutation affected the existing phenotype cannot be ascertained.

3.2.1.3 Xp22.3; Yq12.2 chromosome translocation and its clinical manifestations

Here we report a cytogenetic and molecular investigation in a 8 years old girl referred for chromosomal analysis because mild disproportionate short stature (short neck and pectum excavatum) with an initial diagnosis of TS and karyotipe 46,X,+der(X) in 100% of her blood lymphocytes. By means of FISH and PCR analysis the karyotype of the patient was interpreted as 46,X,der(X)t(X;Y)(qter→p22.3::q11.2→qter).

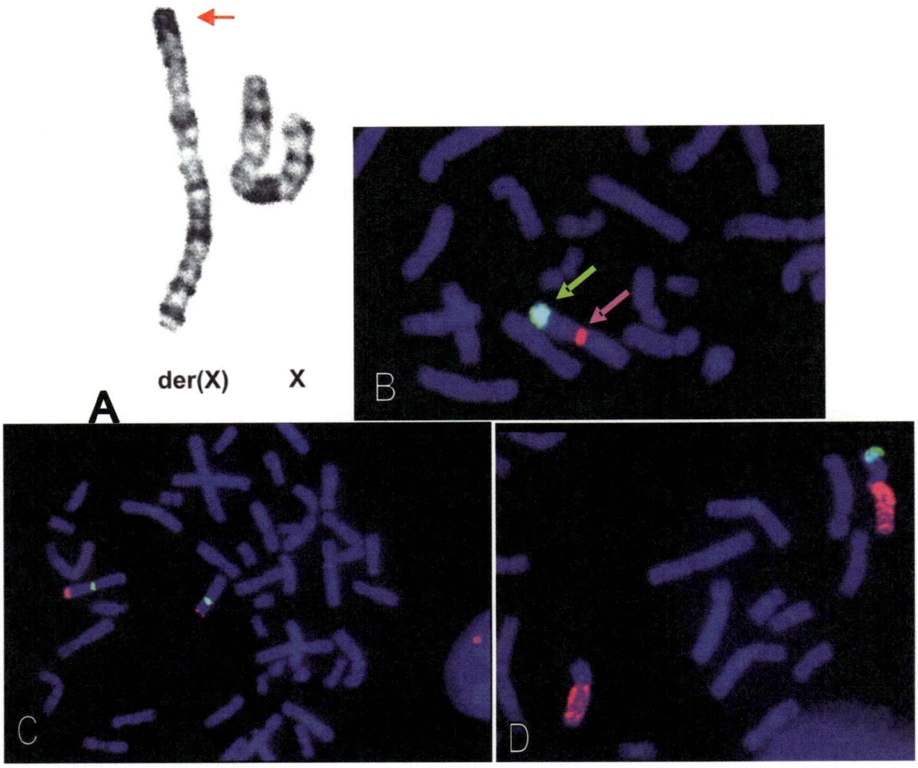

Fig. 4. The der(X;Y) is taught in detail: A.Derivated (X;Y) on the left and X chromosome on the right, with a G-banding pattern. The der(X;Y) appeared to be a metacentric X chromosome with a brightly fluorescing heterocromatin attached to its short arm (red arrow) . B. Partial FISH with the probes DYZ1 (green) and DXZ1 (red). C. Partial FISH with DXZ1 (green) + DYZ1 (red) + SHOX (red). D. Partial FISH with partial painting Yq (green) and partial painting Xq (red) probes

Xp;Yq rearrangements occur rarely in the human population, and result from aberrant recombination between homologous sequences on Xp and Yq (Yen et al., 1991). The distal Xp chromosomal region can be divided into two parts: a pseudoautosomal region which exhibits complete homology with the distal Yp (PAR1) and regularly exchanges with it during male meiosis, and a more proximal region which shares 85-95% similarity with sequences in Yq11 and only occasionally exchanges with Xp22 (Ballabio et al., 1989). Males with Xp;Yq translocations are usually nullisomic for a small portion of Xpter and their phenotype depends on the extent of the Xp deletion. When the deletion is large they can present short stature, bony deformities, ichthyosis, attention problems, generalized epilepsy, etc (Meindl et al., 1993). The phenotype of females carrying a normal X and an Xp;Yq translocation with the concomitant deletion of Xp material is usually normal, except for short stature (Van den Berghe et al., 1977).

The proband is the unique child of non-related healthy young parents. She was born after 39 weeks of gestation with a birth weight of 3,050 gr (36th percentile) and length of 49 cm (3rd percentile). At the age of 7 she initiates the treatment with GH, and after 9 months the growth has been of 10.5 cm/year. Her height is now 119.6 cm and weight 47 kg at the age of 8 years. The bone age correlates well with her chronological age. External genitals were normal. No mental retardation was observed.

Conventional G-banding were performed on cultured blood lymphocytes showing a X/Y translocation in the proband, and a normal karyotype in her parents. All metaphase spreads showed 46 chromosomes with one normal X chromosome and one metacentric derivate 46,X,+der(X) (Figure 4). With DAPI banding, the der(X) appeared to be a metacentric X chromosome with a brightly fluorescing heterocromatin attached to its short arm. The probes DYZ1, DYZ3 and Y painting confirmed that the translocation implicated the Yq arm and that the translocated fragment lacked its centromere. With partial painting probes (Xp, Xq, Yq) there was demostrated that not other chromosomal material was involved in the translocation. All metaphases from the parents were normal. PCR analysis showed the ausence of the genes *SRY* and *SHOX* (hemi- or homozygosity), the ausence of the centromeric Y region, and the presence of the heterocromatic Yq12 region. This translocation probably result from a recombination secondary to DNA homologies within misaligned sex chromosomes in the paternal germline with the derivatives segregating at anaphase I.

Amplification of two microsatellite markers located at the SHOX locus resulted in only one single fragment size at both markers, suggesting hemi- or homozygosity of the SHOX locus. For further analysis, parental DNA was available. By amplification of the parental alleles *SHOX* deletion was confirmed.

Normally, the X and Y chromosomes pair during male meiosis and exchange DNA only within the pseudoautosomal regions at the distal short and long arms of both sex chromosomes (PARs regions). However, it has been suggested that aberrant recombination involving other segments of high homology could be responsible for the production of X/Y translocations.

Sequences in Xp/Yp PAR (PAR1) are identical and, during male meiosis, there is a single and obligatory X-Y crossover within this region (Ellis and Goodfellow, 1989). Recombination assures the homogenization of DNA sequence and like most autosomal genes, those in the PAR1 region are expressed from both X and Y alleles (Disteche, 1995). A formally comparable second pseudoatosomal region, Xq/Yq PAR (PAR2) was discovered during the mapping of the X chromosome (Freije et al., 1992). It constains sequences that had been earlier recovered fron both X and Y, and shows recombination over its entire extent. However, it also shows properties distinct from those of PAR1, thus PAR2 exhibits a much lower frequency of pairing and recombination than PAR1 and is not necessary for fertility (Kuhl et al., 2001).

Occasionally the X-Y interchange occurs outside the pseudoatosomal region. It has been found homologous sequences on the long arm of the X chromosome and the short arm or

the proximal long arm of the Y chromosome. In adition, several loci in the Xpter-Xp22 region were found to share 85-95% similarity with sequences in Yq11 or the pericentric region of the Y chromosome.
The majority of these translocations X/Y occur in Xp22 and Yq11 when analyzed cytogenetically. Some of these translocations are sporadic events, like the patient showed here, whereas others are inherited. The analysis of parent's karyotypes were normal, so in our case the translocation was a de novo product.
Most Xp;Yq translocations in males are associated with a large Xp22.3 deletion and the phenotype can be explained by the extension of the deleted region. Main clinical features include short stature, chondrodysplasia punctata, mental retardation, ichthyosis, deficiency, Kallmann syndrome, etc. On the other hand, most females with Xp;Yq translocation have normal intelligence and gonadal function. Short stature is commonly observed and is attributed to the deletion of the *SHOX* gene in the PAR1 region on Xp22.3.
The low stature observed in the subject is due to the deletion of the SHOX gene in the PAR1 region in Xp22.3. Treatment with the GH is recommended, in spite of not being able to define it as TS. The rest of the X chromosome is apparently intact, hence the little affectation of the phenotype. Due to the absence of a centromere for Y a gonadectomy is not advisable

4. Conclusions

First: The joint application of cytogenetic and molecular techniques has allowed a better definition of chromosomal mosaicism (77.6%). The increase in mosaicism was due mainly to the presence of the 46,XX cell line. This combined use should be routine in the diagnosis of this syndrome.
Second: The data suggest that the frequency of occurrence of the Y chromosome in TS is relatively low (7.29%), but its determination is crucial, hence, a molecular study of the Y chromosome in all women with TS is recommended. The analysis must preferably include the study of the centromeric region for the Y chromosome.
Third: Most of the fragments of the Y chromosome present in TS tend to be isodicentric chromosomes, combined with the 45,X cell line. It is probable that most of these isodicentric chromosomes were formed during spermatogenesis, or during the first cell division after fertilization.
Fourth: The location of the 45,X cell line seems to be fundamental in sex determination, even in the presence of the *SRY* gene.
Fifth: The frequency of karyotypes causing Turner syndrome, in our opinion, is much higher than what was originally believed, 1 in every 1,850 newborn girls (7th International Conference on Turner Syndrome, 2009) due to the phenotypes which are not altered or are so mild that are hidden among the population.

5. References

Alfaro, SK; Saavedra, D; Ochoa, S; Scaglia, H. & Perez-Palacios, G. (1976). Pseudohermaphroditism due to XY gonadal absence syndrome. *J Med Genet,* Vol.13, No.3, pp. 242-6, ISSN 0022-2593.

Alves, ST; Gallicchio, CT; Guimaraes, MM. & Santos, M. (2003). Gonadotropin levels in Turner's syndrome: correlation with breast development and hormone replacement therapy. *Gynecol Endocrinol.,* Vol.17, No.4 , pp. 295-301., ISSN 0951-3590

Ballabio, A; Carrozzo, R; Parenti, G; Gil, A; Zollo, M; Persico, MG; Gillard, E; Affara, N; Yates, J; Ferguson-Smith, MA. & et, al. (1989). Molecular heterogeneity of steroid sulfatase deficiency: a multicenter study on 57 unrelated patients, at DNA and protein levels. *Genomics.,* Vol.4, No.1, pp. 36-40., ISSN 0888-7543

Battin, J. (2003). [Turner syndrome and mosaicism]. *Bull Acad Natl Med.,* Vol.187, No.2, pp. 359-67; discussion 368-70., ISSN 0001-4079

Bergada, C; Coco, R; Santamarina, A. & Chemes, H. (1986). Variants of sexual differentiation in relation to sex chromosomal aberrations. *Acta Endocrinol Suppl (Copenh),* Vol.279, pp. 183-7, ISSN 0300-9750

Berta, P; Hawkins, JR; Sinclair, AH; Taylor, A; Griffiths, BL; Goodfellow, PN. & Fellous, M. (1990). Genetic evidence equating SRY and the testis-determining factor. *Nature.,* Vol.348, No.6300, pp. 448-450., ISSN 0028-0836

Bondy, CA; Matura, LA; Wooten, N; Troendle, J; Zinn, AR. & Bakalov, VK. (2007). The physical phenotype of girls and women with Turner syndrome is not X-imprinted. *Hum Genet.,* Vol.121, No.3-4, pp. 469-74. Epub 2007 Jan 23., ISSN 0340-6717

Cameron, FJ & Sinclair, AH. (1997). Mutations in SRY and SOX9: testis-determining genes. *Hum Mutat,* Vol.9, No.5, pp. 388-95, ISSN 1059-7794

Cohen, MM; MacGillivray, MH; Capraro, VJ. & Aceto, TA. (1973). Human dicentric Y chromosomes. Case report and review of the literature. *J Med Genet.,* Vol.10, No.1, pp. 74-9., ISSN 0022-2593

Cooke, H. (1976). Repeated sequence specific to human males. *Nature.,* Vol.262, No.5565, pp. 182-186., ISSN 0028-0836

Coto, E; Toral, JF; Menendez, MJ; Hernando, I; Plasencia, A; Benavides, A. & Lopez-Larrea, C. (1995). PCR-based study of the presence of Y-chromosome sequences in patients with Ullrich-Turner syndrome. *Am J Med Genet.,* Vol.57, No.3, pp. 393-396, ISSN 0148-7299

Disteche, CM. (1995). Escape from X inactivation in human and mouse. *Trends Genet.,* Vol.11, No.1, pp. 17-22., ISSN 0168-9525

Ellis, N & Goodfellow, PN. (1989). The mammalian pseudoautosomal region. *Trends Genet.,* Vol.5, No.12, pp. 406-410., ISSN 0168-9525

Fernandez-Garcia, R; Garcia-Doval, S; Costoya, S. & Pasaro, E. (2000). Analysis of sex chromosome aneuploidy in 41 patients with Turner syndrome: a study of 'hidden' mosaicism. *Clin Genet.,* Vol.58, No.3, pp. 201-8., ISSN 0009-9163

Fernandez, R; Marchal, JA; Sanchez, A. & Pasaro, E. (2002). A point mutation, R59G, within the HMG-SRY box in a female 45,X/46,X, psu dic(Y)(pter-->q11::q11-->pter). *Hum Genet.,* Vol.111, No.3, pp. 242-6., ISSN 0340-6717

Fernandez, R; Mendez, J. & Pasaro, E. (1996). Turner syndrome: a study of chromosomal mosaicism. *Hum Genet.,* Vol.98, No.1, pp. 29-35., ISSN 0340-6717

Fernandez, R & Pasaro, E. (2006). Molecular analysis of an idic(Y)(qter -->p11.32::p11.32-->qter) chromosome from a female patient with a complex karyotype. *Genet Mol Res,* Vol.5, No.2, pp. 399-406, ISSN 1676-5680

Fernandez, R & Pasaro, E. (2010). Tall stature and gonadal dysgenesis in a non-mosaic girl 45,X. *Horm Res Paediatr,* Vol.73, No.3, pp. 210-4, ISSN 1663-2826

Ford, CE; Jones, KW; Polani, PE; DE Almeida JC. & Briggs, JH. (1959). A sex-chromosome anomaly in a case of gonadal dysgenesis (Turner's syndrome). *Lancet,* Vol.1, No.7075, pp. 711-713, ISSN 0140-6736

Freije, D; Helms, C; Watson, MS. & Donis-Keller, H. (1992). Identification of a second pseudoautosomal region near the Xq and Yq telomeres. *Science.,* Vol.258, No.5089, pp. 1784-1787., ISSN 0036-8075

Gubbay, J; Collignon, J; Koopman, P; Capel, B; Economou, A; Munsterberg, A; Vivian, N; Goodfellow, P. & Lovell-Badge, R. (1990). A gene mapping to the sex-determining region of the mouse Y chromosome is a member of a novel family of embryonically expressed genes. *Nature,* Vol.346, No.6281, pp. 245-50, ISSN 0028-0836

Haddad, NG; Vance, GH; Eugster, EA; Davis, MM. & Kaefer, M. (2003). Turner syndrome (45x) with clitoromegaly. *J Urol.,* Vol.170, No.4 Pt 1, pp. 1355-6., ISSN 0022-5347

Hassold, T; Benham, F. & Leppert, M. (1988). Cytogenetic and molecular analysis of sex-chromosome monosomy. *Am J Hum Genet.,* Vol.42, No.4, pp. 534-41., ISSN 0002-9297

Held, KR; Kerber, S; Kaminsky, E; Singh, S; Goetz, P; Seemanova, E. & Goedde, HW. (1992). Mosaicism in 45,X Turner syndrome: does survival in early pregnancy depend on the presence of two sex chromosomes? *Hum Genet.,* Vol.88, No.3, pp. 288-94., ISSN 0340-6717

Hook, EB. (1977). Exclusion of chromosomal mosaicism: tables of 90%, 95% and 99% confidence limits and comments on use. *Am J Hum Genet,* Vol.29, No.1, pp. 94-7., ISSN 0002-9297

Hook, EB & Warburton, D. (1983). The distribution of chromosomal genotypes associated with Turner's syndrome: livebirth prevalence rates and evidence for diminished fetal mortality and severity in genotypes associated with structural X abnormalities or mosaicism. *Hum Genet,* Vol.64, No.1, pp. 24-27, ISSN 0340-6717

Hsu, LY. (1994). Phenotype/karyotype correlations of Y chromosome aneuploidy with emphasis on structural aberrations in postnatally diagnosed cases. *Am J Med Genet.,* Vol.53, No.2, pp. 108-40., ISSN 0148-7299

Joseph, M; CantÃº, ES; Pai, GS; Willi, SM; Papenhausen, PR. & Weiss, L. (1996). Xp pseudoautosomal gene haploinsufficiency and linear growth deficiency in three girls with chromosome Xp22;Yq11 translocation. *J Med Genet.,* Vol.33, No.11, pp. 906-11., ISSN 0022-2593

Kalousek, DK; Dill, FJ; Pantzar, T; McGillivray, BC; Yong, SL. & Wilson, RD. (1987). Confined chorionic mosaicism in prenatal diagnosis. *Hum Genet,* Vol.77, No.2, pp. 163-7., ISSN 0340-6717

Kirsch, S; Keil, R; Edelmann, A; Henegariu, O; Hirschmann, P; LePaslier, D. & Vogt, PH. (1996). Molecular analysis of the genomic structure of the human Y chromosome in the euchromatic part of its long arm (Yq11). *Cytogenet Cell Genet,* Vol.75, No.2-3, pp. 197-206, ISSN 0301-0171

Kocova, M; Siegel, SF; Wenger, SL; Lee, PA; Nalesnik, M. & Trucco, M. (1995). Detection of Y chromosome sequences in a 45,X/46,XXq--patient by Southern blot analysis of PCR-amplified DNA and fluorescent in situ hybridization (FISH). *Am J Med Genet.,* Vol.55, No.4, pp. 483-488, ISSN 0148-7299

Koopman, P; Gubbay, J; Vivian, N; Goodfellow, P. & Lovell-Badge, R. (1991). Male development of chromosomally female mice transgenic for Sry. *Nature,* Vol.351, No.6322, pp. 117-21, ISSN 0028-0836

Koopman, P; Munsterberg, A; Capel, B; Vivian, N. & Lovell-Badge, R. (1990). Expression of a candidate sex-determining gene during mouse testis differentiation. *Nature*, Vol.348, No.6300, pp. 450-2, ISSN 0028-0836

Kuhl, H; Rottger, S; Heilbronner, H; Enders, H. & Schempp, W. (2001). Loss of the Y chromosomal PAR2-region in four familial cases of satellited Y chromosomes (Yqs). *Chromosome Res.*, Vol.9, No.3, pp. 215-222., ISSN 0967-3849

Meindl, A; Hosenfeld, D; Bruckl, W; Schuffenhauer, S; Jenderny, J; Bacskulin, A ; Oppermann, HC; Swensson, O; Bouloux, P . & Meitinger, T. (1993). Analysis of a terminal Xp22.3 deletion in a patient with six monogenic disorders: implications for the mapping of X linked ocular albinism. *J Med Genet.*, Vol.30, No.10, pp. 838-842., ISSN 0022-2593

Money, J. (1993). Specific neuro-cognitive impairments associated with Turner (45,X) and Klinefelter (47,XXY) syndromes: a review. *Soc Biol.*, Vol.40, No.1-2, pp. 147-51., ISSN 0037-766X

Moorhead, PS; Nowell, PC; Mellman, WJ; Battips, DM. & Hungerford, DA. (1960). Chromosome preparations of leukocytes cultured from human peripheral blood. *Exp Cell Res. 1960* , Vol.20, pp. 613-616, ISSN 0014-4827

Nakagome, Y; Nagafuchi, S; Seki, S; Nakahori, Y; Tamura, T; Yamada, M. & Iwaya, M. (1991). A repeating unit of the DYZ1 family on the human Y chromosome consists of segments with partial male-specificity. *Cytogenet Cell Genet*, Vol.56, No.2, pp. 74-7, ISSN 0301-0171

Pinkel, D; Straume, T. & Gray, JW. (1986). Cytogenetic analysis using quantitative, high-sensitivity, fluorescence hybridization. *Proc Natl Acad Sci U S A.*, Vol.83, No.9, pp. 2934-8., ISSN 0027-8424

Procter, SE; Watt, JL; Lloyd, DJ. & Duffty, P. (1984). Problems of detecting mosaicism in skin. A case of trisomy 8 mosaicism illustrating the advantages of in situ tissue culture. *Clin Genet.*, Vol.25, No.3, pp. 273-7., ISSN 0009-9163

Rao, E; Weiss, B; Fukami, M; Rump, A; Niesler, B; Mertz, A; Muroya, K; Binder, G; Kirsch, S; Winkelmann, M; Nordsiek, G; Heinrich, U; Breuning, MH; Ranke, MB; Rosenthal, A; Ogata, T. & Rappold, GA. (1997). Pseudoautosomal deletions encompassing a novel homeobox gene cause growth failure in idiopathic short stature and Turner syndrome. *Nat Genet.*, Vol.16, No.1, pp. 54-63., ISSN 1061-4036

Robinson, D; Dalton, P; Jacobs, P; Mosse, K; Power, M; Skuse, D. & Crolla, J. (1999). A molecular and FISH analysis of structurally abnormal Y chromosomes in patients with Turner syndrome. *J Med Genet.*, Vol.36, No.4, pp. 279-84., ISSN 0022-2593

Ross, J; Roeltgen, D. & Zinn, A. (2006). Cognition and the sex chromosomes: studies in Turner syndrome. *Horm Res.*, Vol.65, No.1, pp. 47-56. Epub 2006 Jan 4., ISSN 0301-0163

Ross, J; Zinn, A. & McCauley, E. (2000a). Neurodevelopmental and psychosocial aspects of Turner syndrome. *Ment Retard Dev Disabil Res Rev*, Vol.6, No.2, pp. 135-41, ISSN 1080-4013

Ross, JL; Roeltgen, D; Kushner, H; Wei, F. & Zinn, AR. (2000b). The Turner syndrome-associated neurocognitive phenotype maps to distal Xp. *Am J Hum Genet*, Vol.67, No.3, pp. 672-681, ISSN 0002-9297

Salo, P; Kaariainen, H; Petrovic, V; Peltomaki, P; Page, DC. & de la Chapelle, A. (1995). Molecular mapping of the putative gonadoblastoma locus on the Y chromosome. *Genes Chromosomes Cancer.*, Vol.14, No.3, pp. 210-214, ISSN 1045-2257

Schwinger, E; Kirschstein, M; Greiwe, M; Konermann, T; Orth, U. & Gal, A. (1996). Short stature in a mother and daughter with terminal deletion of Xp22.3. *Am J Med Genet.*, Vol.63, No.1, pp. 239-42., ISSN 0148-7299

Seabright, M. (1971). A rapid banding technique for human chromosomes. *Lancet.*, Vol.2, No.7731, pp. 971-972., ISSN 0140-6736

Sinclair, A. (2001). Eleven years of sexual discovery. *Genome Biol,* Vol.2, No.7, pp. REPORTS4017, ISSN 1465-6914

Spranger, S; Kirsch, S; Mertz, A; Schiebel, K; Tariverdian, G. & Rappold, GA. (1997). Molecular studies of an X;Y translocation chromosome in a woman with deletion of the pseudoautosomal region but normal height. *Clin Genet.*, Vol.51, No.5, pp. 346-50., ISSN 0009-9163

Su, H & Lau, YF. (1993). Identification of the transcriptional unit, structural organization, and promoter sequence of the human sex-determining region Y (SRY) gene, using a reverse genetic approach. *Am J Hum Genet.*, Vol.52, No.1, pp. 24-38., ISSN 0002-9297

Tsuchiya, K; Reijo, R; Page, DC. & Disteche, CM. (1995). Gonadoblastoma: molecular definition of the susceptibility region on the Y chromosome. *Am J Hum Genet.*, Vol.57, No.6, pp. 1400-1407, ISSN 0002-9297

Urbach, A & Benvenisty, N. (2009). Studying Early Lethality of 45,XO (Turner's Syndrome) Embryos Using Human Embryonic Stem Cells. *PLoS ONE.*, Vol.4, No.1, pp. e4175, ISSN 1932-6203

Van den Berghe, H; Petit, P. & Fryns, JP. (1977). Y to X translocation in man. *Hum Genet.*, Vol.36, No.2, pp. 129-131., ISSN 0340-6717

Werner, MH; Bianchi, ME; Gronenborn, AM. & Clore, GM. (1995). NMR spectroscopic analysis of the DNA conformation induced by the human testis determining factor SRY. *Biochemistry.*, Vol.34, No.37, pp. 11998-2004., ISSN 0006-2960

Witt, M & Erickson, RP. (1989). A rapid method for detection of Y-chromosomal DNA from dried blood specimens by the polymerase chain reaction. *Hum Genet.*, Vol.82, No.3, pp. 271-4., ISSN 0340-6717

Witt, M & Erickson, RP. (1991). A rapid method for detection of Y-chromosomal DNA from dried blood specimens by the polymerase chain reaction. *Hum Genet.*, Vol.86, No.5, pp. 540., ISSN 0340-6717

Yen, PH; Tsai, SP; Wenger, SL; Steele, MW; Mohandas, TK. & Shapiro, LJ. (1991). X/Y translocations resulting from recombination between homologous sequences on Xp and Yq. *Proc Natl Acad Sci U S A.*, Vol.88, No.20, pp. 8944-8948., ISSN 0027-8424

Yenamandra, A; Deangelo, P; Aviv, H; Suslak, L. & Desposito, F. (1997). Interstitial insertion of Y-specific DNA sequences including SRY into chromosome 4 in a 45,X male child. *Am J Med Genet,* Vol.72, No.2, pp. 125-8, ISSN 0148-7299

Zinn, AR; Roeltgen, D; Stefanatos, G; Ramos, P; Elder, FF; Kushner, H; Kowal, K. & Ross, JL. (2007). A Turner syndrome neurocognitive phenotype maps to Xp22.3. *Behav Brain Funct,* Vol.3, pp. 24-38, ISSN 1744-9081

Zinn, AR & Ross, JL. (1998). Turner syndrome and haploinsufficiency. *Curr Opin Genet Dev,* Vol.8, No.3, pp. 322-7, ISSN 0959-437X

22

Microstomia: A Rare but Serious Oral Manifestation of Inherited Disorders

Aydin Gulses
Gulhane Military Medical Academy, Department of Oral and Maxillofacial Surgery
Turkey

1. Introduction

Microstomia is a term used to describe a small oral aperture (Stedman, 1976). Trauma, ingestion of caustic substances, electrical and thermal burns of perioral tissues and reconstructive lip surgeries can result in undesired cicatricial scar formation and inhibit adequate mouth opening (Smith et al., 1982). Less commonly, microstomia can also occur as a result of systemic and/or inherited disorders.

The orbicularis oris muscle, the primary muscle of the lips, forms the sphincter around the mouth and the philtral columns (Wust, 2006) The muscular layer is separated from the skin by a thin subcutaneous layer and from the mucosa below by a thin submucosal layer that contains the adnexa, sensory end organs, and lymph nodes (Wust, 2006). In acquired cases, perioral facial traumas may result in scarring and contraction caused by the involvement and infiltration of the complex perioral musculature during the healing process depending on the depth of injury (Wust, 2006). However, in genetic disorder related cases, the etiology of the condition is variable and mostly remains uncertain.

Individuals with microstomia may experience several problems related to speech, nutritional needs, dental hygiene, facial expression and social interaction (Mordjikian, 2002). Additionally, airway and ventilation problems and aspiration can induce fatal consequences during general anaesthesia procedures (Jaminet et al., 2009).

Management of microstomia is a complex treatment modality and demands complex functional and aesthetic requirements of soft tissues of circumoral region. Providing well functioning lips should be the main objective of the treatment and relapses should be prevented to obtain stable and long lasting results (Koymen et al., 2009). Treatment of the latter was based on mainly on surgical techniques, non-surgical approaches or combination of both methods.

It is important to highlight the reconstruction of the orbicular sphincter for adequate lip function beside lip symmetry, which is the main objective of microstomia reconstruction.

The aim of this chapter is to review the genetic diseases associated with microstomia and briefly discusses the surgical and non surgical management options of the condition.

2. Inherited disorders associated with microstomia

2.1 Scleroderma

Scleroderma originates from the Greek words *skleros,* meaning "hard", and *derma,* meaning "skin" (Albilia et al., 2007) This pathologic condition is the initial manifestation of a disease process better described as progressive systemic sclerosis (PSS), which was named by (Goetz, 1945). It is a multi-system disorder of the connective tissue characterized by vascular disease and the deposition of collagen and other matrix constituents in the skin and other target organs, *i.e.*, the gut, lung, heart, kidney, joints and muscles (Seibold, 2005). Systemic sclerosis process involves damage to the vascular epithelium, immune activation, and increased matrix production. The clinical manifestations of Systemic sclerosis include Raynaud's phenomenon, as well as fibrotic complications of the skin, skeletal muscles, gastrointestinal tract, pulmonary, renal, and cardiac systems. The disease occurs more commonly in women (estimated female to male ratio, 4:1), and the age of peak onset is 30 to 50 years (Steen&Metsger, 1990). The minimum estimated values of incidence and prevalence are 20/million per year and 1,500/million, respectively (Ferri et al., 2002; Hawk&English, 2001).

Although systemic sclerosis is an uncommon autoimmune rheumatic condition affecting connective tissues, it presents great challenges to both medical and dental professionals and has a profound impact on oral health (Albilia et al., 2007). The current classification of systemic sclerosis is based on the extent and pattern of skin sclerosis and reflects the extent of the involvement of organ systems; however this is not highly specific (Albilia et al., 2007). Systemic Sclerosis is subdivided into limited and diffuse cutaneous subtypes. (Table 1) Survival of people with systemic sclerosis mainly depends on the subtype of the disease. Limited cutaneous systemic sclerosis has a 10-year survival rate of 71%; diffuse cutaneous SS, 21%.18 Pulmonary hypertension and scleroderma renal crisis are important prognostic predictors (Trad et al., 2006).

Localized scleroderma
Linear scleroderma
Localized morphea
Generalized morphea
Systemic sclerosis
Limited cutaneous systemic sclerosis
Diffuse cutaneous systemic sclerosis
Systemic sclerosis sine scleroderma
Environmentally induced scleroderma
Overlap syndromes

Table 1. Classification system for progressive systemic sclerosis (adopted from Albilia et al., 2007)

Patients with limited cutaneous systemic sclerosis typically have skin sclerosis that is restricted to the hands, and sometimes the face and neck. They also have prominent vascular manifestations and frequently exhibit features of CREST syndrome. (Table 2) (adopted from Albilia et al., 2007)

Characteristic	Description
Calcinosis cutis	Calcific deposits, usually within the dermis in the extremities and bony prominences, also in deeper periarticular tissues around or within the joints
Raynaud's phenomenon	Triphasic colour changes in the following order: pallor, cyanosis and erythema, representing vaso-constriction, reduced blood flow and reperfusion, respectively
Esophageal dysmotility	Earliest change in the distal esophagus (primarily smooth muscle); an uncoordinated disorganized pattern of contractions resulting in low amplitude or no peristalsis
Sclerodactyly	Fibrosis of the skin of the fingers or toes, associated with atrophy and ulcerations of the fingertips
Telangiectasias	Nonpulsatile macular areas of hemorrhage

Table 2. Features of CREST syndrome (adopted from Albilia et al., 2007)

2.1.1 Physical findings

The first symptom with scleroderma is deformity in the fingers and the toes, caused by a circulation disorder, called the Raynaud phenomenon. The early skin effects begin with the oedema of the face and extremities. The physical findings in progressive systemic sclerosis are:

2.1.1.1 Esophageal dysmotility

Esophageal dysmotility is the most prominent visceral manifestation of PSS, predisposing these persons to gastroesophageal reflux disease, which may be diagnosed first by a dental practitioner. The dental practitioner may then refer the patient to a gastroenterologist for a ph-Probe Test (Barron et al., 2003; Albilia et al., 2007). A barium swallow test is then used to identify hypomotility of the esophagus. Chronic gastroesophageal reflux disease is an important risk factor for aspiration pneumonitis, and potentially pneumonia, and increases the risk of Barrett metaplasia, which in turn increases the risk of esophageal cancer (Barron et al., 2003; Albilia et al., 2007).

2.1.1.2 Pulmonary disease

Pulmonary disease, the second-most common systemic manifestation of PSS, is documented in over 70% of these patients (Albilia et al., 2007). Eventually pulmonary vascular disease develops and results in pulmonary arterial hypertension and subsequent right-sided myocardial hypertrophy (cor pulmonale). For reasons that are unclear, the incidence of lung cancer is higher in patients with progressive sysytemic sclerosis (Winkelmann et al., 1988).

2.1.1.3 Renal disease

Severe and life-threatening renal disease develops in 10% to 15% of patients with PSS. This form of renal involvement is called "scleroderma renal crisis" and is characterized by significant arteriole thickening and constriction, and interstitial collagen deposition,resulting in acute renal failure, marked hypertension and mild proteinuria (Albilia et al., 2007). Patients who have scleroderma without acute renal failure also have physiologic evidence of compromised renal function, which can be estimated readily from the measurement of serum creatinine levels (Livi et al., 2002).

2.1.1.4 Musculoskeletal findings

Patients may have generalized arthralgias and morning stiffness that may mimic other systemic autoimmune diseases. Hand and joint function may decline over time because of skin tightening, rather than arthropathy, and may have a negative impact on daily activities, including maintenance of oral hygiene (Albilia et al., 2007).

2.1.1.5 Orofacial findings and microstomia

In progressive systemic sclerosis patients, subcutaneous collagen deposition in facial skin results in a characteristic smooth, taut, mask-like facies. Nasal alae may become atrophied and result in "mouse-like" facies (Albilia et al., 2007). Other important orofacial manifestations include fibrosis of the salivary and lacrimal glands, and symptoms consistent with dry mouth or xerostomia. Patients may develop dry eyes with keratoconjunctivitis sicca or xerophthalmia(Albilia et al., 2007). This is particularly problematic because scarring of the eyelids results in a chronic widening of the palpebral fissures and inadequate closure of the eyelid, which causes further drying of already dry eyes (Albilia et al., 2007). Inadequate salivary flow compromises buffering within the oral cavity and allows the acidity produced by bacterial metabolism and GERD to erode the dentition. Classic dental radiographic findings of PSS show a thickening of the periodontal ligament or periodontal ligament space (Albilia et al., 2007). Accentuation of periodontal disease also occurs, believed to be due not only to poor oral hygiene but also to the vascular changes associated with the disease itself. With disease progression may come a uniform widening of the periodontal ligaments of all teeth (Albilia et al., 2007).This change seen in a minority of patients occurs at the expense of alveolar bone (lamina dura) rather than root surface. In addition, in a minority of patients there is mandibular bone resorption in non-tooth bearing areas. The inferior border, the posterior border of the ramus, the mandibular angle, and the coronoid and condylar processes may exhibit radiographic evidence of resorption. A blunting of the angles of the mandible, resembling a "tail of the whale," may be seen on an orthopantograph This is believed to be related to an associated muscle atrophy, pressure of tightening of skin overlying the bone and vascular changes (Yenisey et al., 2005). Infrequently, pathologic fractures of the mandible may develop from the mandibular resorption.

Further, facial and mucosal fibrosis compromises oral access because of microstomia, which limits mouth opening in 70% of these patients (Neville et al., 2002). As a consequence, oral hygiene and fabrication of removable dentures are difficult because of limited access and the obliteration or shallowing of the mucobuccal folds.

Skin sclerosis is often treated with D-penicillamine, a chelating agent that affects unknown mechanisms of collagen formation. Experimental drugs, such as interferon-gamma and cyclophosphamide, and photophoresis have been used with varying degrees of success.

Management of the systemic effects of this disease is not well established, although some large uncontrolled series suggest that D-penicillamine has beneficial effects (Stone &Wigley, 1998). Interferon-gamma is effective, but its use is limited because of inflammatory sequelae.

2.2 Holoprosencephaly

Holoprosencephaly is considered as the most frequent anatomical central nervous system defect in humans (Orioli & Castilla, 2010). However, relatively few epidemiological studies have been performed on holoprosencephaly at older gestational ages, and no definitive risk factor has been clearly proved to be associated with holoprosencephaly. (Orioli & Castilla, 2010). Holoprosencephaly occurs when the prosencephalon fails to cleave sagittally into cerebral hemispheres, transversely into telecephalon and diencephalon, and/or horizontally into olfactory and optic bulbs. Nevertheless, substantial variations of the cerebral defect, as ell as of the accompanying facial anomalies, exist, generating differences in the ascertainment of the involved cases. Severe ear defects, as well as microstomia, were part of the spectrum of the condition. Several studies have excluded, or analyzed separately, the holoprosencephaly cases with chromosome abnormalities, and/or with recognized monogenic syndromes. The chromosome status of a holoprosencephaly patient is not easy to determine, due to their high perinatal mortality rate, and at least 10% of those with normal karyotypes have microdeletions/duplications and remain undetected by usual karyotyping (Orioli & Castilla, 2010; Mastroiacovo et al., 1995).

(Orioli & Castilla, 2010) determined whether craniofacial and noncraniofacial defects in holoprosencephaly cases. They confirmed the observation of Mastroiacovo et al., that among craniofacial defects, severe ear anomalies with atresia of the auditory canal, as well as microstomia, were part of the spectrum of holoprosencephaly (Mastroiacovo et al., 1995). Of the noncraniofacial defects, 24% of the holoprosencephaly cases had genital anomalies, 8% postaxial polydactyly, 5% vertebral defects, 4% limb reduction defects, and 4% had transposition of great arteries; all these defects were significantly associated with holoprosencephaly, while no significant association was found between holoprosencephaly and anencephaly, spina bifida, or encephalocele (Orioli & Castilla, 2010)..

2.3 Richieri-Costa–Pereira syndrome

In 1992 Richieri-Costa and Pereira (Richieri-Costa &Pereira, 1992) described a new syndrome of acrofacial dysostosis, in five unrelated Brazilian females, characterized mainly by Robin sequence, cleft mandible, and limb defects (Favaro et al., 2010). The family history showed parental consanguinity, recurrence in sibs, and increased death rate in males, which led the authors to suggest that this new condition was caused by an autosomal recessive gene(Favaro et al., 2010). Subsequently, the same authors described the first males with this condition (Favaro et al., 2010). The causative gene of this syndrome remains unknown and molecular investigations are in progress. Favaro et al stated the main features and prevalence of this syndrome as follows: microstomia (100%), micrognathia (100%), clinical or radiological abnormal fusion of the mandible (100%), cleft palate/Robin sequence (78.5%), absent central lower incisors (80%), minor ears anomalies (92.8%), hypoplastic thumbs (96.2%), hypoplastic thenar/hypothenar region (83.3%), mesomelic shortening of upper (51.8%) and lower limbs (88.8%), hypoplastic halluces (92.5%), and clubfeet (100%) (Favaro et al., 2010).. Language assessment showed learning disability in 14 cases (84%), and language disorder in 15 (77%). Favaro et al suggested that, due to the high frequency of airway obstruction and feeding difficulties which are common findings in infancy, corroborate that individuals with Richieri-Costa-Pereira syndrome need special support, mainly in first years of life when most of the deaths occur (Favaro et al., 2010).

2.4 Freeman–Sheldon syndrome

Freeman-Sheldon syndrome, also known as distal arthrogryposis, type 2a; OMIM #193700, was first described by Freeman and J.H. Sheldon in 1938 (Corrigan et al., 2006). In 1975, Antley et al introduced the term 'whistling face syndrome' for the condition (Antley et al., 1975). Freeman–Sheldon syndrome is a heterogeneous condition both in its presentation and in its mode of transmission and both sexes are equally affected Freeman–Sheldon is an uncommon, morphologically well-defined syndrome. Orofacial findings of the condition are: A distinctive facial appearance of microstomia, microglossia, a short nose, long philtrum, H-shaped chin dimple, and sunken eyes is described. Extracranially, anomalies of the long bones, scoliosis, hand abnormalities, and joint contractures are found in most of the cases. The syndrome has also been termed 'Windmill–Vane hand' and although rare, is one of the commonest causes of multiple inherited congenital joint contractures(Corrigan et al., 2006). Intelligence is usually normal, although mental disability have been also reported in some cases [4–6]. Congenital respiratory system abnormalities and microstomia related feeding problems have been documented in a number of cases (Song et al., 1996; Corrigan et al., 2006; Antley et al., 1975). Presentation of complications in adolescence has also been reported. Song *et al.* described a 13-year-old with Freeman–Sheldon syndrome who developed late-onset dysphagia and subsequent weight loss. Corrigan et al reported the dental management experience in a patient with Freeman–Sheldon syndrome (Corrigan et al., 2006).

Ohyama *et al.* presented a case in which a mouth expander was used as a nonsurgical method of correcting microstomia (Ohyama et al., 1997). The authors claimed that this therapy produced an increase in mouth width. Corrigan et al suggested that it is debatable whether this change was actually induced by mouth expander use or whether it was simply a result of normal facial growth (Corrigan et al., 2006). No other interventions to improve microstomia have been reported in relation to Freeman– Sheldon syndrome yet.

2.5 De novo duplication of maternal origin of the 15q11.2-q14 pws/ as region [46, xx, dup (15) (q11.2-q14)]

The 15q11-q13 PWS/AS critical region involves genes that are characterized by genomic rearrangements, including interstitial deletions, duplications, and triplications (Browne et al., 1995). Multiple repeat elements within the region mediate rearrangements, including interstitial duplications, interstitial triplications, and supernumerary isodicentric marker chromosomes, as well as the deletions that cause Prader–Willi syndrome and Angelman syndrome. Recently, duplications of maternal origin concerning the same critical region have been implicated in autism spectrum disorders (Kitsiou-Tzeli et al., 2010) presented a 6-month-old girl with a de novo duplication of maternal origin of the 15q11.2-q14 PWS/AS region (17.73Mb in size) [46,XX,dup(15)(q11.2-q14)] detected with a high-resolution microarray-based comparative genomic hybridization (array-CGH) Kitsiou-Tzeli et al., 2010 The features of the condition were described by the same authors as: severe hypotonia, obesity, microstomia, long eyelashes, hirsutism, microretrognathia, short nose, severe psychomotor retardation, and multiple episodes of drug-resistant epileptic seizures, partial corpus callosum dysplasia documented via magnetic resonance imaging. The duplicated region was quite large extending beyond the Prader–Willi–Angelman critical region, containing a number of genes that have been shown to be involved in autism spectrum disorders, exhibiting a severe phenotype, beyond the typical PWS/AS clinical manifestations. Reporting of similar well-characterized clinical cases with clearly delineated breakpoints of the duplicated region will clarify the contribution of specific genes to the phenotype (Kitsiou-Tzeli et al., 2010).

2.6 Hallerman – Streiff syndrome

Hallerman - Streiff syndrome or Francois Syndrome also known as oculomandibulodyscephaly with hypotrichosis was first described by Aubry in 1893. The syndrome was later defined as Hallermann-Streiff Syndrome, underlining the differences with regard to Franceschetti's mandibulofacial dysostosis (Cannistrà et al., 1999).

All individuals with Hallermann- Streiff syndrome have been sporadic, without a sex predilection, but inheritance pattern is still debated (Pizzuti et al., 2004). Concordant monozygotic twins have been described (Van Balen, 1961) and the few cases of Hallermann-Streiff syndrome with children always had unaffected offspring (Hendrix& Sauer, 1991).Oculodentodigital dysplasia is a genetic disorder related to dominant mutations in the connexin 43 gene at chromosome 6q22-23 (Paznekas et al., 2003). Spaepen et al suggested that several clinical features of this autosomal dominant highly penetrant disorder overlap those of the Hallermann- Streiff syndrome (Spaepen et al., 1991). Due to the clinical overlap between Oculodentodigital dysplasia and Hallermann- Streiff syndrome Pizzuti et al tested the work hypothesis they could be allelic disorders, both caused by GJA1 gene mutations and stated that the Homozygous GJA1 Gene Mutation Causes a Hallermann-Streiff/ Oculodentodigital dysplasia Spectrum Phenotype.Hallermann in 1948 and Streiff in 1950 described the cardinal features of the condition as: dyscephaly with bird facies, frontal or parietal bossing, dehiscence of sutures with open fontanelles, hypotrichosis of scalp, eyebrows and eyelashes, cutaneous atrophy of scalp and nose, mandibular hypoplasia, forward displacement of temporomandibular joints, high arched palate, small mouth, multiple dental anomalies and proportionate small stature (Hoefnagel & Benirschke, 1965). Defraia et al assessed the following features from a dentoskeletal point of view: aplasia of the anterior teeth, skeletal Class II malocclusion, narrow upper arch, bilateral posterior crossbite, and anterior open bite (Defraia et al., 2003). Ophthalmic features of the condition are microphthalmia, congenital cataracts, blue sclerae and nystagmus. Individuals with Hallermann-Streiff Syndrome, presence of mandibular hypoplasia and microstomia can result in difficult intubation. Recognition of this syndrome should alert the physician to the possibility of difficulty in airway maintenance (Malde et al., 1994).

2.7 Hutchinson–Gilford progeria

Hutchinson-Gilford progeria syndrome (OMIM 176670) first described by the general practitioner Jonathan Hutchinson in 1886, is a very rare autosomal dominant disorder characterised by growth retardation and progressive, premature senescent changes of the skin, bones and cardiovascular system (Sevenants et al., 2005). According to Polex and Hegele, since 1886 fewer than 100 cases of Hutchinson-Gilford progeria syndrome have been reported, with approximately 40 cases currently diagnosed (Polex & Hegele, 2004).

Feature	Frequency
Prenatal growth delay	0-25 %
Postnatal growth delay	75-100 %
Normal skull growth	50-75 %
Cognitive development	75-100 %
Hair sparse/alopecia	75-100 %
Increased visibility vessels	
Cranium	75-100 %
Nasal bridge	75-100 %
Prominent forehead	25-50 %
Absent eyebrows/eyelashes	50-75 %
Small face	75-100 %
Thin nasal skin	75-100 %
Convex nasal profile	25-50 %
Crowded teeth	50-75 %
Increased dental decay	50-75 %
Absent ear lobule	25-50 %
High voice	75-100 %
Lipodystrophy	75-100 %
Narrow upper thorax	75-100 %
Prominent abdomen	75-100 %
Broadened finger tips	50-75 %
Nail dystrophy	50-75 %
Horse riding stance	50-75 %
Decreased mobility	
Elbows	75-100 %
Wrists	25-50 %
Fingers	75-100 %
Hips	75-100 %
Knees	75-100 %
Ankles	25-50 %

Table 3. Major Findings in 142 Patients With Hutchinson–Gilford Progeria Syndrome (adopted from Domingo et al, 2009)

Fong stated that, most cases are caused by a de novo single-nucleotide substitution in codon 608 of prelamin A (p.G608G (GGC>GGT), p.G608S (GGC>AGC)), leading to the mutated Hutchinson-Gilford progeria syndrome gene product lamin A (LMNA), a structural component of the nuclear membrane (Fong & Meta, 2004). Lamin A contributes to nuclear structural integrity and chromatin regulatory mechanisms (Martin, 2005). Progerin is the mutant form of lamin A and while progerin is expressed at very low levels normally, it is expressed at much greater levels in Hutchinson-Gilford progeria syndrome (Domingo et al, 2009). According to Domingo et al, Progerin accumulation in cells has been associated with instability of the nuclear membrane, progressive nuclear damage, and premature cell death. Polex and Hegele have shown structural nuclear abnormalities in 48% of Hutchinson-Gilford progeria syndrome fibroblast nuclei compared with less than 6% of normal control cells (Domingo et al, 2009). Furthermore, they stated that, Hutchinson-Gilford progeria syndrome fibroblasts undergo hyperproliferation followed by rapid apoptosis.

From the Greek geras, meaning _old age,' progeria is a human disease model of accelerated senescence (Domingo et al, 2009). Affected individuals typically appear normal at birth but begin to demonstrate features of accelerated aging within the first year of life.

Clinically, the main features of Hutchinson-Gilford progeria syndrome include alterations in skin, bone, and cardiovascular tissues, marked retardation of growth, loss of subcutaneous fat, and distinctive bone changes. These main features and their prevalances were shown in Table 3.

Although, microstomia was not reported in majority of the cases, however, sclerodermatous changes which could be the first manifestation of Hutchinson-Gilford progeria syndrome, can result in restriction of the oral aperture.

Among individuals with Hutchinson-Gilford progeria syndrome, death occurs at 13 years of age, most commonly from progressive coronary and cardiovascular atherosclerosis (Pollex&Hegele, 2004).

2.8 Burton skeletal dysplasia

Burton skeletal dysplasia was first described by Burton et al in 1986 (Burton et al., 1986). They reported a pair of sibs suffering from a new skeletal dysplasia with clinical and radiological findings similar to those of Kniest dysplasia but with important differences. They reported the main clinical findings as: sibs with short stature, bowing and shortness of limbs, enlargement of wrists and knee joints, stiffness of knee joints, and a bell-shaped thorax with flare of lower ribs. In addition, they had a small mouth with pursed lips, downward dislocation of the lenses, and myopia. In agreement with Burton et al, Lo et al added the third case to he literature and reported also a small mouth with pursed lips that remained more or less the same size whether she laughed or cried, and a deep philtrum (Lo et al., 1998).

2.9 Fine–Lubinsky syndrome

In 1983, Drs. Fine and Lubinsky described a single patient with craniofacial anomalies, hearing loss, cataracts, microstomia, and developmental delay (Fine & Lubinsky, 1983). In following reports, the main clinical features of the condition was described as: craniosynostosis, prominent frontal bones, flat facial profiles, small noses, microstomia, hearing loss, developmental delay, and abnormal digits (Preus et al., 1984; Suthers et al., 1993; Ayme´ & Philip, 1996; Holder et al., 2007; Schoner et al., 2008; Cole et al., 2010).

Schoner et al reported a female fetus of 24 weeks gestational age with Fine-Lubinsky syndrome and based the diagnosis of Fine-Lubinsky syndrome on growth deficiency, brachycephaly, flat face with associated dysmorphic signs, microstomia and cataract (Schoner et al., 2008).

Cole performed a G-banded chromosome analysis, telomere FISH study, and an array based comparative genome hybridization analysis in a patient with Fine-Lubinsky syndrome (Cole et al., 2010). The genetic evaluation of the individual revealed no abnormalities. However, Holder et al described the first brother and sister sibling pair with features suggestive of Fine- Lubinsky syndrome and the identification of a brother–sister sibling pair with unaffected parents suggested a possible autosomal recessive inheritance pattern with a 25% recurrence risk to future siblings (Holder et al., 2007).

2.10 Leopard syndrome

LEOPARD syndrome, also known as Multiple Lentigines syndrome, Cardio-cutaneous syndrome, Moynahan syndrome, Lentiginosis profusa and Progressive Cardiomyopathic Lentiginosis is a polymalformative disease affecting many organs and systems and was first described by Zeisler and Becker in 1936 (Zeisler& Becker, 1936).

The abnormalities related to Leopard syndrome are: Electrocardiographic anomalies, ocular hypertelorism, pulmonary stenosis. anomalies of genitalia, retardation of growth and deafness(Yam et al., 2001).

The Leopard syndrome follows an autosomal dominant mode of transmission with a wide variability in expression (Ho et al., 1989). However, according to some authors, the syndrome may arise as a result of a spontaneous mutation. Microstomia associated with Leopard syndrome was reported by Yam et al. According to Sarkozy et al, Leopard syndrome may be sporadic or inherited as an autosomal dominant fully penetrant trait (Sarkozy, et., 2008). In approximately 85% of the patients with a definite diagnosis of Leopard syndrome, a missense mutation is found in the *PTPN11* gene, located on chromosome 12q24.1 (Diglio et al., 2002; Sarkozy et al., 2004).

2.11 Auriculo-condylar syndrome

Auriculo-condylar syndrome (OMIM 602483) was first described by Jampol et al in 1998 (Jampol et al., 1998). It is an autosomal dominant disorder of first and second pharyngeal arches, is characterized by malformed ears, prominent cheeks, microstomia, abnormal temporomandibular joint, and mandibular condyle hypoplasia. Comparison of clinical signs of patients with auriculo-condylar syndrome from previous reports were shown in Table IV. Treacher Collins syndrome (OMIM 154500), oculoauriculo- vertebral spectrum (OMIM 164210), and Townes–Brocks syndrome (07480) have several overlapping clinical signs with auriculo-conylar syndrome and should be considered for differential diagnosis of the condition. Masotti et al. (Masotti et al., 2008) stated that, the mapping and identification will certainly bring important contributions to the understanding of the development of embryonic structures derived from these pharyngeal arches, as well as to perform differential diagnosis.

The auriculo-condylar syndrome gene is still unknown. The intra- and inter-familial phenotypic variation in auriculo-condylar syndrome has been noted by several authors. (Guion-Almeida et al., 1999; Storm et al., 2005; Masotti et al., 2008; Jampol et al.,1998) Masotti et al have performed a wide genome search and observed evidence of linkage to 1p21.1–q23.3. They have also stated that an evidence for genetic heterogeneity. (Masotti et al., 2008)

Clinical signs	Cases	Frequency(%)
TMJ abnormality	26/26	100
Micrognathia	33/46	71.7
Microstomia	26/42	61.9
Stenotic ear canals	6/17	35.3
Mild developmental delay	3/13	23.1
Abnormal palate	14/29	48.2
Glossoptosis	11/22	50.0
Ptosis	3/11	27.3
Feeding difficulties	8/30	26.7
Prominent cheeks	29/43	67.4
Respiratory distress	14/34	41.2
Macrocephaly	3/12	25.0
Hearing loss	12/27	44.4
Ear constriction	46/47	97.9

Table 4. Clinical signs and the prevalances of Auriculo- condylar syndrome from previous reports (adopted from Masotti et al., 2008)

2.12 Chromosome 22q11.2 Deletion syndrome (Velocardiofacial/DiGeorge syndrome)

Dr. Angelo DiGeorge described a group of infants with congenital absence of the thymus and parathyroid glands In 1965 (DiGeorge et al., 1965). Facial dysmorphia, conotruncal cardiac malformations, and speech delay were included in the spectrum and various other names came to be applied to this constellation of phenotypic features, including velocardiofacial syndrome, cardiofacial syndrome, and conotruncal anomaly face syndrome(McDonald-McGinn & Sullivan, 2011). Major phenotypic features of the condition were listed in Table 5. According to the review of McDonald-McGinn and Sullivan, the estimated prevalence has been cited as being 1:3000-1:6000 births (McDonald-McGinn & Sullivan, 2011).

Major Phenotypic Features
Cardiac anomaly
Tetralogy of Fallot
Ventriculoseptal defect
Interrupted aortic arch
Truncus arteriosus
Vascular ring
Immune deficiency
T-cell lymphopenia
Thymic aplasia with absent T cells
Delayed IgG production
Palatal defects
Velopharyngeal insufficiency
Submucous cleft palate
Overt cleft palate
Cleft lip and palate

Table 5. Major phenotypic features of Chromosome 22q11.2 Deletion Syndrome (adopted from McDonald-McGinn & Sullivan, 2011)

Cytogenetic and molecular studies have showed that most patients with DiGeorge/ Velocardiofacial syndrome have interstitial or submicroscopic deletions within 22q11 (Driscoll et al., 1992) Clinical findings in Chromosome 22q11.2 Deletion syndrome were shown in Table 6.

Clinical findings
Feeding difficulties
Respiratory infections
Developmental delay
Short stature
Long face, vertical maxillary excess
Abundant hair
Mild, upslanting palpebal fissures
High, wide nasal bridge
Prominent middle nose with hypoplastic nasal alae
Philtrum anomalies
Microstomia
Long recessed chin
Abnormal ears
Short, broad neck
Scoliosis
Heart defect
Umbilical hernia

Table 6. Clinical findings in Velocardiofacial syndrome (adopted from Jaquez et al., 1997)

Microstomia was reported to be one of the clinical findings in Chromosome 22q11.2 Deletion Syndrome. (Jaquez et al., 1997, Martin Mateos et al., 2000) However, the pathogenesis and the frequency of microstomia among individuals with Chromosome 22q11.2 Deletion Syndrome are not known.

2.13 Epidermolysis bullosa

Epidermolysis bullosa is a group of rare, genetically determined disease, which is characterized by cutaneous and mucosal blistering associated with occasional subsequent scarring secondary to minor trauma. It is divided into 3 major types by histological findings, and includes approximately 23 variants, manifested by a spectrum of clinical presentations (Stavropoulos% Abramovicz, 2008; Ozgur et al., 2005).The diagnosis is confirmed by examining the basal membrane with transmission electron microscopy, immunohistochemical analysis, and complementary examinations, such as optical microscopy, immunofluorescence, and enzymatic analysis (Siqueira et al., 2008).
The condition affects approximately 1 in 50,000 to 1 in 500,000 births and encompasses a group of congenital chronic noninflammatory skin disorders. Their common primary

feature is the formation of blisters and erosions at the site of minor mechanical trauma in the skin, mucocutaneous layers of the oral mucosa, and respiratory and digestive tracts (Ergun et al., 1992; Marx&Stern, 2003).
Results of the first gene therapy was reported in 2006 by De Luca and colleagues on a patient with generalized junctional epidermolysis bullosa who had compound heterozygous mutations in the β3 chain of laminin 332 (Fine, 2010) .
Most of the more severe subtypes are associated with clinically significant extracutaneous complications. Some subtypes may lead to death, even in early infancy. Dystrophic epidemolysis bullosa has either an autosomal- dominant or recessive pattern of inheritance and is associated with loss of fibrils of anchorage and increased collagen disintegration on the superficial dermis due to excessive synthesis of collagenase (Silva et al., 2004; de Freitas, 1986). This characteristic may results in limited mouth opening. The recessive subtype of the condition is the more severe form, in which the continuous formation of cicatricial tissue, especially in the hands and feet, leads to the joining of the fingers and toes. The dominant form of epidermolysis bullose presents with bullous eruptions that develop after trauma and heal leaving atrophic scars and milium, which are small white nodules that appear beneath the scars.
According to Stavropoulos and Abramovicz (Stavropoulos& Abramovicz, 2008). oral involvement of epidermolysis bullosa may includes occasional intraoral blistering that heals rapidly and patients may present with severe intraoral blistering and subsequent scar formation which results in restriction of the mouth opening. Spinocellular carcinoma is the most frequent complication of epidermolysis bullosa and morbidity and mortality were frequently reported. (Liversidge et al., 2005).

3. Treatment of Microstomia

The main goal and objective of microstomia treatment are: the reconstruction of the orbicularis sphincter for adequate lip functioning, obtaining lip symmetry and formation of well positioned and undistorted scars. The cause and severity of the perioral restriction and esthetic and functional requirements influence the treatment selection and procedures. Several techniques have been described for the reconstruction of the labial commissures. Surgical possibilities include z-plasties, skin grafts, commissurotomies and local flaps. In addition, a number of nonsurgical methods and designs have been used for maintaining adequate mouth opening. Individuals with restricted mouth opening were considered to be good candidates for intra- and extraoral stretching devices, static and dynamic oral appliances and sectional and collapsible dentures (Wust, 2006).

3.1 Surgical therapy

Basically, an effective surgical treatment for individuals with microstomia must solve two problems: first, to restore the oral opening size by releasing the commissural contracture; and second, to minimize the cosmetic defect caused by oral angle deformation (Griskevich, 2010). Restoration of the oral commissure is always a difficult procedure related to the complex functional and esthetic entity of the circumoral region. idely used methods usually consist of scar 'excision' in the oral angle zone and wound closure with mobilised mucosal flaps (Griskevich, 2010). Dieffenbach.(Dieffenbach, 1829; Jaminet et al., 2009) presented the first technique to correct microstomia by performing advancement of superior, inferior, and lateral mucosal flaps to reconstruct the corner of the mouth after removal of a triangular wedge of scar tissue. The procedure was modified later by Converse (Converse, 1959; Jaminet et al., 2009) and later by Mehra et al (Mehra et al., 1998; Jaminet et al., 2009) by performing either a vermilion advancement or the transposition of the buccal mucosa following the commissurotomy procedure.

Gillies and Millard (Gillies & Millard, 1957, Jaminet et al., 2009) used a vermilion flap to reconstruct the upper lip and an oral mucosal advancement flap for the lower lip. Villoria (Villoria, 1972) transposed inner and outer orbicularis oris muscle flaps and performed an advancement of the oral mucosa to reshape the vermilion. Johns et al (Johns et al., 1998;Jaminet et al., 2009) suggested the success of the triangular pedicled flap for oral commissuroplasty, with good result. Muhlbauer (Muhlbauer, 1970; Jaminet et al., 2009) proposed 2 Z-plasties, using the rotation of 2 small skin flaps into the mucosa of the lip. However, this technique is rarely used as it does not allow restoration of the oral angle if the scars are rough. Sorensen pointed out, "Traditionally, defects are usually closed with a Y-V plasty, but in my opinion the classical Z-plasty is better (Sorensen, 1979)." (Griskevich, 2010). Fairbanks and Dingman reconstructed the oral aperture by obliquely dividing the existing vermilion into 2 diminishing flaps approximated to the new mouth angle (Fairbanks&Dingman, 1972). After contracture release, a trilobed flap is created from the mucosa that is advanced over the defect and sutured into place; the middle part of the flap is used to create the vertical part of the commissure; an overcorrection (2–4 mm) is advisable and a splint is recommended to prevent recurrence of the contracture. After triangular scar excision, mucosal advance- ment Y–V flap, or mucosal rhomboid flaps per side or skin grafts are used (Griskevich, 2010). Takato et al used a free forearm flap for reconstruction of the oral cavity and vermilion flaps at the oral commissure on a patient with severely constricted oral cavity because of mucosal adhesions (Takato et al., 1989). Martins et al reconstructed corners of the mouth via 4 rhomboid flaps rotated from the buccal mucosa (Martins et al., 2003). Ayhan et al described a new technique of reconstructing with a composite graft of the ear-lobule to surgically correct microstomia (Ayhan et al., 2006). Composite auricular lobule grafts, triangular pedicle flaps and bipedicled deep inferior epigastric perforator flaps are seldom used for the reconstruction of the oral commissure.

With the knowledge of the literature review, it can be stated that, no commissure reconstruction without scars of operation has been achieved so far by using the available techniques. Griskevich suggested that most of the commissuroplasties cannot bring good cosmetic results as flaps possess different qualities and the transposition of the flap inwards and placing it within the mucosa deforms the oral angle. For commisurotomy, the red mucosal flap is turned out for wound closure, creating a new angle deformation similar to mucosal ectropion. The oral angle zone becomes deeper, more rounded and wider; the red mucosa remains visible when the mouth is closed, which creates a cosmetic defect. Moreover, the end of the advanced mucosal flap was tightened with sutures, which could impair blood circulation, and it could result in microstomia recurrence. Therefore, an overcorrection and a splint are often recommended after all of microstomia operations (Griskevich, 2010). According to the same author, all techniques mentioned above can provide satisfactory functional outcomes, but the 'aesthetic' results were found only "acceptable (Griskevich, 2010).

The need for a detailed description of anatomical features in their relation to red mucosa after surgery in the newly commissural region still remains. (Griskevich, 2010).

3.2 Non surgical therapy

Compression therapy, mouth splinting, scar massage, contact media, exercise, patient education and neck splinting are standard treatments for the prevention and management of microstomia (Wust, 2006). It has been demonstrated that, effective contracture management needs to provide horizontal, vertical, and circumferential lip stretch.

3.2.1 Static and dynamic mouth splints

Basically, two forms of functional splinting devices exist: passive splints which prevent contraction, and dynamic widening devices which regain lost oral opening. These may be retained by intraoral (fixed or removable) or extraoral devices. The removable splint usually resembles a mouthguard made of acrylic resin and is retained with clasps. The fixed appliance is retained on orthodontic bands placed on the primary maxillary second molars and central incisors. Both devices support acrylic resin posts that maintain the commissural regions equidistant to the midline. Reisberg et al. recommended using an extraoral commissure conformer attached to an orthodontic headgear strap (Reisberg et al., 1983). The amount of tension needed is based on the distance from the midline to the unaffected side when the patient smiles broadly. Many investigators have documented the use of lip and cheek retractors as a splinting device. Silverglade and Ruberg stated that an expansile removable appliance to regain lost lateral dimension due to scar contracture is usefull (Silverglade.& Ruberg, 1986) Two acrylic phalanges are connected to an orthodontic palatal expanding device that expands 0.25 mm with each adjustment. Madjar et al. described a commissure widening device in which a stainless steel wire is bent into the shape of an **fl** and fitted with acrylic resin lip holders such that force is directed laterally and distally (Madjar et al., 1987). Conine et al. evaluated the structural and clinical characteristics of major microstomia orthoses and proposed the Vancouver microstomia orthosis (Conine et al., 1989). They stated an average of 7 mm in the horizontal and 13 mm in the vertical active range of motion within 9 weeks of use.

Dynamic Mouth Splint designed by Van Straten, was considered for trial to improve vertical mouth opening (van Straten, 1991). However, some difficulties were identified. These included:

1. *the thermoplastic material was not designed for intra-oral use,*
2. *the risk of damage to dental structures caused by lack of conformity to the teeth,*
3. *the risk of oral infection caused by possible microbial contamination of the splint lining,*
4. *the fact that the application requires a vertical mouth opening of more than 25 mm.*

Subsequently, a Modified Dynamic Mouth Splint was developed that combines design features of the original Dynamic Mouth Splint with materials designed for intra oral use (Wust, 2006). Wust stated that, good results in functional mouth opening can be obtained by using the Modified Dynamic Mouth Splints (Wust, 2006).

3.2.2 Vertical orthosis

Microstomia devices have been developed to decrease the scarring and contractures imposed by the healing process. Many of these devices are useful for the control of horizontal mouth opening restriction. Recently, another Davis proposed an effective, simple, economical, orthotic device for the enlargement of the vertical mouth diameter and suggested that, patients gave positive feedback for comfort and ease of use, with increased mouth mobility and range of motion (Davis et al., 2006). Additionally, it has been suggested that, from a visual assessment, the vertical orthoses are more comfortable to wear for an extended period because the patient can swallow and, with the lip-based device, talk while it is in place.

3.2.3 Sectional dentures

Without surgical operation it is very difficult to perform prosthetic treatment for patients with microstomia, especially when the severe restriction of the mouth circumference length . Because the smallest diameter of a fully retentive denture and a impression tray may be larger than the greatest diameter of the mouth opening, a sectional impression tray and a sectional denture may be indicated (Suzuki et al., 2000).

Yenisey et al described a technique for the fabrication of mandibular and maxillary sectional trays and a sectional mandibular complete denture fabrication for a patient with microstomia induced by scleroderma a sectional mandibular denture was a suitable treatment to resolve the problem of microstomia caused by scleroderma. They stated that, the cast hinge design reduced the overall costs and simplified the laboratory technique. This technique has proven to be simple, inexpensive and applicable to selected microstomic patients (Yenisey et al., 2005). Watanabe et al reported the use of cast Fe-Pt magnetic attachments to treat an edentulous patient with microstomia induced by scleroderma (Watanabe et al., 2002) and described a cast iron-platinum magnetic attachment system applied to sectional collapsed complete denture. With the use of lingual and palatal midline hinges and an Fe-Pt magnetic attachment, the sectional collapsed complete dentures were successfully and easily inserted and continue to provide adequate function in the patient's mouth. Cura et al described an other technique used to fabricate mandibular and maxillary sectional trays and a folding maxillary complete denture for a patient with limited oral opening caused by systemic sclerosis. For the foldable denture, the anterior teeth had to be arranged on a second base and the hinge fitted at a location higher than the denture base (Cura et al., 2003).

3.3 Exercise programs

Pizzo et al assess the effects of a nonsurgical exercise program on the decreased mouth opening in a group of 10 systemic scleroderma patients with severe microstomia (maximal mouth opening ≤30 mm) (Pizzo et al., 2003). The subjects were instructed to perform an exercise program including both mouth-stretching and oral augmentation exercises. The effects of such exercises were assessed after an 18-week period by measuring the maximal mouth opening of each subject. The exercise program improved the mouth opening of all subjects without significant differences between dentate and edentulous ones. At the end of the 18-week period, all patients commented that eating, speaking and oral hygiene measures were easier. The edentulous subjects also experienced less difficulty inserting their own dentures. These findings suggest that regular application of the proposed exercise program may be useful in the management of microstomia in systemic scleroderma patients (Pizzo et al., 2003)

4. Conclusion

Individuals with microstomia would benefit from early referral to several medical services. Regular follow-up with targeted preventive advice is essential, in view of the potential for disruption of facial growth, genetic disorder pattern and the anatomical limitations faced in providing oral care and restorative treatment in patients with microstomia. The improvement of mouth opening impacts on the patients' quality of life by enabling them to perform activities such as speech, eating, dental hygiene, expression, social interaction, and receiving general anaesthesia via intubation rather than requiring a prolonged tracheostomy. This improved functional performance also impacts positively on psychosocial well being. Management of microstomia is a critical area when treating a patient with burn injuries and should be a priority due to its impact on quality of life (Wust, 2006). Additionally, long-term documentation of such cases and multicentre audit will enhance our understanding and improve our future management of similar rare and interesting genetic disorders.

5. References

Albilia, J.B.; Lam, D.K.; Blanas, N.; Clokie, C.M.& Sándor, G.K. (2007) Small mouths ... Big problems? A review of scleroderma and its oral health implications. *J Can Dent Assoc.* Vol. 73, No. 9, (Nov 2007), pp.831-836, ISSN 1488-2159

Antley, R.M.; Uga, N.; Burzynski, N.J.; Baum, R.S.& Bixler, D. (1975) Diagnostic criteria for the whistling face syndrome. *Birth Defects Orig Artic Ser.* Vol. 11, No. 5, (1975)pp. 161-168, ISSN 0547-6844

Ayhan, M.; Aytug, Z.; Deren, O.; Karantinaci, B.& Gorgu, M.(2006) An alternative treatment for postburn microstomia treatment: composite auricular lobule graft for oral comissure reconstruction. *Burns.* Vol. 32, No. 3, (May 2006), pp. 380-384, ISSN 1879-1409

Aymé, S.& Philip, N. (1996) Fine-Lubinsky syndrome: a fourth patient with brachycephaly, deafness, cataract, microstomia and mental retardation. *Clin Dysmorphol.* , Vol. 5, No. 1, (Jan 1996), pp. 55-60. ISSN 1473-5717

Barron, R.P.; Carmichael, R.P.; Marcon, M.A. & Sandor, G.K. (2003) Dental erosion in gastroesophageal reflux disease. *J Can Dent Assoc* Vol 69, No. 2, (Feb 2003), pp. 84–89, ISSN 1488-2159

Browne, C.E. ; Dennis, N.R. ; Maher, E. ; Long, F.L. ; Nicholson, J.C. ; Sillibourne, J.; Christian, S.L.; Robinson, W.P.; Huang, B.; Mutirangura, A.; Line, M.R.; Nakao, M.; Surti, U.; Chakravarti, A.& Ledbetter, D.H. (1995). Molecular characterization of two proximal deletion breakpoint regions in both Prader-Willi and Angelman syndrome patients. *Am J Hum Genet,* Vol. 57, No. 1, (Jul 1995), pp.40–48, ISSN 1537-6605

Burton, B.K.; Sumner, T.; Langer, L.O. Jr.; Rimoin, D.L.; Adomian, G.E.; Lachman, R.S.; Nicastro, J.F.; Kelly, D.L.&Weaver,R.G. (1986) A new skeletal dysplasia: clinical, radiologic, and pathologic findings. *J Pediatr.*Vol. 109, No. 4, (Oct 1986), pp. 642-648. ISSN 1097-6833

Campos de Freitas, A.C., Mussolino Ribeiro, Z.M.; Tambasco de Oliveira, M.C..& Assed, S. (1986) [Clinical management of a case of epidermolysis bullosa]. *Rev Fac Odontol Ribeiro Preto,* Vol. 23, No. 2, (Jul-Dec 1986), pp. 71-78, ISSN 0102-129X

Cannistrà, C.; Barbet, J.P.; Houette, A.& Iannetti; G. (1999) Temporomandibular region in the Franceschetti's Syndrome. Anatomical study. *Bull Group Int Rech Sci Stomatol Odontol.* Vol. 41, No. 1, (Jan-Mar 1999), pp. 33-38, ISSN 0250-4693

Cole, P.; Hatef, D.A.; Kaufman, Y.& Hollier, L.H. Jr. (2010) Fine-Lubinsky syndrome: managing the rare syndromic synostosis. J Plast Reconstr Aesthet Surg., Vol. 63, No. 1, (Jan 2010), pp(e). 70-72, ISSN 1878-0539

Conine, T.A.; Carlow, D.L.& Stevenson-Moore, P. (1989) The Vancouver microstomia orthosis. *J Prosthet Dent.* , Vol. 61, No. 4, (Apr 1989), pp. 476-483, ISSN 1097-6841

Converse, J.M.& Wood-Smith, D.(1977) Techniques for repair of defects of the lips and cheeks. In J,M, Converse.(ed.) *Reconstructive Plastic Surgery Principles and Procedures in Correction, Reconstruction and Transplantation,* 2nd edition, Volume 3, 1977, pp.1575, WB Saunders, ISBN 0721626815,Philadelphia, USA

Corrigan, L.A.; Duncan, C.A.& Gregg, T.A.(2006) Freeman-Sheldon syndrome: a case report. *Int J Paediatr Dent.* Vol. 16, No. 6, (Nov 2006), pp. 440-443, ISSN 1365-263X

Cura, C.; Cotert, H.S.& User, A.(2003) Fabrication of a sectional impression tray and sectional complete denture for a patient with microstomia and trismus: a clinical report. *J Prosthet Dent.* Vol. 89, No. 6, (Jun 2003), pp. 540-543, ISSN 1097-6841

Davis, S.; Thompson, J.G.; Clark, J.; Kowal-Vern, A.& Latenser, B.A.(2006) A prototype for an economical vertical microstomia orthosis. *J Burn Care Res.,* Vol. 27, No. 3, (May-Jun 2006), pp. 352-356, ISSN 1559-0488

Defraia, E.; Marinelli, A.& Alarashi, M. (2003) Case report: orofacial characteristics of Hallermann-Streiff Syndrome. *Eur J Paediatr Dent.* Vol. 4, No. 3, (Sep 2003), pp. 155-158, ISSN 1591-996X

Dieffenbach, F.(Ed)(1829) *Chirurgische Erfahrungen besonders über die Wiederherstellung zerstörter Teile des menschlichen Körpers nach neuen Methoden.* Enslin, 1829, Berlin, Germany

DiGeorge, A.M. (1965) Discussions on a new concept of the cellular basis of immunology. J Pediatr, Vol. 67 (1998), pp. 907, ISSN 1097-6833

Digilio, M.C.; Conti, E.; Sarkozy, A.; Mingarelli, R.; Dottorini, T.; Marino, B.; Pizzuti, A.& Dallapiccola, B.(2002) Grouping of multiple-lentigines/LEOPARD and Noonan syndromes on the PTPN11 gene. *Am J Hum Genet.,* Vol. 71, No. 2, (Aug 2002), pp. 389-394, ISSN 1537-6605

Domingo, D.L.; Trujillo, M.I.; Council, S.E.; Merideth, M.A.; Gordon, L.B.; Wu, T.; Introne, W.J.; Gahl, W.A.& Hart, T.C. (2009) Hutchinson-Gilford progeria syndrome: oral and craniofacial phenotypes. *Oral Dis.,* Vol. 15, No. 3, (Apr 2009), pp. 187-195, ISSN 1601-0825

Driscoll, D.A.; Budarf, M.L.& Emanuel, B.S. (1992) A genetic etiology for Di- George syndrome: Consistent deletions and microdeletion of 22q11. *Am J Hum Genet* Vol. 50, No. 5, (May 1992), pp. 924–933, ISSN 1537-6605

Ergun, G.A.; Lin, A.N.; Dannenberg, A.J.& Carter, D.M.(1992) Gastrointestinal manifestations of epidermolysis bullosa. *Medicine(Baltimore)* Vol. 71, No. 3, (May 1992), pp. 121-127, ISSN 1536-5964

Fairbanks, G.R.& Dingman, R.O. (1972) Restoration of the oral commissure. *Plast Reconstr Surg.,* Vol. 49, No. 4, (Apr 1972), pp. 411-413, ISSN 1529-4242

Favaro, F.P.; Zechi-Ceide, R.M.; Alvarez, C.W.; Maximino, L.P.; Antunes, L.F.B.B.; Richieri-Costa, A.& Guion-Almeida, M.L. (2010). Richieri- Costa–Pereira syndrome: A unique acrofacial dysostosis type. An overview of the Brazilian cases. *Am J Med Genet Part* Vol. 155, No. 2, (Feb 2010), pp.1–10, ISSN 1552-4833

Ferri, C.; Valentini, G.; Cozzi, F.; Sebastiani, M.; Nichelassi, C.;La Montagna, G.; Bullo, A.; Cazzato, M.; Tirri E.; Storino, F.; Giuggioli, D.; Cuomo, G.; Rasada, M.; Bombardieri, S.; Todesco, S. & Tirri, G. (2002) Systemic sclerosis: demographic, clinical, and serologic features and survival in 1012 Italian patients. *Medicine (Baltimore),* Vol. 81, No. 2, (Mar 2002), pp.139–153, ISSN 1536-5964

Fine, B.A. & Lubinsky, M. (1983) Craniofacial and CNS anomalies with body asymmetry, severe retardation, and other malformations. *J Clin Dysmorphol.,* Vol. 1, No. 4, (Winter 1983), pp. 6-9, ISSN: 0736-4407

Fine, J.D. (2010) Inherited epidermolysis bullosa: past, present, and future. *Ann N.Y. Acad Sci,* Vol. 1194, (Apr 2010), pp. 213-222, ISSN 1749-6632

Fong, LG.; Ng, J.K.; Meta, M.; Coté, N.; Yang, S.H.; Stewart, C.L.; Sullivan, T.; Burghardt, A.; Majumdar, S.; Reue, K.; Bergo, M.O.& Young, S.G. (2004) Heterozygosity for Lmna deficiency eliminates the progeria-like phenotypes in Zmpste 24-deficient mice. *Proc Natl Acad Sci U S A.,* Vol. 101, No. 52, (Dec 2004), pp. 18111-18116, ISSN 1091-6490

Gillies, H.M.& Millard, D.R.(eds) (1957) *Principles of Plastic Surgery.* Little Brown, Boston, USA

Goetz, R.H. (1945) Pathology of progressive systemic sclerosis with special reference to changes in the viscera. *Clin Proc (S. Africa)* Vol. 4, No. 6, pp. 337–342.

Grishkevich, V.M. (2010) Post-burn microstomia: Anatomy and elimination with trapeze-flap plasty. *Burns.* 2010 Dec 10. [Epub ahead of print] doi:10.1016/j.burns.2010.09.003 ISSN 1879-1409

Guion-Almeida, M.L. Kokitsu-Nakata, N.M.; Zechi-Ceide, R.M. & Vendramini, S.(1999) Auriculo-condilar syndrome: further evidence for a new disorder. *Am J Med Genet ,* Vol. 86, No. 2, (Sep 1999), pp. 130– 133, ISSN 1096-8628

Hawk, A.& English, J.C. (2001) Localized and systemic scleroderma. *Semin Cutan Med Surg* Vol 20, No. 1, (Mar 2001), pp. 27–31, ISSN 1558-0768

Hendrix, S.L.& Sauer, H.J. (1991) Successful pregnancy in a patient with Hallermann-Streiff syndrome. *Am J Obstet Gynecol,* Vol. 164, No. 4, (Apr 1991), pp. 1102-1104, ISSN 1097-6868

Ho, I.C.; O'Donnell, D.& Rodrigo, C.(1989) The occurrence of supernumerary teeth with isolated, nonfamilial leopard (multiple lentigines) syndrome: report of case. *Spec Care Dentist.,* Vol. 9, No. 6, (Nov-Dec 1989), pp. 200-202, ISSN 1754-4505

Hoefnagel, D.& Benirschke. K. (1965) Dyscephalia Mandibulo-Oculo-Facialis. (Hallermann-Streiff Syndrome). *Arch Dis Child.* Vol 40, (Feb 1965), pp.57-61, ISSN 1468-2044

Holder, A.M.; Graham, B.H.; Lee, B.& Scott, D.A.(2007) Fine-Lubinsky syndrome: sibling pair suggests possible autosomal recessive inheritance. *Am J Med Genet A.,* Vol. 143A, No. 21, (Nov 2007), pp. 2576-2580, ISSN 1552-4833

Jaminet, P.; Werdin, F.; Kraus, A.; Pfau, M.; Schaller, H.E.; Becker, S.& Sinis, N.(2009) Extreme microstomia in an 8-month-old infant: bilateral commissuroplasty using rhomboid buccal mucosa flaps. *Eplasty.* , Vol. 26, No. 10, (Dec 2009),pp(e) 5, ISSN 1937-5719

Jaminet, P.; Werdin, F.; Kraus, A.; Pfau, M.; Schaller, HE.; Becker, S.& Sinis. N. (2009) Extreme microstomia in an 8-month-old infant: bilateral commissuroplasty using rhomboid buccal mucosa flaps. *Eplasty,* Vol. 26, No. 10, (Dec 2009), pp(e).5, ISSN 1937-5719

Jampol, M.; Repetto, G.; Keith, D.A.; Curtin, H.; Remensynder, J.& Holmes, L.B. (1998) New Syndrome? Prominent constricted ears with malformed condyle of the mandible. *Am J Med Genet,* Vol 75, No. 5, (Feb 1998),pp. 449–452, ISSN 1096-8628

Jaquez, M.; Driscoll, D.A.; Li, M.; Emanule, B.S.; Hernandez, I.; Jaqquez, F.; Lembert, N.; Ramirez, J.&Matalon, R. (1997) Unbalanced 15;22 translocation in a patient with manifestations of DiGeorge and velocardiofacial syndrome, Am J Med Genet., Vol. 70, No. 1, (May 1997), pp. 6-10, ISSN 1096-8628

Johns, F.R.; Sandler, N.A.& Ochs, M.W.(1998) The use of a triangular pedicle flap for oral commisuroplasty: report of a case. *J Oral Maxillofac Surg.,* Vol. 56, No. 2, (Feb 1998), pp.228-231, ISSN 1531-5053

Kitsiou-Tzeli, S.; Tzetis, M.; Sofocleous, C.; Vrettou, C.; Xaidara, A.; Giannikou, K.; Pampanos, A. Mavrou, A.& Kanavakis, E. (2010) De novo interstitial duplication of the 15q11.2-q14 PWS/AS region of maternal origin: Clinical description, array CGH analysis, and review of the literature. *Am J Med Genet Part A* , Vol. 152A, No. 8, (Aug 2010), pp.1925–1932, ISSN1552-4833

Koymen, R.; Gulses, A.; Karacayli, U, Aydintug, YS. (2009). Treatment of microstomia with commissuroplasties and semidynamic acrylic splints. *Oral Surg Oral Med Oral Pathol Oral Radiol Endod.,* Vol. 107, No. 4, (Apr 2009), pp. 503-507, ISSN 1528-395X

Liversidge, H.M.; Kosmidou, A.; Hector, M.P.& Roberts, G.J. (2005) Epidermolysis bullosa and dental developmental age. *Int J Paediatr Dent.,* Vol. 15, No. 5, (Sep 2005), pp. 335-341, ISSN 1365-263X

Livi, R.; Teghini, L.; Pignone, A.; Generini, S.; Matucci-Cerinic, M.& Cagnoni, M. (2002) Renal functional reserve is impaired in patients with systemic sclerosis without clinical signs of kidney involvement. *Ann Rheum Dis* Vol. 61, No. 8, (Aug 2002), pp. 682–686, ISSN 1468-2060

Lo, I.F.; Roebuck, D.J.; Lam, S.T.& Kozlowski, K. (1998) Burton skeletal dysplasia: the second case report. *Am J Med Genet.* , Vol. 79, No. 3, (Sep 1998), pp. 168-171, ISSN 1096-8628

Madjar, D.; Shifman, A.& Kusner, W. (1987) Dynamic labial commissure widening device for the facial burn patient. *Quintessence Int.* , Vol. 18, No. 5, (May 1987), pp.361-363, ISSN 1936-7163

Malde, A.D.; Jagtap, S.R.& Pantvaidya, S.H. (1994) Hallermann-Streiff syndrome: airway problems during anaesthesia. *J Postgrad Med,* Vol. 40, No. 4, (Oct- Dec 1994), pp. 216-218, ISSN 0022-3859

Martin, G.M. (2005) Genetic modulation of senescent phenotypes in Homo sapiens. *Cell.,* Vol. 120, No. 4, (Feb 2005), pp. 523-532. ISSN 1097-4172

Martin Mateos, M.A.; Pérez Dueñas, B.P.; Iriondo, M.; Krauel, J.& Gean Molins, E. (2000) Clinical and immunological spectrum of partial DiGeorge syndrome. *J Investig Allergol Clin Immunol.,* Vol. 10, No. 6, (Nov-Dec2000), pp. 352-360, ISSN 1018-9068

Martins, W.D.; Westphalen, F.H.& Westphalen, V.P.(2003) Microstomia caused by swallowing of caustic soda: report of a case. *J Contemp Dent Pract.* Vol. 4, No. 4, (Nov 2003), pp. 91-99, ISSN 1526-3711

Masotti, C.; Oliveira, K.G.; Poemer, F.; Splendore, A.; Souza, J.; Freitas Rda, S.; Zechi-Ceide, R.; Guion- Almeida, M.L.& Passos-Bueno, M.R. (2008) Auriculo-condylar syndrome: mapping of a first locus and evidence for genetic heterogeneity, *Eur J Hum Genet*, Vol. 16, No.2, (Feb 2008), pp. 145-152, ISSN 1476-5438

Mastroiacovo, P.; Corchia, C.; Botto, L.D.; Lanni, R.; Zampino, G.& Fusco, D. (1995) Epidemiology and genetics of microtia-anotia: a registry based study on over one million births. *J Med Genet.* , Vol. 32, No. 6, (Jun 1995), pp. 453-457, ISSN 1468-6244

Mavilio, F.; Pellegrini, G,; Ferrari, S.; Di Nunzio, F.; Di Iorio,E.; Recchia, A.; Maruggi, G.; Ferrari, G.; Provasi, E.; Bonini, C.; Capurro, S.; Conti, A.; Magnoni, C.; Gianetti, A.& De Luca, M. (2006) Correction of junctional epidermolysis bullosa by transplantation of genetically modified epidermal stem cells. *Nat. Med. Vol.* 12, No. 12, (Dec 2006), pp. 1397–1402, ISSN 1546-170X

McDonald Mc Ginn, D.M.;& Sullivan, K. E. (2011) Chromosome 22q11.2 Deletion Syndrome (DiGeorge Syndrome/Velocardiofacial Syndrome), *Medicine(Baltimore)* ,Vol. 90, No. 1, (Jan 2011), pp. 1-18, ISSN 1536-5964

Mehra, P.; Caiazzo, A.& Bestgen, S.(1998) Bilateral oral commissurotomy using buccal mucosa flaps for management of microstomia: report of a case. *J Oral Maxillofac Surg.*, Vol. 56, No. 10, (Oct 1998), pp. 1200-1203, ISSN 1531-5053

Mordjikian, E. (2002) Severe microstomia due to burn by caustic soda. *Burns.*, Vol. 28, No. 8 (Dec 2002), pp. 802-805, ISSN 1879-1409

Mühlbauer, W.D.(1970) Elongation of mouth in post-burn microstomia by a double Z-plasty. *Plast Reconstr Surg.* , Vol. 45, No. 4. (Apr 1970), pp. 400-402, ISSN 1529-4242

Neville, B.W. Damm, D.D.; Allen, C.M.,& Bouquot, J.E. (Eds) (2002) *Oral and maxillofacial pathology.* 2nd ed., p. 137, W.B. Saunders Co, ISBN 13: 9781416034353, Philadelphia, USA

Ohyama, K.; Susami, T.; Kato, Y.; Amano, H.& Kuroda, T. (1997) Freeman-Sheldon syndrome: case management from age 6 to 16 years. *Cleft Palate Craniofac J.*, Vol. 34, No. 2, (Mar 1997), pp. 151-153, ISSN 1545-1569

Orioli, I.M. & Castilla, E.E. (2010) Epidemiology of holoprosencephaly: Prevalence and risk factors. *Am J Med Genet C Semin Med Genet.* Vol. 154C, No. 1, (Feb 2010), pp. 13-21, ISSN 1552-4876

Ozgur, F.;, Sonmez, E,.& Tuncbilek, G. (2005) Cleft lip and cleft palate closure in 13 month-old female with epidermolysis bullosa. *J Craniofac Surg*, Vol. 16, No. 5, (Sep 2005), pp. 843-847, ISSN 1536-3732

Paznekas, W.A.; Boyadjiev, S.A.; Shapiro, R.E.; Daniels, O.; Wollnik, B.; Keegan, C.E.; Innis, J.W.; Dinulos, M.B,; Christian, C.; Hannibal, M.C.& Jabs, E.W. (2003) Connexin 43 (GJA1) mutations cause the pleiotropic phenotype of oculodentodigital dysplasia. *Am. J. Hum. Genet.* Vol. 72, No. 2, (Feb 2003), pp. 408-418, ISSN 1537-6605

Pizzo, G.; Scardina, G.A.& Messina, P.(2003) Effects of a nonsurgical exercise program on the decreased mouth opening in patients with systemic scleroderma. *Clin Oral Investig.*, Vol. 7, No. 3, (Sep 2003), pp. 175-178, ISSN 1436-3771

Pizzuti, A.; Flex, E.; Mingarelli, R.; Salpietro, C.; Zelante, L.& Dallapiccola, B.(2004) A homozygous GJA1 gene mutation causes a Hallermann-Streiff/ODDD spectrum phenotype. *Hum Mutat.* Vol. 23, No. 3, (Mar 2004), pp. 286, ISSN 1098-1004

Pollex, R.L.& Hegele, R.A. (2004) Hutchinson-Gilford progeria syndrome. *Clin Genet.* Vol. 66, No. 5, (Nov 2004), pp,. 375-381, ISSN 1399-0004

Preus, M.; Cooper, A.R. & O'Leary, E. (1984) Sensorineural hearing loss, small facial features, submucous cleft palate, and myoclonic seizures. *J Clin Dysmorphol.* Vol. 2, No. 1, (Spring 1984), pp. 30-31, ISSN: 0736-4407

Reisberg, D.J.; Fine, L.; Fattore, L.& Edmonds, D.C.(1983) Electrical burns of the oral commissure.*J Prosthet Dent.* , Vol. 49, No. 1, (Jan 1983), pp. 71-76. ISSN 1097-6841

Richieri-Costa, A. & Pereira, S.C.S.(1992) Short stature, Robin sequence, cleft mandible, pre/postaxial hand anomalies, and clubfoot: A new autosomal recessive syndrome. *Am J Med Genet,* Vol. 42, No. 5, (Mar 1992), pp. 681–687, ISSN 1096-8628

Sarkozy, A.; Conti, E.; Digilio, M.C.; Marino, B.; Morini, E.; Pacileo, G.; Wilson, M.; Calabrò, R.; Pizzuti, A.& Dallapiccola, B.(2004) Clinical and molecular analysis of 30 patients with multiple lentigines LEOPARD syndrome. *J Med Genet.* , Vol. 41, No. 5, (May 2004), pp(e). 68, ISSN 1468-6244

Sarkozy, A.; Digilio, M.C.& Dallapiccola, B.(2008) Leopard syndrome. *Orphanet J Rare Dis.* Vol. 27, No. 3, (May 2008), pp. 13, ISSN 1750-1172

Schoner, K.; Bald, R:; Fritz, B.& Rehder, H. (2008) Fetal manifestation of the Fine-Lubinsky syndrome. Brachycephaly, deafness, cataract, microstomia and mental retardation syndrome complicated by Pierre-Robin anomaly and polyhydramnios. *Fetal Diagn Ther.,* Vol. 23, No. 3, (Feb 2008), pp. 228-232, ISSN 1421-9964

Seibold, J.R. (2005). Scleroderma. *In* E.D. JR. Harris, R.C. Budd& G.S. Firestein (Eds.): *Kelley's Textbook 's of Rheumatology,* 7th ed.,1279-1308. Elsevier Saunders, ISBN 13: 9781416032854, Philadelphia, USA

Sevenants, L.; Wouters, C.; De Sandre-Giovannoli, A.; Devlieger, H.; Devriendt, K.; van den Oord, J.J.; Marien, K.; Lévy, N.& Morren, M.A.(2005) Tight skin and limited joint movements as early presentation of Hutchinson-Gilford progeria in a 7-week-old infant. *Eur J Pediatr.* Vol. 164, No. 5, (May 2005), pp. 283-286, ISSN 1432-1076

Silva, L.C.; Cruz, R.A.; Abou-Id, L.R.; Brini, L.N.& Moreira, L.S.(2004) Clinical evaluation of patientswith epidermolysis bullosa: review of the literature and case reports. *Spec Care Dentist* Vol. 24, No. 1, (Jan-Feb 2004), pp. 22-27, ISSN 1754-4505

Silverglade, D.& Ruberg, R.L. (1986) Nonsurgical management of burns to the lips and commissures. *Clin Plast Surg.* , Vol. 13, No. 1, (Jan 1986), pp. 87-94, ISSN 1558-0504

Siqueira, M.A.; de Souza Silva, J.; Silva, F.W.; Diaz-Serrano, K.V.; Freitas, A.C.& Queiroz, A.M. (2008) Dental treatment in a patient with epidermolysis bullosa Spec Care Dentist, Vol.28, No. 3, (May-Jun 2008), pp. 92-95,ISSN 1754-4505

Smith, P.G.; Muntz, H.R.& Thawley S.E. (1982). Local myocutaneous advancement flaps. Alternatives to cross-lip and distant flaps in the reconstruction of ablative lip defects. *Arch Otolaryngol.* Vol.108, No.11, (Nov 1982), pp. 714-718, ISSN 0886-4470

Song, H.R.; Sarwark, J.F.; Sauntry, S.& Grant, J. (1996) Freeman-Sheldon syndrome (whistling face syndrome) and cranio-vertebral junction malformation producing dysphagia and weight loss. *Pediatr Neurosurg.* , Vol. 24, No. 5, (1996), pp. 272-274, ISSN 1423-0305

Sorensen, B. (1979) Contraction of the oral stoma: microstomia. In: I. Feller, W.C. Grabb, (eds) Reconstruction and rehabilitation of the burned patient. 1979, p. 224. Ann Arbor, Michigan, USA

Spaepen, A.; Schrander-Stumpel, C.; Fryns, J.P.; de Die-Smulders, C.; Borghgraef, M.& Van den Berghe H. (1991) Hallermann-Streiff syndrome: clinical and psychological findings in children. Nosologic overlap with oculodentodigital dysplasia? *Am J Med Genet.* Vol. 41, No. 4, (Dec 1991), pp. 517-520, ISSN 1096-8628

Stavropoulos, F.& Abramovicz, S. (2008) Management of the oral surgery patient diagnosed with epidermolysis bullosa: Report of 3 cases and review of the literature, J Oral Maxillofac Surg, Vol. 66, No. 3, (Mar 2008), pp. 554-559, ISSN 1399-0020

Stedman, T.L. (ed) (1976), *Stedman's Medical Dictionary,* 23rd edition, p. 875, The Williams & Wilkins Company, ISBN 0683079247, Baltimore, USA

Steen, V.D.& Medsger, T.A. Jr. (1990) Epidemiology and natural history of systemic sclerosis. *Rheum Dis Clin North Am.* Vol. 16, No. 1, (Feb 1990), pp.1-10. ISSN 1558-3163

Stone, J.H.& Wigley, F.M.(1998) Management of systemic sclerosis: the art and science. *Semin Cutan Med Surg,* Vol. 17, No. 1, (Mar 1998), pp. 55–64, ISSN 1558-0768

Storm, A.L.; Johnson, J.M.; Lammer, E.; Green, G.E.& Cunniff, C. (2005) Auriculo-condylar syndrome is associated with highly variable ear and mandibular defects in multiple kindreds. *Am J Med Genet A* Vol. 138A, No. 2, (Oct 2008), pp. 141–145, ISSN 1552-4833

Suthers, G.K.; Earley, A.E. & Huson, S.M. (1993) A distinctive syndrome of brachycephaly, deafness, cataracts and mental retardation. *Clin Dysmorphol.* Vol. 2, No. 4, (Oct 1993), pp. 342-345, ISSN 1473-5717

Suzuki, Y.; Abe, M.; Hosoi, T.& Kurtz, K.S.(2000) Sectional collapsed denture for a partially edentulous patient with microstomia: a clinical report. *J Prosthet Dent.,* Vol. 84, No. 3, (Sep 2000), pp. 256-259, ISSN 1097-6841

Takato, T.; Ohsone. H.& Tsukakoshi, H. (1989) Treatment of severe microstomia caused by swallowing of caustic soda.*Oral Surg Oral Med Oral Pathol.,*Vol. 67, No. 1, (Jan 1989), pp. 20-24, ISSN 0030-4220

Trad, S.; Amoura, Z.; Beigelman, C.; Haroche, J.; Costedoat, N.; Boutin, le T.H.; Cacoub, P.; Frances, C.; Wechsler, B.; Grenier, P.& Piette, J.C. (2006) Pulmonary arterial hypertension is a major mortality factor in diffuse systemic sclerosis, independent of interstitial lung disease. *Arthritis Rheum.* Vol. 54, No. 1, (Jan 2006), pp.184-191, ISSN 1529-0131.

Van Balen, A.T.M. (1961) Dyscephaly with microphtalmos, cataract and hypoplasia of the mandible. *Ophtalmologica,* Vol. 141, No. 1 (Jan 1961), pp. 53-56, ISSN 1423-0267

Van Straten, O. (1991) A dynamic mouth splint for the patient with facial burns. *J Burn Care Rehabil.* , Vol. 12, No. 2, (Mar-Apr 1991), pp. 174-176, ISSN 0273-8481

Villoria, J.M. (1972) A new method of elongation of the corner of the mouth. *Plast Reconstr Surg.* Vol. 49, No. 1, (Jan 1972), pp. 52-5, ISSN 1529-4242

Watanabe, I.; Tanaka, Y.; Ohkubo, C.& Miller, A.W.(2002) Application of cast magnetic attachments to sectional complete dentures for a patient with microstomia: a clinical report. *J Prosthet Dent.,* Vol. 88, No. 6, (Dec 2002), pp. 573-577, ISSN 1097-6841

Winkelmann, R.K.; Flach, D.B.& Unni, K.K. (1988) Lung cancer and scleroderma. *Arch Dermatol Res,* Vol. 28, No. Suppl., (Feb 1988), pp.(S) 15–18. ISSN 1432-069X

Wust, K.J. (2006). A modified dynamic mouth splint for burn patients. *J Burn Care Res.* Vol 27, No. 1, (Jan-Feb 2006), pp 86-92, ISSN 1559-0488

Yam, A.A.; Faye, M.; Kane, A.; Diop, F.; Coulybaly-Ba, D.; Tamba-Ba, A.; Mbaye, NG.& Ba, I. (2001) Oro-dental and craniofacial anomalies in LEOPARD syndrome. *Oral Dis.*, Vol. 7, No. 1, (May 2001), pp.200-202. ISSN 1601-0825

Yenisey, M.; Külünk, T.; Kurt, S.& Ural, C. (2005) A prosthodontic management alternative for scleroderma patients. *J Oral Rehabil.* Vol. 32, No. 9, (Sep 2005), pp.696-700, ISSN 1365-2842

Zeisler, E.P.& Becker, S.W.(1936) Generalized Lentigo: its relation to systemic nonelevated nevi. *Arch Dermat Syph,* Vol.33, No.2 (1936), pp. 109-125, ISSN 0365-6020